SIXTH EDITION

Family Health Care Nursing

THEORY, PRACTICE, AND RESEARCH

SIXTH EDITION

Family Health Care Nursing

THEORY, PRACTICE, AND RESEARCH

Joanna Rowe Kaakinen, PhD, RN
Professor and Interim Dean
Linfield-Good Samaritan School of Nursing
Linfield College
Portland, Oregon

Deborah Padgett Coehlo, PhD, C-PNP, PMHS, CFLE
Developmental and Behavioral Specialist
Juniper Pediatrics
Faculty Member
Oregon State University Cascades
Bend, Oregon

Rose Steele, PhD, RN
Professor
School of Nursing, Faculty of Health
York University
Toronto, Ontario, Canada

Melissa Robinson, PhD, RN
Associate Professor of Nursing
Linfield-Good Samaritan School of Nursing
Linfield College
Portland, Oregon

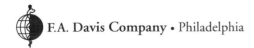
F.A. Davis Company • Philadelphia

F.A. Davis Company
1915 Arch Street
Philadelphia, PA 19103
www.fadavis.com

Printed in the United States of America

Last digit indicates print number: 10 9 8 7 6 5 4 3 2 1

Sponsoring Editor: Jacalyn Sharp
Manager of Project and eProject Management: Catherine H. Carroll
Senior Content Project Manager: Christine M. Abshire
Electronic Project Editor: Katherine E. Crowley
Design and Illustration Manager: Carolyn O'Brien

As new scientific information becomes available through basic and clinical research, recommended treatments and drug therapies undergo changes. The author(s) and publisher have done everything possible to make this book accurate, up-to-date, and in accord with accepted standards at the time of publication. The author(s), editors, and publisher are not responsible for errors or omissions or for consequences from application of the book, and make no warranty, expressed or implied, in regard to the contents of the book. Any practice described in this book should be applied by the reader in accordance with professional standards of care used in regard to the unique circumstances that may apply in each situation. The reader is advised always to check product information (package inserts) for changes and new information regarding dose and contraindications before administering any drug. Caution is especially urged when using new or infrequently ordered drugs.

Names: Kaakinen, Joanna Rowe, 1951– editor. | Coehlo, Deborah Padgett, editor. |
    Steele, Rose, editor. | Robinson, Melissa, editor.
Title: Family health care nursing: theory, practice, and research/
    [edited by] Joanna Rowe Kaakinen, Deborah Padgett Coehlo, Rose Steele, Melissa Robinson.
Description: 6th edition. | Philadelphia: F.A. Davis Company, [2018] |
    Includes bibliographical references and index.
Identifiers: LCCN 2017054122 | ISBN 9780803661660 (pbk.)
Subjects: | MESH: Family Nursing | Family | Family Health
Classification: LCC RT120.F34 | NLM WY 159.5 | DDC 610.73--dc23
    LC record available at https://lccn.loc.gov/2017054122

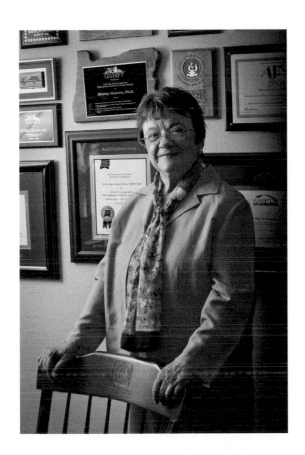

Shirley May Harmon Hanson, RN, PhD, PMHNP/ARNP/FAAN, CFLE, LFMT, is a pioneer in the field of family nursing. Countless family nursing scholars, both nationally and internationally, have been influenced by her work. Dr. Hanson relentlessly pursued her life-long passion for family nursing as she advanced family nursing science, knowledge, and theory.

Dr. Hanson founded a division of Family and Health in the multidisciplinary organization called the National Council for Family Relations in the early 1980s. She recognized the lack of a systematic approach in nursing education with regard to the whole family as a unit of client care. In 1984, Dr. Hanson was awarded a grant to support the first gathering of international nursing faculty to discuss the concept of a family nursing discipline—the precursor to the now well-established International Family Nursing Association.

In the late 1980s, Dr. Hanson was teaching at the Oregon Health & Science University when she noted the need for a comprehensive nursing text that specifically focused student learning on the health needs of the whole family in all specialty aspects of nursing practice. Thus, the first edition of Family Health Care Nursing: Theory, Practice, and Research *was published in 1991. Dr. Hanson continued as lead editor on the second and third editions, then remained on the editorial team for the fourth and fifth editions. The book received the AJN Book of the Year Award in its category for both the 2005 and 2015 editions. Imagine the millions of people, faculty, students, and families who have been positively touched, directly and indirectly, by the work of Dr. Hanson.*

We, the editorial team, are honored to have worked with Dr. Hanson and to carry on her legacy of quality family nursing. We hold Dr. Hanson in the highest esteem.

—In deep gratitude and affection, the editorial team,
  JOANNA, DEBBIE, ROSE, AND MELISSA

OVERVIEW OF THE SIXTH EDITION

Ask anyone about a time they were affected by something that happened to one of their family members and you will be overwhelmed with the intensity of the emotions and the exhaustive details. Every person is influenced significantly by his or her family and the structure, function, and processes within the family. Even people who do not interact with their families have been shaped by their families. The importance and connection between individuals and their families have been studied expansively in a variety of disciplines, including nursing.

The importance of working in partnerships with families in the health care system is evident. Yet many health care providers view dealing with patients' families as an extra burden that is too demanding. Some nurses are baffled when a family acts or reacts in certain ways that are foreign to their own professional and personal family experiences. Some nurses avoid the tensions and anxiety that exist in families during a crisis situation. But it is in just such situations that families most need nurses' understanding, knowledge, and guidance.

The purpose of this book is to provide nursing students, as well as practicing nurses, with the understanding, knowledge, and guidance to practice family nursing. Since the last edition there have been many changes in families, family health, and policy that affect the health of families. Every chapter in this edition reflects those changes with updated, current, evidence-based information.

USE OF THIS BOOK

Family Health Care Nursing: Theory, Practice, and Research, Sixth Edition, is organized so that it can be used on its own and in its entirety to structure a course in family nursing. An alternative approach for the use of this text is for students to purchase the book at the beginning of their program of study so that specific chapters can be assigned for specialty courses throughout the curriculum. The sixth edition complements a concept-based curriculum design. For example, Chapter 16, Family Mental Health Nursing, could be assigned when students take their mental health nursing course, and Chapter 13, Family Child Health Nursing, could be studied during a pediatric course or in conjunction with a life-span–concept curriculum for chronic illness and acute care courses. Thus, this textbook could be integrated throughout the undergraduate or graduate nursing curriculum.

Families in North America are very similar relative to needs and health care outcomes. Though it is true that the United States and Canada have different health care systems, many of the stressors and challenges for families overlap. All of the chapters in this edition include information, statistics, programs, and interventions that address the individual needs of families and family nurses for both Canada and the United States. Where nursing practice and policy differ, specific content is included that addresses these policies and interventions.

ADDITIONS AND DELETIONS

This edition contains one new chapter, Chapter 7, Nursing Care of LGBTQ Families. Since the last edition gay marriage has been legalized in all states. All chapters have been changed and updated significantly so that they reflect the present state of "family," current evidence-based practice, research, and interventions. Chapter 4, Family Policy, is significantly updated and focused more on helping students understand the importance of policy in providing access to health care.

STRUCTURE OF THIS BOOK

Each chapter begins with the critical concepts to be addressed within that chapter. The purpose of placing the critical concepts at the beginning of the chapter is to focus the reader's thinking and learning and offer a preview and outline of what is to come. Another organizing framework for the book is presented in Chapter 2, Theoretical Foundations for the Nursing of Families. This chapter covers the importance of using theory to guide the nursing of families and presents five theoretical perspectives, with a case study demonstrating how to apply these five theoretical approaches in practice. These three family nursing theories, Family Systems Theory, Developmental and Family Life Cycle Theory, and Bioecological Theory, are threaded throughout the book and are applied in many of the chapter case studies. Most of the chapters include two case studies; all of the case studies contain family genograms and ecomaps.

The main body of the book is divided into three units: Unit 1: Foundations in Family Health Care Nursing, which includes Chapters 1 to 5; Unit 2: Families Across the Health Continuum, which includes Chapters 6 to 11; and Unit 3: Nursing Care of Families in Clinical Areas, which includes Chapters 12 to 17.

AVAILABLE ON DAVIS*PLUS*

The *Family Health Care Nursing Active Classroom Instructors' Guide* is an online faculty guide that provides assistance to faculty teaching family nursing or the nursing care of families in a variety of settings. Instructors will also find PowerPoint presentations and test bank questions for each chapter.

The References, Suggested Readings, and Web resources are available for students and instructors. In addition, a bonus chapter, Relational Nursing and Family Nursing in Canada, and Appendix A, The Friedman Family Assessment Model, are on Davis*Plus*.

UNIT 1: FOUNDATIONS IN FAMILY HEALTH CARE NURSING

Chapter 1: Family Health Care Nursing: An Introduction provides foundational materials essential to understanding families and family nursing. The first half of the chapter discusses dimensions of family nursing and defines family, family health, and healthy families. The chapter follows with an explanation of family health care nursing and the nature of interventions in the nursing care of families, along with the four approaches to family nursing (context, client, system, and component of society). The chapter then presents the concepts or variables that influence family nursing, family nursing roles, and obstacles to family nursing practice. The second half of the chapter elaborates on theoretical ideas involved with understanding family structure, family functions, and family processes.

Chapter 2: Theoretical Foundations for the Nursing of Families lays the theoretical groundwork needed to practice family nursing. The introduction builds a case for why nurses need to understand the interactive relationships among theory, practice, and research. It also makes the point that no single theory adequately describes the complex relationships of family structure, function, and processes. The chapter then continues by delineating and explaining relevant theories, concepts, propositions, hypotheses, and conceptual models. Selected for this textbook, and explained in this chapter, are three theoretical/conceptual models specific to family nursing: Family Systems Theory, Developmental and Family Life Cycle Theory, and Bioecological Theory. Using a family case study, the chapter explores how each of the three theories could be used to assess and plan interventions for a family. This approach enables learners to see how different interventions are derived from different theoretical perspectives.

Chapter 3: Family Demography: Continuity and Change in North American Families provides nurses with a basic contextual orientation to the demographics of families and health. This chapter examines changes and variations in North American families in order to understand what these changes portend for family health care nursing. The subject matter of the chapter is structured to provide family nurses with background on changes in the North American family so that they can understand their patient populations. The chapter briefly touches on the implications of these demographic patterns on practicing family nursing.

Chapter 4: Family Policy: The Intersection of Family Policies, Health Disparities, and Health Care Policies explores the many factors and policies that influence the health outcomes for families. Threaded throughout the chapter is the role of the nurse providing care within a framework of family nursing and multiple sociopolitical contexts. Specifically, key theoretical models guide family policies that continue to be challenged by health disparities resulting from negative social stigmatizations, restricted access to health care resources, and a complex political system of cultural beliefs that contribute to continued negative health outcomes. Health disparities are explored in the context of health determinants, family policy, and the nurse's role in advocating for family policies that enhance, rather than discriminate against, positive health care and resulting health outcomes. This chapter also discusses the unique factors that affect health policy and family health across Westernized countries. A case study has been added that demonstrates the role of nurses in advocating for family policies. At the completion of this chapter, the nurse will have developed a broad understanding of family policy and how it can contribute to or mitigate health disparities and health outcomes. Armed with this knowledge, nurses can assist families to adopt health promotion and disease prevention strategies and can advocate for families in their organizations, communities, and nations for policies that minimize disparities and maximize access to resources. This, in turn, will contribute to improved health of families and their members.

Chapter 5: Family Nursing Assessment and Intervention presents a systematic approach to develop a plan of action for the family *with* the family, to address its most pressing needs. This chapter is built on the traditional nursing process model to create a dynamic systematic family nursing assessment approach. Assessment strategies include selecting assessment instruments, determining the need for interpreters, assessing for health literacy, and learning how to diagram family genograms and ecomaps. The chapter also explores ways to involve families in shared decision making and explores analysis, a critical step in the family nursing process that helps focus the nurse and the family on identification of the family's primary concern(s). The chapter uses a family case study as an exemplar to demonstrate the family nursing assessment and intervention.

UNIT 2: FAMILIES ACROSS THE HEALTH CONTINUUM

Chapter 6: Family Health Promotion fosters the health of the family as a unit and encourages families to value and incorporate health promotion into their lifestyles. The purpose of this chapter is to introduce the concepts of family health and family health promotion. The chapter presents models to represent these concepts, including the Family Health Model, the Family Resilience Framework, the McMaster Model of Family Functioning, the Family Health Promotion Model, the Developmental Model of Health and Nursing, and the Model of the Health-Promoting Family. The chapter also examines internal and external factors through a lens of the bioecological systems theory that influences family health promotion, family nursing intervention strategies for health promotion, and two family case studies demonstrating how different theoretical approaches can be used for assessing and intervening in the family for health promotion.

Chapter 7: Nursing Care of LGBTQ Families is a new chapter for this edition. Families with LGBTQ members are working to achieve the same socially prescribed functions of all families to rear responsible and independent children, provide emotional and instrumental support to one another, and provide family member health care across the life span. Nurses care for families with members with unique gender identities, sexual orientations, and family structures in a variety of settings and circumstances with increasing visibility and frequency. The purpose of this chapter is to provide nurses with an evidence-based foundation and to facilitate the delivery of culturally competent family nursing care, thus decreasing health risks and disparities among this most vulnerable population. In this chapter, historical, political, sociocultural, religious, and economic contexts are explored that influence the meaning of gender, gender identities, and gender expressions. Language and social ideas about gender are ever evolving; therefore, a glossary of terms and pronouns is presented to assist nurses in using correct terminology to create safe and respectful dialogue from the position of learner when caring for LGBTQ individuals and their families. The chapter presents LGBTQ family structures and family processes that are unique to LGBTQ families, which are explored across the life span. Health challenges and disparities in LGBTQ families also are presented using a life-span approach. A case study demonstrates evidence-based family nursing practice.

Chapter 8: Genomics and Family Nursing Across the Life Span describes nursing responsibilities for families of persons who have, or are at risk for having, genetic conditions. The ability to apply an understanding of genetics in the care of families is a priority for nurses and for all health care providers. As a result of genomic research and the rapidly changing body of knowledge regarding genetic influences on health and illness, more emphasis has been placed on involving all health care providers in this field, including family nursing. Genetic conditions are life-long, so families living with genetic conditions need ongoing care and support. These responsibilities are described for families working with individuals and families across the life span. The goal of the chapter is to describe the relevance of genetic information within families when there is a question about genetic aspects of health or disease for members of the family. The chapter begins with a brief introduction to genomics and genetics, and then goes on to explain how families react to finding out they are at risk for genetic conditions and decide how and with whom to disclose genetic information. The critical aspect of confidentiality is then discussed. The chapter outlines the components of conducting a genetic assessment and history and offers interventions that include education and resources. Several specific case examples and a detailed case study illustrate nurses working with families that have a member(s) with a genetic condition.

Chapter 9: Families Living With Chronic Illness describes ways for nurses to think about the impact of chronic illness on families and to consider strategies for helping families manage chronic illness. The chapter begins with the importance of integrating ethnoculture in family health care and the impact of chronic illness on family life. Four theoretical approaches are introduced for assisting nurses to think about the best way to assist the family living with chronic illness. The rest of the chapter captures a variety of possible nursing actions to assist these families. Two case studies are presented in this chapter: one family who has a family member living with type 1 diabetes and another family helping an older parent and grandparent managing Parkinson's disease. Although every family and illness experience is completely individual, many of the trials that these two families demonstrate are universal to other families supporting members living with different chronic illnesses.

Chapter 10: Families in Palliative and End-of-Life Care details the key components to consider in providing palliative and end-of-life care, as well as

families' most important concerns and needs when a family member experiences a life-threatening illness or is dying. It also presents some concrete strategies to assist nurses in providing optimal palliative and end-of-life care to all family members. More specifically, the chapter begins with a brief definition of palliative and end-of-life care, including its focus on improving quality of life for patients and their families. The chapter then outlines principles of palliative care and ways to apply these principles across all settings, regardless of whether death results from chronic illness or a sudden or traumatic event. Three evidence-based, palliative care and end-of-life case studies conclude the chapter.

Chapter 11: Trauma and Family Nursing helps nurses develop knowledge about trauma and family nurses' key role in the field of trauma. It emphasizes the importance of prevention, early treatment, encouraging family resilience, and helping the family to make meaning out of negative events. This chapter also stresses an understanding of secondary trauma or the negative effects of witnessing the trauma of others. This discussion is particularly salient for family nurses, because they are some of the most likely health care providers to encounter traumatized victims in their everyday practice. Two case studies explicate family nursing when working with families who are experiencing the effects of traumatic life events.

UNIT 3: NURSING CARE OF FAMILIES IN CLINICAL AREAS

Chapter 12: Family Nursing With Childbearing Families focuses on family relationships and the health of all family members in childbearing families. Therefore, nurses involved with childbearing families use family concepts and theories as part of developing the plan of nursing care. A review of literature provides current evidence about the processes families experience when deciding on and adapting to childbearing, including theory and clinical application of nursing care for families planning pregnancy, experiencing pregnancy, adopting and fostering children, struggling with infertility, and coping with illness during the early postpartum period. This chapter starts by presenting theoretical perspectives that guide nursing practice with childbearing families. It continues with an exploration of family nursing with childbearing families before conception through the postpartum period. The chapter covers specific issues that childbearing families may experience, including postpartum depression, attachment concerns, and postpartum illness. Nursing interventions are integrated throughout this chapter to demonstrate how family nurses can help childbearing families prevent complications, increase coping strategies, and adapt to their expanded family structure, development, and function. The chapter concludes with two case studies that explore family adaptations to stressors and changing roles related to childbearing.

Chapter 13: Family Child Health Nursing builds on the major task of families to nurture children to become healthy, responsible, creative adults who can develop meaningful relationships across the life span. Families experience the stress of normative transitions with the addition of each child and situational transitions when children are ill. Knowledge of the family life cycle, child development, and illness trajectory provides a foundation for offering anticipatory guidance and coaching at stressful times. Family life influences the promotion of health and the experience of illness in children, and is influenced by children's health and illness. This chapter provides a brief history of family-centered care of children and then presents foundational concepts that will guide nursing practice with families with children. The chapter goes on to describe nursing care of well children and families with an emphasis on health promotion, nursing care of children and families in acute care settings, nursing care of children with chronic illness and their families, and nursing care of children and their families during end of life. Case studies illustrate the application of family-centered care across settings.

Chapter 14: Family Nursing in Acute Care Adult Settings discusses how the hospitalization of an adult family member for an acute illness, injury, or exacerbation of a chronic illness is stressful for patients and their families. The ill adult enters the hospital, usually in a physiological crisis, and the family most often accompanies the ill or injured family member into the hospital; both the patient and the family are usually in an emotional crisis. Families with members who are acutely or critically ill are seen in adult medical-surgical units, intensive care or cardiac care units, or emergency departments. The purpose of this chapter is to describe family nursing in acute care settings, including families in the CCUs and medical-surgical units.

The chapter begins with a review of literature that captures the major stressors families face during hospitalization of an adult family member: the transfer from one unit to another, being discharged home, participation in cardiopulmonary resuscitation (CPR), withdrawing life support therapy, and organ donation. This chapter concludes with a family case study that (1) highlights the issues families experience and adapt to when an adult member is ill; and (2) applies the Family Systems Theory in order to demonstrate one theoretical approach for working with families.

Chapter 15: Family Health in Mid- and Later Life examines families using a variety of different theoretical approaches, including Family Systems Theories, Developmental and Family Life Cycle Theory, and a Bioecological Model. The chapter presents evidence-based practice on working with adults in mid- and later life, including a review of living choices for older adults with chronic illness, and the importance of peer relationships and intergenerational relationships to quality of life. This chapter includes extensive information about family caregiving for and by older adults, including spouses, adult children, and grandparents. Two case studies conclude the chapter. One family case study illustrates the integrated generational challenges facing older adults today. The second case study addresses care of an older adult family member who never married and has no children. This case presents options for caregiving and the complexity of living healthy.

Chapter 16: Family Mental Health Nursing begins with a brief demographic overview of the pervasiveness of mental health conditions (MHCs) in both Canada and the United States. The remainder of the chapter focuses on the impact a specific MHC can have on the individual with the MHC, individual family members, and the family as a unit. Although the chapter does not go into specific diagnostic criteria for various conditions, it does offer nursing interventions to assist families. One case study explores the impact and treatment of substance abuse. The second presents how a family nurse can work with a family to improve the health of all family members when one family member lives with paranoid schizophrenia.

Chapter 17: Families and Community and Public Health Nursing offers a description of community health nursing in promoting the health of families in communities. It begins with a definition of community health nursing and follows with a discussion of concepts and principles that guide the work of these nurses, the roles they enact in working with families and communities, and the various settings in which they work. This discussion is organized around a visual representation of community health nursing. The chapter ends with a discussion of current trends in community and public health nursing. A case study is presented on working with a homeless family.

ANNETTE BAILEY, PhD, RN
Associate Professor
Ryerson University
Toronto, Ontario, Canada

MARY E. BARTLETT, DNP, APRN,
 FNP-BC, AAHIVs
Assistant Professor
Linfield-Good Samaritan School of Nursing
Linfield College
Portland, Oregon

HENNY BREEN, PhD, RN, CNE, COI
Associate Professor of Nursing
Linfield-Good Samaritan School of Nursing
Linfield College
Portland, Oregon

JULIANA C. CARTWRIGHT, PhD, RN
Associate Professor
School of Nursing
Oregon Health & Science University
Portland, Oregon

LYNNE M. CASPER, PhD
Professor of Sociology
University of Southern California
Los Angeles, California

DEBORAH PADGETT COEHLO, PhD, C-PNP,
 PMHS, CFLE
Developmental and Behavioral Specialist
Juniper Pediatrics
Faculty Member
Oregon State University Cascades
Bend, Oregon

ALLI CORITZ, PhD CANDIDATE
PhD Candidate, Sociology
University of Southern California
Los Angeles, California

DAWN DOUTRICH, PhD, RN
Associate Professor Emeritus
College of Nursing
Washington State University
Vancouver, Washington

LINDA L. EDDY, PhD, RN, ARNP
Associate Dean and Associate Professor
College of Nursing
Washington State University
Vancouver, Washington

LOUISE FLEMING, PhD, RN
Assistant Professor
School of Nursing
University of North Carolina at Chapel Hill
Chapel Hill, North Carolina

TAMMY L. HENDERSON, PhD, CFLE
Professor and Department Chair
Family and Consumer Sciences
Lamar University
Beaumont, Texas

JOANNA ROWE KAAKINEN, PhD, RN
Professor and Interim Dean
Linfield-Good Samaritan School of Nursing
Linfield College
Portland, Oregon

YEOUNSOO KIM-GODWIN, PhD, MPH,
 CNE, RN
Professor
School of Nursing
University of North Carolina Wilmington
Wilmington, North Carolina

KIMBERLY E. KINTZ, DNP, ANP-BC, RN
Associate Professor
Linfield-Good Samaritan School of Nursing
Linfield College
Portland, Oregon

CHUCK LESTER, MPH CANDIDATE
Grant Coordinator
Oklahoma State University
Stillwater, Oklahoma

JUDITH A. MACDONNELL, BScN, RN,
  MED, PhD
Associate Professor
School of Nursing, Faculty of Health
York University
Toronto, Ontario, Canada

JOYCE M. O'MAHONY, RN, PhD
Assistant Professor
School of Nursing
Thompson Rivers University
Kamloops, British Columbia, Canada

CAROLE A. ROBINSON, PhD, RN
Professor
School of Nursing
University of British Columbia Okanagan
Kelowna, British Columbia, Canada

MELISSA ROBINSON, PhD, RN
Associate Professor of Nursing
Linfield-Good Samaritan School of Nursing
Linfield College
Portland, Oregon

LAURA S. RODGERS, PhD, PMHNP-BC
Professor
Linfield-Good Samaritan School of Nursing
Linfield College
Portland, Oregon

MARIA ELENA RUIZ, PhD, RN, FNP-BC
Associate Adjunct Professor
School of Nursing
Coordinator, International Scholarly Activities
  Mexico-Cuba Programs
Affiliate Faculty: Chicano Studies Research Center;
  Latin America Institute
University of California Los Angeles
Los Angeles, California

PAUL S. SMITH, PhD, RN, CCRN, CNE
Assistant Professor
Linfield-Good Samaritan School of Nursing
Linfield College
Portland, Oregon

ROSE STEELE, PhD, RN
Professor
School of Nursing, Faculty of Health
York University
Toronto, Ontario, Canada

AARON TABACCO, PhD, RN
Director of Pre-Licensure Program
Linfield-Good Samaritan School of Nursing
Linfield College
Portland, Oregon

MARCIA VAN RIPER, PhD, RN, FAAN
Professor
Chair of Family Health Division
University of North Carolina at Chapel Hill
Chapel Hill, North Carolina

LINDA VELTRI, PhD, RN
Associate Professor
RN to BSN Program Director
Northwest Christian University
Eugene, Oregon

JACQUELINE F. WEBB, DNP, FNP-BC, RN
Associate Professor
Linfield-Good Samaritan School of Nursing
Linfield College
Portland, Oregon

DIANA L. WHITE, PhD
Senior Research Associate
Institute on Aging
Portland State University
Affiliate Faculty
School of Nursing
Oregon Health and Science University
Portland, Oregon

KIMBERLEY A. WIDGER, PhD, RN,
  CHPCN(C)
Assistant Professor
Lawrence S. Bloomberg School of Nursing
University of Toronto
Toronto, Ontario, Canada

KARLINE WILSON-MITCHELL, DNP, MSN,
  CNM, RN, RM
Associate Professor
Midwifery Education Program
Ryerson University
Toronto, Ontario, Canada

Christine Aramburu Alegria, PhD, APRN, FNP-BC
Associate Professor
Orvis School of Nursing
University of Nevada, Reno
Reno, Nevada

Jennifer Casperson, MSN, RN, CPN, CHSE
Nursing Instructor
Everett Community College
Everett, Washington

Joan Clites, EdD, RN
Associate Professor of Nursing
California University of Pennsylvania
California, Pennsylvania

Patricia E. Freed, MSN, EdD, CNE
Associate Professor, Faculty
School of Nursing
Saint Louis University
St. Louis, Missouri

Mary Ann Glendon, PhD, RN
ACE and RN to BSN Program Coordinator
Professor of Nursing
Southern Connecticut State University
New Haven, Connecticut

Sue K. Goebel, RN, MS, WHNP, SANE
Associate Professor of Nursing
Colorado Mesa University
Grand Junction, Colorado

Beverley Jones, RN, MScN, MPA
Professor BScN Collaborative Program
St. Clair College
Windsor, Ontario
Canada

Jean M. Klein, PhD, PMHCNS, BC
Associate Professor Emerita
Widener University
Chester, Pennsylvania

Brenda G. Kucirka, PhD, PMHCNS-BC, CNE
Assistant Professor
Widener University
Chester, Pennsylvania

Victoria Kyarsgaard, DNP, RNC, PHN, CNE
Associate Professor
Crown College
St. Bonifacius, Minnesota

Krista Lussier, RN, BScN, MSN
Senior Lecturer
Thompson Rivers University
Kamloops, British Columbia
Canada

Nicole McCain, MSN, RN, CNE, CNL
Assistant Professor
Jefferson College of Health Sciences
Roanoke, Virginia

Kim Pickett, MS, APRN, BC-ADM, CDE/PhD(c)
Nurse Practitioner
Center for Family Medicine Residency Program
Spartanburg Regional Healthcare System
Spartanburg, South Carolina

Judith Quaranta, PhD, RN, CPN, AE-C, FNAP
Assistant Professor
Decker School of Nursing
Binghamton University
Binghamton, New York

Theresa Turick-Gibson, EdD(c), MA, PNP-BC, RN-BC
Professor
Hartwick College
Oneonta, New York

Susan S. VanBeuge, DNP, APRN,
  FNP-BC, CNE, FAANP
Associate Professor in Residence
University of Nevada, Las Vegas
Las Vegas, Nevada

Kelli D. Whittington, PhD, RN, CNE
Chair, Division of Nursing
Assistant Professor
McKendree University
Lebanon, Illinois

Contents

Available online at davisplus.fadavis.com:
References
Bonus Chapter: Relational Nursing and Family Nursing in Canada
Appendix: The Friedman Family Assessment Model (Short Form)

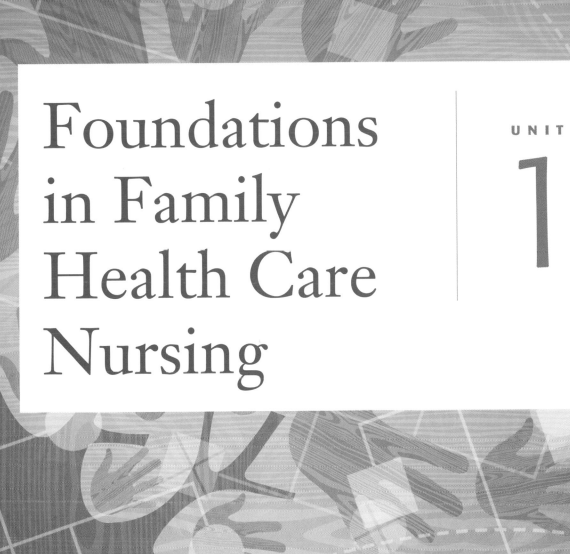

Foundations in Family Health Care Nursing

Chapter 1

Family Health Care Nursing
An Introduction

Joanna Rowe Kaakinen, PhD, RN

Critical Concepts

- Family health care nursing is an art and a science that has evolved as a way of thinking about and working with families.
- The term *family* is defined in many ways, but the most salient definition is, *The family is who the members say it is.*
- Health and illness are family events.
- Health and illness affect all members of families.
- Families influence the process and outcome of health care.
- Understanding families enables nurses to assess the family health status, ascertain the effects of the family on individual family member's health status, predict the influence of alterations in the health status of the family system, and work with members as they plan and implement action plans customized for improved health for each individual family member and the family as a whole.
- Knowledge about each family's structure, function, and process informs the nurse in how to optimize nursing care in families and provide individualized nursing care, tailored to the uniqueness of every family system.

Family health care nursing is an art and a science, a philosophy and a way of interacting with families about health care. It has evolved since the early 1980s as a way of thinking about, and working with, families when a member experiences a health problem. This philosophy and practice incorporates the following assumptions:

- Health and illness affect all members of families.
- Health and illness are family events.
- Families influence the process and outcome of health care.

All health care practices, attitudes, beliefs, behaviors, and decisions are made within the context of larger family and societal systems.

Families vary in structure, function, and processes. The structure, functions, and processes of the family influence and are influenced by each individual family member's health status and the overall health status of the whole family. Families even vary within given cultures because every family has its own unique culture. People who come from the same family of origin create different families over time. Nurses need to be knowledgeable about the theories of families

3

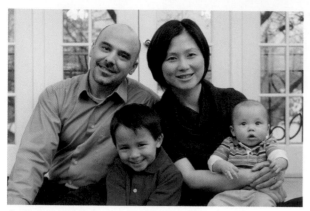

© iStock.com/YinYang

as well as the structure, function, and processes of families to assist them in achieving or maintaining a state of health.

When families are considered the unit of care—as opposed to individuals—nurses have much broader perspectives for approaching health care needs of both individual family members and the family unit as a whole (Kaakinen & Hanson, 2015). Understanding families enables nurses to assess the family health status, ascertain the effects of the family on individual family members' health status, predict the influence of alterations in the health status of the family system, and work with members as they plan and implement action plans customized for improved health for each individual family member and the family as a whole.

Recent advances in health care, such as changing health care policies and health care economics, ever-changing technology, shorter hospital stays, and health care moving from the hospital to the community/family home, are prompting changes from an individual person paradigm to the nursing care of families as a whole. This paradigm shift is affecting the development of family theory, practice, research, social policy, and education, and it is critical for nurses to be knowledgeable about and at the forefront of this shift. The centrality of family-centered care in health care delivery is emphasized by the American Nurses Association (2015) in its publication, described in the *American Nurses Association Guide to Nursing's Social Policy Statement* (Fowler, 2015). In addition, ANA's *Nursing: Scope and Standards of Practice* mandates that nurses provide family care (ANA, 2015). The *National Strategy for Quality Improvement in Health Care* is the first policy to set national goals to improve the quality of health care (Department of Health and

Human Services [DHHS], 2015). It sets standards and regulations to measure the quality of health care and its impacts on public health. The *National Quality Strategy* (DHHS, 2015), the Nursing Alliance for Quality Care (NAQC, 2013), and the Agency for Health care Research and Quality (2015) place a priority on ensuring that each person and the family as a whole are engaged as partners in their health care. "Nurses have an ethical and moral obligation to involve families in their health care practices" (Wright & Leahey, 2013, p. 1).

The overall goal of this book is to enhance nurses' knowledge and skills in the theory, practice, research, and social policy surrounding nursing care of families. This chapter provides a broad overview of family health care nursing. It begins with an exploration of the definitions of family and family health care nursing, as well as the concept of healthy families. Next are described four approaches to working with families: family as context, family as client, family as system, and family as a component of society. The chapter presents the varied, but ever-changing, family structures and explores family functions relative to reproduction, socialization, affective function, economic issues, and health care. Finally, the chapter discusses family processes, so that nurses know how their practice makes a difference when families experience stress because of the illness of individual family members.

THE FAMILY AND FAMILY HEALTH

Three foundational components of family nursing are (1) determining how family is defined, (2) understanding the concepts of family health, and (3) knowing the current evidence about the elements of a healthy family.

What Is the Family?

Family life is a universal human experience and no two individuals have the exact same experience within a family (Galvin, Braithwaite, & Bylund, 2015). However, there is no universally agreed-upon definition of family. Now more than ever, the traditional definition of family is being challenged and is shifting. Canada enacted the Civil Marriage Act in 2005, becoming the fourth country to legalize same-sex marriage (Hogg, 2006). Spain had legalized same-sex marriage less than a month earlier. In June 2015, the United States became the 21st country to legalize same-sex marriage nationwide (Pew Research Center, 2015). *Family* is a word that conjures up different images for each individual and group, and the word has evolved in its meaning over time. Definitions differ by discipline; for example:

- *Legal:* relationships through blood ties, adoption, guardianship, or marriage
- *Biological:* genetic biological networks among and between people
- *Sociological:* groups of people living together with or without legal or biological ties
- *Psychological:* groups with strong emotional ties

Historically, early family social science theorists (Burgess & Locke, 1953, pp. 7–8) adopted the following traditional definition in their writing:

The family is a group of persons united by ties of marriage, blood, or adoption, constituting a single household; interacting and communicating with each other in their respective social roles of husband and wife, mother and father, son and daughter, brother and sister; and creating and maintaining a common culture.

The U.S. Census Bureau basically has held the same definition of family since 1930 (Pemberton, 2015). It defines *family* as two or more people living together who are related by birth, marriage, or adoption. This traditional definition continues to be the basis for the implementation of many social programs and policies. Yet, this definition excludes many diverse groups who consider themselves to be families and who perform family functions, such as economic, reproductive, and affective functions, as well as child socialization. Depending on the social norms, all the following examples could be viewed as "family": married or remarried couples with biological or adoptive children, cohabiting same-sex couples (gay and lesbian families), single-parent families with children, kinship care families such as two sisters living together, or grandparents raising grandchildren without the parents.

The definition of *family* adopted by this textbook and that applies from the previous edition (Kaakinen & Hanson, 2015) is as follows: *Family refers to two or more individuals who depend on one another for emotional, physical, and economic support. The members of the family are self-defined.* Nurses who work with families should ask clients who they

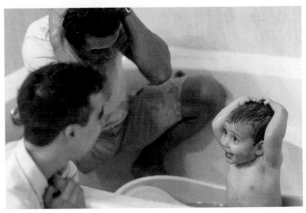

© *iStock.com/Juanmonino*

consider to be members of their family and should include those persons in health care planning with the patient's permission.

What Is Family Health?

The World Health Organization (WHO, 2016) notes that there are more than 400 million people in the world who lack essential health care. In response to this growing need, the WHO developed the Framework on Integrated People-Centered Health Services. This framework states that care should be coordinated around the needs of the people; respect their preferences; and be safe, effective, timely, affordable, and of acceptable quality. It is important to note that this framework is not about patient-centered care, which focuses on the individual, but is about people-centered care that expands the care to individuals, families, communities, and society. The term *family health* is often used interchangeably with the terms *family functioning, healthy families,* or *familial health.* To some, family health is the composite of individual family members' physical health, because it is impossible to make a single statement about the family's physical health as a single entity.

The definition of *family health* adopted in this textbook and that applies from the previous edition (Kaakinen & Hanson, 2015) is as follows: *Family health is a dynamic, changing state of well-being, which includes the biological, psychological, spiritual, sociological, and cultural factors of individual members and the whole family system.* This definition and approach combines all aspects of life for individual members, as well as for the whole family. An individual's health (on the wellness-to-illness continuum) affects the entire family's functioning; in turn, the family's ability to function affects each individual member's health.

Assessment of family health involves simultaneous data collection on individual family members and the whole family system (Kaakinen & Hanson, 2015).

What Is a Well-Functioning Family?

Although it is possible to define family health, it is more difficult to describe characteristics of a family that is well-functioning. Characteristics used to describe functional versus dysfunctional families have varied throughout time in the literature. Krysan, Moore, and Zill (1990) described "healthy families" as "successful families" in a report prepared by the U.S. DHHS. Otto (1963) was the first scholar to develop psychosocial criteria for assessing family strengths, and emphasized the need to focus on positive family attributes instead of the pathological approach that accentuated family problems and weaknesses. Pratt (1976) introduced the idea of the "energized family" as one whose structure encourages and supports individuals to develop their capacities for full functioning and independent action, thus contributing to family health. Curran (1985) investigated not only family stressors but also traits of healthy families, incorporating moral and task focus into traditional family functioning. These traits are listed in Box 1-1.

Olson and Gorall (2005) conducted a longitudinal study on families in which they merged the concepts of marital and family dynamics in the Circumplex Model of Marital and Family Systems. They found that the ability of the family to demonstrate flexibility is related to its ability to alter family leadership roles, relationships, and rules, including control, discipline, and role sharing. Functional, healthy families have the ability to change these factors in response to situations. Dysfunctional families, or unhealthy families, have less ability to adapt and flex in response to changes. See Figures 1-1 and 1-2, which depict the differences in functional and dysfunctional families in the Circumplex Model. Balanced families will function more adequately across the family life cycle and tend to be healthier families. The family communication skills enable balance and help families to adjust and adapt to situations. Couples and families modify their levels of flexibility and cohesion to adapt to stressors, thus promoting family health.

Building on the work of Olson and Gorall (2005), Metegevic, Todorovic, and Javanovic (2014) conducted a study that explored patterns of family function related to parenting style. Their work supports the idea that balanced cohesion and balanced flexibility are the dominant patterns of family functioning. Well-functioning families have tremendous diversity in the ways they cope with predictable and unpredictable stressors and changes (Bush, Price, Price, & McKenry, 2015).

FAMILY HEALTH CARE NURSING

The specialty area of family health care nursing has been evolving since the early 1980s. Some question how family health care nursing is distinct from other specialties that involve families, such as maternal-child health nursing, community health nursing, and mental health nursing. The definition and framework for *family health care nursing* adopted by this textbook and that applies from the previous edition (Kaakinen & Hanson, 2015) is as follows:

> *The process of providing for the health care needs of families that are within the scope of nursing practice. This nursing care can be aimed toward the family as context, the family as a whole, the family as a system, or the family as a component of society.*

At the same time, it cuts across the individual, family, and community for the purpose of promoting, maintaining, and restoring the health of families. This framework illustrates the intersecting concepts of the individual, the family, nursing, and society (Figure 1-3).

BOX 1-1
Traits of a Healthy Family

- Communicates and listens
- Fosters table time and conversation
- Affirms and supports each member
- Teaches respect for others
- Develops a sense of trust
- Has a sense of play and humor
- Has a balance of interaction among members
- Shares leisure time
- Exhibits a sense of shared responsibility
- Teaches a sense of right and wrong
- Abounds in rituals and traditions
- Shares a religious core
- Respects the privacy of each member
- Values service to others
- Admits to problems and seeks help

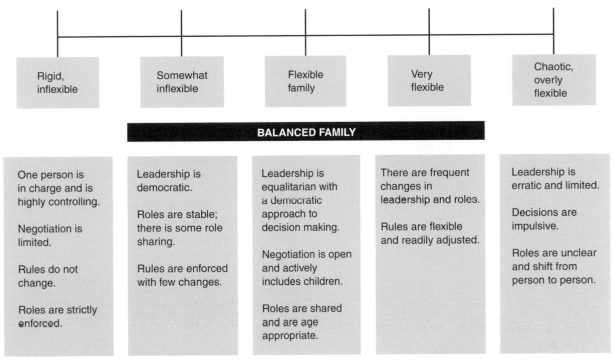

FIGURE 1-1 Family Flexibility Continuum

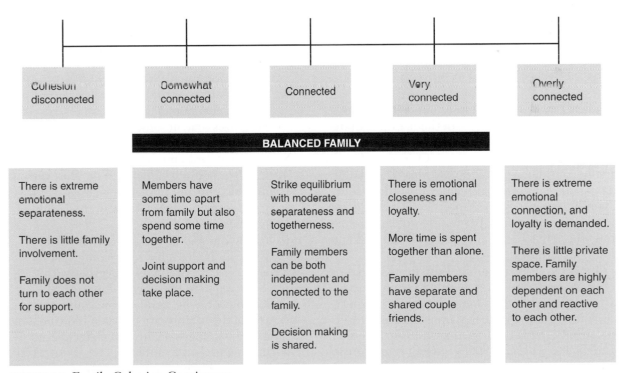

FIGURE 1-2 Family Cohesion Continuum

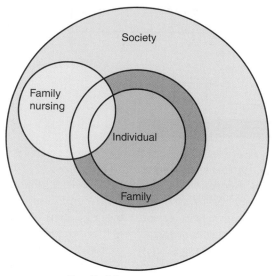

FIGURE 1-3 Family Nursing Conceptual Framework

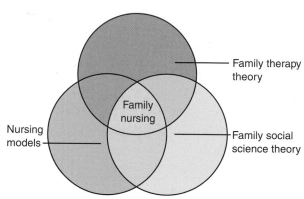

FIGURE 1-4 Family Nursing Practice

Table 1-1	Family Nursing Competencies: Generalist

1. Enhance and promote family health.

2. Focus nursing practice on family's strengths, the support of family and individual growth, the improvement of family self-management abilities, the facilitation of successful life transitions, the improvement and management of health, and the mobilization of family resources.

3. Demonstrate leadership and systems thinking skills to ensure the quality of nursing care with families in everyday practice and across every context.

4. Commit to self-reflective practice based on examination of nurse actions with families and family responses.

5. Practice using an evidence-based approach.

Source: International Family Nursing Association. (2015). *IFNA position statement on generalist competencies for family nursing practice.* Retrieved from http://internationalfamilynursing.org/wordpress/wp-content/uploads/2015/07/GC-Complete-PDF-document-in-color-with-photos-English-language.pdf

Another way to view family nursing practice is conceptually, as a confluence of theories and strategies from nursing, family therapy, and family social science as depicted in Figure 1-4. Over time, family nursing continues to incorporate ideas from family therapy and family social science into the practice of family nursing. See Chapter 2 for a discussion about how theories from family social science, family therapy, and nursing converge to inform the nursing of families.

The International Family Nursing Association (IFNA, April 24, 2017) represents 33 countries with the mission to transform family health by serving as a unifying force and voice for family nursing globally. The IFNA (2015) developed a position statement that defines five specific family nursing competencies for generalist nurses, which are found in Table 1-1.

The following 10 interventions are used by family nurses to provide structure to working with families

regardless of the theoretical underpinning of the nursing approach. These are enduring ideas that support the practice of family nursing (Kaakinen & Hanson, 2015):

1. Family care is concerned with the experience of the family over time. It considers both the history and the future of the family group.

2. Family nursing considers the community and cultural context of the group. The family is encouraged to receive from, and give to, community resources.

3. Family nursing considers the relationships between and among family members, and recognizes that, in some instances, all individual members and the family group will not achieve maximum health simultaneously.

4. Family nursing is directed at families with both healthy and ill members, regardless of the severity of the illness in the family member.

5. Family nursing is often offered in settings where individuals have physiological or psychological problems. Together with competency in treatment of individual health problems, family nurses must recognize the reciprocity between individual family member's health and collective health within the family.

6. Family nursing requires the nurse to manipulate the environment to increase the likelihood of family interaction. The

physical absence of family members, however, does not preclude the nurse from offering family care.

7. The family system is influenced by any change in its members. In family nursing the focus includes the individual as well as how the family system and all family members are affected by the health event. Family nursing requires the nurse to manipulate the environment to increase the likelihood of family interaction. The physical absence of family members, however, does not preclude the nurse from offering family care.

8. The family nurse recognizes that the person in a family who is most symptomatic may change over time; this means that the focus of the nurse's attention will also change over time.

9. Family nursing focuses on the strengths of individual family members and the family group to promote their mutual support and growth.

10. Family nurses must define with the family which persons constitute the family and where they will place their therapeutic energies.

These are the distinctive intervention statements specific to family nursing that appear continuously in the care and study of families in nursing, regardless of the theoretical model in use.

APPROACHES TO FAMILY NURSING

As noted earlier, four different approaches to care are inherent in family nursing: (1) family as the context for individual development, (2) family as a client, (3) family as a system, and (4) family as a component of society (Kaakinen & Hanson, 2015). Figure 1-5 illustrates these approaches to the nursing of families. Each approach derived its foundations from different nursing specialties: maternal-child nursing, primary care nursing, psychiatric/mental health nursing, and community health nursing, respectively. All four approaches have legitimate implications for nursing assessment and intervention. The approach that nurses use is determined by many factors, including the health care setting, family circumstances, and nurse resources. Figure 1-6 shows how a nurse can view

all four approaches to families through just one set of eyes. It is important to keep all four perspectives in mind when working with any given family.

Family as Context

The first approach to family nursing care focuses on the assessment and care of an individual client in which the family is the context. Alternate labels for this approach are *family centered* or *family focused*. This is the traditional nursing focus, in which the individual is foreground and the family is background. The family serves as context for the individual as either a resource or a stressor to the individual's health and illness. Most existing nursing theories or models were originally conceptualized using the individual as a focus. This approach is rooted in the specialty of maternal-child nursing and underlies the philosophy of many maternity and pediatric health care settings. A nurse using this focus might say to an individual client: "Who in your family will help you with your nightly medication?" "How will you provide for child care when you have your back surgery?" or "It is wonderful for you that your wife takes such an interest in your diabetes and has changed all the food preparation to fit your dietary needs."

Family as Client

The second approach to family nursing care centers on the assessment of all family members. The family nurse is interested in the way all the family members are individually affected by the health event of one family member. In this approach, all members of the family are in the foreground. The family is seen as the sum of individual family members, and the focus concentrates on each individual. The nurse assesses and provides health care for each person in the family. This approach is seen typically in primary care clinics in the communities where primary care physicians (PCPs) or nurse practitioners (NPs) provide care over time to all individuals in a given family. From this perspective, a nurse might ask a family member who has just become ill: "How has your diagnosis of juvenile diabetes affected the other individuals in your family?" "Will your nightly need for medication be a problem for other members of your family?" "Who in your family is having the most difficult time with your diagnosis?" or "How are the members of your family adjusting to your new medication regimen?"

Family as Context

Individual as foreground
Family as background

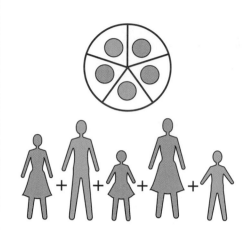

Family as Client

Family as foreground
Individual as background

Family as System

Interactional family

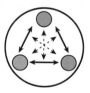

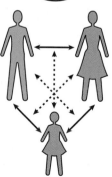

Family as Component of Society

Legal

Family   Education

              Health

Religion   Social

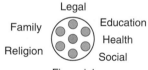

Financial

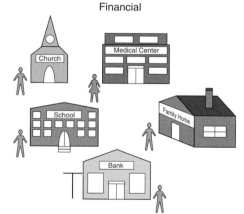

FIGURE 1-5 Approaches to Family Nursing

Family as System

The third approach to care views the family as a system. The focus in this approach is on the family as a whole as the client; here, the family is viewed as an interactional system in which the whole is more than the sum of its parts. In other words, the interactions between family members become the target for the nursing interventions. The interventions flow from the assessment of the family as a whole. The family nursing system approach focuses on the individual

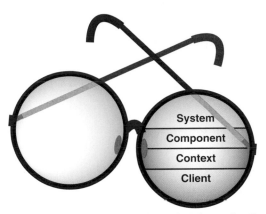

FIGURE 1-6 Four Views of Family Through a Lens

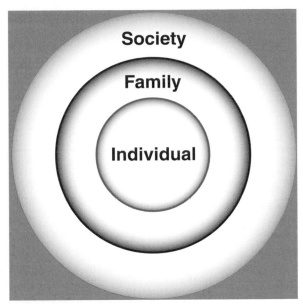

FIGURE 1-7 Family as Primary Group in Society

and family simultaneously. The emphasis is on the interactions between family members; for example, the direct interactions between the parental dyad or the indirect interaction between the parental dyad and the child. The more children there are in a family, the more complex these interactions become.

This interactional model had its start with the specialty of psychiatric and mental health nursing. The systems approach always implies that when something happens to one part of the system, the other parts of the system are affected. Therefore, if one family member becomes ill, it affects all other members of the family. Examples of questions that nurses may ask in a systems approach include the following: "What has changed between you and your spouse since your child was diagnosed with juvenile diabetes?" or "How has the diagnosis of juvenile diabetes affected the ways in which your family is functioning and getting along with each other?"

Family as Component of Society

The fourth approach to care looks at the family as a component of society, in which the family is viewed as one of many institutions in society, similar to health, educational, religious, or economic institutions. The family is a basic or primary unit of society, and it is a part of the larger system of society (Figure 1-7). The family as a whole interacts with other institutions to receive, exchange, or give communication and services. Family social scientists first used this approach in their study of families in society. Community health nursing has drawn many of its tenets from this perspective as it focuses on the interface between families and community agencies. Questions nurses may ask in this approach include the following: "What issues has the family been experiencing since you made the school aware of your son's diagnosis of HIV?" or "Have you considered joining a support group for families with mothers who have breast cancer? Other families have found this to be an excellent resource and a way to reduce stress."

VARIABLES THAT INFLUENCE FAMILY NURSING

Family health care nursing has been influenced by many variables that are derived from both historical and current events within society and the profession of nursing. Examples include changing nursing theory, practice, education, and research; new knowledge derived from family social sciences and the health sciences; national and state health care policies; changing health care behavior and attitudes; and national and international political events. Chapters 2 and 4 provide detailed discussions of these areas.

Figure 1-8 illustrates how many variables influence contemporary family health nursing, making the point that the status of family nursing is dependent on what is occurring in the wider society—family as community. A recent example of this point is that health practices and policy changes are underway because of the recognition that current costs of health

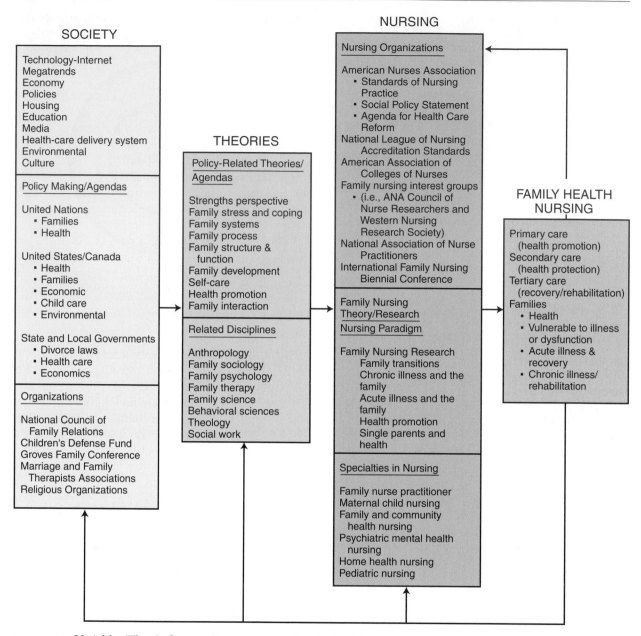

FIGURE 1-8 Variables That Influence Contemporary Family Health Care *(Adapted from Bomar, P. J. [Ed.]. [2004]. Promoting health in families: Applying family research and theory to nursing practice [3rd ed., p. 17]. Philadelphia, PA: Saunders/Elsevier, with permission.)*

care are escalating and, at the same time, greater numbers of people are underinsured or uninsured and have lost access to health care. The goal of this health care reform is to make access and treatment available for everyone at an affordable cost. That will require a major shift in priorities, funding, and services. A major movement toward health promotion and family care in the community will greatly affect the evolution of family nursing.

FAMILY NURSING ROLES

Families are the basic unit of every society, but it is also true that families are complex, varied, dynamic, and adaptive, which is why it is crucial for all nurses to be knowledgeable about the scientific discipline of family nursing, and the variety of ways nurses may interact with families (Kaakinen & Hanson, 2015).

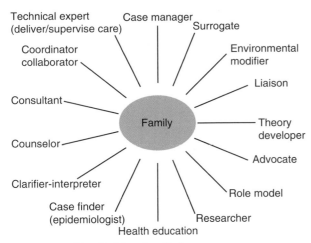

FIGURE 1-9 Family Nursing Roles

The roles of family health care nurses are evolving along with the specialty. Figure 1-9 lists the many roles that nurses can assume with families as the focus. This figure was constructed from some of the first family nursing literature that appeared, and it is a composite of what various scholars believe to be some of the current roles of nurses. Keep in mind that the health care setting affects roles that nurses assume with families.

Health Teacher: The family nurse teaches about family wellness, illness, relations, and parenting, to name a few topics. The teacher-educator function is ongoing in all settings in both formal and informal ways. Examples include teaching new parents how to care for their infant and giving instructions about diabetes to a newly diagnosed adolescent boy and his family members.

Coordinator, Collaborator, Navigator, and Liaison: The family nurse coordinates the care that families receive, collaborating with the family to plan care. For example, if a family member has been in a traumatic accident, the nurse would be a key person in helping families to access resources—from inpatient care, outpatient care, home health care, and social services to rehabilitation. Nurse navigators provide a holistic approach to care delivery by working with patients and families as a care coordinator and patient advocate with the purpose of giving each patient/family under their care a consistent point of connection in a highly fragmented, complex health care industry. Nurse navigators help patients and

their family access the health care system and overcome barriers to receiving care, as well as facilitate the provision of timely, quality care in a culturally sensitive manner.

"Deliverer" and Supervisor of Care and Technical Expert: The family nurse either delivers or supervises the care that families receive in various settings. To do this, the nurse must be a technical expert both in terms of knowledge and skill. For example, the nurse may be the person going into the family home on a daily basis to consult with the family and help take care of a child on a respirator.

Family Advocate: The family nurse advocates for families and empowers family members to speak with their own voices, or the nurse speaks out for the family. An example is a school nurse advocating for special education services for a child with attention deficit-hyperactivity disorder.

Consultant: The family nurse serves as a consultant to families whenever asked or whenever necessary. For example, a clinical nurse specialist in a hospital may be asked to assist the family in finding the appropriate long-term care setting for their sick grandmother. The nurse comes into the family system by request for a short period and for a specific purpose.

Counselor: The family nurse has a therapeutic role in helping individuals and families solve problems or change behavior. An example from the mental health arena is a family that requires help with coping with a long-term chronic condition, such as when a family member has been diagnosed with schizophrenia.

"Case-Finder" and Epidemiologist: The family nurse gets involved in case-finding and becomes a tracker of disease. For example, consider the situation in which a family member has been recently diagnosed with a sexually transmitted infection. The nurse would engage in sleuthing out the sources of the transmission and in helping other sexual contacts to seek treatment. Screening families and subsequent referral of the family members may be a part of this role.

Environmental Specialist: The family nurse consults with families and other health care providers to modify the environment. For example, if a man with paraplegia is about to be discharged from the hospital to home, the nurse assists the family in modifying the home environment so that the patient can move around in a wheelchair and engage in self-care.

Clarifier and Interpreter: The nurse clarifies and interprets data to families in all settings. For example, if a child in the family has a complex disease, such as leukemia, the nurse clarifies and interprets information pertaining to the diagnosis, treatment, and prognosis of the condition to parents and extended family members.

Surrogate: The family nurse serves as a surrogate by substituting for another person. For example, the nurse may stand in temporarily as a loving parent to an adolescent who is giving birth to a child by herself in the labor and delivery room.

Researcher: The family nurse should identify practice problems and find the best solution for dealing with these problems through the process of scientific investigation. An example might be collaborating with a colleague to find a better intervention for helping families cope with incontinent older adults living in the home.

Role Model: The family nurse is continually serving as a role model to other people. A school nurse who demonstrates the right kind of health in personal self-care serves as a role model to parents and children alike.

Case Manager: Although case manager is a contemporary name for this role, it involves coordination and collaboration between a family and the health care system. For example, a family nurse working with seniors in the community may become assigned to be the case manager for a patient with Alzheimer's disease.

OBSTACLES TO FAMILY NURSING PRACTICE

There are several obstacles to practicing family nursing. A vast amount of literature is available about families, but there has been little taught about families in the nursing curricula until the past three decades. Most practicing nurses have not had exposure to family theory or concepts during their undergraduate education and continue to practice using the individualist paradigm. Even though there are several family assessment models and approaches, families are complex, so no one assessment approach fits all family situations.

Nursing also has strong historical ties with the medical model, which has traditionally focused on the individual as client, rather than the family. At best, families have been viewed in context, and many times families were considered a nuisance in health care settings—an obstacle to overcome to provide care to the individual.

Another obstacle is the fact that the traditional charting system in health care has been oriented to the individual. For example, charting by exception focuses on the physical care of the individual and does not address the whole family or members of families. Likewise, the medical and nursing diagnostic systems used in health care are disease centered, and diseases are focused on individuals and have limited diagnostic codes that pertain to the family as a whole. To complicate matters further, most insurance companies require that there be one identified patient, with a diagnostic code drawn from an individual disease perspective. There are some ICD-10 diagnostic codes that include family diagnosis, such as Problems With Primary Support System, but insurance companies often do not cover these diagnoses.

Thus, even if health care providers are intervening with entire families, companies require providers to choose one person in the family group as the identified patient and to give that person a physical or mental diagnosis, even though the client is the whole family. Although there are family diagnostic codes that address care with families, insurance companies may not pay for care for those codes, especially if the care is more psychological or educational in nature. See Chapter 5 for a detailed discussion on diagnostic classification systems.

The established hours during which health care systems provide services pose another obstacle to focusing on families. Traditionally, office hours take place during the day, when family members cannot accompany other family members. Recently, some urgent care centers and other outpatient settings have incorporated evening and weekend hours into their schedules, making it possible for family members to come in together. But many clinics and physician offices still operate on traditional Monday through Friday, 9:00 a.m. to 5:00 p.m. schedules, thus making it difficult for all family members to attend together. Some hospitals and residential care centers still have limited visiting hours for family members, and often do not include family members in treatment meetings, even if the care has an impact on family members. These obstacles to family-focused nursing practice are slowly changing; nurses should continue to lobby for changes that are more conducive to caring for the family as a whole.

FAMILY STRUCTURE, FUNCTION, AND PROCESS

Knowledge about family structure, functions, and processes is essential for understanding the complex family interactions that affect health, illness, and well-being (Kaakinen & Hanson, 2015). Knowledge emerging from the study of family structure, function, and process suggests concepts and a framework that nurses can use to provide effective assessment and intervention with families. Many internal and external family variables affect individual family members and the family as a whole. One of the major influences on how the family responds to health care needs and how nurses provide care to the family is the dimension and complexity involved in caring for people from diverse cultural backgrounds. Internal family variables include unique individual characteristics, communication, and interactions, whereas external family variables include location of family household, social policy, and economic trends. Family members generally have complicated responses to all these factors. Although some external factors may not be easily modifiable, nurses can assist family members to manage change, conflict, and care needs. For instance, a sudden downturn in the economy could result in the family breadwinner becoming underemployed or unemployed. Although nurses are unable to alter this situation directly, understanding the implications on the family situation provides a basis for planning more effective interventions that may include financial support programs for families. Nurses can assist members with coping skills, communication patterns, location of needed resources, effective use of information, or creation of family rituals or routines (Kaakinen & Hanson, 2015).

Nurses who understand the concepts of family structure, function, and process can use this knowledge to educate, counsel, and implement changes that enable families to cope with illness, family crisis, chronic health conditions, and mental illness. Nurses prepared to work with families can assist them with needed life transitions (Kaakinen & Hanson, 2015). For example, when a family member experiences a chronic condition such as diabetes, family roles, routines, and power hierarchies may be challenged. Nurses must be prepared to address the complex and holistic family problems resulting from illness, as well as to care for the individual's medical needs.

Family Structure

Family structure is the ordered set of relationships within the family, without respect to roles and function. The family form or structure does not indicate how healthy the family is or how it functions.

In terms of family nursing, it is logical to begin with the "who" of families before moving to the "how" or "why." In determining the family structure, the nurse needs to identify the following:

- The individuals who comprise the family
- The relationships between them
- The interactions between the family members
- The interactions with other social systems

Families in the past were more homogeneous than they are today. In the past, the norm in predominantly white families was a two-parent family (traditional nuclear family) living together with their biological children. Today there are a multitude of family forms. For example, a new type of family structure is "living together apart," where couples share living space and may share financial, household, or parenting responsibilities even though they have no romantic attachment to each other. This new family form should not be confused with a more recent trend in family relationships called "living apart together," where couples are forgoing cohabitation entirely, preferring to keep their separate homes (Duncan & Phillips, 2010; Duncan, Phillips, Roseneil, Carter, & Stoilova, 2013).

Different family types have their strengths and limitations, which directly or indirectly affect individuals and family health. Many families still adhere to more customary forms and patterns, but many of today's families fall into categories more clearly labeled as nontraditional (Table 1-2).

Table 1-2	Variations of Family and Household Structures
Family Type	**Composition**
Single family	Living alone, never married
Nuclear dyad/childless	Married couple, no children
Nuclear	Two generations of family, parents, and their own or adopted children residing in the same household
Binuclear	Two postdivorce families with children as members of both
Extended/Multigenerational	Two or more adult generations and one that includes grandparents and grandchildren living in the same household
Blended/Reconstituted	One or more of the parents have been married previously and they bring with them children from their previous marriage
Single parent/lone family	One parent and child(ren) residing in one household
Commune	Group of men, women, and children
Cohabitation (domestic partners)	Unmarried couple sharing a household who are involved in an emotional and/or sexually intimate relationship
Living together apart	Couples share living space and may share financial, household, or parenting responsibilities even though they have no romantic attachment to each other; this form of a structure lives in the same household
Living apart together	Two people with or without children forgoing cohabitation entirely, preferring to keep their separate homes

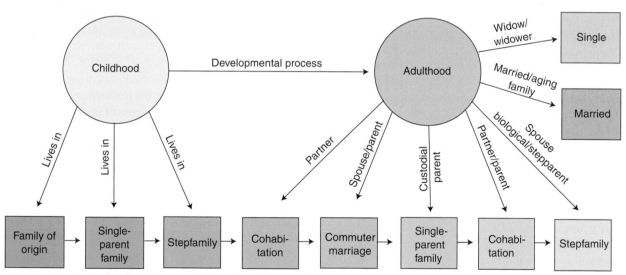

FIGURE 1-10 An Individual's Potential Family Life Experiences

With greater life expectancy, four- and five-generation families are not uncommon (Walsh, 2016b). The average person born today will experience many family forms during his or her lifetime. Figure 1-10 depicts the variety of familial forms that a person can live through today. Nurses will encounter families structured differently from their own families of origin, which may conflict with personal versus professional value systems.

So not only does structure influence the way the family meets the needs of its members, but it also brings stressors and strengths from how the family came to be that structure. There are multiple ways to think about family structure besides these more common structures (Golombok, 2015). For example, there are coparenting families, families with some children adopted and some biological, open marriage and open families, dual career families, commuter families, or multiadult households.

There is some evidence that children can be raised well in a variety of family structures (Lansford, Ceballo, Abby, & Stewart, 2001). Recent studies show that children in cohabitating households have poorer health outcomes than children in married households regardless of the sex composition of their parents (Krueger, Jutte, Franzini, Elo, & Hayward, 2015; Lee & McLanahan, 2015; Reczek, Spiker, Liu, & Crosnoe, 2016). Research clearly shows that children in gender-variant families fare as well as those with heterosexual parents, although they are challenged by social stigma (Biblarz & Stacey, 2010; Brodzinsky, Green, & Katuzny, 2012). What this recent research is suggesting is that what matters most for healthy child development is living in a family that has caring committed relationships that last over time and effective family processes (Lansford, Ceballo, Abby, & Stewart, 2001; Lee & McLanahan, 2015; Walsh, 2016b).

For nurses to work effectively with families, they must maintain open and inquiring minds. Nurses are not only experiencing this proliferation of variation in their own personal lives, but also with the individuals and families with whom they work in the health care settings (Kaakinen & Webb, 2015). Understanding family structure enables nurses assisting families to identify effective coping strategies for daily life disturbances, health care crises, wellness promotion, and disease prevention (Ferrara, Corsello, Sbordone, Cutrona, & Pettoello-Mantavani, 2016; Kaakinen & Hanson, 2015). In addition, nurses are central in advocating and developing social policies relevant to family health care needs. For example, taking political action to increase the availability of appropriate care for children could reduce the financial and emotional burden of many working and single-parent families when faced with providing care for sick children. Similarly, caregiving responsibilities and health care costs for acutely and chronically ill family members place increasing demands on family members. Nurses well informed about different family structures can identify specific needs of unique families, provide appropriate clinical care to enhance family resilience, and act as change agents to enact social policies that reduce family burdens.

Family Functions

A functional perspective has to do with the ways families serve their members. One way to describe the functional aspect of family is to see the unit as made up of intimate, interactive, and interdependent persons who share some values, goals, resources, responsibilities, decisions, and commitment over time (Steinmetz, Clavan, & Stein, 1990). Family function relates to the larger purposes or roles of families in society at large.

It is important to be clear that there is a distinction between the concepts of family function (the prescribed social and cultural obligations and roles of family in society) and family functioning (the processes of family life). Family functioning has been described as "the individual and cooperative processes used by developing persons as to dynamically engage one another and their diverse environments over the life course" (Denham, 2003, p. 277). Family function includes the ways a family reproduces offspring, interacts to socialize its young, cooperates to meet economic needs, and relates to the larger society.

Nurses should ask about specific characteristics that factor into achieving family or societal goals, or both. Families' functional processes such as socialization, reproduction, economics, and health care provision are areas nurses can readily assess and address during health care encounters. Nursing interventions can enhance the family's protective health function when teaching and counseling is tailored to explicit learning needs. Family cultural context and individual health literacy needs are closely related to functional needs of families. Nurses become therapeutic agents as they assist families to identify social supports and locate community resources during times of family transitions and health crisis. Five specific family functions are worth deeper investigation here: reproductive, socialization, affective, economic, and health care.

Reproductive Functions of the Family

The survival of a society is linked to patterns of reproduction. Sexuality serves the purposes of pleasure and reproduction, but associated values differ from one society to another. Traditionally, the family has been organized around the biological function of reproduction. Reproduction was viewed as a major concern for thousands of years during which efforts to populate the world were continually threatened by famine, disease, war, and other life uncertainties.

Norms about sexual intercourse affect the fertility rate. Fertility rate is "the average number of children that would be born per woman if all women lived to the end of their childbearing years and bore children according to a given fertility rate at each age" (World Factbook, 2015). In general, global fertility rates are in decline, with the most pronounced decline being in industrialized countries, especially Western Europe (World Factbook, 2015). Global concerns about overpopulation and environmental threats, as well as personal views of morality and financial well-being, have been reasons for limiting numbers of family births.

Since the 1980s, the reproductive function has become increasingly separated from the family (Kaakinen & Hanson, 2015). As mores and norms change over time, it is not deemed "unacceptable" in many industrialized countries for birth to occur outside of marriage. Abstinence, various forms of contraception, tubal ligation, vasectomy, family planning, artificial insemination, and abortion have various degrees of social acceptance as means to control reproduction. Many aspects of reproduction continue to be the subject of social and ethical controversy. Nurses working with families find themselves at the forefront of practical issues related to providing care in this complex context.

The ethical dilemmas surrounding abortion, for example, seem compounded by technological advances that affect reproduction and problems of infertility. Reproductive technologies are guided by few legal, ethical, or moral guidelines. Artificial insemination by husband or donor, in vitro fertilization, surrogate mothers, and artificial embryonization, in which a woman other than the woman who will give birth to and raise the child donates an egg for fertilization, create financial and moral dilemmas. Although assistive reproductive technologies can provide a biological link to the child, some families are choosing to adopt children. Many are wrangling over the issues implicit in cross-racial and cross-cultural adoptions. Reproductive technologies and adoption are being considered by all family types to add children to the family unit. Religious, legal, moral, economic, and technological challenges will continue to cause debates in the years ahead about family control over reproduction, such as gender selection of the child.

Socialization Functions of the Family

The family is the first and one of the most influential settings for socialization. Families are the primary source of individual development and the primary setting in which children begin to acquire their beliefs, attitudes, values, and behaviors considered appropriate to society (Ogwo, 2013). A major function for families is to teach children to be well-integrated and participating members of society. Socialization also includes how children acquire culture through language and the modeling of others in the family. Individuals learn and usually adopt cultural norms through the socialization process.

Families have great variability in the ways they address the physical and emotional needs, moral values, and economic needs of children, and these patterns are influenced specifically by the role of parenting and somewhat by the larger society (Grusec, 2011). Children are born into families without knowledge of the values, language, norms, morals, communication, or roles of the society in which they live. A major function of the family continues to be to socialize them about family life and ground them in the societal identity of which they are a part. The function of the family relative to socialization includes protection, mutual reciprocity or interdependence between family members, control, guided learning, and group participation, and all these functions are assumed to be operative in all cultures (Grusec, 2011).

Although the family is not the only institution of society that participates in socialization of children, it is generally viewed as having primary responsibility for this function. When children fail to meet societal standards, it is common to blame this on family deficits and parental inadequacies; however, it is important to keep in mind that the issues are more complex.

Today, patterns of socialization require appropriate developmental care that fosters dependence and leads to independence (Denham, 2005). Socialization is the primary way children acquire the social and psychological skills needed to take their place in the adult world. Parents combine social support and social control as they equip children to meet future life tasks. Parental figures interact in multiple roles such as friends, lovers, child-care providers, housekeepers, financial providers, recreation specialists, and counselors. Children growing up within families learn the values and norms of their parents and extended families.

Another role of families in the socialization process is to guide children through various rites of passage. Rites of passage are ceremonies that announce a change in status in the ways members are viewed. Examples include events such as a baptism, communion, circumcision, puberty ritual, graduation, wedding, and death. These occasions signal to others changes in role relationships and new expectations. Understandings about families' unique rites of passage can assist nurses working with diverse health care needs.

Affective Functions of the Family

Affective function is one of the basic functions of family. Fulfilling this function and positive emotional relationships among family members are essential for creating a harmonic and stable environment that is optimal for healthy child development and for the satisfaction of all family members. Affective function has to do with the ways family members relate to one another and those outside the immediate family boundaries. Well-functioning families are able to maintain a consistent level of involvement with one another, yet at the same time not become too involved in each other's lives (Peterson & Green, 2009). Well-functioning families have empathetic interaction where family members care deeply about each other's feelings and activities, and are emotionally invested in each other. Families with a strong affective function are the most effective type of families (Peterson & Green, 2009). All families have boundaries that help to buffer stresses and pressure of systems outside the family on its members. Well-functioning families protect their boundaries, but at the same time give members room to negotiate their independence. Achieving this balance is often difficult in our fast-paced culture. It is also particularly difficult in families with adolescents (Peterson & Green, 2009). Emotional involvement is a key to successful family functioning. Researchers have identified several characteristics of strong families. Among these are expressions of appreciation, spending time together, strong commitment to the family, good communication, and positive conflict resolution (Peterson & Green, 2009). When family members feel that they are supported and encouraged and that their personal interests are valued, family interaction becomes more effective.

Families provide a sense of belonging and identity to their members. This identity often proves to be vitally important throughout the entire life cycle. Within the confines of families, members learn dependent roles that later serve to launch them into independent ones. Families serve as a place to learn about intimate relationships and establish the foundation for future personal interactions. Families provide the initial experience of self-awareness, which includes a sense of knowing one's own gender, ethnicity, race, religion, and personal characteristics. Families help members become acquainted with who they are and experience themselves in relationships with others. Families provide the substance for self-identity, as well as a foundation for other-identity. Within the confines of families, individual members learn about love, care, nurturance, dependence, and support of the dying.

Resilience implies an ability to rebound from stress and crisis, the capacity to be optimistic, solve problems, be resourceful, and develop caring support systems. Although unique traits alter potential for emotional and psychological health, individuals exposed to resilient family environments tend to have greater potential to achieve normative developmental patterns and positive sibling and parental relationships (Denham, 2005).

Variables such as the quality of couples' relationships, the ways families' conflicts are handled, whether abuse or violence has previously occurred in the households or members' lives, frequency of children's contact with nonresidential parents, shared custody arrangements, and emotional relationships between parents and children appear to be important predictors of family affective functions.

Affective functions can best be understood by gathering information from all the various members involved within a household. Shared or discrepant views among family members have an important influence on the overall functioning of families' management of illness (Knafl, Breitmayer, Gallo, & Zoeller, 1996; Knafl, Deatrick, & Gallo, 2008).

Economic Functions of the Family

Families are the means whereby children are supplied with necessities such as food, shelter, and clothing. Families have an important function in keeping both local and national economies viable. Economic conditions significantly affect families. When economies become turbulent, it affects families' structures, functions, and processes. People make decisions about when to enter the labor force, when to marry, when to have children, and when to retire or come out of retirement based on economic factors. For a detailed discussion on family and economics, see Chapter 2.

Family income provides a substantial part of family economics, but an equally important aspect has to do with economic interactions and consumerism related to household consumption and finance. Money management, housing decisions, consumer spending, insurance choices, retirement planning, and savings are some of the issues that affect the family's capacity to care for the economic needs of its members (Lamanna & Reidmann, 2011). These values and skills are passed down to children within the family structure. Financial vulnerability and bankruptcy have increased for middle-class families (Denham, 2005). The ability of the family to earn a sufficient income and to manage its finances wisely is a critical factor related to economic well-being.

In order to meet their own economic needs and maintain family life and health, family members take upon themselves several contributory roles for obtaining and utilizing the wages. Family nurses should explore the types of resources available or lacking as families engage in providing health care functions to their members.

Health Care Functions of the Family

The family is the primary source where individuals learn how to maintain health, protect health, and restore health. Families are expected to provide care for sick family members. Families influence well-being, prevention, illness care, maintenance care associated with chronic illness, and rehabilitative care. Individuals regularly seek services from a variety of health care providers, but the family is the primary social context in which health issues are addressed. It is within the family that decisions are made about health care, such as when to seek professional treatment and whether to follow or ignore treatment options. Families can become particularly vulnerable when they encounter health threats, and family-focused nurses are in a position where they can provide education, counseling, and assistance with locating resources. Family-focused care implies that when a single individual is the target of care, the entire family is still viewed as the unit of care (Denham, 2003).

Health care functions of the family include many aspects of family life. Family members have different ideas about health and illness, and often these ideas are not discussed within families until problems arise. Availability and cost of health care insurance is a concern for many families, but many families lack clarity about what is and is not covered until they encounter a problem. Lifestyle behaviors, such as healthy diet, regular exercise, and alcohol and tobacco use, are areas that family members may not associate with health and illness outcomes. Risk reduction, health promotion and maintenance, rehabilitation, and caregiving are areas where families often need information and assistance. Family members spend far more time taking care of health issues of family members than professionals do.

Family Processes

Family process refers to the interactions between members of a family, including their relationships, communication patterns, time spent together, and satisfaction with family life (World Family Map, 2015). In part, family process makes every family unique within its own particular culture. Families with similar structures and functions may interact differently. Family process, at least in the short term, appears to have a greater effect on the family's health status than family structure as it influences how a family functions. In any illness situation, processes within families are affected by alterations in health status. Families mobilize and organize their resources, buffer stresses, and at times reorganize who does what in the family to fit the changing conditions (Walsh, 2016b).

Alterations in family processes most likely occur when the family faces a transition brought about by normative (expected) developmental changes and nonnormative (uncommon, untimely, or unexpected) changes in the family such as adding or subtracting family members, an illness or accident, or other potential crisis situations, such as natural disasters, wars, or personal crises. The family's current modes of operation may become ineffective, and members are confronted with learning new ways of coping with change. For example, when coping with the stress of a chronic illness, families experience alterations in role performance. When individuals are unable to perform their usual roles in the family, those roles need to be assumed either by other family members or by an outside person or microsystem. During times of change, family nurses can assist family members to restabilize by helping the family determine how to accomplish daily routines (family roles), facilitate communication, locate needed resources, and use a shared decision-making approach to foster family resilience and coping.

Nursing interventions that promote resiliency in family processes vary with the degree of strain faced by the family. Families have complex needs related to adaptation, goal attainment, integration, pattern, and tension management. When family processes are ineffective or disrupted, the families and their members may be at risk for problems pertinent to health outcomes, and the family itself could be in danger of disintegrating.

Following is a discussion of a few family processes that nurses can influence through their relationships with families in caregiving situations. The family processes covered here include family coping, family roles, family communication, family decision making, and family rituals and routines.

Family Coping

In any kind of crisis families function best when the whole family can come together in offering support, resources, and nurturance (Walsh, 2015, 2016b). "Informal kin and chosen family members can be lifelines for resilience, especially for under-resourced single parents, immigrants, refugees, and migrant workers" (Walsh, 2016b, p. 77).

Every family has its own repertoire of coping strategies, which may or may not be adequate in times of stress, such as when a family member experiences an altered health event. Even families who function at optimal levels with well-established coping strategies may experience difficulties when stressful events pile up (Walsh, 2015, 2016b). Coping consists of "constantly changing cognitive and behavioral efforts to manage specific external and/or internal demands that are appraised as taxing or exceeding the resources of the person" (Lazarus & Folkman, 1984, p. 141). Families with support can withstand and rebound from difficult stressors or crises (Walsh, 2016b), which is referred to as *family resilience*. "Family resilience refers to the capacity of the family system to withstand and rebound from adversity, strengthened and more resourceful. More than coping with or surviving an ordeal, resilience involves positive adaptation, (re)gaining the ability to thrive, with personal and relational transformation and positive growth forged through the experience" (Walsh, 2016a, p. 616).

Not all families have the same ability to cope because of multiple reasons. There is no universal list of key effective factors that contribute to family resiliency, but a review of research and literature by Black and Lobo (2008) found the following similarities across studies for those families that cope well: a positive outlook, spirituality, family member accord, flexibility, communication, financial management, time together, mutual recreational interests, routines and rituals, and social support

(Black & Lobo, 2008). According to Walsh (2016a, 2016b) some key processes in family resiliency include belief system, organizational patterns, and family communication. The family's belief system involves making meaning of adversity, maintaining a positive outlook, and being able to transcend adversity through a spiritual/faith system (Walsh, 2016a, 2016b). The families' organization patterns, which speak to their flexibility, connectedness, and social and economic resources, help the family maintain resilience. Finally, families who communicate with clarity, allow open emotional expression, and have a collaborative problem-solving approach facilitate family resiliency (Walsh, 2016a, 2016b).

Nurses have the ability to support families in times of stress and crisis through empowering processes that work well and are familiar to the family. Using a strengths-based approach, family nurses help families to adjust and adapt to stressors (Walsh, 2015, 2016b). Table 1-3 lists some competencies of

Table 1-3	**Core and Associated Competencies of Cancer Nurse Navigators**

Cancer nurse navigators perform the following competencies:

- Facilitate a collaborative approach by helping the patient/family and the health care providers to work as a team
- Be a conduit of information between the patient and health care team
- Work with one family member or the whole family-as-client to understand and manage the care plan and associated side effects, symptoms, and complications
- Provide individualized information and education, based on their need, education level, and situation using evidence-based strategies to help patients and families cope
- Engage in conversations comfortably about different needs, feelings, fears, concerns, and losses that the individual and family may encounter throughout their illness story
- Prepare the patient/family to self-manage and anticipate problems and issues associated with treatment side effects and symptoms of standard treatments
- Use evidence-based interventions to prevent or minimize problems/symptoms as they occur
- Facilitate a coordinated approach by using assessment skills to identify and address changing health and supportive care needs .

Adapted from Cook, S., Fillion, L., Fitch, M., Veillette, A-M., Matheson, T., Aubin, M., . . . Rainville, F. (2013). Core areas of practice and associated competencies for nurses working as professional cancer navigators. *Canadian Oncology Nursing Journal, 23*(1), 44–52.

nurse navigators in the area of cancer that can be used by all family nurses to assist families in coping with illness.

Family Roles

All families have a variety of different kinds of roles. A role is an expected pattern or set of behaviors associated with a particular position or status. Roles in the family are defined as formal when they are associated with position and structure. Roles can be defined according to the job that a role performs to help the family function on a daily basis. Other roles are informal and often fall under the aspect of being related to the family member's personality. All roles help the family function.

Within the family, regardless of structure, each family position has several attached roles, and each role is accompanied by expectations. The following formal roles defined by family structure are typically present in all families in some fashion: parent, child, brother, sister, spouse/partner, grandparent, aunt/uncle, and grandchild. The *family genogram* is a format for diagramming a family tree that records information about family members and relationships over at least three generations (McGoldrick, 2016). It provides a quick overview of family complexities that provide the nurse opportunities to explore with the family about possible resources. Family genograms are discussed in detail in Chapter 5.

Functional roles help the family accomplish tasks that keep the family organized in getting the work of the family done. Some of these roles include the tasks of provider (breadwinner), housekeeper, child care, cook, shopper, fix-it repair person, chauffer, caregiver, financial manager, laundry person, lawn mower, kinship, organizer/planner, and decision maker. When a new family member is added, such as with the birth of a child or adoption of a child, new roles are necessary to support the functioning of the family. When a family member becomes ill, he or she struggles to perform the family roles that support family functioning. When the disruption is experienced during a short illness such as a broken wrist, the family can adapt quite well to the role(s) not being performed or not being performed as well as expected. However, when the disruption is caused by chronic illness, the changes brought about by non-role performance require more creativity to reduce the family stress. When a family member dies from a sudden acute event, roles are shifted

unexpectedly, thus potentially setting off a cascade of family crises. When death is caused by a long haul chronic situation, the family must still adjust to the permanent change in structure and roles. Each family defines the sick role in that family and the expected behavior of the ill person.

Individuals learn health and illness behaviors in their family of origin. Health behaviors are related to the primary prevention of disease, and include health promotion activities to reduce susceptibility to disease and actions to reduce the effects of chronic disease. Kasl and Cobb (1966) identified three types of health behaviors in families:

- Health behavior is any activity a person believes promotes, protects, or maintains health.
- Illness behavior is any activity undertaken by a person who feels ill to define the state of his health and to discover a suitable remedy.
- Sick-role behavior is any activity undertaken for the purpose of getting well, by those who consider themselves ill.

Once a family member becomes ill, he or she demonstrates various illness behaviors or enacts the "sick role." Parsons (1951) defines four characteristics of a person who is sick:

- While sick, the person is temporarily exempt from carrying out normal social and family roles. The more severe the illness, the freer one is from role obligations.
- In general, the sick person is not held responsible for being ill.
- The sick person is expected to take actions to get well, and therefore has an obligation to "get well."
- The sick person is expected to seek competent professional medical care and to adhere to medical advice on how to "get well."

Voluminous research has been conducted on the theoretical concepts of the sick role. Some criticisms of the Parsons perspective of the sick role are as follows: (1) Some individuals reject the sick role; (2) some individuals are blamed for their illness, such as alcoholics or individuals with AIDS; and (3) sometimes independence is encouraged in persons who have a chronic illness as a way to "get well." Regardless of the theoretical debates about the sick role, individuals in families experience acute and chronic illness. Each family, depending on its family processes, defines the sick role differently. Most "sick" people require some level of care; someone needs to assume the family caregiver role. The caregiving role may be as simple as a stop at the store on the way home to buy chicken soup or pick up medicines, or as involved as providing around-the-clock care for someone. The female individuals in our society still provide the majority of the care required when family members become sick or injured.

Family roles are affected, some more than others, when a family member becomes ill. Usually the women in the family add the role of family caregiver to their other roles. Nurses have a crucial role in helping families adjust to illness by discussing and exploring role strain, role conflict, and role overload. Nurses can facilitate family adaptation by helping to problem-solve role negotiations and helping families access outside resources.

Lack of competence in role performance may be a result of role strain. Some researchers have found that sources of role strain are cultural and interactional. Interactional sources of role strain are related to difficulties in the delineation and enactment of familial roles. Heiss (1981) identifies five sources of difficulties in the interaction process that place strain on a family system:

- Inability to define the situation
- Lack of role knowledge
- Lack of role consensus
- Role conflict
- Role overload

The inability to define the situation creates ambiguity about what one should do in a given scenario. Continual changes in family structures and gender roles means that members increasingly encounter situations in which guidelines for action are unclear. Single parents, stepparents, nonresident fathers, and cohabiting partners deal daily with situations for which there are no norms. What right does a stepparent have to discipline the new spouse's child? Is a nonresident father expected to teach his child about AIDS? What name or names go on the mailbox of cohabiting partners? Who can sign for consent when divorced parents share custody?

Regardless of whether the issues are substantive, they present daily challenges to the people involved. Some choose to withdraw from the situation, and others choose to redefine the situation when they are uncertain how to act. For instance, a blended

family might want to operate in the same way as a traditional family but may experience conflict when thinking about which members to include in family decision making. When a solution cannot be found, family members suffer the consequences of role strain.

Role strain sometimes results when family members lack role knowledge, or they have no basis for choosing between several roles that might seem appropriate. In America, most people are not taught how to be parents, and much learning is observational and experiential. Socialization related to caregiving of a chronically ill family member seldom occurs, and many individuals are unfamiliar with and unprepared to assume the roles necessary for providing care. When an individual is learning how to be a parent or a caregiver, role training may be required. Knowledge may be acquired by peer observation, trial and error, or explicit instruction. Parents may have limited opportunities to observe peers, and other family members may not have the knowledge necessary to help. Thus, the family may need to seek external resources or obtain needed information using other means such as child-care classes, self-help groups, or instruction from health care providers. When individuals are unable to figure out their roles in a situation, it limits their problem-solving abilities.

Family members may lack role consensus, or be unable to agree about the expectations attached to a role. One family role that is often the source of family disagreement is the housekeeping role, especially for dual-career couples. Men who have been socialized into more traditional male roles are less inclined to accept responsibility for household tasks readily and may limit the amount of time they are willing to spend on these activities. When active participation does not meet the wife's expectations, she tends to assume responsibility for the greater number of household tasks. If she has been socialized into thinking that women are accountable for traditional housekeeping roles, she may feel guilty or neglectful if she asks for help. Lack of agreement about the role sometimes results in familial discord and impedes satisfaction with the partner. Negotiation is likely the most effective way to reach consensus about things that can be done.

Role conflict occurs when expectations about familial roles are incompatible. For example, the therapeutic role might involve becoming a caregiver to an elderly parent, but expectations of this new role may be incompatible with that of provider, housekeeper, sexual partner, and child-care provider. Does one go to the child's baseball game or to the doctor with the older adult parent? Role conflict may occur when roles present conflicting demands. Individuals and families often have to set priorities. Demands of caregiver and provider roles may be conflicting and may conflict with other therapeutic familial tasks. The caregiver may withdraw from activities that, in the short term, seem superfluous, but in the long term are sources of much-needed energy. Family nurses are likely to encounter members facing many strains because of role conflict, and may need to assist by providing information and suggesting ways the family could negotiate roles to discover meaningful solutions.

A source of role strain closely related to role conflict is role overload. In role overload, the individual lacks resources, time, and energy to meet role demands. As with role conflict, the first option usually considered is to withdraw from one of the roles. Maintaining a balance between energy-enhancing and energy-depleting roles reduces role strain. An alternative to withdrawing from a role might be to seek time away from some role responsibilities. For example, a friend of the family member could relieve the primary caregiver for several hours. Nurses could arrange for a home-health aide to assist with personal care hygiene. The dependent family member can be temporarily cared for in a residential facility while the other family members go on a vacation, which is called respite care.

It is within this aspect of family roles that nurses have the greatest ability to help families manage stress that is created when these functional roles are not being met in times of stress. Nurses can help families to adapt roles, negotiate roles, give up expectations about how roles are met or who does them, or find additional resources to fill the roles that are not being conducted. Each chapter in this book addresses ways nurses can assist families relative to changes it experiences with illness. See Chapter 5 for a discussion of general interventions about family roles nurses can use to assist the family.

Family Communication

Communication is an ongoing, complex, changing activity and is the means through which people create, share, and regulate meaning in a transactional process to make sense of their world (Dance, 1967). In all families, communication is continuous in that it defines their present reality and constructs family relationships (Dance, 1967; Galvin et al., 2015). It is through communication that families find ways to adapt to changes as they seek family stability. In well-functioning families, members invest energy and effort to maintain open communication patterns in order to maintain relationships (Galvin, Braithwaite, & Bylund, 2015).

Family communication affects family physical and mental health and is incredibly complex. Most programs and intervention strategies for improving family communication are beyond the role and experience of nurses with undergraduate education. The role of the nurse is to facilitate family communication, which may include a family conference for a specific discussion topic or teaching listening skills, reflective skills, and summarizing skills at times when families are stressed by changes that occur with its members, such as birth of an infant, growth and development issues of children, when family members become ill, or the death of family members. It is the role of the nurse to assist family communication to achieve healthful outcomes. Many of the interventions in Chapter 5 inherently include strategies that facilitate communication among and between family members.

Family Decision Making

Communication and power are family processes that influence decision making. Family decision making is not an individual effort but a joint one that is steeped in culture and that family's history. Therefore, each family has its own style of making decisions for the whole family as well as for its members.

Relative to health care, individuals rarely make decisions alone or only from their perspective. Individuals and family make multiple decisions about health care that do not involve the formal health care provider or system. However, it is crucial that the health care provider work with the family to provide information and options. Shared decision making is a process where health care providers work together with the individual and family to make health care choices. There are five stages comprising shared decision making (McCaffery, Smith, & Wolf, 2010):

1. Understanding the nature of the disease or condition
2. Being aware of the clinical services available and likely consequences such as risks, limitations, benefits, alternatives, and uncertainties

3. Considering personal preferences
4. Participating in decision making at the level the individual chooses to participate
5. Making decisions consistent with personal preference and values or electing to defer the decisions to another

Decision aides provide structured guidance in the steps of decision making for a health-related event. They provide information about options and help patients and their families to construct, clarify, and communicate personal values they associate with the different options. See Chapter 5 for a detailed discussion on shared decision making and how nurses use several instruments to assist families in making health care decisions.

Family Rituals and Routines

All families have unique rituals and routines that provide organization, give meaning to family life, and help families cope when in crisis. Routines are patterned behaviors or interactions that provide a sense of continuity through daily or regular activities, such as bedtime procedures, mealtimes, greetings, and treatment of guests (Kiser, 2015; Walsh, 2016b).

Routines are about what needs to be done, when the activities need to occur, and who does it (roles) to keep the family functioning (Fiese & Spagnola, 2013). They are typically repeated over time without much variation. Families use routines to provide structure and order so that the family works together to serve the needs of the family as a whole and for each member. Some purposes that family routines accomplish for families appear in the following list (Kiser, 2015, p. 26):

- Accomplish tasks in order to meet basic needs
- Provide structure
- Clarify roles
- Stipulate rules
- Establish boundaries around who is part of the family
- Support family communication and cohesion
- Establish an identity by denoting how things are done in this family
- Provide predictability within the family, which in turn provides comfort

Rituals involve symbolic communication among the family members that provides for a feeling of belonging (Fiese & Spagnola, 2013). Rituals are actions family members undertake individually and collectively as a family for a specific purpose; they provide meaning to who that family is, reveal what the members believe, and identify what is important to that family. Rituals can be created about any aspect of life, but often are associated with formal celebrations, cultural or family traditions, and religious and spiritual observances with symbolic meaning that all provide a shared meaning of life events.

When family rituals and routines are disrupted by illness, the family system as a whole is affected; therefore, it can affect the health of each family member and the family as a whole (Buchbinder, Longhofer, & McCue, 2009; Walsh, 2016b).

Family rituals and routines are important aspects that influence positive health outcomes in chronic illness. Crespo et al. (2013) conducted a systematic review of 39 studies that investigated the impact of rituals and routines for individuals and families living with chronic illness. The following findings about routines and rituals emerged from this systematic review on chronic illness (p. 729):

- Established family routines and rituals were performed less as the illness interfered with the timing or ability of members to participate.
- New routines and rituals were established to help the family adapt to changing needs.
- Routines and rituals provided opportunities for family members to emotionally support each other.
- Rituals and routines offered the family a sense of normalcy amid the challenges posed by chronic conditions.
- Rituals and routines supported positive health and adaptation outcomes for both patients and family members.

Assessing rituals and routines related to specific health or illness needs provides a basis to envision distinct family interventions and to devise specific plans for health promotion and disease management, especially when adherence to medical regimens is critical or caregiving demands are burdensome to the families (Denham, 2016). Family nurses who support families in conducting their routines help families have a sense of normalcy in the face of stress from a family member's illness. Nurses can help families establish new routines that provide structure and meet the needs of the family (Denham, 2016). Nurses can facilitate family rituals by navigating organizational obstacles that may prevent the family from conducting or participating in an important family ritual. Nurses can assist families to establish daily routines that support the functioning of the family. Specific ways to work with families relative to routines and rituals are discussed in Chapter 5.

SUMMARY

This chapter provides an introduction and broad overview to family health care nursing. The following major concepts were discussed in this chapter:

- Family health care nursing is an art and a science that has evolved as a way of thinking about and working with families.
- Family nursing is a scientific discipline based in theory.
- Health and illness are family events.
- The term *family* is defined in many ways, but the most salient definition is, *The family is who the members say it is.*

- An individual's health (on the wellness-to-illness continuum) affects the entire family's functioning; in turn, the family's ability to function affects each individual member's health.
- Family health care nursing knowledge and skills are important for nurses who practice in generalized and in specialized settings.
- The structure, function, and processes of families have changed, but the family as a unit of analysis and service continues to survive over time.
- Nurses should intervene in ways that promote health and wellness, as well as prevent illness risks, treat disease conditions, and manage rehabilitative care needs.
- Knowledge about each family's structure, function, and process informs the nurse in how to optimize nursing care in families and provide individualized nursing care, tailored to the uniqueness of every family system.

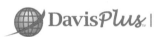 | For additional resources and information, visit **http://davisplus.fadavis.com**. References can be found on Davis*Plus*.

Chapter 2

Theoretical Foundations for the Nursing of Families

Joanna Rowe Kaakinen, PhD, RN

Critical Concepts

- Theories inform the practice of nursing. Practice informs theory and research. Theory, practice, and research are interactive, and all three are critical to the profession of nursing and family care.

- The major purpose of theory in family nursing is to provide knowledge and understanding that improves the quality of nursing care of families.

- By understanding theories and models, nurses are prepared to think more creatively and critically about how health events affect family clients. Theories and models provide different ways of comprehending issues that may be affecting families and offer choices for action.

- The theoretical/conceptual frameworks and models that provide the foundations for nursing of families have evolved from three major traditions and disciplines: family social science, family therapy, and nursing.

- No single theory, model, or conceptual framework adequately describes the complex relationships of family structure, function, and process. Nor does one theoretical perspective give nurses a sufficiently broad base of knowledge and understanding to guide assessment and interventions with families. No one theoretical perspective is better, more comprehensive, or more correct than another. Nurses who use an integrated theoretical approach build on the strengths of families in creative ways. Nurses who use a singular theoretical approach to working with families limit the possibilities for families they serve. By integrating several theories, nurses acquire different ways to conceptualize problems, thus enhancing thinking about interventions.

By understanding theories and models, nurses are prepared to think creatively and critically about how health events affect the family client. The reciprocal or interactive relationship between theory, practice, and research is that each aspect informs the other, thereby expanding knowledge and nursing interventions to support families. Theories and models extend thinking to higher levels of understanding problems and circumstances that may be affecting families and, thereby, offer more choices and options for nursing interventions.

Currently, no single theory, model, or conceptual framework adequately describes the complex relationships of family structure, function, and process. Nor does one theoretical perspective give nurses a sufficiently broad base of knowledge and understanding to guide assessment and interventions with families. No one theoretical perspective is better,

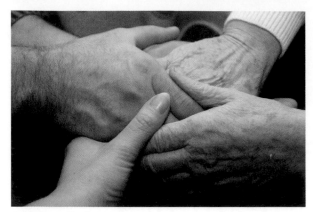

© iStock.com/diephosi

more comprehensive, or more correct than another (Doane & Varcoe, 2015; Kaakinen & Hanson, 2015). The goal for nurses is to have a deep understanding of the stresses that families experience when their family clients have a health event and to support and implement family interventions based on theoretical perspectives that best match the needs identified by the family.

Many theoretical approaches exist to help understand families. The purpose of this chapter is to demonstrate how families who have members experiencing a health event are conceptualized differently depending on the theoretical perspective. In this chapter, nurses seek different data depending on which theory is being used, both to understand the family experience and to determine the interventions offered to the family to help bring them back to a state of stability.

This chapter begins with a brief review of the components of the three chosen theories and how the components contribute to the nursing of families. It then presents three theoretical approaches for working with families, ranging from a broader to a more specific perspective:

- Family Systems Theory
- Developmental and Family Life Cycle Theory
- Bioecological Theory

The chapter utilizes a case study of a family with a member who is experiencing progressive multiple sclerosis (MS) to demonstrate these three different theoretical approaches to nursing care of families.

RELATIONSHIP BETWEEN THEORY, PRACTICE, AND RESEARCH

In nursing, the relationship of theory to practice constitutes a dynamic feedback loop rather than a static linear progression. Theory, practice, and research are mutually interdependent. Theory grows out of observations made in practice and is tested by research; then tested theory informs practice; practice, in turn, facilitates the further refinement and development of theory. Figure 2-1 depicts the dynamic relationship between theory, practice, and research.

Theories do not emerge all at once. Rather, they build slowly over time as data are gathered through practice, observation, and analysis of evidence. Relating together the various concepts that emerge from observation and evidence occurs through a purposeful, thoughtful reasoning process. *Inductive reasoning* is a process that moves from specific pieces of information toward a general or broader idea; it is thinking about how the parts create the whole. *Deductive reasoning* goes in the opposite direction from inductive reasoning. Deductive reasoning occurs when the broader ideas of a given theory generate more specific questions. These specific questions further clarify the theory, and filter back into the cycle. Deductive reasoning helps refine understanding of the specific details of the theory and how to apply the theory to practice (Smith & Hamon, 2016; White, Klein, & Martin, 2014).

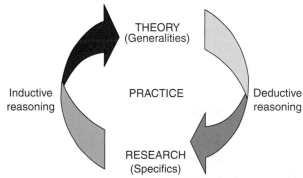

FIGURE 2-1 Relationship Between Theory, Practice, and Research *(Adapted from Smith, S. R., Hamon, R. R., Ingoldsby, B. B., & Miller, J. E. [2008]. Exploring family theories [2nd ed.]. New York, NY: Oxford University Press.)*

Theories are designed to make sense of the world by showing how one concept is related to another and how together they make a meaningful pattern that can predict the consequences of certain clusters of characteristics or events. Theories are abstract, general ideas that are subject to rules of organization. Theories provide a general framework for understanding data in an organized way, as well as showing us how to predict patterns and more accurately intervene to prevent, stabilize, or treat problems. We live in a time when tremendous amounts of information are readily available and quickly accessible in multiple forms. Therefore, theories provide ways to transform this large volume of information into organized knowledge and to integrate the information in order to help us make better sense of the world (White et al., 2014). Ideally, nursing theories represent logical and intelligible patterns that make sense of the observations nurses make in practice and enable nurses to predict what is likely to happen to clients based on observed patterns (Polit & Beck, 2016). Theories can be used as a level of evidence in which to base nursing practice (Fawcett & Desanto-Madeya, 2012). The major function of theory in family nursing is to provide knowledge and understanding that improves nursing services to families.

Another important aspect of theories is that they explain what is happening; they provide answers to "how" and "why" questions, help to interpret and make sense of complex phenomena, and predict what could happen in the future based on careful thought and study about what has happened in the past. All scientific theories use the same components: *concepts*, *relationships*, and *propositions*. Theories also construct hypotheses (i.e., what is expected to happen) and conceptual models (i.e., relationships between several concepts).

Concepts, the building blocks of theory, are words that create mental images or abstract representations of phenomena of study. Concepts, the major ideas expressed by a theory, may exist on a continuum from empirical (concrete) to abstract (Masters, 2015). The more concrete the concept, the easier it is to figure out when it applies or does not apply (White et al., 2014). For example, one concept in Family Systems Theory is that families have boundaries. A highly abstract aspect of this concept is that the boundary reflects the energy between the environment and the system. A more concrete aspect of this concept is that families open or close their boundaries, or their willingness to let others into their lives, in times of stress.

Propositions are statements about the proposed relationship between two or more concepts (Masters, 2015). A proposition might be a statement such as the following: Families as a whole influence the health of individual family members. The word *influence* proposes a link between the two concepts of "families as a whole" and "health of individual family members." Propositions suggest a relationship between the subject and the object. Propositions may lead to hypotheses. Theories are generally made up of several propositions that suggest the relationships among the concepts in that specific theory.

A *hypothesis* is a way of stating an expected relationship between concepts or an expected proposition (Masters, 2015). The concepts and propositions in the hypothesis are derived from and driven by the original theory. For example, using the concepts of family and health, one could hypothesize that there is an interactive relationship between how a family is coping and the eventual health outcome of family members. In other words, the family's ability to cope with stress affects the health of individual family members; in turn, the health of an individual family member influences the family's ability to cope. The proposed relationship, or hypothesis, is that the concept of coping is related to the concept of health in families. This hypothesis may be tested by a research study that measures family coping strategies and family members' health over time and that uses statistical procedures to look at the relationships between the two concepts.

A *conceptual model* is a set of general propositions that integrate concepts into meaningful configurations or patterns (Fawcett & Desanto-Madeya, 2012). Conceptual models in nursing are based on the observations, insights, and deductions that combine ideas from several fields of inquiry. Conceptual models provide a frame of reference and a coherent way of thinking about nursing phenomena. A conceptual model is more abstract and more comprehensive than a theory. Similar to a conceptual model, a conceptual framework is a way of integrating concepts into a meaningful pattern; however, conceptual frameworks are often less definitive than models. They provide useful conceptual approaches or ways to look at a problem or situation, rather than a definite set of propositions about relationships between concepts.

In this book, the terms *conceptual model or framework* and *theory or theoretical framework* are often used interchangeably. In part, this is because no single theoretical base exists for the nursing of families. Rather, nurses typically draw from many theoretical conceptual foundations using a more pluralistic and eclectic approach. The interchangeable use of these various terms reflects the fact that there is considerable overlap among ideas in the various theoretical perspectives and conceptual models/ frameworks and that many "streams of influence" are important for family nurses to understand, consider, and incorporate into practice. As might be expected, a substantial amount of cross-fertilization among disciplines has occurred, such as between social science and nursing, and concepts originating in one theory or discipline have been translated into similar concepts for use in another discipline. Currently, no one theoretical perspective or one discipline gives nurses a sufficiently broad base of knowledge and understanding to guide assessment and interventions with families.

THEORETICAL AND CONCEPTUAL FOUNDATIONS FOR THE NURSING OF FAMILIES

Nursing is a scientific discipline; thus, nurses are concerned about the relationships between ideas and data. Nurse scholars explain empirical observations by creating theories that can be used as evidence in evidence-based practice (Fawcett & Garity, 2008). From a nursing perspective, Melnyk, Fineout-Overholt, Stillwell, and Williamson (2010) define evidence-based practice as "a problem-solving approach to the delivery of health care that integrates best evidence from studies and patient care data with clinician expertise and patient preferences and values (p. 51)." Nurse researchers investigate and test the models and relationships. Nurses in practice use theories, models, and conceptual frameworks to decide on interventions that will help clients achieve the best outcomes (Kaakinen & Hanson, 2015). In nursing, evidence, in the form of theory, is used to explain and guide practice. The theoretical foundations, theories, and conceptual models that explain and guide the practice of nursing families have evolved from three major traditions and disciplines: family social science theories, family therapy theories, and

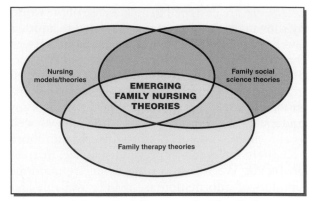

FIGURE 2-2 Theoretical Frameworks That Influence the Nursing of Families

nursing models and theories. Figure 2-2 shows the theoretical frameworks that influence the nursing of families.

Family Social Science Theories

Of the three sources of theory, *family social science theories* are the best developed and informative about family phenomena. Examples of such theories include the following: family function, the environment-family interchange, interactions and dynamics within the family, changes in the family over time, and the family's reaction to health and illness. Table 2-1 summarizes the basic family social science theories and provides some classic references where these theories originate. It is challenging to use the purist form of family social science theories as a basis for nursing assessment and intervention because of their abstract nature. Despite this challenge, in recent years nursing and family scholars have made strides in extrapolating and morphing these theories for use in clinical work (Fine & Fincham, 2013; Kaakinen & Hanson, 2015).

Family Therapy Theories

Family therapy theories are newer than and not as well developed as family social science theories. Table 2-2 lists these theories and the names of some foundational scholars who first developed them. These theories emanate from a practice discipline of family therapy, rather than from an academic discipline of family social science. Family therapy theories were developed to work with troubled families and, therefore, focus primarily on family

Table 2-1	Family Social Science Theories Used in Family Nursing Practice
Family Social Science Theory	**Summary**
Structural Functional Theory Artinian (1994) Friedman, Bowden, & Jones (2003) Nye & Berardo (1981)	The focus is on families as an institution and how they function to maintain the family and social network.
Symbolic Interaction Theory Hill & Hansen (1960) Nye (1976) Rose (1962) Turner (1970)	The focus is on the interactions within families and the symbolic communication.
Developmental Theory and Family Life Cycle Theory Carter & McGoldrick (2005) Duvall (1977) Duvall & Miller (1985) Goldberg (2010) Pelton (2011) Falicov (2016)	The focus is on the life cycle of families and representing normative stages of family development. Expanding the family life cycle to address the needs of lesbian and gay parents and their children. Expanding the family life cycle to address needs of voluntary childfree couples. Expanding the family life cycle to address needs of migrant families.
Family Systems Theory von Bertalanffy (1950, 1968)	The focus is on the circular interactions among members of family systems, which result in functional or dysfunctional outcomes.
Family Stress Theory Hill (1949, 1965) McCubbin & McCubbin (1993) McCubbin & Patterson (1983)	The focus is on the analysis of how families experience and cope with stressful life events.
Change Theory Maturana (1978) Maturana & Varela (1992) Watzlawick, Weakland, & Fisch (1974) Wright & Leahey (2013) Wright & Watson (1988)	The focus is on how families remain stable or change when there is change within the family structure or from outside influences.
Transition Theory White (2005) White, Klein, & Martin (2014)	The focus is on understanding and predicting the transitions families experience over time by combining Role Theory, Family Development Theory, and Life Course Theory.

Table 2-2	Family Therapy Theories Used in Family Nursing Practice
Family Therapy Theories	**Summary**
Structural Family Therapy Theory Minuchin (1974)	This systems-oriented approach views the family as an open sociocultural system that is continually faced with demands for change, both from within and from outside the family. The focus is on the whole family system, its subsystems, boundaries, and coalitions, as well as family transactional patterns and covert rules.
Minuchin & Fishman (1981)	
Minuchin, Rosman, & Baker (1978)	
Nichols (2004)	
International Family Therapy Theory Jackson (1965)	This approach views the family as a system of interactive or interlocking behaviors or communication processing. Emphasis is on the here and now rather than on the past. Key interventions focus on establishing clear, congruent communication and clarifying and changing family rules.
Satir (1982)	
Watzlawick, Beavin, & Jackson (1967)	
Family Systems Therapy Theory Freeman (1992)	This approach focuses on promoting differentiation of self from family and promoting differentiation of intellect from emotion. Family members are encouraged to examine their processes to gain insight and understanding into their past and present. This therapy requires a long-term commitment.
Kerr & Bowen (1988)	
Toman (1961)	

pathology. Nevertheless, these conceptual models describe family dynamics and patterns that are found, to some extent, in all families. Because these models are concerned with what can be done to facilitate change in "dysfunctional" families, they are both descriptive and prescriptive. That is, they not only describe and explain observations made in practice, but also suggest treatment or intervention strategies.

Nursing Conceptual Frameworks

Finally, of the three types of theories, *nursing conceptual frameworks* are the least developed "theories" in relation to the nursing of families. Table 2-3 lists several of the theories and theorists from within the nursing profession. During the 1960s and 1970s, nurses placed great emphasis on the development of nursing models. Other than the Neuman Systems Model (Neuman & Fawcett, 2010) and the Behavioral Systems Model for Nursing (Johnson, 1980), both of which were based on family social science theories, the majority of the classic nursing theorists from the 1970s focused on individual patients and not on families as a unit of care/analysis. The nursing models, in large part, represent a deductive approach to the development of nursing science (general to specific). Although they embody an important part of our nursing heritage, these nursing conceptual frameworks and their deductive approach are viewed more critically today. As the science of nursing has evolved, more inductive approaches to nursing theory have developed (specific to the general) and are now being used in everyday nursing practice.

Table 2-4 shows the differences between family social science theories, family therapy theories, and nursing models/theories as they inform the practice of nursing with families. The following case study is used to demonstrate how the three different theoretical approaches may guide a nurse's work with one family. Box 2-1 compares these three theories as they apply to the Jones family case study.

Table 2-3	Nursing Theories and Models Used in Family Nursing Practice

Nursing Theories and Models	Summary
Nightingale Nightingale (1859)	Family is described as having both positive and negative influences on the outcome of family members. The family is seen as a supportive institution throughout the life span for its individual family members.
Rogers's Science of Unitary Human Beings Casey (1996) Rogers (1970, 1986, 1990)	The family is viewed as a constant open system energy field that is ever-changing in its interactions with the environment.
Roy's Adaptation Model Roy (1976) Roy & Roberts (1981)	The family is seen as an adaptive system that has inputs, internal control, and feedback processes and output. The strength of this model is an understanding of how families adapt to health issues.
Johnson's Behavioral Systems Model for Nursing Johnson (1980)	The family is viewed as a behavioral system composed of a set of organized interactive interdependent and integrated subsystems that adjust and adapt with internal and external forces to maintain stability.
King's Goal Attainment Theory King (1981, 1983, 1987)	The family is seen as the vehicle for transmitting values and norms of behavior across the life span, which includes the role of a sick family member. Family is responsible for addressing the health care function of the family. Family is seen as both an interpersonal and a social system. The key component is the interaction between the nurse and the family as client.
Neuman's Systems Model Neuman (1983, 1995)	The family is viewed as a system. The family's primary goal is to maintain its stability by preserving the integrity of its structure by opening and closing its boundaries. It is a fluid model that depicts the family in motion and not a static view of family from one perspective.
Orem's Self-Care Deficit Theory Gray (1996) Orem (1983a, 1983b, 1985)	The family is seen as the basic conditioning unit in which the individual learns culture, roles, and responsibilities. Specifically, family members learn how to act when one is ill. The family's self-care behavior evolves through interpersonal relationships, communication, and culture that is unique to each family.
Parse's Human Becoming Theory Parse (1992, 1998)	The concept of family and who makes up the family is viewed as continually becoming and evolving. The role of the nurse is to use therapeutic communication to invite family members to uncover their meaning of the experience, to learn what the meaning of the experience is for each other, and to discuss the meaning of the experience for the family as a whole.
Friedemann's Framework of Systemic Organization Friedemann (1995)	The family is described as a social system that has the expressed goal of transmitting culture to its members. The elements central to this theory are family stability, family growth, family control, and family spirituality.

(continued)

Table 2-3	Nursing Theories and Models Used in Family Nursing Practice *(cont.)*
Nursing Theories and Models	**Summary**
Denham's Family Health Model Denham (2003)	Family health is viewed as a process over time of family member interactions and health-related behaviors. Family health is described in relation to contextual, functional, and structural domains. Dynamic family health routines are behavioral patterns that reflect self-care, safety and prevention, mental health behaviors, family care, illness care, and family caregiving.

Table 2-4	Family Social Science Theories, Family Therapy Theories, and Nursing Models/Theories		
Criteria	**Family Social Science Theories**	**Family Therapy Theories**	**Nursing Models/Theories**
Purpose of theory	Descriptive and explanatory (academic models); to explain family functioning and dynamics.	Descriptive and prescriptive (practice models); to explain family dysfunction and guide therapeutic actions.	Descriptive and prescriptive (practice models); to guide nursing assessment and intervention efforts.
Discipline focus	Interdisciplinary (although primarily sociological).	Marriage and family therapy; family mental health; new approaches focus on family strengths.	Nursing focus.
Target population	Primarily "normal" families (normality-oriented).	Primarily "troubled" families (pathology-oriented).	Primarily families with health and illness problems.

BOX 2-1

Comparison of Theories as They Apply to the Jones Family

Family Systems Theory

Conceptual

Family is viewed as a whole. What happens to the family as a whole affects each individual family member, and what happens to individuals affects the totality of the family unit. Focus is on the circular interactions among members of the family system, resulting in functional or dysfunctional outcomes.

Assessment

The family may be assessed together or individually. Assessment questions relate to the *interaction* between the individual and the family, and the *interaction* between the family and the community in which the family lives.

Intervention Examples

- Complete a family genogram to understand patterns and relationships over several generations over time.
- Complete a family ecomap to see how individuals/family relate to the community around them.
- Collect data about the family as a whole and about individual family members.
- Conduct care-planning sessions that include family members.

Strengths

Focus is on family as a whole, its subsystems, or both. It is a generally understood and accepted theory in society.

Weaknesses

Theory is broad and general. It does not give definitive prescriptions for interventions.

Application to the Jones Family

All members of the Jones family are affected by the mother's progressive chronic health condition and changes. Family structure, functions, and processes of the family are influenced, changing family roles and dynamics. Everyone in the family has his or her own concerns and needs attention from health care professionals.

Family Developmental and Life Cycle Theory

Conceptual

Family is viewed as a whole over time. All families go through similar developmental processes starting with the birth of the first child to death of the parents. Focus is on the life cycle of families and represents normative stages of family development.

(continued)

BOX 2-1
Comparison of Theories as They Apply to the Jones Family *(cont.)*

Assessment

The family may be assessed together or individually. Assessment questions relate to the normative predictable events that occur in family life over time. It also includes nonnormative, unexpected events.

Intervention Examples

- Conduct a family interview to determine where the family is in terms of cognitive, social, emotional, spiritual, and physical development.
- Complete a family genogram and ecomap.
- Determine the normative and nonnormative events that have occurred to the family as a whole or to individuals within the family.
- Analyze how an individual's growth and developmental milestones may affect the family developmental trajectory.

Strengths

Focus is on the family as a whole. The theory provides a framework for predicting what a family will experience at any given stage in the family life cycle so that nurses can offer anticipatory guidance.

Weaknesses

The traditional linear family life cycle is no longer the norm. Modern families vary widely in their structure and roles. Divorce, remarriage, gay parents, and never-married parents have changed the traditional trajectory of growth and developmental milestones. The theory does not focus on how the family adapts to the transitions from one stage to the other; rather, it simply predicts what transitions will occur.

Application to the Jones Family

The Jones family is in the stages of "families with adolescents" and "launching young adults." The nonnormative health condition of the mother is changing the predictable normative course of development for the individuals and for the family as a whole. These health events will change the cognitive, social, emotional, spiritual, and physical development as the family shifts to integrate new roles into their lives as family members.

Bioecological Systems Theory

Conceptual

Bioecological systems theory combines children's biological disposition and environmental forces that come together to shape the development of human beings. This theory has a basis in both developmental theory and systems theory to understand individual and family growth. It combines the influence of both genetics and environment from the individual and family with the larger economic/political structure over time. The basic premise is that individual and family development are contextual over time. The different levels of the theory that apply to the family at any one point in time vary depending on what is happening at that time. Therefore, the interaction of the systems vary over time as the situation changes.

Assessment

Assess all levels of the larger ecological system when interviewing the family. Determine the microsystem, mesosystem, exosystem, macrosystem, and chronosystem of the individual and of the family as a whole.

Intervention Examples

- Conduct a family interview to determine the family's status in relationship to four locational/spatial contexts and one time-related context.
- Complete a family genogram and ecomap.
- Determine how individuals are doing in relationship to their entire environment, which includes immediate family, extended family, home, school, and community.
- Analyze the family in its smaller and larger contextual aspects.

Strengths

Focus is on a holistic approach to human/family development. A bio/psycho/socio/cultural/spiritual approach to understanding how individuals and families develop and change/adapt over time in their society is a more complete approach.

Weaknesses

This holistic approach is not specific enough to define contextual changes over time. Nor can the larger context in which individuals/families are embedded be predicted or controlled.

Application to the Jones Family

- *Microsystem:* The Jones family consists of school-age children living at home. The parental roles have been traditional until recent health events.
- *Mesosystem:* Family has much interaction with schools, church, and extended family.
- *Exosystem:* Family influenced by father's work at the factory and other institutions in the community.
- *Macrosystem:* Family consistent with community culture, attitudes, and beliefs. Their community is largely Caucasian, middle class, and Christian.
- *Chronosystem:* At this time in the illness story of the Jones family with the mother's illness changing, the family situation changes and moves between stability and crisis.

Family Case Study: Jones Family

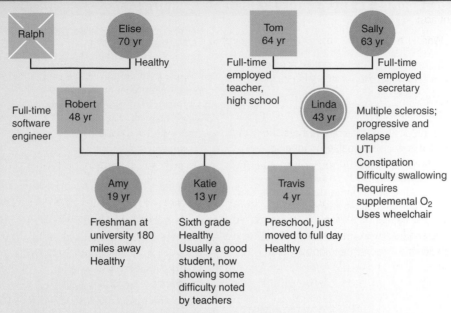

FIGURE 2-3 Jones Family Genogram

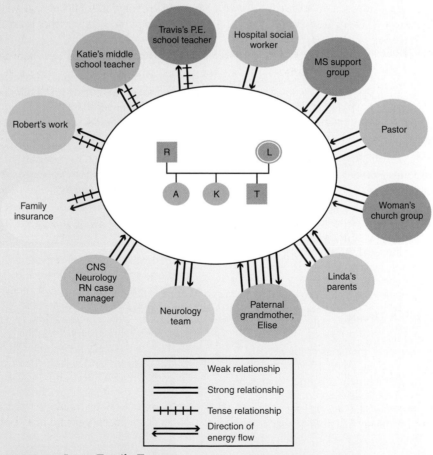

FIGURE 2-4 Jones Family Ecomap

Family Case Study: Jones Family *(cont.)*

Setting: Inpatient acute care hospital.

Nursing Goal: Work with the family to assist them in preparation for discharge that is planned to occur in the next 2 days.

Family Members:

The Jones family is a nuclear family. The Jones family genogram and ecomap are illustrated in Figures 2-3 and 2-4.

- Robert: 48 years old; father, software engineer, full-time employed.
- Linda: 43 years old; mother, stay-at-home homemaker, has progressive MS, which recently has worsened significantly.
- Amy: 19 years old; oldest child, daughter, freshman at university in town 180 miles away.
- Katie: 13 years old; middle child, daughter, sixth grade, usually a good student.
- Travis: 4 years old; youngest child, son, just started attending an all-day preschool because of his mother's illness.

Jones Family Story:

Linda was diagnosed with MS at age 30 when Katie was 3 months old. After she was diagnosed with MS, Linda had a well-controlled, slow progression of her illness. Travis was a surprise pregnancy for Linda at age 39, but he is described as "a blessing." Linda and Robert are devout Baptists, but they did discuss abortion in light of the fact that Linda's illness could progress significantly after the birth of Travis. Their faith and personal beliefs did not support abortion. They made the decision to continue with Linda's pregnancy, knowing the risk that it might exacerbate and speed up her MS. Linda had an uncomplicated pregnancy with Travis. She felt well until 3 months postpartum with Travis when she noted a significant relapse of her MS.

During the last 4 years, Linda has experienced development of progressive relapsing MS, which is a progressive disease from onset with clear, acute relapses without full recovery after each relapse. The periods between her relapses are characterized by continuing progression of the disease. She now has secondary progressive MS because of her increased weakness. Robert and Linda are having sexual issues with decreased libido and painful intercourse for Linda. Both are experiencing stress in their marital roles and relationship.

Currently, Linda has had a serious relapse of her MS. She is hospitalized for secondary pneumonia from aspiration. She has weakness in all limbs, left foot drag, and increasing ataxia. Linda will be discharged with a wheelchair (this aid is new as she has used a cane up until this admission). She has weakness of her neck muscles and cannot hold her head steady for long periods. She has difficulty swallowing, which probably caused her aspiration. She has numbness and tingling of her legs and feet. She has severe pain with flexion of her neck. Her vision is blurred. She experiences vertigo at times and has periodic tinnitus. Constipation is a constant problem, together with urinary retention that causes periodic urinary tract infections.

Health Insurance:

Robert receives health insurance through his work that covers the whole family. Hospitalizations are covered 80/20, so they have to pay 20% of their bills out of pocket. Although Robert is employed full-time, this cost adds heavily to the financial burden of the family. Robert has shared with the nurses that he does not know whether he should take his last week of vacation when his wife comes home, or whether he should save it for a time when her condition worsens. Robert works for a company that offers family leave, but without pay.

Family Members:

Robert reports being continuously tired from caring for his wife and children, as well as working full-time. He asked the doctor for medication to help him sleep and decrease his anxiety. He said he is afraid that he may not hear Linda in the night when she needs help. He is open to his mother moving in to help care for Linda and the children. He begins counseling sessions with the pastor in their church.

Amy is a freshman at a university that is 180 miles away in a different town. Her mother is proud of Amy going to college on a full scholarship. Amy does well in her coursework but travels home weekends to help the family and her mother. Amy is considering giving up her scholarship to transfer home to attend the local community college. She has not told her parents about this idea yet.

Katie is in the sixth grade. She is typically a good student, but her latest report card showed that she dropped a letter grade in most of her classes. Katie is quiet. She stopped having friends over to her home about 6 months ago when her mother

(continued)

began to have more ataxia and slurring of speech. Linda used to be very involved in Katie's school but is no longer involved because of her illness. Katie has been involved in Girl Scouts and the youth group at church.

Travis just started going to preschool 2 months ago for full days because of his mother's illness. This transition to preschool has been difficult for Travis because he had been home full-time with Linda until her disease

worsened. He is healthy and developmentally on target for his age.

Linda's parents live in the same town. Her parents, Tom and Sally, both work full-time and are not able to help. Robert's widowed mother, Elise, lives by herself in her own home about 30 minutes out of town and has offered to move into the Jones' home to help care for Linda and the family.

Discharge Plans: Linda will be discharged home in 2 days.

THEORETICAL PERSPECTIVES AND APPLICATION TO FAMILIES

The case of the Jones family is used throughout the rest of this chapter to demonstrate how assessments, interventions, and options for care vary based on the particular theoretical perspective chosen by nurses caring for this family.

Family Systems Theory

Family Systems Theory has been the most influential of all the family social science frameworks (Kaakinen & Hanson, 2015; Wright & Leahey, 2013). Much of the understanding of how a family is a system derives from physics and biology perspectives that organisms are complex, organized, and interactive systems (Bowen, 1978; von Bertalanffy, 1950, 1968). Nursing theorists who have expanded the concept of systems theory include Hanson (2001), Johnson (1980), Neuman (1995), Neuman and Fawcett (2010), Smith and Parker (2014), Walker (2005), and Wilkerson and Loveland-Cherry (2005).

The Family Systems Theory is an approach that allows nurses to understand and assess families as an organized whole and/or as individuals within family units who form an interactive and interdependent system (Kaakinen & Hanson, 2015). Family Systems Theory is constructed of concepts and propositions that provide a framework for thinking about the family as a system. Typically, in family nursing we look at three-generational family systems (Goldenberg, Stanton, & Goldenberg, 2017).

One of the major assumptions of Family Systems Theory is that family system features are designed to maintain stability, although these features may be

adaptive or maladaptive. At the same time, families change constantly in response to stresses and strains from both the internal and external environments. Family systems increase in complexity over time and increase their ability to adapt and to change (Smith & Hamon, 2016; White et al., 2014). The family systems theoretical perspective encourages nurses to see individual clients as participating members of a larger family system. Figure 2-5 depicts a mobile showing how family systems work. Any change in one member of the family affects all members of the family. As it applies to the Jones family, nurses who use this perspective would assess the impact of Linda's illness on the entire family as well as the effects of family functioning on Linda. The goal of nurses is to help maintain or restore the stability of the family, in order to help family members achieve the highest level of functioning that they can. Therefore, emphasis should be on the whole, rather than on an individual. Some of the concepts of systems theory that help nurses working with families are explained in the following sections.

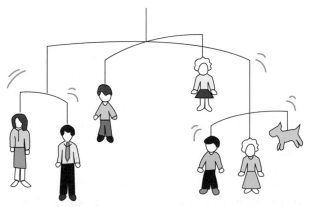

FIGURE 2-5 Mobile Depicting Family System

Concept 1: All Parts of the System Are Interconnected

What influences one part of the system influences all parts of the system. When an individual in a family experiences a health event, all members are affected because they are connected. The effect on each family member varies in intensity and quality. In the Jones case study, all members of the Jones family are touched when Linda's health condition changes, requiring her to be hospitalized. Linda takes on the role of a sick person and must give up some of her typical at-home mother roles; she is physically ill in the hospital. She feels guilty about not being at home for her family. Robert is affected because he has to assume the care of Katie and Travis. These tasks require getting them ready for school, transporting them to school and other events, and making lunches. Katie gives up some after-school activities to help Travis when he gets home from preschool. Travis misses the food his mother prepared for him, his afternoon alone time with his mother when they read a story, and being tucked into bed at night with songs and a back rub. Amy, who is a freshman in college, finds it difficult to concentrate while reading and studying for her college classes. The formal and informal roles of all these family members are affected by Linda's hospitalization. What affects Linda affects all the members of the Jones family in multiple ways.

Concept 2: The Whole Is More Than the Sum of Its Parts

The family as a whole is composed of more than the individual lives of family members. It goes beyond parents and children as separate entities. Families are not just relationships between the parent and child but are all relationships seen together. As we look at the Jones family, it is a nuclear family—mother, father, and three children. They are a family system that is experiencing the stress of a chronically ill mother who is deteriorating over time; each of them is individually affected, but so is the family as a whole affected by this unexpected (nonnormative) family health event. The individuals in this family may, at times, wonder what will happen to them as a family (whole) when Linda dies.

One way of visualizing the family as a whole is to think of how the Jones family has built the concept of the "Jones Family Easter." Even though Linda always decorates the house and bakes several special dishes for the family for this holiday, this year she has been too ill to decorate or cook for Easter. The family as a whole feels stressed by the loss of routine and ritual as it represents a change in their family tradition and beliefs. Thus, the family loss is larger than individual loss of this tradition.

Concept 3: All Systems Have Some Form of Boundaries or Borders Between the System and Its Environment

Families control the inflow of information and people coming into its family system to protect individual family members or the family as a whole. Boundaries are physical or abstract imaginary lines that families use as barriers or filters to control the impact of stressors on the family system (Smith & Hamon, 2012; White et al., 2014). Family boundaries include levels of permeability in that they can be closed, flexible, or too open to information, people, or other forms of resources. Some families have closed boundaries as exemplified by statements such as, "We as a family pull together and don't need help from others," or "We take care of our own." For example, if the Jones family were to have a *closed boundary*, they would not want to meet with the social worker or, if they did, they would reject the idea of a home-health aide and respite care.

Some families have *flexible boundaries*, which they control and selectively open or close to gain balance or adapt to the situation. For example, the Jones family welcomes a visit from the pastor but turns down visits from some of the women in Linda's Bible study group. Some families have *too open boundaries* in which they are not discriminating about who knows their family situation or the number of people from whom they seek help. Open boundaries can invite chaos and unbalance if the family is not selective in the quantity or quality of resources. If the Jones family were to have truly *open boundaries*, it may reach out to the larger community for resources and have different church members come stay with the children every evening. The permeability of boundaries resides on a continuum and varies from family to family.

Concept 4: Systems Can Be Further Organized into Subsystems

In addition to conceptualizing the family as a whole, nurses can think about the subsystems of the family, which may include husband to wife, mother to child, father to child, child to child, grandparents to parents, grandparents to grandchildren, and so forth. These subsystems consider the three dimensions of families discussed in Chapter 1: structure, function (including roles), and processes (interconnection and dynamics). By understanding these three dimensions, family nurses can streamline interventions to achieve specific family outcomes. For example, the Jones family has the following subsystems: parents, siblings, parent-child, a daughter subsystem, an in-law subsystem, and a grandparent subsystem. The nurse may work to decrease family stress by focusing on the marital spouse subsystem to help Linda and Robert continue couple time, or the nurse may focus on the sibling subsystem of Katie and Travis and their after-school activities.

Application of Family Systems Theory to the Jones Family

The focus of the nurses' practice from this perspective is family as the client. Nurses work to help families maintain and regain stability. Assessment questions of family members are focused on the family as a whole. While planning for Linda's discharge that is scheduled in the next couple of days, a nurse would ask questions such as the following to explore with Linda or with Linda and Robert:

- Who are members of your family? (See Concept 1.)
- How do you see your family being involved in your care once you go home? (See Concept 1.)
- Who in your family will experience the most difficulty coping with the changes, especially now that you will be using a wheelchair? (See Concept 1.)
- How are the members of your family meeting their personal needs at this time? (See Concept 1.)
- The last time your condition worsened, what was the most help to your family? (See Concept 2.)
- The last time your condition worsened, what was the least help to your family? (See Concept 2.)
- Who outside of your immediate family do you see as being a potential person to help your family during the next week when you go home? (See Concept 3.)
- How do you feel your family would react to having a home-health aide come to help you twice a week? (See Concept 3.)

- Are there some friends, church members, or neighbors who might be able to help with some of the everyday management issues, such as carpooling to school, or providing some after-school care for Travis so Katie could go to her after-school activities? (See Concepts 3 and 4.)
- What are your thoughts about how the children will react to having Grandma Elise here to help the family? (See Concept 4.)
- Interventions by family nurses must address individuals, subsystems within the family, and the whole family all at the same time. One strategy would be to assess family process and functioning and then offer intervention strategies to assist the family in its everyday functioning. Nurses could ask the following types of questions about functioning:
  - Linda and Robert, from what you have told me, it appears that your oldest daughter, Amy, has been able to help take on some of the parental jobs in the family by being the errand runner, chauffeur, and grocery shopper. Now that Amy is off to college, which of your family roles will need to be covered by someone else for a while when you and Linda first come home: cooking, laundry, chauffeur, cleaning the house? Who do you think could cover these roles?
  - Because you both shared with me that your family likes to go bowling on family night out, how do you think Linda being in a wheelchair might affect family night out?
  - Robert and Linda, have the two of you discussed legal durable power of attorney for health care so Robert can make health care decisions when the time comes that Linda may not be able to do this for herself? Linda, who would you prefer to make health care decisions for you, should you not be able to do so? Let's discuss what those health care decisions might involve.
  - Tell me about your personal/sexual relationship that you, Linda, are experiencing now that you are more disabled.

The goal of using a family systems perspective is to help the family reach stability by building on their strengths as a family, using knowledge of the family as a social system, and understanding how the family is an interconnected whole that is adapting to the changes brought about by the health event of a given family member.

Strengths and Weaknesses of Family Systems Theory

The strengths of the general systems framework are that this theory covers a large array of phenomena and views the family and its subsystems within the context of its suprasystems (the larger community in which it is embedded). Moreover, it is an interactional and holistic theory that looks at processes within the family, rather than at the content and relationships between the members. The family is viewed as a whole, not as merely a sum of its parts. Another strength of this approach is that it is an excellent data-gathering method and assessment strategy, such as using a family genogram to gather a snapshot of the family as a whole; the genogram and other family system assessment instruments are discussed in Chapter 4.

Systems theory also has its limitations (Smith & Hamon, 2016). Because this theoretical orientation is so global and abstract, it may not be specific enough for beginners to define family nursing interventions. It is important for family nurses to be able to understand conceptually how important the family as a whole is to the practice of family nursing. As health care systems continue to emphasize the autonomy of the individual, it takes time and practice to develop ways to deeply understand how a family, as a whole, is greater than the members of the family.

Developmental and Family Life Cycle Theory

Developmental and Family Life Cycle Theory provides a framework for nurses to understand normal family changes and experiences over the members' lifetimes; the theory assesses and evaluates both individuals and families as a whole because individual family members and the family as a whole develop and change over time. This approach views the evolving needs and priorities of family members and the family. Developmental stages for individuals are seen as a system in that what happens at one level has powerful ramifications at other levels of the system. Families are seen as the basic social unit of society and as the optimal level of intervention.

The family developmental theories are specifically geared to understanding families and not individuals (Smith & Hamon, 2016; White et al., 2014). Families, similar to individuals, are in constant movement and change throughout time—the family life cycle. Family

developmental theorists who inform the nursing of families include Duvall (1977); Duvall and Miller (1985); McGoldrick, Garcia Preto, & Carter (2015), and Walsh (2015, 2016). The original work of Duvall (1977), and later Duvall and Miller (1985), examined how families were affected or changed cognitively, socially, emotionally, spiritually, and physically when all members experienced developmental changes. The relationships among family members are affected by changes in individuals, and changes in the family as a whole affect the individuals within the family. These theorists recognized that families are stressed at common and predictable stages of change and transition and need to undergo adjustment to regain family stability. This early theoretical work was primarily based on the experiences of white Anglo middle-class nuclear families, with a married couple, children, and extended family.

McGoldrick et al. (2015) expanded on the original Developmental and Family Life Cycle Theory because they recognized the dramatically changing landscape of family structure, functions, and processes that was making it increasingly difficult to determine normal predictable patterns of change in families. They replaced the concept of "nuclear family" with "immediate family," which takes into consideration all family structures, such as stepfamilies, gay families, and divorced families. Instead of addressing the legal aspects of being a married couple, they viewed the concept of couple relationships and commitment as a focal point for family bonds. There is much value in nurses studying the normative sequential new experiences, challenges, and opportunities regardless of the type of family as all these normative stressors will be affected when a family also experiences events that are not expected, such as illness, death, or disability. Walsh studied the ability of the family to withstand and rebound from adversity (2015, 2016). Walsh (2015, 2016) explored the life cycle perspective on family development to increase understanding of family resilience over time. For example, an earlier experience with overcoming an adverse situation is not indicative that the family will manage the current situation with ease or resiliency.

What are thought of as normal development and family life are largely influenced by socially constructed subjective worldviews from the historical era of the oldest family members. These normative milestones are associated with chronological ages of family members and the family (Duvall, 1977; Duvall & Miller, 1985). McGoldrick et al. (2015) and Walsh (2015, 2016) recognized that previous "normative changes" do not apply, especially related to chronological ages (i.e., a woman can have her first child at 16, and then marry, divorce, and restart a family at age 35). Many previous family "phases" repeat themselves with blended families and grandparents raising grandchildren.

Walsh studied the ability of the family to withstand and rebound from adversity, known as family resilience (2015, 2016). By examining the life cycle perspective of family development, Walsh noted how individual family members and the family as a whole manage stresses and conflict and disruptive life changes by using short-term and long-term adaptive strategies.

Concept 1: Families Develop and Change Over Time

According to Developmental and Family Life Cycle Theory, family interactions among family members change over time in relation to structure, function (roles), and processes. The stresses created by these changes in family systems are somewhat predictable for different stages of family development.

The first way to view family development is to look at predictable stresses and changes as they relate to the expected age of the family members at certain transitions (i.e., societal expectation that most couples marry before turning 30 years old) and the social norms the individuals experience throughout their development. The classic traditional work of Duvall (1977) and Duvall and Miller (1985) identifies overall family tasks that need to be accomplished for each stage of family development, as related to the developmental trajectory of the individual family members. It starts with couples getting married and ends with one member of the couple dying. Refer to Table 2-5 for a detailed list of the traditional family life cycle stages and developmental tasks.

Table 2-5 Traditional Family Life Cycle Stages and Developmental Tasks	
Stages of Family Life Cycle	**Family Developmental Tasks**
Married couple	Establishing relationship as a married couple.
	Blending of individual needs; developing conflict-and-resolution approaches, communication patterns, and intimacy patterns.
Childbearing families with infants	Adjusting to pregnancy and then infant.
	Adjusting to new roles as mother and father.
	Maintaining couple bond and intimacy.
Families with preschool children	Understanding normal growth and development.
	If more than one child in family, adjusting to different temperaments and styles of children.
	Coping with energy depletion.
	Maintaining couple bond and intimacy.
Families with school-age children	Working out authority and socialization roles with school.
	Supporting child in outside interests and needs.
	Determining disciplinary actions and family rules and roles.
Families with adolescents	Allowing adolescents to establish their own identities but still be part of the family.
	Thinking about the future, education, jobs, and working.
	Increasing roles of adolescents in family, cooking, repairs, and power base.
Families with young adults: launching	After member moves out, reallocating roles, space, power, and communication.
	Maintaining supportive home base.
	Maintaining parental couple intimacy and relationship.
Middle-aged parents	Refocusing on marriage relationship.
	Ensuring security after retirement.
	Maintaining kinship ties.
Aging families	Adjusting to retirement, grandparent roles, death of spouse, and living alone.

According to this theory, families have a predictable natural history. The first stage involves the couple pairing; the family group then becomes more complex over time with the addition of new members. When the younger generation leaves home to take jobs, attend college, or marry, the original family group changes in roles, expectations, and adjustment back to a smaller core within the household home.

The second way to view family development is to assess the predictable stresses and changes in families based on the stage of family development and how long the family is in that stage. For example, suppose each of the following couples have made a choice to be childless: a newly married couple, a couple who have been married for 3 years, and a couple who have been married for 15 years (White et al., 2014). The stresses each couple experiences from this decision would be different because of societal expectations of childbearing and child rearing.

Concept 2: Families Experience Transitions From One Stage to Another

Disequilibrium occurs in the family during the transitional periods from one stage of development to the next stage. When transitions occur, families experience changes in kinship structures, family roles, social roles, and interaction. Family stress is considered to be greatest at the transition points as families adapt to achieve stability, redefine their concept of family in light of the changes, and realign relationships because of the changes (McGoldrick et al., 2015; Walsh, 2015, 2016). For example, marriage changes the status of all family members, creates new relationships for family members such as including extended family into the married dyad, and joins two different complex family systems.

Family developmental theorists explore whether families make these transitions "on time" or "off time" according to cultural and social expectations (Smith & Hamon, 2016; White et al., 2014). For example, it is "off time" for a couple in their forties to have their first child. It is considered "on time" in North America to have a couple be married before the birth of a child, but that norm may be changing given the increasing numbers of babies born to couples who are not married before the birth of their first child. (See Chapter 3 for statistics about cohabitation.)

Although some family developmental needs and tasks must be performed at each stage of the family life cycle, developmental tasks are general goals, rather than specific jobs that must be completed at that time. Achievement of family developmental tasks enables individuals within families to realize their own individual tasks. According to Developmental and Family Life Cycle Theory every family is unique in its composition and in the complexity of its expectations of members at different ages and in different roles. Families, similar to individuals, are influenced by their history and traditions and by the social context in which they live. Furthermore, families change and develop in different ways because their internal/external demands and situations differ. Families may also arrive at similar developmental levels using different processes. For example, the launching phase in one family might have a child attend community college and live at home whereas another may have their college-age child live in the dorm in the same town in which they live or the college student may attend a college across the country. How the child launches is different but many of the tasks of the family are the same. Another example would be a family with a stay at home mother caring for an infant and another family with a working mother needing day care for their infant.

Despite their differences, however, families have enough in common to make it possible to chart family development over the life span in a way that applies to most families (Friedman, Bowden, & Jones, 2003). Families experience stress when they transition from one stage to the next. The predictable changes that are based on these family developmental steps are called *normative* changes. When changes occur in families out of sequence, "off time," or are caused by a different family event, such as illness, they are called *nonnormative*. For example, it is expected to lose a parent to death during the seventh to ninth decade of life. If a parent dies during his or her forties, then that is considered an "off time" or *nonnormative* event.

In contrast with Duvall's (1977) and later Duvall and Miller's (1985) traditional developmental approach, Carter and McGoldrick (1989) and McGoldrick et al. (2015) built on this work by approaching family development from the perspective of family life cycle stages. They explored what happens within families when family members enter or exit their family group; they focus on specific family experiences, such as disruption in family relationships, roles, processes, and family structure. Examples of a family member leaving would be divorce, illness, a miscarriage, incarceration, or death of a family member. Examples of family members entering would include birth, adoption, marriage, or other formal union. Examples of family structures would include traditional, blended, lesbian and gay male, cohabitation, single parent, multiple generations in one household, grandparents raising grandchildren, or living apart but feeling together (i.e., deployed adults causing separation from their family).

Today, the Developmental and Family Life Cycle Theory remains useful as long as it is viewed generally for use with families, despite all the current variations of families. McGoldrick et al.

(2015) expanded the family life cycle to incorporate the changing family patterns and broaden the view of both development and the family. McGoldrick et al. (2015) expanded the traditional Developmental and Family Life Cycle Theory to address changes in the family that undergoes a divorce. Table 2-6 outlines the emotional process of a family undergoing a divorce and describes the developmental tasks the family deals with at different stages.

Table 2-6	Family Life Cycle for Divorcing Families	
Phase	**Emotional Process of Transition: Prerequisite Attitude**	**Developmental Issues**
Divorce		
The decision to divorce	Acceptance of inability to resolve marital tensions sufficiently to continue relationship.	Acceptance of one's own part in the failure of the marriage.
Planning the breakup of the system	Supporting viable arrangements for all parts of the system.	a. Working cooperatively on problems of custody, visitation, and finances. b. Dealing with extended family about the divorce.
Separation	a. Willingness to continue cooperative coparental relationship and joint financial support of children. b. Work on resolution of attachment to spouse.	a. Mourning loss of intact family. b. Restructuring marital and parent-child relationships and finances; adaptation to living apart. c. Realignment of relationships with extended family; staying connected with spouse's extended family.
The divorce	More work on emotional divorce: overcoming hurt, anger, and guilt, among other emotions.	a. Mourning loss of intact family. b. Retrieval of hopes, dreams, and expectations from the marriage. c. Staying connected with extended families.
Postdivorce Family		
Single parent (custodial household or primary residence)	Willingness to maintain financial responsibilities, continue parental contact with ex-spouse, and support contact of children with ex-spouse and his or her family.	a. Making flexible visitation arrangements with ex-spouse and family. b. Rebuilding own financial resources. c. Rebuilding own social network.
Single parent (noncustodial)	Willingness to maintain financial responsibilities and parental contact with ex-spouse, and to support custodial parent's relationship with children.	a. Finding ways to continue effective parenting. b. Maintaining financial responsibilities to ex-spouse and children. c. Rebuilding own social network.

Source: Adapted from Carter, B., & McGoldrick, M. (2005). The divorce cycle: A major variation in the American family life cycle. In B. Carter & M. McGoldrick (Eds.), *The expanded family life cycle: Individual, family, and social perspectives* (3rd ed.). New York, NY: Allyn & Bacon.

Goldberg (2010) explored the family life cycle tasks that are specific to lesbian and gay men families. Once lesbian and gay men make the decision to pursue parenthood, the decision then becomes how to become parents (Goldberg, 2010). These options may include sexual relations of a lesbian female with a male, surrogacy, alternative insemination, adoption, pursuit of custody from previous heterosexual partnerships, or foster care. Each one of these choices has a cascade of decisions that accompany the choice similar to decisions heterosexual parents must determine in the path to start or maintain parenthood. For example, for lesbians who elect alternative insemination, a common question is: Which parent should carry the child (Goldberg, 2010)? Another decision this couple faces is the donor type such as acquaintance, friends, or anonymous semen donors. Then they have to decide the extent of involvement of the donor. These families must decide what to name and call each parent that assumes a parental role.

Another life cycle stressor for lesbian and gay men parents is the victimization and stigma both the parents and their children experience and determining how to teach their children to handle these homophobic encounters (Chabot & Ames, 2004; Lassiter, Dew, Newton, Hays, & Yarbrough, 2006). Lesbian and gay men families must negotiate parental roles that are usually thought of based on gender-related views as mother and father (Dunne, 2000). In some cases, lesbian and gay men parents report that they blend traditional mother and father roles to create new, hybrid degendered parenting roles (Gianino, 2008; Goldberg, 2010).

In 2011, Pelton described specific stressors and tasks relative to heterosexual couples that elect to remain childfree or childless by choice. The first task is making the decision to not have children. The second task for this couple is to manage the stigma and pressure that family, friends, acquaintances, and society place on them. In fact, this stress is one the couple will face until the woman is no longer biologically able to have children. The third task for the childfree couple is defining their identity that does not include children. During this task couples may elect to focus on their chosen career, determine how to spend their leisure time, and decide if there are projects in which they would like to volunteer their time and expertise. The fourth major task of a childfree couple is to build a support system with other couples who do not have children. During this task the members of the childfree couple work together to determine the legacy they will leave to future generations. Childless couples approach the developmental stage of generativity in different ways. For example, childless couples often choose careers that involve children (teachers, counselors, etc.), or they consciously seek to give to the next generation through writing or art.

Falicov (2016) noted that normal developmental tasks and stressors are likely intensified by cultural contrasts in situations such as migration to a new country. For example, in the case of immigration, parents may be separated from their children. Young adults may elect to not leave the family to venture out on their own in the same time frame, which places them in a nonnormative developmental progression. If the children are more savvy with language acquisition, there may be a reverse of roles, with decision making and power within the family given to the children rather than the parents.

Application of Developmental and Family Life Cycle Theory to the Jones Family

When conducting family assessments using the developmental model, nurses begin by determining the family structure and where this family falls in the family life cycle stages. Using the developmental tasks outlined in the developmental model, the nurse has a ready guide to anticipate stresses the family may be experiencing or to assess the developmental tasks that are not being accomplished or are being accomplished "off time."

According to Duvall and Miller (1985), the Jones family is in the *Families With Young Adults: Launching Phase* because Amy left home and is now a freshman at a college. She is living away from home for the first time. Although the Jones family is experiencing a nonnormative event (unexpected, developmental stressor) because Linda, the mother, is now in the hospital, the family is also experiencing the normative or expected challenges for a family when the oldest child leaves home. This family is undergoing the Launching Phase at the same time that they are raising an adolescent and a toddler. Although Duvall (1977; Duvall & Miller, 1985) recommended focusing on the older child, later researchers noted this does not work, as transitions for each child have an impact on all family members.

This is a good example of where major individual and whole family events coincide and present challenges for families. Questions to explore with the family relative to Amy might include the following:

1. How has the family addressed the reallocation of family household physical space since Amy left for school (for example, the allocation of bedrooms or the arrangement of space within the bedroom if Katie and Amy shared the bedroom)?
2. How has Amy developed as an indirect caregiver (such as calling home to chat with Dad and see how he is doing, talking with the siblings and teasing or supporting their efforts, or sharing with parents her school life to reduce their worry about her adjustment)?
3. How have family roles changed since Amy left for school? What roles did Amy perform for the family that someone else needs to pick up now? For example, who will perform such roles as chauffeur, grocery shopper, errand runner, and babysitter now that Linda is not able and Amy is gone?
4. How has the power structure of the family shifted now that Katie is more responsible for the care of Travis?
5. How has the parents' couple time changed since Amy went off to college?

Questions to explore about Travis, the 4-year-old preschool child, include:

1. Children at this age need to develop increasingly complex social relationships. As Travis is struggling with being suddenly introduced to being in a preschool, can the transition be designed so that he attends preschool only 2 days a week for now and gradually increase as he becomes adjusted to this new experience?
2. Are there any extended family members who have children the same age as Travis that he can interact with?
3. Could it be arranged that Travis has some special time with Mom when he gets home from preschool so that he feels like he is still center stage with his mother's attention?
4. What type of ritual and routine would help provide Travis with stability and change?

Finally, questions that might be explored relative to 13-year-old Katie follow. Katie's position in the family

is between the school-age child and the teenager. Katie wants to move toward more independence at the same time she is being asked to babysit with Travis. Questions for Katie might include:

1. Can the family negotiate allowing Katie to have special time when she is not responsible at home to hang out with her friends, to go to youth camp with the Girl Scouts, or to be with the youth group at church?
2. Is there a way that both Travis and Katie can attend individual groups at the church, but go there together?
3. Are there other ways that Katie can help support the family rather than provide child care for Travis?
4. Would it be helpful for the school counselor to reach out to Katie about her stress or explore having a child-life specialist work with Katie?

With the developmental approach, nursing interventions may include helping the family to understand individual and family developmental tasks. Interventions could also include helping the family understand the normalcy of disequilibrium during these transitional periods. Another intervention is to help the family mitigate these transitions by capitalizing on family rituals. Family rituals serve to decrease the anxiety of changes in that they help link the family to other family members and to the larger community (Imber-Black, 2005).

Family nurses must recognize that every family must accomplish both individual and family developmental tasks for every stage of the Developmental and Family Life Cycle. Events at one stage of the cycle have powerful effects at other stages. Helping families adjust and adapt to these transitions is an important role for family nurses. It is important for nurses to keep in mind the needs and requirements of both the family as a whole and the individuals who make up the family.

Strengths and Weaknesses of the Developmental and Family Life Cycle

A major strength of the developmental approach is that it provides a systematic framework for predicting what a family may be experiencing at any stage in the family life cycle. Family nurses can assess a family's stage of development, the extent to which the family has achieved the tasks associated with that stage of family development, and problems that may or may not exist. It is a superb theoretical approach for assisting nurses who are working with families on health promotion. Family strengths and available resources are easier to identify because they are based on assisting families to achieve developmental milestones.

A primary criticism of family development theory is that it best describes the trajectory of intact, two-parent, heterosexual nuclear families. The original eight-stage model was based on a nuclear family, assumed an intact marriage throughout the life cycle of the family, and was organized around the oldest child's developmental needs. It did not consider divorce, death of a spouse, remarriage, unmarried parents, childless couples, the developmental needs of subsequent children, or cohabitating or gay and lesbian couples. It normalized one type of family and ignored others (Smith & Hamon, 2016). Today's families vary widely in their structure and related roles. The traditional view of families moving in a linear direction from getting married, tracking children from preschool to launching, middle-aged parents, and aging families is no longer the majority family structure or development, and therefore is questionably applicable. Carter (2005), Carter and McGoldrick (1989, 2005), and McGoldrick et al. (2015) expanded the family developmental model to include stresses in the remarried family. A serious shortcoming of these models is that they ignore the importance of cultural diversity and health disparities in families, and the impact on family development (Falicov, 2016). As family structures continue to change in response to cultural factors and the ecologic system, trajectories of families likely will not fit within the traditional developmental framework (White et al., 2014). Future theory development and research need to expand understanding of family development across time while considering changes and diversity within family development.

Bioecological Systems Theory

Urie Bronfenbrenner was one of the world's leading scholars in the field of developmental psychology (Bronfenbrenner, 1972a, 1972b, 1979, 1981, 1986, 1997; Bronfenbrenner & Morris, 1998). He contributed greatly to the ecological theory of human development, which concentrated on the interaction and interdependence of humans—as biological and social entities—within the environment. Originally this idea was called the *Human Ecology Theory*, then

it was changed to *Ecological Systems Theory*, and it finally evolved into the *Bioecological Systems Theory* (Bronfenbrenner & Lerner, 2004; Rosa & Tudge, 2013). The Bioecological System is the combination of children's biological disposition and environmental forces coming together to shape the development of human beings. This theory combines both Developmental Theory and Systems Theory to understand individual and family growth.

Before Bronfenbrenner, child psychologists studied children, sociologists examined families, anthropologists analyzed society, economists scrutinized the economic framework, and political scientists focused on political structures. Through Bronfenbrenner's groundbreaking work in "human ecology," environments from the individual and family to larger economic/political structures have come to be viewed as part of systems interacting across the life course from infancy through adulthood. This "bioecological" approach to human development crosses over barriers among the social sciences and builds bridges among the disciplines, allowing for better understanding to emerge about key elements in the larger social structure that are vital for optimal human development (both individual and family) (Rosa & Tudge, 2013).

The human ecology framework brings together other diverse influences. From evolutionary theory and genetics comes the view that humans develop as individual biological organisms with capacities limited by genetic endowment (*ontogenetic development*) that lead to hereditary familial characteristics. From population genetics comes the perspective that populations change by means of natural selection. For the individual, this means that individuals/families demonstrate their fitness by adapting to ever-changing environments. From ecological theories come the notion that human and family development is "contextualized" and "interactional" over time (Rosa & Tudge, 2013; White et al., 2014). All this leads to the ongoing debate related to the dual nature of humans as constructions of both biology and culture; hence, the argument of nature versus nurture. Although this debate has not been resolved, scientists have moved beyond debate to the realization that the development of most human traits depends on a nature/nurture interaction rather than on one influence having priority over the other (White et al., 2014). Thus, Bronfenbrenner moved his own theory and ideas from the concept and terminology of ecology (environment) to bioecology (both genetics and society) as a way of embracing two developmental origins for this theory (Rosa & Tudge, 2013). His Bioecological Systems Theory emphasizes the interaction of both the biological/genetics (ontologic/nature) and the social context (society) characteristics of development (Rosa & Tudge, 2013; Smith & Hamon, 2016; White et al., 2014).

The human bioecological perspective consists of a framework of four locational/spatial contexts and one time-related context (Rosa & Tudge, 2013; White et al., 2014). A primary feature of this theory is the premise that individual and family development is contextual over time. According to Bronfenbrenner (1986), individual development is affected by five types or levels of environmental systems (Figure 2-6). Family Bioecological Theory describes the interactions and influences on the family from systems at different levels of engagement.

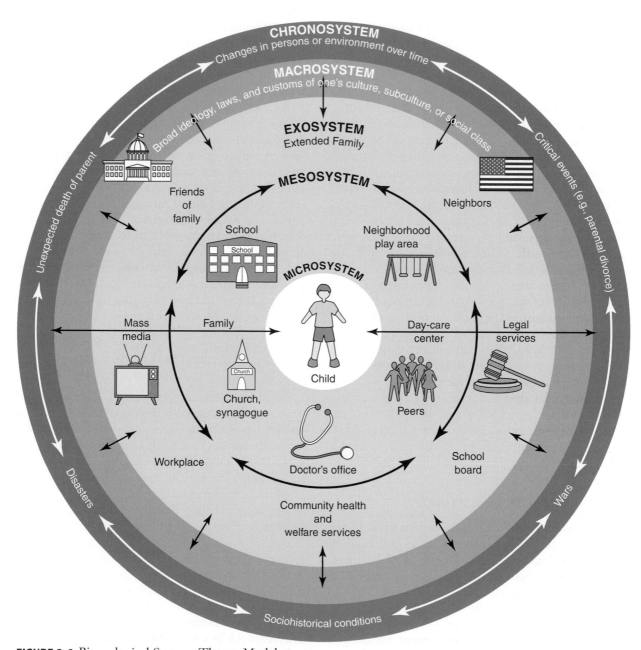

FIGURE 2-6 Bioecological Systems Theory Model

Microsystems are the settings in which individuals/ families experience and create day-to-day reality. They are the places people inhabit, the people with whom they live, and the things they do together. In this level, people fulfill their roles in families, with peers, in schools, and in neighborhoods where they are in the most direct interaction with agents around them.

Mesosystems are the relationships among major microsystems in which persons or families actively participate, such as families and schools, families and religion, and families with peers. For example, how does the interaction between families and schools affect families? Can the relationship between families and their religious/spiritual communities be used to help families?

Exosystems are external environments that influence individuals and families indirectly. The person may not be an active participant within these systems, but the system has an effect on the persons/families. For example, a parent's job experience affects family life which, in turn, affects the children (parent's job's travel requirements, job stress, salary). Furthermore, governmental funding to other microsystems environments—schools, libraries, parks, health care, and day care—affects the experiences of children and families.

Macrosystems are the broad cultural attitudes, ideologies, or belief systems that influence institutional environments within a particular culture/subculture in which individuals/families live. Examples include the Judeo-Christian ethic, democracy, ethnicity, and societal values. Mesosystems and exosystems are set within macrosystems, and together they are the "blueprints" for the ecology of human and family development.

Chronosystems are time-related contexts where changes occur over time and have an effect on the other four levels/systems of development mentioned earlier. Chronosystems include the patterning of environmental events and transitions over the life course of individuals/families. These effects are created by time or critical periods in development and are influenced by sociohistorical conditions, such as parental divorce, unexpected death of a parent, or a war. Individuals/families have no control over the evolution of such external systems over time.

Within each one of these levels are roles, norms, and rules that shape the environment. Bronfenbrenner's model of human/family development acknowledges that people develop not in isolation, but rather in relation to their larger environment: families, home, schools, communities, and society. All these interactive, ever-changing, and multilevel environments over time are key to understanding human/family development.

Bronfenbrenner uses the term *bidirectional* to describe the influential interactions that take place between children and their relationships with parents, teachers, and society. All relationships among humans/ families and their environment are bidirectional or interactional. The environment influences individuals and families; in turn, individuals/families influence what happens in their own environments. This interaction is also basic to the Family Systems Theory.

Within the bioecological framework, what happens outside family units is as important as what happens inside individual members and family units. Developing families are on center stage as an active force shaping their social experiences for themselves. The ecological perspective views children/families and their environments as mutually shaping systems, each changing and adapting over time (again, also included in the Family Systems' perspective). The bioecological approach addresses both opportunities and risks. Opportunities refer to what the environment offers families, such as material, emotional, and social encouragement compatible with their needs and capacities. Risks to family development are composed of direct threats or the absence of opportunities, such as poverty, mental health challenges, or social isolation.

Application of the Bioecological Systems Theory to the Jones Family

Assessment using the *Biological Systems Theory* consists of looking at all levels of the system when interviewing the family in a health care setting. Assessment of the *microsystem* reveals that the Jones family consists of five members: two parents and three children. They live in a two-story home with four bedrooms in an older suburban section of the town. Mother Linda had been a full-time homemaker before experiencing health problems related to her diagnosis of MS. The *mesosystem* assessment for the family consists of identifying the schools the children attend, neighborhood/friends, extended family, and religious affiliation. The oldest daughter is a college student who travels home on weekends to help the family. The second daughter is in a local middle school and can walk back and forth to her school. The youngest child, a boy, attends an all-day preschool and is transported by his parents or other parents from the preschool. The family has attended a Protestant church in the neighborhood. The family lives in a house in an older established neighborhood, and has made friends through the schools, church, and neighborhood contacts. Part of the extended family (grandparents) live nearby, and all the family members get together for the holidays; neither parent has siblings who live nearby. The *exosystem* assessment shows that father Robert works 40 hours a week for an industrial plant at the edge of town, and he drives back and forth daily. The father has some job stress, because he is in a middle-management position. His salary is average for middle-class families in the United States. State and county funding to the area schools, libraries, and recreational facilities are always a struggle in this community. The town has physicians/clinics of all specialties and has one community hospital. An assessment of the *macrosystem* shows that this community is largely white, with only 10% of residents from other backgrounds. Most people in the community embrace a Christian ethic.

The community value system includes a family focus and a strong work ethic. Many of the people prefer the Democratic Party. In terms of the time-related contexts of the *chronosystem*, a few things are notable. These time-related events put more stress on the family than usual nonnormative events. Linda's disease process with MS has exacerbated in recent times, placing additional strain on the family system. Robert's own dad died in the past year, leaving him extra responsibility for his widowed mother in addition to his responsibility for his own children and now ill wife. The economy in the country and region is going through a recession, leading people to feel some fear about their economic futures. Robert had hoped that his wife could go to work part-time when their youngest child went to school, but that no longer seems to be a possibility. The family assessment would include how the family at each of the earlier-mentioned levels is influenced by the changes brought about by Linda's progressing debilitative disease and recent hospitalization. The family is experiencing disturbance at many of these levels.

Interventions include the following possibilities. In general, nurses can also look for additional systems that the family could interact with to help support family functioning during this family illness event. Nurses could make home visits to assess the living arrangements of the family and to determine how the home could be changed to accommodate a wheelchair/walker. The nurses should talk with the parents about their relationship to the schools, church, and extended family support systems. The parents might be advised to inform the school(s), church, workplace, and grandparents of what is happening to their family. The nurses could make suggestions relative to Travis's current behavior with having to go to all-day preschool. The nurses also could explore with the family the larger external environment, including community resources (e.g., Multiple Sclerosis Society, visiting nurse service, or counseling services). The nurses should contact the medical doctor(s) and discharge planning nurse at the hospital to obtain information to interpret the diagnosis, prognosis, and treatment of MS to the family. The nurses might talk to the family about how their faith can be of help during these tough times and what their primary concerns are as a family. The nurses should get in touch with the social workers at the hospital to coordinate care and social well-being strategies for the posthospitalization period, as well as in the future. Strategies may involve application to Social Security for the disabled. A family care planning meeting should be set up to involve as many caretakers and stakeholders as possible.

Evaluation of the interventions would consist of follow-up with the family through periodic home visits and telephone contact. The nurses would explore how the family is adapting to its situation, how the father is dealing with the extra responsibility, how the children are coping, and the physical and mental health of the mother. Because MS is a chronic progressive relapsing disorder, a plan would be put into place for periodic evaluations that might involve changing the plan of care.

Strengths and Weaknesses of the Bioecological Systems Theory

The strength of the bioecological perspective is that it represents a comprehensive and holistic view of human/family development—a bio/psycho/socio/cultural/spiritual approach to the understanding of how humans and families develop and adapt to the larger society. It includes both the *nature* (biological) and *nurture* (environmental contexts) aspects of growth and development for both individuals and families. It directs our attention to factors that occur within as well as to the layered influences of factors that occur outside individuals and families. The bioecological perspective provides a valuable complement to other theories that may offer greater insight into how each aspect of the holistic approach affects individuals and families over time.

The strength of this theory is also part of the weakness of this approach. The different systems show nurses what to think about that may affect the family, but the direction of how the family adapts is not specifically delineated in this theory. In other words, the bio/psycho/socio/cultural/spiritual aspects of human/family growth and development are not detailed enough to define how individuals/ families can accomplish or adapt to these contextual changes over time. Aspects of the theory require further delineation and testing, that is, the influence of biological and cognitive processes and how they interact with the environment.

SUMMARY

Theory is used in all aspects of nursing care and assists the practicing nurse in organizing, understanding, and analyzing information. Essentially, theory provides a systematic, consistent way of thinking about nursing care. Nurses who understand the relationship between theory and practice use multiple approaches in their practice with families, and thereby can explore more options for families in providing health care. By understanding theories and models, nurses are better prepared to think creatively and critically about how health events affect the family. This chapter introduced nurses to the concept of theory-guided, evidence-based family nursing practice. It presented the relationship between theory, practice, and research, and explained crucial aspects of theory. The chapter then explored three theories for the nursing care of families and applied the theories to the case study in the chapter:

- Family Systems Theory
- Developmental and Family Life Cycle Theory
- Bioecological Theory

The chapter revealed how nurses can practice family nursing differently with the Jones family according to the different theoretical perspectives.

The following points highlight critical concepts that are addressed in this chapter:

- No single theory, model, or conceptual framework adequately describes the complex relationships of family.
- No one theoretical perspective gives nurses a sufficiently broad base of knowledge and understanding to guide assessment and interventions with all families.
- No one theoretical perspective is better, more comprehensive, or more correct than another.
- Nurses who draw from multiple theories are more effective in tailoring their nursing practice and family interventions to reach the optimal outcomes. Using multiple theories substantially increases the likelihood that the family will be able to achieve stability and health as a family unit.
- Theories that inform the nursing of families should be the "gold standard" of nursing practice (Segaric & Hall, 2005); hence, family nursing is a theory-guided, evidence-based practice.

This chapter presents ways of providing excellent family health care nursing that is theory driven and evidence based. By using different lenses to view family care problems, different solutions and options for care and interventions become available. Clearly, no one theoretical perspective gives all nurses in all settings a sufficiently broad base of knowledge on which to assess and intervene with the complex health events experienced by families. What is crucial is that nurses use multiple theoretical perspectives to guide their practice with the nursing care of families.

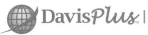 | For additional resources and information, visit **http://davisplus.fadavis.com**. References can be found on Davis*Plus*.

Chapter 3

Family Demography
Continuity and Change in North American Families

Lynne M. Casper, PhD

Alli Coritz, PhD Candidate

Critical Concepts

- Economic, social, and cultural changes have increased family diversity in North America. More families are maintained by single mothers, single fathers, cohabitating couples, and grandparents than in the past.

- Increases in women's labor force participation, especially among mothers, have reduced the amount of nonwork time that families have to attend to health care needs.

- North Americans are more likely to live alone than they were a few decades ago. Thus, people are less likely to have family members living with them who can assist them when they become ill or injured.

- Recurring recessions, tight job markets, slow wage growth, and soaring housing costs increase the likelihood that young adults will remain or return to their parent's home after graduating from college. Many of them cannot find a stable job that pays enough for them to live on their own. In the United States, many young adults do not have health insurance and, thus, do not seek health care regularly.

- More North Americans are immigrants than was the case a few decades ago. Family nurses provide care for an increasingly ethnically, culturally, and linguistically diverse population.

- Single-mother families are particularly vulnerable. They are more likely to live in poverty than are other families. These mothers are usually the sole wage earners and care providers in their families. Thus, these families are more likely than other families both to be monetarily poor and to face stringent time constraints.

- Single-father families have been increasing in recent decades and fathers are spending more time caring for their children. Nurses will be increasingly likely to encounter fathers who bring their children in for checkups or medical treatments.

- Cohabitation among opposite- and same-sex couples continues to rise in North America. In the United States, because cohabiting relationships are not legally sanctioned in many states and localities, partners may not have the right to make health care decisions on behalf of each other or for the other partner's children.

- Couples who are having trouble conceiving are increasingly turning to the medical profession for help. Births resulting from assisted reproductive technologies (ARTs) are on the rise in North America. The ART process is expensive, time consuming, and often increases health risks for the women and children involved.

(continued)

Critical Concepts *(cont.)*

■ Many children in North America are adopted. These children need time to adjust to their new circumstances and are more likely than other children to have special health care needs.

■ Stepfamilies are common among North American families. Legal arrangements in these families can be complicated; it is not always clear who has the right to make health care decisions for children in these families.

■ Many children are raised by or receive regular care from their grandparents. These grandparents may or may not have legal responsibility for their grandchildren, but may seek medical care for them.

■ The aging of the population, as well as the impending retirement of the baby-boom generation, presents significant challenges for both informal caregivers and the health care system. The need for nurses who specialize in caring for elderly persons will continue to increase.

■ Most young children spend at least some time every week in child care outside of their nuclear family. Child-care arrangements are diverse and change frequently. Child care may increase health issues, such as colds and respiratory infections, as well as increase exposure to undervaccinated peers.

If there is one "mantra" about family life in the last half century, it is that the family has undergone tremendous change. The United States population as a whole had increased 0.79% to 321.1 million during July 1, 2014 and July 1, 2015 (U.S. Census Bureau, 2015). No other institution elicits as contentious debate as the North American family. Many argue that the movement away from marriage and traditional gender roles has seriously degraded family life. Others view family life as amazingly diverse, resilient, and adaptive to new circumstances (Cherlin, 2009; Popenoe, 1993; Stacey, 1993).

Any assessment of the general health of family life in North America and the health and well-being of family members, especially children, requires a look at what is known about the demographic and socioeconomic trends that affect families. Unlike the way in which statistics and references are used in most nursing articles and textbooks, the sources used in this chapter need to represent the population and not just be from a single study or another source where the data do not reflect the population. Therefore, all the statistics in this chapter are current for populations. Furthermore, researchers in demography/sociology tend to cite seminal references that are important in explaining and interpreting changes over time, even though those references may be decades old. Therefore, the older references in this chapter are included because of their necessary function in elucidating the demographic and socioeconomic trends that affect families.

A pragmatic approach to family nursing requires an understanding of the broader changes in family within the population. The latter half of the 20th century was characterized by tumultuous change in the economy, civil rights, and sexual freedom and by dramatic improvements in health and longevity. Marriage and family life felt the reverberations of these societal changes.

In the first decades of the 21st century, as North Americans reassess where they have come from and where they are going, one issue stands out—rhetoric about the dramatically changing family may be a step behind the reality. Recent trends suggest a quieting of changes in the family in Canada, as well as the United States, or at least of the pace of change. Little change has occurred in the proportions of two-parent or single-parent families since the mid-1990s (Casper & Bianchi, 2002; U.S. Census Bureau, 2015i). After a significant increase in the proportion of children living with unmarried parents, the living arrangements of children stabilized, as did the living arrangements of young adults and older adults. The divorce rate increased substantially in the mid-1960s and 1970s, reached its peak in 1980, and has declined only slightly since then. In the United States, between 43% and 46% of marriages contracted today are expected to end in divorce (Schoen & Canudas-Romo, 2006). In Canada, divorce rates also increased during the 1970s and 1980s, peaked slightly later in 1987, but have declined slightly since then. In 2008, 41% of marriages were expected to end in divorce within the first 30 years (Statistics Canada, 2012c). The rapid growth in cohabitation among unmarried adults has also slowed.

Yet, family life is still evolving. Young adults have often postponed marriage and children to complete higher education before attempting to enter labor markets that have become inhospitable to poorly educated workers. Accompanying this delay in marriage was the continued increase in births to unmarried women. By 2014, 40% of all births in the United States were to unmarried women (Hamilton, Martin, Osterman, Curtin, & Mathews, 2015).

Within marriage or marriage-like relationships, the appropriate roles for each partner are shifting as North American societies accept and value more equal roles for men and women. The widening role of fathers has become a major agent of change in the family. More father-only families exist than in the past, and after divorce fathers are more likely to share custody of children with the mother. Within two-parent families, fathers are also more likely to be involved in the children's care than in the past (Dotti Sani & Treas, 2016). In addition, the number of same-sex couples has been increasing, and a larger proportion of them are now raising children. Family roles in same-sex couples are more likely to be negotiated than in opposite-sex families (Matos, 2015).

Whether the slowing, and in some cases cessation, of change in family living arrangements is a temporary lull or part of a new, more sustained equilibrium will only be revealed in the next decades of the 21st century. New norms may be emerging about the desirability of marriage, the optimal timing of children, and the involvement of fathers in child rearing and mothers in breadwinning. Understanding the evolution of North American families and the implications these changes have for family nursing requires taking the pulse of contemporary family life.

This chapter examines changes and variations in North American families in order to understand what these changes portend for family health care nursing during the first half of this century. This chapter draws on information pertaining to family demography from a variety of data sources (Box 3-1). The reader should note that family nursing is not the major focus of this chapter. The subject matter of the chapter is structured to provide family nurses with background on changes in the North American family so that they can understand their patient populations. The chapter does briefly touch upon the implications of these demographic patterns for practicing family nursing.

Where possible, statistics have been reported for both the United States and Canada, but comparable data for Canada were not always readily accessible for the topics covered in this chapter. Readers should note that data are not always collected in the same year and that some family indicators are defined and measured differently across the two countries.

A CHANGING ECONOMY AND SOCIETY

Consider the life of a North American young woman reaching adulthood in the 1950s or early 1960s. Such a woman was likely to marry straight out of high school or to take a clerical or retail sales job until she married. She would have moved out of her parents' home only after she married to form a new household with her husband. This young woman was likely to marry by about age 20 in the United States (U.S. Census Bureau, 2015c), age 22 in Canada, and begin a family soon thereafter. If she were working when she became pregnant, she would probably have quit her job and stayed home to care for her children and husband while her husband had a steady job that paid enough to support the entire family. Thus, usually someone was at home who had the time to care for the health needs of family members, to schedule routine checkups with doctors and dentists, and to take family members to these appointments.

Fast-forward to the first decades of the 21st century. A young woman reaching adulthood in the first decades of the 21st century is not likely to marry before her 27th birthday. She will probably attend higher education and is likely to live by herself, with a significant other, or with roommates before marrying. She may move in and out of her parents' house several times before she gets married. Similar to her counterpart reaching adulthood in the 1950s, she is likely to marry and have at least one child, but the sequence of those events may well be reversed. She probably will not drop out of the labor force after she has children, although she may curtail the number of hours she is employed. She is much more likely to divorce, and possibly even to remarry, compared with a young woman in the 1950s or 1960s. Because she is more likely to be a single mother and to be working outside of the home, she is also not as likely to have the time necessary to devote to caring for the health of family members.

A dramatic change in women's participation in the labor market occurred after 1970, as mothers with young children began entering the labor force in greater numbers. Historically, unmarried mothers (either never married or formerly married) of young children had higher labor force participation rates than married mothers. These women often were the only earners in their families. One notable change

BOX 3-1

Sources of Information on Demography and Public Health

Current Population Surveys

Many of the statistics discussed in this chapter draw on information from the Current Population Surveys (CPS) collected by the U.S. Census Bureau.

■ This is a continuous survey of about 60,000 households, selected at random to be representative of the national population.
■ Each household is interviewed monthly for two 4-month periods. During February through April of each year, the CPS collects additional demographic and economic data, including data on health insurance coverage, from each household.
■ This Annual Demographic Supplement is the most frequently used source of data on demographic and economic trends in the United States and is the data source for the majority of statistics presented in this chapter regarding changes in the family.

Decennial Census

For estimates for small areas or subgroups of the population, demographers often used data from the "long form" of the decennial census, which collected data from one-sixth of all households.

■ The census collects a range of economic and demographic information, including incomes and occupations, housing, disability status, and grandparent responsibility for children.
■ The census cannot match the detail found in more specialized surveys. For example, only four short questions measure disability for children; surveys designed for precise and complete estimates of disabilities will usually have dozens of such questions. Since 2004, the American Community Survey replaced the sample data from the census and now provides a more continuous flow of estimates for states, cities, counties, and even towns and rural areas, for which estimates were made only once a decade.

National Center for Health Statistics

Several large health-related surveys are conducted by the National Center for Health Statistics.

■ *National Health Interview Survey (NHIS):* The NHIS is a large, continuous survey of about 43,000 households per year, covering the civilian, noninstitutionalized population of the United States. The NHIS is the major source of information on health status and disability, health-related behaviors, and health care utilization for all age groups.
■ *National Health and Nutrition Examination Survey (NHANES):* The NHANES includes physical examinations, mental health questionnaires, dietary data, analyses of urine and blood, and immunization status from a random sample of Americans (about 10,000 in each 2-year cycle). NHANES also collects some basic demographic and income data. It is the major source of information on trends in obesity, cholesterol status, and a host of other conditions in the national population, and in particular age groups and racial/ethnic groups.
■ *National Survey of Family Growth (NSFG):* The NSFG is the primary source of information on marriage and divorce trends, pregnancy, contraceptive use, and fertility behaviors, and the ways in which they vary among different groups and over time. Birth and death certificates, sent by hospitals and funeral homes to state offices of vital events registration, provide the raw material for calculating fertility and mortality rates and life expectancy. The data are collected from the states and analyzed by the National Center for Health Statistics.

National Population Health Survey, Canada

In Canada, the National Population Health Survey has interviewed a panel of respondents every 2 years since 1994 to track changes in health-related behaviors, risk factors, and health outcomes.

has been the increase in the combination of paid work and mothering among married mothers. In 1960, for example, in the United States, only 19% of married mothers with children younger than age 6 were in the labor force. By 2015, the proportion increased to 64% (U.S. Census Bureau, 2015k). In Canada, 28% of women with children under the age of 3 were employed in 1976 compared with 64% in 2009. Among Canadian mothers with children under the age of 16 living at home, the proportion is even

higher at 73% (Uppal, 2015). Another truly remarkable change in the United States has been the increase in the labor force participation of single mothers from 44% to 69% between 1980 and 2015 (U.S. Census Bureau, 2015f). In Canada, the proportion of single mothers who were employed in 1976 was 48% and increased to 69% in 2014 (Statistics Canada, 2015c). What does this trend imply for family nursing? The majority of North American families with young children in the mid-20th century had mothers who were home full-time to care for the health needs of family members, whereas at the beginning of the 21st century such families were in the minority.

Changes in the Economy

Economic conditions have an influence on young people's decisions about when to enter the labor force, when to marry, and when to have children (and how many children to have). After World War II, the United States and Canada enjoyed an economic boom characterized by rapid economic growth, full employment, rising productivity, higher wages, low inflation, and increasing earnings. A man with a high-school education in the 1950s and 1960s could secure a job that paid enough to allow him to purchase a house, support a family on one income, and join the swelling ranks of the middle class.

The economic realities of the 1970s and 1980s were quite different. The two decades after the oil crisis, which began in 1973, were decades of economic change and uncertainty marked by a shift away from manufacturing and toward services, stagnating or declining wages (especially for less-educated workers), high inflation, and a slowdown in productivity growth. The 1990s were just as remarkable for the turnaround: sustained prosperity, low unemployment, and economic growth that seemed to reach many in the poorest segments of society (Farley, 1996; Levy, 1998). The Great Recession, which began in 2008, reversed this trend, and many men and women joined the ranks of the unemployed and underemployed.

When the economy is on such a roller coaster, family life often takes a similar ride. Marriage occurred early and was nearly universal in the decades after World War II; mothers remained in the home to rear children as the baby-boom generation was born and nurtured. When baby boomers hit working age in the 1970s, the economy was not as hospitable as it had been for their parents. They postponed marriage, delayed having children, and found it difficult to establish themselves in the labor market.

Many of the baby boomers' own children began reaching working age in the 1990s and 2000s, when individuals' economic fortunes were increasingly dependent on their educational attainment. Those who attended higher education were much more likely to become self-sufficient and to live independently from their parents (Rosenfeld, 2007). High-school graduates who did not continue for higher education discovered that jobs with high pay and benefits were in relatively short supply. In the United States, a high-school graduate in full-time work earned about 25% (allowing for inflation) less than a comparable new worker would have earned 20 years earlier (Farley, 1996). The increasing relative benefits of further education encouraged more young men and women to delay marriage and attend higher education.

Partly because of these changes in the economy, both men and women are remaining single longer and are more likely to leave home to pursue higher education, to live with a partner, and to launch a career before taking on the responsibility of a family of their own. The traditional gender-based organization of home life (in which mothers have primary responsibility for care of the home and children and fathers provide financial support) has not disappeared, but young women today can expect to be employed while raising children, and young men are more likely to share in some child-rearing and household tasks. Thus, in the first decades of this century, men are more likely to play a role in looking after the health of family members than they were in previous decades.

Before World War II, most men worked nearly to the end of their lives. Retirement was a privilege for the wealthy or the fortunate workers whose companies provided pensions. Currently, with increases in life expectancy and healthier lives, the passage of the Social Security Acts in 1936 and 1938 in the United States, and the institution of provincial (in the 1920s) and federal (since 1952) pensions in Canada, most workers can look forward to at least a modest guaranteed income for themselves and their spouses and minor children. Social Security benefits constitute more than half of the household income for two-thirds of Americans older than 65. The increased availability of public pensions made possible a growing period of retirement for most workers, a steady decrease in poverty rates for older people, and an increase in the proportion of older people maintaining their own households separately from their adult children.

Changing Family Norms

In 1950, in North America, there was one dominant and socially acceptable way for adults to live their lives. Those who deviated could expect to be censured and stigmatized. The "ideal" family was composed of a homemaker-wife, a breadwinner-father, and two or more children. Americans shared a common image of what a family should look like and how mothers, fathers, and children should behave. These shared values reinforced the importance of the family and the institution of marriage (McLanahan & Casper, 1995). This vision of family life showed amazing staying power, even as its economic underpinnings were eroding. For this 1950s-style family to exist, North Americans had to support distinct gender roles, and the economy had to be vibrant enough for an average man to support a family financially on his own.

Government policies and business practices perpetuated this family type by reserving the best jobs for men and discriminating against working women when they married or had a baby. Beginning in the 1960s, though, women and people from minority backgrounds gained legal protections in the workplace and discriminatory practices began to recede.

A transformation in attitudes toward family behaviors also took place. People became more accepting of divorce, cohabitation, and sex outside marriage; less sure about the universality and permanence of marriage; and more tolerant of blurred gender roles and of mothers working outside the home (Bianchi, Raley, & Casper, 2012; Casper & Bianchi, 2002; Cherlin, 2009). Society became more open-minded about a variety of living arrangements, family configurations, and lifestyles.

Although the transformation of many of these attitudes occurred throughout the 20th century, the pace of change accelerated in the 1960s and 1970s. These years brought many political, social, and medical upheavals affecting gender issues and views of the family. The feminist movement included a highly publicized, although unsuccessful, attempt to pass the Equal Rights Amendment (ERA) to the U.S. Constitution. New and effective methods of contraception were introduced in the 1950s and 1960s. In 1973, the U.S. Supreme Court ruled that state laws banning abortion were unconstitutional. In Canada, abortion was illegal until 1969 when the law was changed to allow abortions for health reasons. Popular literature and music heralded the sexual revolution and an era of "free love." In all industrialized countries, a new ideology was emerging during these years that stressed personal freedom, self-fulfillment, and individual choice in living arrangements and family commitments (Bianchi et al., 2012; Casper & Bianchi, 2002; Cherlin, 2009). People began to expect more out of marriage and to leave marriages that failed to fulfill their expectations. Certainly not all Americans approved of all these changes in beliefs and behaviors. The general North American culture changed, though, as divorce and single parenting became more widespread realities.

An Aging Society

For Americans born in 1900, the average life expectancy was fewer than 50 years. But the early decades of the 20th century brought the discovery of antibiotics and such tremendous advances in the control of communicable diseases of childhood that life expectancy at birth increased to 70 years by 1960. Rapid declines in mortality from heart disease—the leading cause of death—significantly lengthened life expectancy for those aged 65 or older after 1960 (Treas & Torrecilha, 1995). By 2014, life expectancy at birth was nearly 78.8 years for Americans (National Center for Health Statistics, 2014) and 82.5 years for Canadians (World Health Organization, 2015). Further, an American woman who reached age 60 in 2016 could expect to live an additional 26 years, on average, and a 60-year-old American man would live another 23 years. For Canadians, life expectancy at age 60 is the same—another 26 years for women and another 23 years for men. Women continue to outlive men in North America, though the gender gap in recent years has shrunk somewhat, primarily because of the delayed effects of smoking trends (men have always been more likely to smoke than women, but they have reduced smoking much more than women in recent decades). The gap in life expectancy between men and women means that women tend to outlive their husbands and women predominate in the older age groups. About 60% of the population 75 years and older in the United States and Canada are women (Statistics Canada, 2016e; U.S. Census Bureau, 2013a).

Partly because more North Americans are surviving until older ages, and partly because of a long-term decline in fertility rates, the proportion of the population aged 65 or older has grown. In 1900, only 1 of every 25 Americans was aged 65 or older (nearly 3% of the total population). By 2013, the proportion was more than 3 in 25 (14% of the total population). In 2011, the first of some 78 million baby boomers reached their 65th birthdays, and the rate of increase of the population of older adults began to accelerate. By 2030, it is expected that one in five Americans will be aged 65 or older. The scenario for Canada is similar, although Canada has a slightly higher proportion of the population aged 65 and older; in 2016, 16.5% of Canada's population was 65 years and older compared with 14% of U.S. residents in 2013 (Statistics Canada, 2016e; U.S. Census Bureau, 2012; U.S. Census Bureau, 2015q).

People do not suddenly become old on their 65th birthday, of course. Together with improvements in life expectancy have come improvements in the disability rates at older ages, so that North Americans are not only living longer than in the past but also enjoying more years of life without chronic illness or disabilities. In the United States, 65 is still a convenient marker for "old age" in health policy terms, because it is the age at which most Americans become eligible for medical and hospital insurance funded mainly by the federal government through Medicare. In Canada, at the age of 65 people become eligible for the Old Age Security (OAS) pension (Service Canada, 2016). By 65, most workers (both men and women) have left full-time work, though many continue to work part-time, or for part of the year, often at different jobs than those they pursued during most of their careers.

The aging of the population is often considered a major cause of increasing demand for medical services and of the growth in medical expenditures. Population aging is, indeed, one factor, because older people in every country consume more medical care than younger adults. The major causes of increased health expenditures in industrialized countries, however, have been rising incomes and changes in medical technology, including increased use of pharmaceuticals, rather than the simple growth of the population of older adults (World Health Organization, 2011).

Increased life expectancy translates into extended years spent in family relationships. A couple who marry in their twenties could spend the next 50 years together, assuming they remain married. Couples in the past were much more likely to experience the death of one spouse earlier in their adult years. Longer lives (together with lower birth rates) also mean that people spend a smaller portion of their lives parenting young children. More parents live long enough to be part of their grandchildren's and even great-grandchildren's lives (Seltzer & Bianchi, 2013). Many adults are faced with the demands of caring for extremely elderly parents about the time they reach retirement age and begin to experience health limitations of older age themselves.

Immigration and Ethnic Diversity

In 1965, the U.S. Congress amended the Immigration and Naturalization Act to create a fundamental change in the nation's policy on immigration. Visas for legal immigrants were no longer to be based on quotas for each country of origin; instead, preference would be given to immigrants joining family members in the United States. The legislation also removed limitations on immigration from Latin America and Asia. The numbers of legal immigrants to the United States increased to an average of 900,000 persons per year in the 1990s and to 1 million in 2014. Immigration has likewise increased in Canada from about 140,000 in 1980 to 260,404 in 2014. In 2014, 63.5% of legal immigrants were admitted to the United States because family members already living there petitioned the government to grant them entry (Mossaad, 2016). For Canada, the corresponding figure is 26% (Citizenship and Immigration Canada, 2014a). Immigrant visas were also granted for economic reasons, usually after employers petitioned the government for admission of persons with special skills or for humanitarian reasons, including asylum granted to refugees because of well-founded fear of persecution in their home countries. In the United States and Canada, immigration laws provide refugees with resettlement assistance including temporary health care services. The goal of these programs is to promote and improve the health of refugees, as well as to control the potential spread of any contagious diseases brought into the country by these immigrants. The benefits of these health programs are restricted to the prevention and treatment of disease that poses a risk to the public health and safety (Citizenship and Immigration Canada, 2014b; U.S. Centers for Disease Control and Prevention, 2012).

In addition to legal immigrants, an estimated 11.4 million undocumented immigrants lived in the United States in 2012, either because they entered without detection or because they stayed longer than allowed by a temporary visa (Baker & Rytina, 2013). In 2013, the U.S. Census Bureau estimated that there were 40 million U.S. residents born outside the country, nearly 13% of the total population (U.S. Census Bureau, 2013b). Because immigrants tend to arrive in the United States early in their working careers, they are younger, on average, than the overall U.S. population and account for a larger share of young families. In 2010, for example, 20% of all births in the United States were to mothers born outside the country (U.S. Census Bureau, 2010). Undocumented immigrants are ineligible for any type of federal public benefits including welfare, Social Security, and health services such as Medicaid and Medicare (U.S. Department of Health and Human Services, 2009). Importantly, undocumented immigrants are less likely to seek care for themselves or for their children, even when their children are citizens, for fear of detection and deportation (Glick, 2010).

Estimates based on U.S. American Community Survey data reveal that 60 million people older than age 5 speak a language other than English at home, the most common being Spanish (37 million) and Chinese (2.9 million) (U.S. Census Bureau, 2015b). In the United States, half of adults 18 to 40 years old who speak Spanish at home reported that they could not speak English well (Shin & Kominski, 2010). Keep in mind, however, that the overwhelming majority of those who do not speak English well are recent immigrants. Around 81% of the native born who speak Spanish at home report that they can speak English well (Ryan, 2013). In Canada, although English and French are still dominant, more than 200 languages are now spoken in the country. In 2011, 6.6 million people, representing nearly 20% of the Canadian population, reported speaking a language other than English or French at home. Of them, a third, or 2.1 million, reported speaking *only* a language other than English or French at home, primarily Asian languages. The 10 most common foreign languages spoken in 2011 in Canada were Punjabi, Chinese (not specified), Cantonese, Spanish, Tagalog, Arabic, Mandarin, Italian, Urdu, and German (Statistics Canada, 2012b).

The majority of foreign-born U.S. residents live in states that are the traditional "gateways" for immigration: California, New York, Florida, Texas, and Illinois. In recent decades, however, significant increases have occurred in the immigrant populations of most parts of the country, including the rural South and the Upper Midwest, which had seen few immigrants for most of the 20th century (Migration Policy Institute, 2017).

Implications for Health Care Providers

The aging and the growing diversity of the American and Canadian populations, combined with shifts in the economy and changing norms, values, and laws, have altered the context for the nursing care of families. As the population ages, the demand will increase for nurses who specialize in caring for older adults, and even those who do not choose a geriatric specialty will find that older people constitute an increasing portion of the patient population. Improvements in health and physical functioning among those aged 60 to 70 reduce the need for care among this group. Yet rates of population growth are greatest for those aged 80 and older, implying an increased demand for care among the "oldest old" who are likely to suffer from poorer health and require substantial care. Because women continue to outlive men, on average, nurses are more likely to be dealing with the health care needs of older women than of men. Extended lives and delayed childbearing have increased the chances that middle-aged adults will experience the double whammy of having to provide care and financial support for their children and their parents. Families in these situations can face considerable time and money pressures.

At the same time that changing gender roles point to more men in families taking on caregiving duties, more women are in the labor force and unavailable to care for family members and it is doubtful that the increase in men's time in caregiving will fully compensate for the decrease in women's time. Individuals and families are increasingly turning to extended kin and informal care providers to meet their caregiving needs. Societal changes also influence individuals' life-course trajectories. All these changes in individual lives and family relationships are transforming North American households and families and, in turn, changing the context in which health needs are defined and both formal and informal health care and caregiving are provided. Nurses are more likely to encounter fathers seeking health care for their children and individuals whose health needs are met by extended kin or untrained caretakers, especially among the fragile and older populations.

Increased immigration throughout both the United States and Canada has meant that patient populations in many regions are more linguistically, racially, and ethnically diverse than in the past. Working with a diverse pool of immigrant and refugee populations, health care providers may encounter health conditions and diseases unusual in North America. Nurses in North America work with families whose cultural backgrounds, perceptions of sickness, and expectations of healers may be different from those with which they are familiar. Everyone providing health care can expect to face both the challenges and the professional rewards of adapting to a diverse patient population.

LIVING ARRANGEMENTS

The demographic changes for individuals discussed earlier in this chapter are reflected in changes in living arrangements, which have become more diverse over time. For most statistical purposes, a family is defined as two or more people living together who are related by blood, marriage, or adoption (Casper & Bianchi, 2002). Most households (defined by the U.S. Census Bureau as one or more people who occupy a house, apartment, or other residential unit, as opposed to "group quarters" such as nursing homes or student dormitories) are maintained by families. Demographic trends, including late marriage, divorce, and single parenting, have resulted in a decrease in the "family share" of U.S. and Canadian households. In 1960, in the United States, 85% of households were family households; by 2015, just 66% were family households (U.S. Census Bureau, 2015f). Married-couple family households with children under 18 constituted 44% of all households in 1960, but only 29% of all households in 2015 (U.S. Census Bureau, 2015d). Nonfamily households, which consist primarily of people who live alone or who share a residence with roommates or with a partner, have been on the rise. The fastest growth was among persons living alone, although much of this growth occurred during the 1960s and 1970s. The proportion of households with just one person more than doubled from 13% to 27% between 1960 and 2012 (Vespa, Lewis, & Kreider, 2013). Thus, fewer Americans live with family members who can help care for them when they are ill or injured.

In Canada, in 1981, two-thirds of households were single-family households maintained by married or cohabiting couples, but by 2011 the percentage declined to 56% (Statistics Canada, 2011b). As in the United States, the percentage of households that contained two parents with children declined from 36% in 1981 to 22% in 2014. The proportion of Canadian households that contained one person grew from 20% in 1981 to 28% in 2011. Single-person households are the fastest growing type of household and projections indicate this trend will continue well into the 21st century (Canadian Housing Observer, 2013). With the diversity of family forms that have emerged, nurses are increasingly likely to encounter patients who are living alone and have no one to help them in the home should they become seriously ill. Nurses will come into contact with more single-mother families who are more likely than other types of families to be time poor and cash strapped. In fact, most families with children today do not conform to the traditional notion of a breadwinner/homemaker family.

Living Arrangements of Older Adults

Improvements in the health and financial status of older Americans helped generate a revolution in lifestyles and living arrangements among older persons. Older North Americans now are more likely to spend their later years with their spouse or live alone, rather than with adult children as in the past. The options and choices differ between older women and older men, however, in large part because women live longer than men, yet have fewer financial resources.

At the beginning of the 20th century, more than 70% of Americans aged 65 or older resided with kin (Ruggles, 1994). In part because of increased incomes of older adults but also because of declining numbers of children and increased divorce rates, the proportion of older adults living alone has increased dramatically. Just 15% of widows aged 65 or older lived alone in 1900, whereas 66% lived alone in 2011 (Ruggles, 1996; U.S. Census Bureau, 2011a). In 2015, 43% of the population aged 65 and older lived alone (U.S. Census Bureau, 2015q).

A woman is likely to spend more years living alone after a spouse dies than will a man because life expectancy is about 3 years longer for an older woman than for an older man, and because women usually marry men older than themselves. Therefore, older American women are nearly twice as likely as men to be living alone (36% vs. 19%) (West, Cole, Goodkind, & He, 2014). This pattern is similar in Canada; for example, in 2011 among Canadians aged 65 and older, 32% of women lived alone compared with only 16% of men (Statistics Canada, 2011a). Just under half of all American women aged 75 and older live by themselves (U.S. Census Bureau, 2011a). Living alone can mean delays in getting attention for illness or injury and can complicate arrangements for informal care or transportation to formal care when needed.

Older American women are also more than twice as likely as men to be living with someone other than their spouse (16% vs. 7%), in part because they tend to live longer and reach advanced ages when they are most likely to need the physical care and the financial help others can provide (authors' calculations from U.S. Census Bureau, 2015g, 2015h). In the United States, 43% of adults older than 65 will reside in assisted living facilities at some point in their lives. In Canada, a larger proportion of women (33%) than men (22%) aged 85 and older lived in institutional settings in 2011 (Statistics Canada, 2011a). Older men who need help with activities of daily living (ADLs) such as eating, bathing, or getting around generally receive informal care from their wives, whereas older women with disabilities are more likely to rely on assistance from grown children, to live with other family members, or to enter a nursing home (Silverstein, Gans, & Yang, 2006).

To explain trends in living arrangements among older persons, researchers have focused on a variety of constraints and preferences that shape people's living arrangement decisions (Bianchi, Hotz, McGarry, & Seltzer, 2008; Casper & Bianchi, 2002). The number and sex of children generally affect the likelihood that an older person will live with relatives. The greater the number of children, the greater the chances that there will be a son or daughter who can take care of an older parent. Daughters are more likely than sons to provide housing and care for an older parent, presumably as an extension of the traditional female caretaker role and stronger norms of filial responsibility. Geographical distance from children is also a key factor; having children who live nearby promotes coresidence when living independently is no longer feasible for the older person (Haxton & Harknett, 2009; Silverstein et al., 2006).

Older Americans with higher income and better health are more likely to live independently (Klinenberg, 2012). In the United States, since 1940, the growth in Social Security benefits accounts for a proportion of the increase in independent living among older persons, though the exact amount is disputed (Ruggles, 2007). However, older Americans in financial need are more likely to live with relatives (Klinenberg, 2012).

Social norms and personal preferences also determine the choice of living arrangements for older persons (Casper & Bianchi, 2002; Seltzer, Lau, & Bianchi, 2012; Silverstein et al., 2006). Many older adults are willing to pay a substantial part of their incomes to maintain their own residence, which suggests strong personal preferences for privacy and independence (Klinenberg, 2012). Social norms involving family obligations and ties may be especially important when examining racial and ethnic differences in the living arrangements of older persons. Immigrants and ethnic minorities are more likely than whites to live with an older relative not only because of their often limited economic circumstances, but also because their cultural norms and values stipulate moral obligations to care for the oldest members of a culture (Seltzer & Bianchi, 2013).

Despite the trend toward independent living among older Americans, many of them are not able to live alone without assistance. Many families who have older kin in frail health provide extraordinary care. The overwhelming majority (at least 90%) of adults older than 65 who need help with daily tasks receive help informally from friends or family (National Alliance for Caregiving [NAC] & AARP Public Policy Institute, 2015). The majority of these informal caregivers are women (60%), most frequently daughters or spouses, and they compose the largest time-shares of informal care (31%), (NAC & AARP Public Policy Institute, 2015).

On average, adult caregivers have been providing care for 4 years, with a quarter doing so for 5 years or longer and spending more than 20 hours a week providing care. Nearly half of all informal caregivers report that there are negative aspects to informal caregiving, including time and resource strains, and the same amount report that they had no choice in taking on the caregiving role (NAC & AARP Public Policy Institute, 2015). Some evidence suggests that people who spent the greatest number of hours in informal caregiving and those who felt they had no choice in providing care report experiencing lower levels of emotional and physical health (NAC & AARP Public Policy Institute, 2015). Research has shown that even relatively low-cost interventions, such as support groups and telephone counseling, to assist informal caregivers can greatly reduce the harmful effects of such stress on caregivers' health (Belle & REACH II Investigators, 2006).

Living Arrangements of Young Adults

The young-adult years (ages 18 to 30) have been described as "demographically dense" because these years involve many interrelated life-altering transitions (Rindfuss, 1991). Between these ages, young people usually finish their formal schooling, leave home, develop careers, marry, and begin families, but these events do not always occur in this order. Delayed marriage extends the period during which young adults can experiment with alternative living arrangements before they adopt family roles. Young adults may experience any number of independent living arrangements before they marry as they change jobs, pursue education, and move into and out of intimate relationships. They may also return to their parents' homes for periods of time, if money becomes tight or at the end of a relationship.

In 1890, half of American women had married by age 22, and half of American men had married by age 26. The ages of entry into marriage dipped to an all-time low during the post–World War II baby-boom years, when the median age at first marriage reached 20 years for women and 23 years for men in 1956. Age at first marriage then began to increase and reached 27 years for women and 29 years for men by 2015 (U.S. Census Bureau, 2015c). In Canada, the average age at marriage increased from 25 years in 1972 to 31 years in 2008 for men and from 23 years to 30 years for women in 2008 (Statistics Canada, 2015b). In 1960, it was unusual for a woman to reach age 25 without marrying; only 10% of women aged 25 to 29 had never married (Casper & Bianchi, 2002). In 2015, 54% of women aged 25 to 29 in the United States and 67% of men in the same age group had never been married (U.S. Census Bureau, 2015j).

This delay in marriage has shifted the family and living arrangement behaviors in young adulthood in three important ways. First, later marriage coincides with a greater diversity and fluidity in living arrangements in young adulthood. Second, delaying marriage has accompanied an increased likelihood of entering a cohabitating union before marriage. Third, the trend to later marriage affects childbearing; it tends to delay entry into parenthood and, at the same time, increases the chances that a birth (sometimes planned but more often unintended) occurs before marriage (Cherlin, 2010).

Many demographic, social, and economic factors influence young adults' decisions about where and with whom to live (Casper & Bianchi, 2002; Cherlin, 2010). Family and work transitions are influenced greatly by fluctuations in the economy, as well as by changing ideas about appropriate family life and roles for men and women. Since the 1980s, the transition to adulthood has been hampered by

recurring recessions, tight job markets, slow wage growth, and soaring housing costs, in addition to the confusion over roles and behavior sparked by the gender revolution. Even though young adults today may prefer to live independently, they may not be able to afford to do so (Rosenfeld, 2007). Many entry-level jobs today offer low wages, yet housing costs have soared, putting independent living out of reach for many young adults. Higher education, increasingly necessary in today's labor market, is expensive, and living at home may be a way for families to curb higher education expenses. In Canada, the average student debt accrued by college/university students who report education debt is more than $25,000 (Hart Research Associates, 2015) and in the United States it is more than $30,000 (Board of Governors of the Federal Reserve System, 2016). These debts delay life course events such as marriage, home buying, and having children. Even when young adults attend school away from home, they still frequently depend on their parents for financial help and may return home after graduation if they cannot find a suitable job.

The percentage of young men living in their parents' homes was 59% in 2011, about the same as in 1970, whereas the percentage increased for young women from 39% to 50% (U.S. Census Bureau, 2011d). In Canada, the proportion of young adults 20 to 29 years old who resided with their parents increased dramatically from 27% in 1981 to 42% in 2006 (Statistics Canada, 2016f).

Young adults who leave home to attend school, join the military, or take a job have always had, and continue to have, high rates of "returning to the nest" and have become known as "boomerang children." Those who leave home to get married have had the lowest likelihood of returning home, although returns to the nest have increased over time even in this group.

American parents often take in their children after they return from the military or school, or when they are between jobs. In the past, however, many American parents apparently were reluctant to take children in if they had left home simply to gain "independence." This is not true today. Before the 1970s, leaving home for simple independence was probably the result of friction within the family, whereas today leaving and returning home seems to be a common part of a successful transition to adulthood (Klinenberg, 2012; Rosenfeld, 2007). In the past, a young adult may have been reluctant to move back in with parents because a return home implied failure; fewer stigmas are attached to returning home these days (Casper & Bianchi, 2002). In fact, by age 27 nearly half of all young millennials (born 1980 to 1984) returned to their parental home at some point after moving out, making this a common phenomenon (U.S. Department of Labor, 2014).

Changing demographic behaviors among young adults and their living arrangements have implications for family health care nursing. In contrast to the situation in Canada, in the United States, young adults often lack health insurance and, in many cases, are not financially independent, reducing the likelihood that they will receive routine checkups or seek medical care when the need arises (Twietmeyer, Brindis, Adams, & Park, 2016). Though insurance coverage among this age group has increased under the Affordable Care Act (ACA), around 15% of those aged 20 to 30 years remained uninsured in 2015 (Barnett & Vornovitsky, 2016). The increasing numbers of people seeking care in emergency rooms and urgent care settings put additional pressure on the health care providers, especially nurses. Also, the acuity level of the medical problems in these young adults is greater because they did not seek earlier treatment.

Unmarried Opposite-Sex Couples

One of the most significant household changes in the second half of the 20th century in North America was the increase in men and women living together without marrying. The increase of cohabitation outside marriage appeared to counterbalance some of the delay of marriage among young adults and the overall increase in divorce. Unmarried-couple households made up fewer than 1% of U.S. households in 1960 and 1970 (Casper & Cohen, 2000). Heterosexual partner families increased to just more than 2% by 1980, and to nearly 6.7% by 2011, representing 8.3 million family groups (U.S. Census Bureau, 2015j). Unmarried-couple households also are increasingly likely to include children. In 1978, 24% of unmarried-couple households included children younger than age 15; by 2015, 39% of unmarried-partner family groups included children. Although the percentage of U.S. households consisting of an unmarried couple is small, many Americans have lived with a partner outside marriage at some point (U.S. Census Bureau, 2015n). A recent study shows that by age 30, 74% of women had cohabited

(Copen, Daniels, & Mosher, 2013). Nearly 62% of the couples who married between 1997 and 2002 had lived together before marriage, up from 49% in 1985 to 1986, and a big jump from just 8% of first marriages in the late 1960s (Bumpass & Lu, 2000; Kennedy & Bumpass, 2008).

In Canada, cohabiting couples are known as common-law couples. The 2001 Canadian Census showed that increasing proportions of families were headed by common-law couples, from 5.6% in 1981 to 13.8% in 2001. By 2011 this figure increased to 17% (Statistics Canada, 2012d). As in the United States, more Canadian children are living with common-law (cohabitating) parents. Nearly 44% of common-law couples in 2011 had children under age 24 residing with them. In 2011, about 910,700 children aged 0 to 14 (16.3% of the total) lived with common-law parents, up from 12.8% in 2001 (Statistics Canada, 2012d). In both countries, the pace of the increase in cohabitation has slowed somewhat since the rapid rise in the 1970s and 1980s.

Why has cohabitation increased so much? Researchers have offered several explanations, including increased uncertainty about the stability of marriage, the erosion of the stigma associated with cohabitation and sexual relations outside of marriage, the wider availability of reliable birth control, economic changes, and increased individualism and secularization (Bianchi et al., 2012; Cherlin, 2009). Youths reaching adulthood in the past two decades are much more likely to have witnessed their parents' divorce than any generation before them. Some have argued that cohabitation allows a couple to experience the benefits of an intimate relationship without committing to marriage. If a cohabiting relationship is not successful, one can simply move out; if a marriage is not successful, one suffers through a sometimes lengthy and difficult divorce.

Nevertheless, most adults in the United States eventually do marry. In 2015, 89% of women aged 50 to 54 had been married at least once (U.S. Census Bureau, 2015j). Considerable differences exist by race/ethnicity; for example, recent figures for women born between 1957 and 1964 show that only 68% of African American women compared with 90% of white women married by the time they were 46 in 2011 (U.S. Department of Labor, 2013). The meaning and permanence of marriage may be changing, however. Marriage used to be the primary demographic event that marked the formation of new households, the beginning of sexual relations, and the birth of a child. Marriage also implied that an individual had one sexual partner, and it theoretically identified the two individuals who would parent any child born of the union. The increasing social acceptance of cohabitation outside marriage has meant that these linkages can no longer be assumed. Couples began to set up households that might include the couple's children, as well as children from previous marriages or other relationships (Casper & Bianchi, 2002). Similarly, what it meant to be single was no longer always clear, as the personal lives of unmarried couples began to resemble those of their married counterparts.

Cohabiting households can pose unique challenges for health care providers, especially in the United States. Because cohabiting relationships are not legally sanctioned in most states, partners may not have the right to make health care decisions on behalf of each other or of the other's children (Casper & Haaga, 2005). Cohabiting couples report poorer health and have lower incomes than do married couples, on average (Hardie & Lucas, 2010). Thus, although they are more likely to need health care services, they may be less likely to have the financial ability to secure them.

Same-Sex Couples

The number of same-sex couples has increased substantially in North America during the past couple of decades. A conservative estimate shows that the number of same-sex couples in the United States doubled from 358,390 in 2000 to 783,100 in 2014 (U.S. Census Bureau, 2014e). In Canada, the number of same-sex couples increased by 42.4% from 45,345 in 2006 to 64,575 in 2011, of which nearly a third were married couples (Statistics Canada, 2012d). The vast majority of same-sex couples live in common-law or cohabiting relationships. Before 2000, same-sex marriage was not legally recognized. In 2005, however, after the Netherlands, Belgium and Canada both legalized same-sex marriage in 2005. Following legalization, the number of same-sex married couples in Canada almost tripled from 7465 in 2006 to 21,015 in 2011 (Statistics Canada, 2012d). In the United States, the first state to allow same-sex marriage was Massachusetts in 2003, and in 2015 same-sex marriage became legal across the nation. Though same-sex marriage was not legal in all states in 2014, 43% of all same-sex households were marriages (U.S. Census Bureau, 2014e). With

the federal legalization of same-sex marriage this proportion has undoubtedly increased.

Although the division of labor for parenting and household chores in same-sex families tends to be more egalitarian than among opposite-sex couples, same-sex couples are not as "genderless" as has been previously suggested. This equality often changes as couples transition to parenthood, when one of the partners usually becomes more involved in child rearing, assumes more responsibility for housework, and often becomes the partner in charge of caring for the health of the children and seeking health services for them (Matos, 2015).

PARENTING

Even with the increase in divorce and cohabitation, postponement of marriage, and decline in childbearing, most North American adults have children, and most children live with two parents. In 2015, in the United States, 64% of families with children were two-parent, married families and an additional 5% were two-parent, unmarried families (U.S. Census Bureau, 2015a). In Canada, in 2011, the level was comparable: 62% of Canadian families with children were married two-parent families, 14% were two-parent common-law families, and 24% were lone-parent (single-parent) families (authors' calculations from Statistics Canada, 2011b). In 2015, 26% of American families were mother-only families and only 5% were father-only families. "Lone-parent families" in Canada increased from 9% of all families (including those with no children) in 1971 to about 16% in 2011, including 13% lone mothers and 3% lone fathers. The changes in marriage, cohabitation, and nonmarital childbearing during the past few decades have had a profound effect on North American families with children and are changing our images of parenthood.

This section discusses individuals' and couples' transitions into parenthood, beginning with current trends in fertility, the increased use of ARTs to achieve parenthood, and trends and patterns in adoption. As individuals become parents, different types of family forms emerge. The section explores single motherhood, fathering, and child rearing within cohabitation and same-sex couple families. The section concludes with a discussion of the important role grandparents are playing in rearing and caring for grandchildren.

Fertility

In the United States and Canada, fertility has exhibited a trend of long-term decline for more than a century, interrupted by the baby-boom period and other small fluctuations. In recent decades, fertility rates in most developed countries have fallen below the level required to replace the population. Replacement-level fertility refers to the required number of children each woman in the population would have to bear on average to replace herself and her partner, and it is conventionally set at 2.1 children per woman for countries with low mortality rates. This threshold is set slightly above 2 in order to account for a negligible rate of childhood mortality and a small proportion of individuals who do not survive to their reproductive age (Poston & Bouvier, 2010).

The U.S. fertility decline has not been very drastic; thus, the United States is an atypical case among developed countries. Figure 3-1 shows the trends in fertility rates since the 1930s for the United States and Canada, respectively. As this graph shows, both countries experienced a post-WWII baby boom during the 1950s and 1960s, after which fertility began to decline again. Since the 1980s, the United States has exhibited fertility rates close to replacement level. In 2014, according to vital statistics data, the total U.S. fertility rate was 1.86 children per woman (Hamilton et al., 2015). In Canada, however, the fertility decline has been of greater magnitude; in 2013, the fertility rate was 1.59 (Statistics Canada, 2016a). Persistent levels of below replacement level fertility have raised concerns regarding population shrinkage. Fewer births also imply a subsequent contraction of the working-age population that, coupled with increases in life expectancy, reduces the tax base that supports health care and retirement benefits for the aging population (Reznik, Shoffner, & Weaver, 2007). In the United States and Canada, a significant proportion of population growth during recent decades has come from immigration.

Fertility varies by demographic characteristics. In the United States, except for Asians, immigrants tend to exhibit higher fertility rates than the native-born population. In 2014, native-born women aged 45 to 50 had given birth to 1.9 children on average; the comparable figure for foreign-born women was 2.2 children (U.S. Census Bureau, 2014b). Fertility also varies by race and ethnicity. In 2014 in the United States, the total fertility rate was the highest among Hispanic women (2.13), followed by African Americans and whites (1.87), and the lowest rate was observed among Asian women (1.71) (Hamilton et al., 2015). The differences are greater by educational level. U.S. Census Bureau data indicate that women aged 45 to 50 with less than a high school education had on average 2.62 births, whereas women with a graduate or professional degree had only 1.64 births (U.S. Census Bureau, 2014b).

The causes behind the secular trends in fertility decline can be grouped into socioeconomic, ideological, and institutional factors. Among socioeconomic factors are the increase in women's opportunity costs and the rising cost of rearing children. The

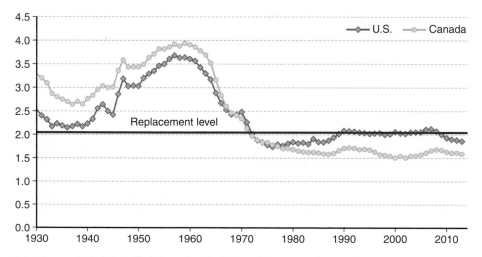

FIGURE 3-1 Total Fertility Rate for the United States and Canada: 1930–2013 *(Data from Statistics Canada, 2011c, 2016a; World Bank, 2016.)*

socioeconomic position of women has drastically changed since the 1960s. Economic changes have also made it more difficult to maintain a family on the income of a single earner. Women's education and labor force participation increased considerably during this period. In addition, changes in laws and civil rights have reduced discriminatory practices against women. All these changes have resulted in increases in women's wages, although they have not yet reached parity with men's. As women's incomes and career opportunities have improved, women's opportunity costs of not participating in the labor market have increased, thus reducing women's fertility intentions. At the same time, higher educational expectations for children and rising living standards have substantially increased the costs of raising children (Lino, Kuczynski, Rodriguez, & Schap, 2017).

Cultural and ideological changes, such as the growth in individualism and the desire for self-realization, have decreased the appeal of long-term commitments, including childbearing (Bianchi et al., 2012; Cherlin, 2009). The accentuation of individual autonomy and the rise of feminism have increased the desirability for more symmetrical gender roles. However, institutions dealing with family life still exhibit high levels of gender inequality. Equal opportunities for women in education and employment are often curtailed within families as women continue to pay a penalty for having children in the form of reduced career involvement and income prospects. This asymmetry accentuates the incompatibility of childbearing and labor force participation (Correll, Benard, & Paik, 2007).

In addition, in the 1960s more effective birth control methods became available, providing couples with better means to control their fertility. Moreover, favorable attitudes toward nonmarital sex and cohabitation have also weakened the link between sex, marriage, and childbearing (Casper & Bianchi, 2002; Lesthaeghe, 2014). Thus, most developed countries have experienced a considerable rise in nonmarital births to single and cohabiting mothers. In 2010, 41% of all births in the United States were to unmarried women, of which 58% were to cohabiting women (Martin et al., 2012). In Canada, births to unmarried women have also increased, representing 28.9% of all births in 2013 (Statistics Canada, 2016d).

The birth rate for teenagers has decreased substantially in both countries, although in the United States this rate is more than twice that observed in Canada. In Canada in 2013, only 3% of all births were to women ages 15 to 19, compared with 6.3% in the United States in 2014 (Statistics Canada, 2016c). The birth rate for teenagers in Canada was 12.6 births per 1000 women in 2011, down from 26.1 in 1981 (Milan, 2011; Statistics Canada, 2015a). The U.S. teenage birth rate for women ages 15 to 19 was 24.2 births per 1000 women in 2014, down from 52.2 in 1981 (Hamilton et al., 2015). The United States still exhibits one of the highest rates of teenage pregnancy in the industrialized world.

Nonetheless, women increasingly have been delaying childbearing since the 1960s; thus, the average age at first birth has risen in both countries. In 2014, the average age at first birth in the United States was 26.3 (Hamilton et al., 2015). In 2008, in Canada, the average age at first birth was 28.5, up from 23.5 in the mid-1960s (Milan, 2013). However, the onset of fertility varies by race/ethnicity in the United States. Whereas the average age at first birth for African American and Hispanic women was slightly above 24 years in 2014, for white women it was 27. Asian and Pacific Islanders exhibited the highest average age at first birth at 29.5 (Hamilton et al., 2015). Thus, childbearing for middle-class whites and Asians is increasingly becoming concentrated in the late twenties and early thirties.

Overall, these trends imply not only that women are having fewer children, but also that they are increasingly having children at older ages. Nurses are more likely to encounter more educated and mature mothers and pregnant women. However, as women wait longer to have their first child, complications in pregnancies and deliveries will become more common. Moreover, age-related infertility will be more likely to affect these women, increasing the rate of involuntary infertility. As delays in fertility continue, a larger pool of women approaching the end of their reproductive years will seek the services of ARTs.

Assisted Reproductive Technologies

Although various definitions have been used for ARTs, the current definition used by the U.S. Centers for Disease Control and Prevention (CDC) is based on the 1992 Fertility Clinic Success Rate and Certification Act. According to this definition, ARTs include all fertility treatments in which both eggs and sperm are handled. In general, ART procedures involve surgically removing eggs from a woman's ovaries, combining them with sperm in the laboratory, and returning them to the woman's body or donating them to another woman. According to this definition, treatments in which only sperm are handled are not included (i.e., intrauterine—or artificial—insemination), nor are procedures in which a woman takes medications only to stimulate egg production without the intention of having eggs retrieved (U.S. Centers for Disease Control and Prevention, 2014).

ARTs have been used in the United States since 1981 to help women become pregnant, most commonly through the transfer of fertilized human eggs into a woman's uterus (in vitro fertilization [IVF]). Deciding whether to undergo this expensive and time-consuming treatment can be difficult. Worldwide, it is estimated that between 1% to 3% of women face challenges conceiving their first child (primary infertility) and approximately 9% to 13% have difficulties conceiving children after having at least one live birth (secondary infertility) (Mascarenhas, Flaxman, Boerma, Vanderpoel, & Stevens, 2012). In the United States, approximately 6% of married couples reported at least 12 months of unprotected intercourse without conception, whereas slightly more than 2% of women reported having visited an infertility-related clinic within the past year (Chandra, Copen, & Stephen, 2013, 2014). In Canada, the estimated percentage of couples experiencing infertility in 2010 ranged from 11.5% to 15.7%, depending on the definition of infertility used. Infertility treatment costs sum up to significantly more than $3 billion annually in the United States (Myers et al., 2008). As women wait longer to have their first child, the likelihood of age-related infertility increases. Although there is some controversy about whether the proportion of the population with self-reported infertility is increasing, stable, or decreasing, there has been a clear increase in the use of ARTs (Stephen & Chandra, 2006; Sunderam et al., 2012).

The number of IVF cycles performed in the United States increased from approximately 30,000 in 1996 (Myers et al., 2008) to 208,604 in 2014, resulting in 57,323 live births (deliveries of one or more living infants) and 70,354 infants (U.S. Centers for Disease Control and Prevention, 2014). During this time, the proportion of deliveries in the United States resulting from ARTs has increased from 0.37% in 1996 to 1.4% in 2014. Because of the frequency of multiple births, in 2014 ARTs accounted for 1.7%

of U.S. births despite accounting for only 1.4% of deliveries (U.S. Department of Health and Human Services, 2016b). In Canada 6988 babies were born through ARTs in 2012 (Gunby, 2014). ARTs often result in multiple births, such as twins, triplets, and so on, which increase health risks for children and mothers. In the United States, nearly 27% of all ART births resulted in multiple births in 2012 (Kissim et al., 2015). In Canada, multiple births have decreased from 32% to 18.4% as of 2012 because of the Assisted Human Reproduction Canada (AHRC) agency's goal to reduce the rate of multiple births resulting from ARTs owing to the high costs and increased health risks (AHRC, 2011; Gunby, 2014).

A growing number of same-sex couples seeking to become parents are also turning to ARTs to achieve this goal: in the case of lesbians, usually through the use of a sperm donor and artificial insemination; and in the case of gay men, through the use of an egg donor and/or a surrogate. It is worth noting that male same-sex couples face greater challenges than female same-sex couples to become parents, not only because fertility centers are less likely to accept male gay patients, but also because the procedure is more expensive as it involves obtaining both an oocyte donor and a gestational surrogate, that is, a woman who will carry the zygote and take the pregnancy to term (Greenfeld, 2007).

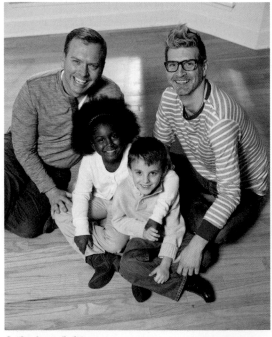

© iStock.com/kali9

Based on the available literature, there are no differences in parenting skills when comparing singleton pregnancies resulting from ART to spontaneous conceptions (Myers et al., 2008). In fact, mothers of infants resulting from ART appear to have better outcomes. Some of the differences found in these studies may well be caused by systematic variations in the ages of mothers in the two groups; mothers who conceived using ARTs are older on average. By contrast, there is some evidence that fathers may do worse on some scales. The multiple gestations and preterm births that frequently result with ART significantly increase stress and depressive symptoms, especially for mothers of infants with chronic disabilities.

Births resulting from ART are more likely to involve multiple births, pregnancy complications, preterm delivery, and low birth weight, which may all pose substantial risks to the health of mothers and infants. Additionally, children born because of ART experience relatively worse neurodevelopmental outcomes, higher rates of hospitalization, and more surgeries than other children. There is little evidence, however, that the relatively worse outcomes for ART babies are a direct result of infertility treatments; infertility treatments are more likely to be used by couples with a history of subfertility—difficulty achieving and sustaining pregnancy without medical assistance—and worse outcomes typically result for the children of these couples, irrespective of whether they have received infertility treatments (Myers et al., 2008).

In sum, family nurses will likely encounter a growing number of opposite-sex couples seeking infertility treatment, as well as same-sex couples who wish to become parents. This process is time consuming, expensive, and stressful for all the parties involved. Unsuccessful attempts to become pregnant are likely to be met with sorrow, anger, and regret. Nurses should be aware of the delicate circumstances surrounding this type of care. They should also be aware of the heightened risk of multiple births, potential birth defects, and increased women's health risks.

Adoption

Accurate trends on adoption in the United States are difficult to obtain, but U.S. Census Bureau data indicate that the number of adopted children increased in the 1990s from about 1.6 million in

1991 to 2.1 million in 2004 and then decreased to 1.5 million in 2010 (Kreider & Ellis, 2011; Kreider & Lofquist, 2014). Other data show that in 2007 there were approximately 1.7 million adopted children under the age of 18 living in the United States (Vandivere, Malm, & Radel, 2009). Box 3-2 illustrates the three primary forms of adoption in the United States: foster care adoption, private domestic adoption, and international adoption.

According to the U.S. Administration for Children and Families, the number of adoptions from foster care has ranged from 50,600 to 57,200 annually between 2005 and 2014, with some fluctuations and no clear trend (U.S. Department of Health and Human Services, 2014). By 2007, 661,000 children had been adopted from foster care, representing 37% of all adopted children. Of foster care–adopted children, 23% were adopted by relatives, 40% were adopted by someone who knew them before the adoption (including relatives), and 69% were adopted by someone who was previously their foster parent (Vandivere et al., 2009). Because these children were removed from their homes because of abuse or neglect, they were more likely than other children, and even than those adopted through different means, to have special health care needs—in 2007, 54% had special needs.

Similarly, by 2007, about 677,000, or 38% of, adopted children had been adopted privately from sources other than foster care. Of these, 41% were adopted by relatives and 44% were adopted by someone who knew them before the adoption (including relatives). Almost one-third of these children have special health care needs. The majority of children adopted privately in the United States were placed with their adoptive family as newborns or when they were younger than 1 month old (62%).

International adoptions increased from about 15,700 in 1999 to about 23,000 children in 2004. Since 2004, they have been decreasing steadily to 5648 in 2015 because of stricter laws and regulations (U.S. Department of State, 2015). Internationally adopted children make up the smallest group, numbering about 444,000, or 25% of all adopted children. Of these adopted children, 29% have special health care needs. More than 6 in 10 internationally adopted children in 2015 came from just five countries—China (42%), Ethiopia (6%), South Korea (6%), Ukraine (5%), and Uganda (4%). In Canada, international adoptions also have decreased slightly from an average of 2000 adoptions per year during the 1990s

BOX 3-2

Three Primary Forms of Adoption in the United States

Foster Care Adoption

Children adopted from foster care are those who were removed from their families because of their families' inability or unwillingness to provide appropriate care and were placed under the protection of the state by the child protective services system. Public child welfare agencies oversee such adoptions, although they sometimes contract with private adoption agencies to perform some adoption functions.

Private Domestic Adoption

These children were adopted privately from within the United States and were not part of the foster care system at any time before their adoption. Such adoptions may be arranged independently or through private adoption agencies.

International Adoption

This group includes children who originated from countries other than the United States.

■ Typically, adoptive parents work with private U.S. adoption agencies, which coordinate with adoption agencies and other entities in children's countries of origin.
■ Changes in international adoption laws have made it more difficult to adopt children from abroad.
■ Starting in 2008, the Hague Convention on Protection of Children and Co-operation in Respect of Intercountry Adoption has been regulating adoptions from several countries. Its purpose is to protect children and to

ensure that placements made are in the best interests of children.
■ For adoptions from countries not part of the Hague Convention, U.S. law dictates that children have to be orphans in order to immigrate into the United States.
■ The Hague Convention seems to have contributed to the decrease in international adoptions.
  ● For example, in 2007, 24% of all international adoptions of children under age 18 were from Guatemala, but in March 2008, the U.S. Department of State announced that it would not process new Guatemalan adoptions until further notice, because of concerns about the country's ability to adhere to the guidelines of the Hague Convention.
  ● Additionally, in 2008, Guatemala stopped accepting any new adoption cases (U.S. Department of State, 2015).
■ Other countries have also implemented stricter regulations for international adoptions.
  ● For example, as of May 2007, China enacted a rigorous policy requiring adoptive parents to be heterosexual married couples between the ages of 30 and 50 with assets of at least $80,000 and in good health (including not being overweight).
  ● In January 2013, Russian federal law banned adoptions of Russian children to U.S. citizens (U.S. Department of State, 2015).
  ● In addition, China and other countries, such as Russia and Korea, are attempting to promote domestic rather than international adoption (Barnes, 2013; Lee, 2007).

and early 2000s; in 2014, 905 children were adopted from abroad. In the same year, 55% of international adoptions to Canada came from China (17%), the United States (14%), the Philippines (8%), Vietnam (6%), South Korea (6%), and India (4%) (Hague Conference on Private International Law, n.d.).

Since 2008, the Hague Convention on Protection of Children and Co-operation in Respect of Inter-country Adoption has been regulating adoptions from approximately 75 countries. The stricter law adopted by the Hague Convention has probably contributed to the decline in international adoption (see Box 3-2). In the past several years, many countries have changed their adoption requirements, thus making it harder to adopt. All these legal changes have reduced the number of international adoptions in the United States and Canada.

Social and demographic changes coupled with changing laws have altered the context of adoption. Recent developments in reproductive medicine, such as intrauterine insemination and IVF, seem to have contributed to the decline in adoption in recent years by reducing the demand for adoption. At the same time, never-married mothers have become less likely to put their infants up for adoption—in 1973, 9% of births were placed for adoption compared with just 1% in the 1990s and 2000s, reducing the supply of infants for domestic adoptions (Jones, 2008).

Researchers found in a study conducted at the U.S. Department of Health and Human Services that, overall, 87% of adopted children have parents who said they would "definitely" make the same decision to adopt their child, knowing everything then that they now know about their child. More than 90%

of adopted children ages 5 and older have parents who perceived their child's adoption experience as "positive" or "mostly positive" (Vandivere et al., 2009).

Further, overall, 40% of the adopted children are in transracial adoptions; either one or both adoptive parents are of a different race, culture, or ethnicity than their child. The majority of adopted children have non-Hispanic white parents but are not themselves non-Hispanic white. Transracial adoptions are most common for children whose families adopted internationally (Vandivere et al., 2009). Overall, about half of adopted children are male (49%)—39% of internationally adopted children are male, whereas around 51% of children adopted from foster care are male (U.S. Department of Health and Human Services, 2016a; U.S. Department of State, 2015; Vandivere et al., 2009). Adopted children are less likely than biological children in the general population to live in households below the poverty line (12% compared with 18%). However, nearly half of children adopted from foster care (46%) live in households with incomes no higher than two times the poverty threshold. More than two-thirds of adopted children (69%) live with two married parents; they are just as likely to do so as children in the general population (Vandivere et al., 2009).

The majority of adoptive children engage in enrichment activities with their families, and in fact they are more likely to have some of these positive experiences than all children in the population (Vandivere et al., 2009). As youngsters, adopted children are more likely than all children to be read to every day (68% compared with 48%), to be sung to or told stories every day (73% compared with 59%), and to participate in extracurricular activities as school-age children (85% compared with 81%). A small percentage of adopted children have parents who report parental aggravation (for example, feeling the child was difficult to care for, or feeling angry with the child). Parental aggravation is more common among parents of adopted children than among all parents (11% compared with 6%).

This socioeconomic and demographic portrait of adopted children has implications for family nursing. First, although most adoptive children fare well with regard to health, educational achievement, and social and cognitive development, those who are adopted through foster care are disproportionately disadvantaged. Second, because most parents of adopted children do not share with them their genetic endowment and because the medical histories of the biological parents are often unknown, diagnosis for these children can be more challenging than for biological children. Third, the substantial proportion of transracial adoptive families requires special attention. For decades, adoptive parents who were of a different race than their child were taught to be color blind regarding their adoptive children and to raise them according to the culture of the parent. More recently, adoption social workers have encouraged adoptive parents to embrace the child's culture of origin and to help their children develop positive racial and ethnic identities. As most of these parents are white, however, they may be unaware of the nuances of the culture the child is coming from and may not have the capacity to teach their children how to deal with bias and discrimination (Barn, 2013). Nurses should be sensitive to these differences and help guide the parents in understanding how to help their children.

Finally, unlike biological families, many adoptive families emerge out of loss for all members—for example, foster parents who are not able to have biological children; biological parents who are relinquishing their children; and adoptive children who are losing or have lost their biological parents. This unique family form requires an adjustment period for all those involved. Separations of adoptive children from biological parents at birth deprive children of the bioregulatory channels that exist between a mother and her baby—from breathing, to respiration, to heart rate and blood pressure. Taking away a baby at birth cuts off this regulation and may cause children to cry more often, become angry or confused, or behave badly simply because they do not understand the separation (Verrier, 1993/2011). Nurses should be aware that unusual behaviors such as these among adoptive children may not stem from illness or health-related causes.

Single Mothers

How many single mothers are there? This turns out to be a more difficult question to answer from official statistics than it would first appear. Over time, it is easiest to calculate the number of single mothers who maintain their own residence. In the United States between 1950 and 2015, the number of such single-mother families increased from 1.3 million to 8.6 million (U.S. Census Bureau, 2015d). These estimates do not include single mothers living in other persons' households but do include single mothers who are cohabitating with a male partner. The most dramatic increase was during the 1970s, when the number of single-mother families was increasing at 8% per year. The average annual rate of increase slowed considerably during the 1980s and was near 0% after 1994 (Casper & Bianchi, 2002). By 2015, single mothers who maintained their own households accounted for 24% of all families with children, up from 6% in 1950 (U.S. Census Bureau, 2015e). Almost 1.3 million more single mothers lived in someone else's household, bringing the total number of single mothers to 9.9 million (U.S. Census Bureau, 2015d). In 2011, in Canada, there were 1.2 million lone mothers and 328,000 lone fathers with children of any age living with them (Statistics Canada, 2012d).

Single mothers with children at home face a multitude of challenges. They usually are the primary breadwinners, disciplinarians, playmates, and caregivers for their children. They must manage the financial and practical aspects of a household and plan for the family's future. Many mothers cope remarkably well, and many benefit from financial support and help from relatives and from their children's fathers.

Women earn less than men, on average, and because single mothers are usually younger and less educated than other women, they are often at the lower end of the income curve. Never-married single mothers are particularly disadvantaged; they are younger, less well educated, and less often employed than are divorced single mothers and married mothers. Single mothers often must curtail their work hours to care for the health and well-being of their children.

Despite the fact that the majority of American single mothers are not poor, they are much more likely to be poor than other parents. Single-parent families are officially defined as poor if they have incomes under the poverty line, which for a single mother with two children translates into an annual income of lower than $19,096 in 2015. Overall, 20% of U.S. children lived in poverty in 2015 (Proctor, Semega, & Kollar, 2016). Children in two-parent families had the lowest rate at 7.5%, followed by children living in father-only families at 22.1%. Children in mother-only families had the highest poverty rate at 36.5% (U.S. Census Bureau, 2016b). Poverty and family structure are highly correlated with race in the United States. White non-Latino families with children experienced poverty rates of 10.5% in

2015, compared with 28.4% for African American, 25% for Latino, and 9.9% for Asian families with children. However, these numbers increase greatly for single-mother households: 34.8% of white non-Latino single-mother households live in poverty, compared with 40% of African American, 42% of Latino, and 24.3% of Asian single-mother families. Of all families with children, white non-Latino married couples experience the lowest poverty rates at 4.4%, with poverty being highest for African American and Latina single mothers.

The family income of children who reside with a never-married single mother is, on average, significantly lower than for all other family forms, including divorced single mothers (McKeever & Wolfinger, 2011). Almost two of every three children who live with a never-married mother are poor. Mothers who never married are much less likely to get child support from the father than are mothers who are divorced or separated. Whereas 46% of divorced mothers with custody of children younger than 21 received some child support from the children's father, fewer than 26% of never-married mothers reported receiving regular support from their child's father (U.S. Census Bureau, 2014a). Children who live with a divorced mother tend to be much better off financially than are children of never-married mothers. Divorced mothers are substantially better educated and more often employed than are mothers who are separated or who never married. Even so, divorce increases inequality and the risk of poverty significantly for mothers (Ananat & Michaels, 2008).

In 2014, 3.4 million Canadians lived in low-income families (Statistics Canada, 2016b) and about 546,000, or 8.8%, of children younger than 18 lived in low-income families (Statistics Canada, 2013). Canadian lone-parent families with children younger than 18 are much more likely to have low incomes, and thus, are more likely to be poor (First Call: BC Child and Youth Advocacy Coalition, 2011). Among children living in female lone-parent families, 187,000, or 23%, were low income, whereas the incidence of low income was 5.9% among children living in two-parent families (Statistics Canada, 2013).

In the United States, single mothers with children in poverty are particularly affected by major welfare reform legislation such as the Personal Responsibility and Work Opportunity Reconciliation Act (PRWORA) (Box 3-3, see DavisPlus). President Clinton claimed in his 1993 State of the Union Address that the 1996 law would "end welfare as we know it," and the changes embodied in PRWORA—time limits on welfare eligibility and mandatory job-training requirements, for example—seemed far-reaching (Casper & Bianchi, 2002; Hays, 2003). Some argued that this legislation would end crucial support for poor mothers and their children; several high-level government officials resigned because of the law. Others heralded PRWORA as the first step toward helping poor women gain control of their lives and making fathers take responsibility for their children. Many states had already begun to experiment with similar reforms. The success of this program is open to dispute because it has been and continues to be such a political issue.

Why have mother-child families increased in number and as a percentage of North American families? Explanations tend to focus on one of two trends. First is women's increased financial independence. More women entered the labor force and women's incomes increased relative to those of men, and welfare benefits for single mothers expanded during the 1960s and 1970s. Women today are less dependent on a man's income to support themselves and their children, and many can afford to live independently rather than stay in an unsatisfactory relationship. Second, the job market for men has tightened, especially for less-educated men. As the North American economy experienced a restructuring in the 1970s and 1980s, the demand for professionals, managers, and other white-collar workers expanded, whereas wages for men in lower-skilled jobs declined in real terms (Casper & Bianchi, 2002). During the past two decades, this pattern has continued because of technological advances and outsourcing displacing manufacturing and other lower-skilled jobs (Bianchi et al., 2012). Men still earn more than women, on average, but the earnings gap narrowed steadily between the 1970s and 2000 as women's earnings increased and men's earnings remained flat or declined. In the past decade, the gender-earnings gap has been relatively constant because both men's and women's average earnings have stagnated. In 2014 in the United States, full-time, year-round female workers earned 82.5 cents for every dollar earned by full-time, year-round male workers (U.S. Department of Labor, 2015).

In the early years of the 20th century, higher mortality rates made it more common for children to live with only one parent (Uhlenberg, 1996). As declining death rates reduced the number of widowed single parents, a counterbalancing increase in

single-parent families occurred because of divorce. For example, at the time of the 1960 U.S. Census, almost one-third of American single mothers living with children younger than 18 were widows (Bianchi, 1995). As divorce rates increased precipitously in the 1960s and 1970s, most single-parent families were created through divorce or separation. Thus, at the end of the 1970s, only 11% of American single mothers were widowed and two-thirds were divorced or separated. In 1978, about one-fifth of single American mothers had never married but had a child and were raising that child on their own (Bianchi & Casper, 2000). By 2015, 49.2% of single mothers had never married (U.S. Census Bureau, 2015m).

The remarkable increase in the number of single-mother households with women who have never married was driven by a dramatic shift to childbearing outside marriage. The number of births to unmarried women grew from fewer than 90,000 per year in 1940 to nearly 1.6 million per year in 2014 (Hamilton et al., 2015). Fewer than 4% of all births in 1940 were to unmarried mothers compared with 40% in 2014. The rate of nonmarital births—the number of births per 1000 unmarried women—increased from 7.1 in 1940 to 43.9 in 2014. The nonmarital birth rate peaked in 1994 at 46.2, leveled out in the latter 1990s, and has increased slightly since the mid-2000s (Bianchi & Casper, 2000; Martin et al., 2012). Births to unmarried women have increased in Canada as well, from 12.8% in 1980 to 29% of all births in 2013 (Statistics Canada, 2016d).

The proportion of births that occur outside marriage is even higher in some European countries than in the United States and Canada. But unmarried parents in European countries and Canada are more likely to be living together with their biological children than are unmarried parents in the United States (Perelli-Harris et al., 2012). In the United States, the tremendous variation in rates of unmarried childbearing among population groups suggests that there may be a constellation of factors that determine whether women have children when they are not married. In 2014, the percentage of births to unmarried mothers was the highest for African Americans at 71%, followed by American Indian (66%), Hispanics (53%), and white non-Hispanics (29%). Asian and Pacific Islanders reported the lowest percentage at 16% (Hamilton et al., 2015, Table 15). Overall, 25% of all family groups with children under 18 are maintained by single mothers. The percentage of mother-only family groups is much higher for African American families (51%) than for Hispanic (28%), white non-Hispanic (18%), and Asian (12%) families (U.S. Census Bureau, 2015e).

Single-mother families present challenges for family health care nurses providing care to this vulnerable group. Single mothers today are younger and less educated than they were a few decades ago. This presents problems because these mothers have less experience with the health care system and are likely to have more difficulty reading directions, filling out forms, communicating effectively with doctors and nurses, and understanding their care instructions. In the United States, these mothers are also more likely to be poor and uninsured, making it less likely they will seek care and more likely they will not be able to pay for it. Consequently, when the need arises, these women are more likely to resort to emergency rooms for noncritical illnesses and injuries. Time is also in short supply for single mothers. With the advent of welfare reform in the United States, more of them are working, which conceivably reduces the time they used in the past to care for themselves and their children (see Box 3-3, see DavisPlus online).

Fathers and Fathering

A new view of fatherhood emerged out of the feminist movement of the late 1960s and early 1970s. The new ideal father was a co-parent who was responsible for and involved in all aspects of his children's care. The ideal has been widely accepted throughout North American society; people today, as opposed to those in earlier times, believe that fathers should be highly involved in caregiving (Hook, 2010). In the United States and Canada, although mothers still spend nearly twice as much time caring for children than fathers do, fathers are spending more time with their children and are doing more housework than in earlier decades. In 1998, married fathers in the United States reported spending an average of 4 hours per day with their children, compared with 2.7 hours in 1965 (Bianchi, 2000). As a primary task, men spent an average of 24 minutes on child care in 1965 (Bianchi, 2000) compared with 51 minutes for full-time employed fathers and 87 minutes for nonemployed fathers in the early 2010s (U.S. Department of Labor, 2016). In 2010, in Canada, fathers spent on average 24.4 hours per week (3.5 hours per day) taking care of children (Statistics Canada, 2012e). These estimates

vary by employment status of both parents and by the children's age. Fathers spend more time caring for children when mothers are employed and when children are young.

At the same time, other trends increasingly remove fathers from their children's lives. When the mother and father are not married, for example, ties between fathers and their children often falter. Fathers' involvement with children differs by marital status and living arrangements. Among fathers residing with their children, biological married fathers spend more time with their children, followed by fathers in cohabiting relationships. Stepfathers exhibit the lowest level of involvement among all resident fathers. Nonresidential fathers exhibit the lowest involvement in child rearing. They also provide less financial support to their children (Carlson, VanOrman, & Turner, 2012). Family demographer Frank Furstenberg (1998, 2011) used the label "good dads, bad dads" to describe the parallel trends of increased commitment to children and child rearing on the part of some fathers at the same time that there seems to be less connection to and responsibility for children on the part of other fathers.

Fathers' involvement is associated with improved child well-being, including better cognitive development, fewer behavioral problems, and better emotional health. However, fathers' involvement and child support significantly decrease when parents separate, especially if the father or mother forms a new family or if the custodial mother poses obstacles for a father's contact with his children (Carlson & McLanahan, 2010). Thus, union disruption not only hurts children's cognitive and emotional well-being, but also reduces children's contact with fathers, decreasing the parental and financial resources available to children (Amato & Dorius, 2010). Nonetheless, when fathers re-partner and acquire stepchildren, they usually assume new responsibilities and provide for their stepchildren, a fact that is often overlooked when assessing fathers' involvement (Manning & Brown, 2006).

How many years do men spend as parents? Demographer Rosalind King (1999) estimated the number of years that American men and women will spend as parents of biological children or stepchildren younger than 18 if the parenting patterns of the late 1980s and early 1990s continue throughout their lives; her estimations have not been refuted to date. Almost two-thirds of the adult years will be "child-free" years in which the individual does not have biological children younger than 18 or responsibility for anyone else's children. Men will spend, on average, about 20% of their adulthood living with and raising their biological children, whereas women will spend more than 30% of their adult lives, on average, raising biological children. Whereas women, regardless of race, spend nearly all their parenting years rearing their biological children, men are more likely to live with stepchildren or a combination of their own children and stepchildren. Among men in the United States, white men will spend about twice as much time living with their biological children as African American men.

One of the new aspects of the American family in the last 50 years has been an increase in the number of single fathers. Between 1950 and 2015, the number of households with children that were maintained by an unmarried father increased from 229,000 to 2.4 million (U.S. Census Bureau, 2015d). During the 1980s and 1990s, the percentage of single-father households nearly tripled for white and Hispanic families and doubled for African American families (Casper & Bianchi, 2002). Although still a very small subset of married couple families, the rate of stay-at-home dads has tripled between 1994 and 2015 in the United States and has grown even more rapidly in Canada (Uppal, 2015; U.S Census Bureau, 2015o). The increase in single fathers and stay-at-home dads has resulted in more fathers being in charge of their children's health and interacting with the health care system. As child rearing is often viewed as a feminine task, single fathers and stay-at-home dads may experience parenthood differently from mothers. They may have difficulty tapping into the same social networks that mothers use, such as play groups, which may preclude them from receiving health and child-care information that is shared between mothers (Marsiglio, 2009). Not only might this have an impact on their children's health, but the social exclusion experienced by these fathers often has negative physical and psychological repercussions on the men's health as well (Rochlen, McKelley, & Whittaker, 2010).

Studies indicate that single fathers are less likely to take their children for regular preventative health care. However, they do not delay health care that is immediately necessary, largely because of a lack of financial concerns (Gorman & Braverman, 2008). The delay for preventative care may be attributed to gender differences in how men and women perceive health, as adult men are also less likely to seek preventative treatment for themselves as compared with women. Children in families with stay-at-home dads are, therefore, more likely to be seen preventatively as compared with the children of single fathers because there is a mother in the home to encourage going to the primary health care provider. Beyond physician and nurse practitioner appointments, fathers shape their children's health outcomes through their own health behaviors. For example, fathers' smoking, lack of exercise, and alcohol drinking predict the same behaviors among their adolescent children. Obesity is also more common among children whose fathers (or mothers) are obese (Marsiglio, 2009).

Recent demographic trends in fathering have changed the context of family health care nursing. The growth in single fatherhood and joint custody, together with the increased tendency for fathers to perform household chores, means that family health care nurses are more likely today than in decades past to be interacting with the fathers of children.

Unmarried Parents Living Together

In the United States, changes in marriage and cohabitation tend to blur the distinction between one-parent and two-parent families. The increasing acceptance of cohabitation as a substitute for marriage, for example, may reduce the chance that a premarital pregnancy will lead to marriage before the birth (Cherlin, Cross-Barnet, Burton, & Garrett-Peters, 2009). Greater shares of children today are born to a mother who is not currently married than in previous decades. Some of those children are born to cohabiting parents and begin life in a household that includes both their biological parents. Data from the 2006–2010 National Survey of Family Growth show that 58% of recent nonmarital births were to cohabiting women (Martin et al., 2012). Cohabitation increased for unmarried mothers in all race and ethnic groups, but especially among whites. Cohabiting couples account for up to 13% of all single-parent family groups. In 2015, 8% of white single parents were actually cohabiting compared with 8.6% of African American, 3.9% of Asian, and 10.1% of Hispanic single parents (U.S. Census Bureau, 2015p). In 2011 in Canada, 17% of all families consisted of common-law couples, and among families with children under age 14, 14% were common-law families (Statistics Canada, 2012d).

Same-Sex Couple Families

An increasing number of same-sex couples are now raising children. In the United States, 17% of same-sex couples had children in 2014 (U.S. Census Bureau, 2014d). In Canada, 9.4% of same-sex couples were raising children in 2011 (Statistics Canada, 2012d). Same-sex couples, especially gay male couples, face considerable obstacles and need to overcome negative public attitudes to become parents (Biblarz & Savci, 2010). Female couples are more likely than male couples to be parents (Statistics Canada, 2012d; U.S. Census Bureau, 2014d). Many same-sex couples bring children into their households from previous heterosexual relationships; others become parents through the use of ART and surrogacy, yet an increasing number of them become parents through adoption as same-sex couples obtain legal adoption rights (Biblarz & Savci, 2010; Greenfeld, 2007).

Although some people have raised concerns about the parenting styles of same-sex parents and the potential negative effect for children's outcomes and well-being, recent research has found that, for the most part, the parental skills of same-sex couples are comparable to if not better than those of heterosexual couples (Biblarz & Savci, 2010). This finding is partly explained by the fact that although many same-sex couples are very eager to become parents, they face several obstacles that require them to invest more time, money, and effort to achieve this goal. Their higher initial investments make them more likely to devote a great deal of time to their children when they finally become parents (Biblarz & Savci, 2010).

Research on children's outcomes has focused on different dimensions of well-being, including psychological well-being, emotional development, social behavior, and school performance. Overall, these studies have found that children of same-sex parents fare relatively as well, if not better, compared with children raised by heterosexual couples. The gender of the child is an important moderating factor. Sons of same-sex couples are more likely to experience disapproval from their peers and face greater homophobic teasing than girls; boys may be at greater risk of experiencing emotional distress. This effect seems to depend on the level of social tolerance in their surrounding environments (Biblarz & Savci, 2010).

Nurses and health care providers should be aware that same-sex couples often face particular challenges to safeguarding their well-being and that of their children. Although children raised by same-sex couples generally exhibit similar outcomes and levels of well-being, these children may be more sensitive to judgmental attitudes of individuals with whom they interact, including health care providers.

Stepfamilies

Stepfamilies are formed when parents bring together children from a previous union. By contrast, remarriages or cohabiting unions in which neither partner brings children into the marriage are conceptualized and measured similarly to first marriages. The U.S. Census Bureau uses the term *blended families* to denote families with children that are formed when remarriages occur or when children living in a household share only one or no biological parents. The presence of a stepparent, stepsibling, or half-sibling designates a family as blended; these families can include adoptive children who are not the biological child of either parent if there are other children present who are not related to the adoptive child. In 2009, 13.3% of households with children under 18 were blended-family households, numbering 5.3 million (Kreider & Ellis, 2011). Almost 16% of U.S. children (11.7 million) lived in blended families in 2009. Blended families were the least common among Asian children (7%) and the most common among African American and Hispanic children (17% each). Although the number of children living in blended families has increased by almost 2 million since 1991, the percentage increase has been negligible (from 15% to 16%) (Furukawa, 1994; Kreider & Ellis, 2011). In 2011, the Census of Population in Canada identified stepfamilies for the first time. Nearly 13% of couple families with children were stepfamilies, and almost 10% of children aged 14 and under were living in stepfamilies in 2011 (Statistics Canada, 2012a).

Parental and financial responsibilities for biological parents are upheld by law, customs, roles, and rules that provide a cultural map of sorts for parents to follow in raising their children. Because no such map is available for stepfamilies, stepparents' roles, rules, and responsibilities must be defined, negotiated, and renegotiated by stepparents. Through these negotiations, many different types of stepfamilies are formed, resulting in a variety of configurations and different patterns of everyday living. The ambiguity surrounding roles in stepfamilies and the lack of a shared family history and kinship system provide opportunities to build new traditions and family rituals; however, they also open the door for greater conflict. Consider the following scenarios.

When asked by researchers, members of families who are all related by either blood or partnership (marriage or cohabitation) can very easily tell you and agree upon who is in their family. By contrast, members within stepfamilies often do not share a common definition of who is included in their family. Common omissions include stepchildren, biological children not living in the household, biological parents not living in the household, and stepparents (Brown & Manning, 2009). Even biological siblings can have different ideas regarding who they consider to be family members depending on the degree of closeness they feel toward stepparents, biological parents, biological siblings, half-siblings, and stepsiblings, especially if the biological siblings are living in different households; a girl living with her biological mother and stepfather may consider her brother living with his biological father and a stepmother as a separate family.

Negotiations must occur with ex-spouses or ex-partners, as well as with former in-laws. Researchers have found that the ex-spouse relationship can play an important role in the well-being of stepfamilies (Ganong, Coleman, & Hans, 2006) and may affect the relationship between the new stepparents, especially in the beginning of the relationship. Couples' relationships in stepfamilies and remarriages are informed and shaped by experiences in previous unions, leading to increased expectations in the remarriage. Remarried women expect and have more say in decision making than women in first marriages. In stepfamilies, the division of labor in the household is more egalitarian between spouses, as are economic roles and responsibilities (Ganong et al., 2006).

Step-relationships in particular are often weak or ambivalent, and stress arises around various issues such as perceptions of playing favorites, or jealousy among biological children, of former spouses, and of stepchildren toward stepparents. These tensions arise because in some families, stepparents are not viewed by stepchildren as real parents (King, 2009). The level of conflict also depends on the age of children, increasing as children approach adolescence, and whether or not the stepparent cohabits with or has married the biological parent. Unlike in biological families where the role of parent emerges with the birth of the child (ascribed), stepparent roles must

be earned (achieved). Therefore, discipline in stepfamilies is often a problem. Additionally, it is more difficult to be a stepparent than a biological parent because new family cultures are being developed.

Similar to children growing up in single-parent families, children with stepparents have lower levels of well-being than children growing up with biological parents (Hofferth, 2006). Thus, it is not simply the presence of two parents, but the presence of two biological parents that seems to promote children's healthy development. Despite these challenges, positive changes can occur when stepfamilies are formed. For example, a stepfather's income can compensate for the negative economic slide that tends to occur for divorced mothers, and a stepparent can alleviate the demands of single parenting (Hofferth, 2006).

Because stepfamilies comprise a significant proportion of families with children, nurses are likely to deal with parents whose roles and responsibilities are not well defined and with children who have behavioral problems, especially among recently formed blended families. Obtaining legal authorization for medical procedures can be challenging when legal obligations are unclear. Family nurses should take care to identify which parent(s) have legal responsibility for medical decision making. Health care providers should be aware that they may also need to notify nonresidential parents when their children require medical attention as these parents may share the legal right to make medical decisions.

Grandparents

One moderating factor in children's well-being in single-parent families can be the presence of grandparents in the home. Although the image of single-parent families is usually that of a mother living on her own and trying to meet the needs of her young child or children, many single parents live with their parents. For example, in the United States in 2016, about 11% of children of single mothers lived in the homes of their grandparents, as did 10% of children of single fathers (U.S. Census Bureau, 2016a). An additional 6% of children of single mothers had a grandparent living with them compared with 4% of children of single fathers. This is a snapshot at one point in time, however. A much higher percentage of single mothers with children born between 1998 and 2000 (60%) lived in their parents' home *at some point* after their child was born (Pilkauskas, 2012). African American single mothers with children at home are more likely than are others to live with a parent at some time.

Several studies have shown that the presence of grandparents has beneficial effects on children's outcomes and can buffer some of the disadvantages of living in a single-parent family (Casper, Florian, Potts, & Brandon, 2016; Sun & Li, 2014). This beneficial effect, however, seems to be more pronounced among whites than among African Americans, probably because white grandparents in the United States have more education and resources than African American grandparents (Dunifon & Kowaleski-Jones, 2007). The involvement of grandparents in the lives of their children has even become an issue for court cases, as there have been several rulings in recent years on grandparents' visitation rights. The 2000 U.S. Census included a new set of questions on grandparents' support of grandchildren. Children whose parents cannot take care of them for one reason or another often live with their grandparents. In 1970, 2.2 million, or 3.2% of all American children, lived in their grandparents' households. By 2014, this number increased to nearly 5 million, or 6.6% of all American children (U.S. Census Bureau, 2014c). Since the Great Recession in 2008 the number of children living with grandparents increased by 11%, from 4.3 million in 2008 to nearly 5 million in 2014. In 2011, in Canada, 4.8% of children aged 0 to 14 resided with at least one grandparent, up from 3.3% in 2001 (Statistics Canada, 2012d). In addition, in 2010 in the United States, grandparents were the regular child-care providers for 13% of grade-schoolers and 23% of preschoolers (U.S. Census Bureau, 2011b, 2011c).

The prevalence of grandparent families is a result of demographic factors, socioeconomic conditions, and cultural norms. Increases in life expectancy have expanded the supply of potential kin support across generations, resulting in more multigenerational households (Casper et al., 2016). At the same time, changes in work and family life have increased parents' need for child care, which, coupled with pressing economic circumstances, has made multigenerational households a strategic symbiotic arrangement, especially among single-mother, low-income, and immigrant families (Hook, 2010). Grandparents often provide financial, emotional, child care, and residential support and, in turn, receive emotional and physical support (Powell, Hamilton, Manago, & Cheng, 2016). Nonetheless, after practical and economic factors are taken into account, racial and ethnic differences in

the prevalence of grandparent households remain. Strong kinship ties and family norms also seem to explain the prevalence of grandparent households, especially among African American, Native American, Hispanic, and immigrant families (Casper et al., 2016; Florian & Casper, 2011; Haxton & Harknett, 2009). Thus, norms stressing familial obligations may also be an important factor explaining differences in the formation of grandparent families.

Emerging research reveals that grandparents play an important role in multigenerational households, which is at odds with the traditional image of grandparents as family members who themselves require financial and personal support. Although early studies assumed that financial support flowed from adult children to their parents, more recent research suggests that the more common pattern is for parents to give financial support to their adult children (Bianchi et al., 2008). In multigenerational households, it is more common for adult children and grandchildren to move into a house that grandparents own or rent. In 2007, in the United States, 64% of multigenerational households were headed by grandparents (Florian & Casper, 2011). Nearly 33% of all the grandparent-maintained families are skipped generation, that is, grandparents living with their grandchildren without the children's parents (authors' calculations based on data from U.S. Census Bureau, 2014c). A little more than 3%, or 413,490, of all households in Canada contained a grandparent in 2011. Of these households, 53% also contained both parents, 32% contained a lone parent (mostly the mother), and 12% were skipped-generation households comprised of children residing with their grandparents without a parent (Statistics Canada, 2012d).

Grandparents who own or rent homes that include grandchildren and adult children are younger, healthier, and more likely to be in the labor force than are grandparents who live in a residence owned or rented by their adult children (Casper et al., 2016; Keene & Batson, 2010). Grandparents who maintain multigenerational households are also better educated (more likely to have at least a high-school education) than are grandparents who live in their children's homes (Ellis & Simmons, 2014). Nevertheless, supporting grandchildren can drain grandparents' resources. One study indicated that grandfathers who are primary caretakers of grandchildren are at higher risk of experiencing poverty if they are in a skipped-generation household, are ethnic minorities, or are not married (Keene, Prokos, & Held, 2012).

The structure of grandparent households differs by nativity. Although coresidential grandparent families are more common among immigrant families, immigrant grandparent families are less likely to be maintained by grandparents and less likely to be skipped generation. Thus, although the flow of support in native-born multigenerational families more often runs from older to younger generations, in immigrant grandparent families support more often flows from adult children to their older parents (Casper et al., 2016; Florian & Casper, 2011).

Parents who support both dependent children and dependent parents have been referred to as the "sandwich" generation, because they provide economic and emotional support for both the older and younger generations. Although grandparents in parent-maintained households tend to be older, in poorer health, and not as likely to be employed, many are in good health and are, in fact, working (Ellis & Simmons, 2014). These findings suggest that, at the very least, the burden of maintaining a coresidential "sandwich family" household may be somewhat overstated in the popular press. Many of the grandparents who are living in the houses of their adult children are capable of contributing to the family income and helping with the supervision of children.

Many grandparents step in to assist their children in times of crisis. Some provide financial assistance or child care, whereas others are the primary caregivers for their grandchildren. Although grandmothers comprise the majority of grandparent caregivers, a sizable number of grandfather caregivers exist who are likely to experience more challenges than grandmothers as primary caregivers (Keene et al., 2012).

The recent increase in the numbers of grandparents raising their grandchildren is particularly salient to health care providers because both grandparents and grandchildren in this situation often suffer health problems (Dunifon, Ziol-Guest, & Kokpo, 2014). Researchers have documented high rates of asthma, weakened immune systems, poor eating and sleeping patterns, physical disabilities, and hyperactivity among grandchildren being raised by their grandparents (Kelley, Whitley, & Campos, 2011). Grandparents raising grandchildren tend to be in poorer health than their counterparts. They have higher levels of stress, higher rates of anxiety and depression, poorer self-rated health, and more multiple chronic health problems, especially if the grandchildren exhibit behavioral problems (Leder,

Grinstead, & Torres, 2007). Other studies suggest, however, that these negative outcomes may not necessarily be a result of caring for grandchildren; instead, they may reflect grandparents' preexisting health conditions and economic circumstances before they began to raise their grandchildren (Hughes, Waite, LaPierre, & Luo, 2007). It is important to keep in mind that, although many of the grandparents who live in their adult children's homes are in good health, some of these grandparents require significant care. Nurses should also be aware that there are also adult children who provide care for their parents who are not living with them. Adults who provide care for both generations are likely to face both time and money concerns.

Child Care

Families consider many factors when deciding on how best to take care of their children: whether one or both parents should work for pay, whether to engage in full-time or part-time employment, and what type of child care to use. Financial constraints, career goals, and the quality, price, and availability of child care are all considered (Casper & Bianchi, 2002). The substantial growth of employed mothers with young children—both married and single—has increased the need, availability, and acceptance of child care. As a consequence of changing labor force participation, unprecedented numbers of children spend at least some part of their week in the care of someone other than their parents. In Canada, the majority of parents (86%) report using child-care arrangements on a regular basis, particularly for younger children (Sinha, 2014). In 2011, 61% of American children under the age of 5 spent time in a regular child-care arrangement (Laughlin, 2013).

There are two broad types of child care: informal, such as a family member, and formal, including day-care centers (Casper & Bianchi, 2002). Grandparents are used as child care mainly for children under age 5 (Laughlin, 2013). In fact, for children under 5, grandparents may be the single most frequent (24%) child-care arrangement (Laughlin, 2013). Another quarter of preschoolers who are in a regular arrangement are cared for in organized facilities such as day-care centers, nursery or preschools, or Head Start programs. Formal child care is linked with positive cognitive outcomes and school readiness for children (Augustine, Crosnoe, & Gordon, 2013). Despite these benefits, many children are unable to attend center-based care because of their mother's work hours, as centers are time-inflexible (Press, Fagan, & Laughlin, 2006). There is a middle ground, however, as many children do not experience only one type of care arrangement at the same time or throughout their childhood. Multiple child-care arrangements are becoming increasingly common, especially for parents who need to ensure child-care coverage during shift-work (Morrissey, 2013). One-third of preschoolers whose mothers work a non-day shift have multiple care arrangements as compared with only one quarter whose mothers work day shifts (Laughlin, 2013).

The conversations around child care often focus on mothers and maternal employment, not because child care is exclusively the mother's job, but because it is mothers rather than fathers whose labor force participation has changed. In fact, fathers' care of children has increased over time. For example, the number of fathers who report providing "any care" to their children increased between 1988 and 2011 (Laughlin, 2013). With the increased expectation that fathers provide child care, some couples have one parent work evenings or overnight in order to decrease reliance on nonparental child care (Joshi & Bogen, 2007).

Women's employment is only part of the increased demand for child care. For many parents, formal center-based child care offers enrichment opportunities for their children, socially and educationally, which is why even among families with a stay-at-home parent child-care usage has increased (Laughlin, 2013; Morrissey, 2008). For example, in 2011, 13% of preschoolers whose mothers were not working received formal center-based care on a regular basis (Laughlin, 2013). Often as children age, their use of "child care" decreases, as it is replaced with formal schooling and after-school, extracurricular activities.

An increase in child care can affect health in many ways. Children are spending more time outside of the nuclear family; thus, they are dependent on more people to notice health issues that may arise and to tend to their needs. The quality of care children receive varies across types of child-care arrangements, although the different types only have modestly different effects on child health up to age 4 and a half (U.S. Department of Health and Human Services, 2006). Importantly, quality of child care is difficult to link directly to health outcomes because very few children are in consistent child-care arrangements,

in part because of the frequency of multiple care arrangements, and in part because of changes in parental work (Hynes, 2008). Because children frequently change child care, few remain in consistently high or low quality care; rather, most children are clustered over time in a mix of arrangements that have varying quality (Hynes, 2008). This variation makes it difficult to disentangle direct outcomes of child-care quality. On the one hand, studies suggest cognitive and linguistic benefits linked to center-based care compared with home care (Abner, Gordon, Kaestner, & Korenman, 2013). On the other hand, extended time in child-care arrangements before the age of 4 and a half has been linked to increased behavioral issues (U.S. Department of Health and Human Services, 2006). Child care has also been linked to an increased rate of common colds and respiratory infections, though this is most common for children in care centers who tend to be around many other children (Morrisey, 2008).

Increasingly, in both Canada and the United States, children in group settings such as nurseries and schools mingle with unvaccinated or undervaccinated peers. In a recent report by UNICEF (2013), Canada was ranked below most developed countries, including the United States, for the immunization rates of children aged 12 to 23 months. Neither country mandates vaccines, leaving regulations up to individual states, provinces, or local health and education departments. This means that vaccination coverage ranges widely across the two nations. For the United States, the combined 7-vaccine series coverage in 2015 for children aged 19 to 35 months ranged from 64.4% in Virginia to 80.6% in Connecticut (U.S. Centers for Disease Control and Prevention, 2016). Especially given the increase in childhood diseases because of some parents not having their children immunized, it remains important for health care providers to discuss the benefits and risks of immunizations with parents and to encourage them to keep their children's immunizations up-to-date before entering child-care arrangements.

SUMMARY

Families change in response to economic conditions, cultural change, and shifting demographics, such as the aging of the population and immigration. North America has gone through a particularly tumultuous period in the last few decades, resulting in rapid changes in family structure, functions, and processes. Families have grown more diversified.

- More single-mother families, single-father families, same-sex parent families, and families with both parents in the labor force exist today than in the past. This translates into less time for parents to take care of the health needs of family members.
- Most young children spend at least some time every week in child care outside of their nuclear family in arrangements that are diverse and frequently changing. The associated increase in health issues adds a burden to families.
- Single mothers may find it particularly challenging to meet the health care needs of their families because they tend to have the least time and money to do so.
- More fathers are taking responsibility for being primary caretakers of their children and will be more likely than in the past to be the parent with whom nurses will interact.
- Changes in childbearing behaviors have also altered family life.
- Persistent levels of below replacement fertility in Canada have raised concerns about the future contraction of the population, which would reduce the tax base to support children and the growing number of senior citizens.
- As more couples delay childbearing, they are more likely to seek assistance to conceive from health care providers.
- The growing number of same-sex couples who aspire to become parents has further increased the demand for ART.
- Nurses should be aware that this is a stressful time in families' lives, as more adults and children live in nontraditional family forms.
- Nurses also should be aware that the roles of parents and responsibility for children in these households may be ambiguous.
- Many North American families adopt children. These children are likely to face a period of adjustment and are also more likely than other children to have special health care needs.

- More grandparents are raising their grandchildren, and these grandchildren may suffer from more health problems compared with other children.
- Many families maintained by grandparents are in poverty, and many of the grandparents in these families suffer from poor health themselves. Nurses will increasingly be likely to provide care to grandparent families, and they should be aware of the unique health and financial challenges these families face.
- As mortality rates at older ages continue to improve, and as baby boomers move into their retirement years, the proportions of the population of older adults will continue to increase. This demographic shift will increase the need for nurses who specialize in caring for older persons.
- More adults will have children and parents for whom they must care, increasing the need for care in both directions, that of the younger and the older.
- Working with health care needs of both generations will be a challenge for health care providers, especially nurses who are on the front line in most health care systems.
- Today, more North Americans come from other countries than in the past.
- Health care providers will be serving a more ethnically and culturally diverse population.
- Many of these individuals speak a language other than English.
- Economics and family relationships remain intertwined. Family issues growing in importance include balancing paid work with child rearing, income inequality between men and women, fathers' parenting roles, the expected increase in the number of frail elderly persons, and intergenerational relationship changes because of the increase in life expectancy.
- The Great Recession of 2008 has put economic strain on many families, increasing the likelihood of stress-related illness and decreasing the ability to afford appropriate care.
- Families have been amazingly adaptive and resilient in the past; one would expect them to be so in the future.

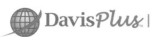 **DavisPlus** | For additional resources and information, visit **http://davisplus.fadavis.com**. References, as well as Suggested Readings and Websites can be found on Davis*Plus*.

Chapter 4

Family Policy
The Intersection of Family Policies, Health Disparities, and Health Care Policies

Deborah Padgett Coehlo, PhD, C-PNP, PMHS, CFLE

Tammy L. Henderson, PhD, CFLE

Chuck Lester, MPH Candidate

Critical Concepts

- The health outcomes of families continue to be challenged by health disparities that result from deeply rooted social issues, including racism and stigma, as well as from a variety of factors including poverty, racism, negative social stigmatizations, restricted access to health care resources, and a complex political system of cultural beliefs.

- Providing health care to families based on a human rights and legal perspective may promote health equity by transforming and developing policies, programs, and laws that inhibit the limited or restricted access to health care services to families.

- Policy decisions made by a society or government about families and what constitutes legal relationship and how health care is delivered, have a profound effect on families and their health.

- Health care policies are currently being challenged in the United States owing to conflict over the ongoing debate of private versus public health care, competing views toward individual responsibility and personal behaviors, and the meanings attached to laws. Currently, there are no policies that guarantee the right to health care in the United States with the exception of the social insurance program of Medicare and need-based programs and policies. Canada has boasted universal, federally funded health care access for physicians' services, hospital care, and diagnostics since 1966.

- The meanings that a family, the government, or the health care system attaches to family shapes the health of the person by impacting access to government-funded programs.

- For effective outcomes, health policies and health promotion programs must consider the social determinant of health as the foundational concepts influencing health.

(continued)

■ Today, most front-line nurses in the United States and Canada function primarily in the acute care setting which is a practice that fosters an inadequate perspective and understanding of the social determinants of health and an associated limitation in advocacy.

■ Advancing health care will require a cultural shift in the expectations of the nursing profession regarding education, practice, and advocacy for vulnerable populations.

INTRODUCTION

Understanding the foundation for the concepts underlying the substance of this chapter regarding the intersection of family policies and health, and social determinants of health and health disparities is an important step in understanding the nurse's role in family policy. As with the meanings attached to families and family policy, these terms set the stage for understanding health disparities, followed by understanding health care policies, and the role of nurses.

Social determinants of health are factors that contribute to and/or determine the health status, health care delivery, or health equity of a person, community, or group; including family and personal culture, educational level, socioeconomic status, location of birth and where individuals live and work, access to resources, and cultural beliefs and practices (Jones, 2014). Social determinants of health directly influence the health of individuals, families, and communities (World Health Organization [WHO], 2012). WHO (2012) defines *social determinants of health* as "the conditions in which people are born, grow, live, work and age, including the health system. These circumstances are shaped by the distribution of money, power and resources at global, national and local levels" (paragraph 1). More specifically, determinants include a person's demographic characteristics, such as gender, race, ethnicity, able-bodiness, and age, which cannot be changed. Social determinants organize the world and shape societal responses, which are and may be altered.

Social determinants also include characteristics that can be changed. These changeable characteristics are considered behavioral or social. Behavioral determinants include activities such as eating habits, smoking, substance use, physical activity, and coping skills. Social determinants include physical, social, educational, and economic environments, which further break down into income, housing, education,

employment, access to health care, public safety, transportation, and availability of community-based resources (Hunter, Neiger, & West, 2011; Mikkonen & Raphael, 2010; U.S. Department of Health and Human Services, 2013a). Along with demographic and behavioral characteristics, social determinants have a strong, deep-seated influence on the health of families and will continue to contribute to health disparities within family and community systems. An uneven distribution of the social determinants of health, including access to health care and healthy environments, is often reported as the root problem of health disparities. Without the necessary financial resources for a healthy lifestyle, for example, it is difficult or even impossible to overcome such disparities.

Health disparities are defined as differences in health outcomes that are closely tied to social, economic, racial, ethnic, gender, disability, religious, environmental, and geographic disadvantage. Health disparities adversely affect groups of people who have systematically experienced greater obstacles to health because of stigmatization as part of a culturally identified oppressed group or other characteristics linked to discrimination or exclusion (USDHHS, 2013a). Health literacy is important in preventing health disparities. Health literacy is the extent to which individuals have the capacity to understand, process, and obtain basic health care information and needed services (U.S. Department of Health and Human Services, 2017; Office of Disease Prevention and Health Promotion, 2017).

Health disparities arise from complex interaction between family policies, personally mediated racism, and internal racism, or the acceptance by stigmatized groups of people that they have inferior abilities (Jones, 2014).

■ Institutional racism refers to deferential access to resources and opportunities that impede the health and well-being of individuals, families, and communities.

- Personally mediated racism refers to prejudice (e.g., differential assumptions) and discrimination (e.g., negative actions) practiced by individuals, families, and communities across societies, which undermines the humanity of others (Jones, 2014).
- Internalized racism refers to the acceptance and adoption of socially constructed negative messages about one's abilities, character, lower status, and the resulting loss of civil and social rights (Jones, 2000).

In this chapter health disparities are explored in the context of health determinants, family policy, and the nurse's role in advocating for family policies that enhance, rather than discriminate against, positive health care and resulting health outcomes. This chapter also discusses the unique factors that affect health policy and family health across Westernized countries.

This chapter explores the many factors and policies that influence health outcomes for families. Threaded throughout the chapter is the role of the nurse providing care within a framework of family nursing and multiple sociopolitical contexts. Specifically, key theoretical models are presented that guide family policies. The health outcomes of families continue to be challenged by health disparities that result from a variety of factors including negative social stigmatizations, restricted access to health care resources, and a complex political system of cultural beliefs.

Health care policies are currently being challenged in the United States owing to conflict over the ongoing debate of private versus public health care, competing views toward individual responsibility and personal behaviors, and the meanings attached to laws (Levitsky, 2013). However, the resulting health risks faced by stigmatized groups of people unveil the influence of access to health care and related needed services. Finally, this chapter explores nursing involvement in the development of health policy from either professional organizations or individual perspectives.

At the completion of this chapter, the nurse will have a broad understanding of family policy and how it can contribute to or mitigate health disparities and health outcomes. Armed with this knowledge, nurses can assist families to adopt health promotion and disease prevention strategies and can advocate for families in their organizations, communities, and

nations to adopt policies that minimize disparities and maximize access to resources. This, in turn, will contribute to improved health of families and their members.

FAMILY POLICY

Family policy, explicit and implicit laws, codes, programs, and policies are designed to promote and protect children, families, and communities (Bogenschneider, 2014). The notion of "family" is not explicitly noted in the U.S. Constitution. Federal, state, and local governments are charged to protect the individual rights of citizens. Individual rights must be balanced against the common good of all citizens (Etzioni, 2015). Policies indirectly influence the health and overall well-being of children and families, including zoning ordinances as well as traffic, criminal, environmental, corporate, and voting laws. Explicit family policies, programs, and laws center around marriage, divorce, adoption, child care, family leave, reproductive rights, and more.

Ideally, family policies support and help parents and families to effectively manage paid work and family caregiving, reduce poverty, and improve children's development (Adema, 2012; Hengstebeck, Helms, & Crosby, 2016). Policies, laws, and programs influence everyday life, including affecting a person's ability to form intimate partnerships, render economic support to family members, parent and care for children, and engage in family caregiving of infants, children, spouses, siblings, older adults, individuals with intellectual and other disabilities, and others (Bogenschneider, 2014).

The Definition of Family

Today's nurse advocacy role is shaped by the social and legal meanings of family to provide quality care and services. The definition of family in the context of family policy is created and shaped by policies, laws, and programs. Policy decisions made by a society or government about families and how they are legally defined, and the meaning of what constitutes a legal relationship, have a profound effect on families, their health care options, and their health outcomes.

The influence of family policies, laws, and codes on the health and development of children, youth, families, and communities begins with the fact that "family" is not included in the U.S. Constitution. The meaning of and protections afforded to families have emerged from legislative, administrative, and judicial decision making. For example, the fundamental right to personal and family relationships and the right to life, liberty, and the pursuit of happiness (liberty interests) are woven into the U.S. Constitution and U.S. Supreme Court decisions (*Loving v. Virginia*, 1967; *Moore v. the City of East Cleveland*, 1977). In the case of *Loving v. Virginia* (1967), the U.S. Supreme Court determined that the Virginia law that prohibited African Americans and whites from marrying violated the marital autonomy rights, among other rights, of Richard and Mildred Loving.

For the most part, family has been socially defined as two heterosexual parents with children, creating the cultural expectation for the traditional family in the United States (Coontz, 1992) and carving out a hierarchy of legal protections. In the decision of *Moore v. the City of East Cleveland* (1977), the U.S. Supreme Court determined that an intergenerational household—a grandmother, her son, and two grandchildren—functioned similar to a traditional family. Therefore, this family deserved to live in an area zoned for single-family units. This functional definition of family is complemented by structural meanings such as single-parent, blended, divorced, and long-term foster families or same-sex partners and cohabiting couples. More recently, the U.S. Census Bureau (2015a) defined a *family* as two or more people living together who are related by birth, marriage, or adoption. Although this definition expands policies that support families, individuals living together as a family but without legal protection based on this definition remain vulnerable. For example, two adults living together but not married cannot obtain the same benefits as two adults who are legally married.

Contemporary demographic trends reflect shifts in the meaning of families that correspond to the growth of intergenerational and other diverse families. In 2015, an estimated 5.8 million children younger than 18 years of age in the United States resided with a grandparent and 2.6 million grandparents were responsible for the basic needs of one or more grandchildren younger than 18 years of age (U.S. Census Bureau, 2016). Similarly, in the *United States v. Windsor* (2013) decision, the Supreme Court determined that Section 3 of the Defense of Marriage Act (DOMA, 1996) defining

"marriage" as the legal union "between one man and one woman as husband and wife" and "spouse" as "a person of the opposite sex who is a husband or a wife" unconstitutional. DOMA stigmatized and created a disadvantaged and separate status for same-sex couples. In essence, the law violated the Fifth Amendment's guarantee of equal protection under the law, similar to the *Loving v. Virginia* case (1967).

Looking specifically at the context of health care, members of a "family" can be given or denied access to health insurance, housing, social, and health programs based on whether they meet the federal definition of family. In the United States, the Administration for Children and Families (2016), is part of the U.S. Department of Health and Human Services that oversees federal programs that support the economic and social well-being of children and families. Such programs include, for example, Temporary Assistance to Needy Families (TANF) (Office of Family Assistance, 2017), The Healthy Marriage Initiative (Office of Family Assistance, 2012), and Head Start (USDHHS, 2017). But because of how families are legally defined, many individuals who consider themselves part of a family unit would be ineligible for these programs. In fact, a limited legal definition of family can have devastating results. Consider, for example, one instance in Black Jack City, Missouri, where a family composed of two parents and three children was denied an occupancy permit simply because the parents were not legally married and the male parent was not the biological father of the oldest child residing in the household (Burkeman, 2006).

The meanings that a family, the government, or the health care system attaches to family shapes the health of the person by impacting access to government-funded programs. For example, to qualify for Medicaid an individual needs to check his or her state code because of ongoing changes in the laws governing Medicaid. Legislators in Washington, DC, and about 29 other states expanded the cap for Medicaid (see Medicaid and the Children's Health Insurance Program (CHIP) (n.d.) https://www.healthcare.gov/medicaid-chip/getting-medicaid-chip/). Looking at states that expanded their Medicaid coverage, an individual may qualify for Medicaid if he or she earns $16,243 or less per year; a family of four may have a total annual income of $24,300 per year (U.S. Centers for Medicare & Medicaid Services, 2016).

An International View From Canada

The definition of family most directly influences who is able to access health care and social support resources and who is not across the providences of Canada. The most recent Canadian definition of family according to the Vanier Institute of the Family (2017) is "any combination of two or more persons who are bound together over time by ties of mutual consent, birth and/or adoption or placement and who, together, assume responsibilities for variant combinations of some of the following" (paragraph 1):

- Physical maintenance and care of group members
- Addition of new members through procreation or adoption
- Socialization of children
- Social control of members
- Production, consumption, distribution of good and service
- Affective nurturance—love

This board definition is based on the functions of the family (see Chapter 1) and not on the gender or legal relationship of people in the group.

Canada's progressive views on family policies include provisions for other family forms. The provinces, with the exception of the Province of Quebec, legally recognize the common-law family, meaning two people cohabitating without being officially married (Statistics Canada, 2011). In 1967, former Prime Minister Pierre Elliott Trudeau, then justice minister, declared: "The state has no business in the bedrooms of the nation" (cited by Overall, 2004, p. 1). Today, same-sex marriage is legally recognized in that "a couple may be of the opposite or same sex" (Statistics Canada, 2015). Canada's recognition of both same-sex and common-law families results in major implications for access to spousal benefits and pensions, child custody, and other traditionally family-oriented rites of inheritance. Previously, only traditionally married couples of the opposite sex were recognized as beneficiaries, leaving many non-traditional spouses destitute after their life partners died or the relationship dissolved. Legal definitions of family in the United States will continue to be blurred as families continue to evolve through adoption, guardianship, same-sex marriage, cohabitation, blended families, and other ways nonrelated adults and children continue to form families.

THE INTERSECTION BETWEEN FAMILY POLICIES AND HEALTH DISPARITIES

Family policy refers to explicit and implicit laws, codes, programs, and policies developed to promote and protect children, families, and communities (Bogenschneider, 2014); however, in the United States the government works to protect the individual rights of citizens and balance those rights against the common good of all citizens. An exploration of health determinants and health disparities logically begins with a discussion of family policy and its impact on families. Family policies are those policies that protect social rights, including health, food and water, education, housing, employment, and a healthy environment. Different than civil rights, which protect a citizen's right to participate in political decisions (i.e., voting and public forums), legal rights, and civil protection, social rights are controversial because of a generational belief that social rights are largely the responsibility of the individual (Levitsky, 2013). Family policies have been developed for the purpose of preventing health problems on a societal scale (i.e., immunization programs and clean water policies) and to *mitigate* health disparities. This section will explore examples of family policies that have had an impact on family health and on health disparities.

Theoretical Background for the Intersection of Family Policies and Health Disparities

A discussion of the intersection of family policy and health cannot be fully understood without an understanding of theoretical models that help explain the complexity of health disparities. Health disparities are best understood using Jones' Three Levels of Racism Model (2000) and Bronfenbrenner's Ecological Systems Model (1985, 1999, 2001, 2005; Bronfenbrenner & Morris, 1998). The term *racism* can be interspersed with other groups that are stigmatized, "not by a biological construct, but rather a social construct" (Jones, 2014, p. 1), including those stigmatized by religion, gender, sexual orientation or identity, socioeconomic status, or ability.

Jones' Three Levels of Racism Model
Jones (2000) identifies three levels of racism in her model: institutional, personally mediated, and internalized.

Institutional racism refers to deferential access to resources and opportunities, including health care, educational opportunities, gainful employment, healthy food and clean water, adequate housing, and living in a healthy environment. Each of these resources and opportunities in turn impacts health and is commonly listed as a health determinant. Institutional racist practices are often normalized by a particular society and often protected by laws and policies within that society. For example, previous laws that prohibited gay men and women from participating in parts of the military also limited vocational opportunities (Berube, 1990). Institutional racism often influences practices and customs across generations, as we have observed with African Americans and indigenous populations in many countries.

Personally mediated racism refers to prejudice and discrimination practiced by individuals, families, and communities across societies (Jones, 2000). Prejudice refers to differential assumptions about the "abilities, motives, and intentions of others" (Jones, 2000, p. 2) according to their identified, stigmatized group affiliation. Discrimination refers to the action toward the differentiated groups that negatively impacts their well-being. These actions include lack of respect, unwarranted suspicion (i.e., not sitting next to a person based on prejudiced beliefs), devaluation (i.e., not choosing a qualified person for a job based on the person's stigmatized characteristics), and scapegoating (i.e., punishing an entire group of people based on the rumored actions of one in the group). See *A Documented History of the Incident Which Occurred at Rosewood, Florida, in January 1923* (Jones, 1993) for a clear example of this process. This tragedy involved an entire town being burned and an undocumented number of African Americans killed based on a rumor that a white woman was sexually assaulted by an African American man. The incident occurred in 1923, and yet it took until 1994 for any retribution to be awarded to the nine survivors.

Finally, *internalized racism* refers to stigmatized individuals accepting negative messages about their abilities and their inherent lower status, leading to loss of civil and social rights (Jones, 2000). Many individuals who are placed in a stigmatized group begin to accept labels placed on them by other groups and accept disparities in resources as their "due." This pattern is similar to a rape victim blaming herself for the rape, labeling herself as "asking for it" based on the clothes she was wearing at the time of the rape.

Jones (2000, 2014) provides clear metaphors to illustrate the negative impact of each of the three levels of racism on health. Her first metaphor describes the difference in perception of moths as they fly in and out of colored lights. The metaphor emphasizes that the moths do not change in color or ability as they fly, but rather the surrounding lights change the perception of their appearance. This is similar to certain groups of people that are stigmatized in one setting, yet welcomed and valued in another setting based on perception rather than any inherent change in the identified group. For example, a Native American is welcomed within his cultural celebrations but may be shunned in a predominantly white celebration.

Jones' second metaphor is that of a closing restaurant. The people already in the restaurant are able to enjoy the resources, yet those locked on the outside can only observe the enjoyment. This is often illustrated by a stigmatized group being unable to access a service but being able to observe the privileged groups enjoying that resource, such as quality health care.

Finally, the most compelling metaphor Jones offers is noticing the difference in growth of two plants: One plant is given rich soil and an abundance of water to grow and the other plant is given poor soil and barely enough water to survive. The first plant will obviously flourish, whereas the second plant will grow slowly and never reach its true potential. If one is observing these two plants and not considering the impact of the environment on the difference in growth, one could easily decide that the first plant was inherently superior. This metaphor describes the common practice of observing an oppressed group of individuals who are surrounded by an unhealthy environment and assuming they are inherently inferior to those growing up in a rich and healthy environment (Jones, 2014).

Using Jones' model to understand and change family policy is valuable for nurses. If nurses consider the three levels of racism they are more likely to identify these trends and participate in changing policies that continue to oppress vulnerable populations. Nurses can intervene on an individual, institutional, and cultural level by promoting change through education, involvement, and no longer accepting racism as an tolerable value. Understanding Jones' model and how her model interacts within the ecological systems is a way to understand where to place health promotion across systems.

Bronfenbrenner's Ecological Systems Model

Bronfenbrenner's Ecological Systems Model describes the interacting systems between micro-, meso-, macro-, and exo-levels, adding the system of time or the chrono-level. The microsystem or individual system includes internal systems (i.e., the most intimate system of development or health status of the individual). The mesosystem refers to the family system, including roles, responsibilities, boundaries, and communication patterns within the family and toward the outside world. The macrosystem refers to the surrounding community, including neighborhood culture and structure, schools, parks, churches, and other community resources. The exosystem refers to the larger government and culture, including laws and policies. See Chapters 2 and 11 for a more in-depth description of this theory.

When considering family policy development, the use of an ecological model has broadened our focus from an individualist model to a multisystem model (Fielding, Teutsch, & Breslow, 2010). Historically, the United States made a major shift in overall health through family policies that improved sanitation, air quality, and local environments, as well as overall access to health care. With the growth in biomedical science, however, there was a shift away from family policy changes from broad environmental policies to individual health care. The life expectancy grew an average of 3 years per decade as biomedical research improved the treatment for hypertension, diabetes, heart disease, and cancers. This trend caused a marked increase in the development of the current individual insurance program rather than social programs to pay for health care. This change resulted in increased health care spending dollars by 97% over a 30-year period from 1970 to 2000 (Fielding et al., 2010). The individualized approach focused on the individual's responsibility to maintain health, find providers to treat health problems, and pay for care to support health.

Application of Theoretical Models of Health Disparities

Both Jones' Three Levels of Racism Model and Bronfenbrenner's Ecological Systems Model consider the individual, families, communities, and the broad economic, social, cultural, and physical environment and how each system improves both our understanding of and treatment of disease and promotion of health. These models emphasize the importance of environments, such as Jones' metaphor of the plants growing differently dependent on the health of their environments. From a public health viewpoint, Bronfenbrenner's Ecological Systems Model considers multiple levels of health. Family policies tend to target the exo-level health practices, such as economic (i.e., living wage), social (i.e., Family and Medical Leave Act of 1993 (2006)), and physical environments (i.e., Clean Air Act of 1963 (1990)). Focusing on individuals alone cannot create healthy communities, and without healthy communities individuals cannot be healthy. Individualism promotes individual care and the continued advancement of biomedical treatments for health. Individualism, however, also has its risks, including higher health care costs and higher disparity between the rich and the poor, with the United States having up to 17.6% of families living in poverty and 23% of children living in poverty (Gould & Wething, 2012). Further, only 47% of U.S. workers earn 10% above the living wage, compared with 67.8% of Canadian workers and 72% of Irish workers (Gould & Wething, 2012). These statistics are important because living wages are directly correlated with health outcomes (Institute for Research on Poverty, 2016). Those with lower wages have lower standards of living, including lowered access to health care. Low wages are, in part, responsible for the 17.3% of U.S. citizens living in poverty, compared with 8.8% in France and 6.3% in Denmark. The three levels of racism offered by Jones impact each of the three levels of systems described by Bronfenbrenner.

From a family policy viewpoint, it is important to consider how a government transfers tax dollars to social service programs that reduce the overall poverty rate because the poverty rate directly impacts the health of citizens and health of communities. The United States ranks at the bottom of 27 peer countries, with tax-supported programs reducing the poverty rate by 9.7% compared with 25.4% in France. North America also ranks lowest in the percentage of the gross domestic product (GDP) spent on social programs: The United States spends 16.2% of their GDP compared with other Westernized countries that average spending 21.3% (Gould & Wething, 2012). By understanding these figures, nurses can better understand the importance of assessing exo-level variables that impact macro-level family health. For example, whereas the death certificate of a 60-year-old male might state the cause of death as heart disease, from an ecological viewpoint the cause of death includes smoking and a sedentary lifestyle (micro), a loss of support from family members following divorce (meso-level), inadequate resources in the community (i.e., macro-level; support groups, education, and access to health care), and living in poverty without qualifications to receive governmental support (i.e., exo-level; under 65 years of age, and therefore does not qualify for Medicare).

Social Determinants and Resulting Health Disparities

Health disparities are a continuing problem in the United States, causing negative health outcomes for stigmatized groups of individuals and families. Because of this continued problem, Congress ordered the Institute of Medicine (IOM) to investigate and develop a report on the subject. The landmark IOM report, *Unequal Treatment: Confronting Racial and Ethnic Disparities in Health Care* (Smedley, Stith, & Nelson, 2003), detailed the long-standing and deeply rooted inequalities in health care directly related to race and ethnicity. Despite the IOM providing a comprehensive review of the contributing factors to health disparities and recommendations to promote health equity, a 2012 evaluation on the progress toward reducing health disparities revealed continued health disparities (IOM, 2011, 2012). For instance, African Americans continue to experience higher rates of death from heart disease and cancer than white Americans, and children of color who live in urban areas are more likely to have asthma than children living in less population dense areas as well as white children in both rural and urban communities (IOM, 2012). These health disparities continue to correlate with the following: certain environments that lack adequate resources such as limited access to health care, exposure to environmental toxins in impoverished environments, personal behaviors related to substance abuse, inadequate nutrition, lack of physical exercise, and lack of treatment for mental illnesses (IOM, 2012). This section will apply Jones' Three Levels of Racism Model and Bronfenbrenner's Ecological Systems Model to social determinants of continued health disparity.

Poverty

Social determinants of health are interrelated and mutually reinforcing. Poverty is likely the most fundamental social determinant contributing to health disparities (Institute for Research on Poverty, 2016). Poverty influences the other social determinants that have a negative impact on family health such as housing, food and job security, education, and life-style choices. Racism continues to strongly influence who is victim to poverty and can be analyzed from examining multiple interacting ecological systems. It is impossible to discuss individual lifestyle choices, for example, without discussing family cultures, community access to education about healthy lifestyles, and governmental policies that fund and support, through family policies, healthy lifestyle promotion. Likewise, poor-quality housing or overcrowding—a result of poverty—affects health by contributing to stress (individual or micro-level) and safety issues (micro- and macro-level). When considering chronic illnesses such as asthma, using medications can decrease symptoms, but medications can only be used if the individual has access to health care. Mildew and dampness (community environment) might trigger asthma and be beyond an individual or family's ability to correct. Unemployment or employment insecurity, which can result in poverty, limits the choice of affordable housing, and living in a low-resource community further adds to unhealthy lifestyle choices. For example, areas where affordable housing is located tend to lack public transportation and grocery stores; therefore, citizens using low-income housing end up having less access to fresh fruits and vegetables, which makes shopping for, and eating, healthy foods difficult. The only choice for these families is often to buy unhealthy processed foods from the local variety stores, frequently at high prices (Hilmers, Hilmers, & Dave, 2012).

Poverty creates serious issues when it comes to housing and can result in homelessness for many families who live below the poverty level. There are 2.5 million homeless children in the United States, which is one in every 30 children (Bassuk, DeCandia, Beach, & Berman, 2014). Homeless children are three times more likely to have been born to a single mother than their nonhomeless counterparts (Bassuk, DeCandia, Beach, & Berman, 2014). The major causes of homelessness in children include (Bassuk, DeCandia, Beach, & Berman, 2014):

- National high poverty rate
- Lack of affordable housing
- Racial disparities
- Challenges of single parenting

■ History of a traumatic experience, especially domestic violence

One of the most significant outcomes for young children who experience homelessness is the potential for devastating changes in the brain that can interfere with learning, emotional self-regulation, cognitive skills and social relationships (Bassuk, DeCandia, Beach, & Berman, 2014).

Family nurses should work with homeless families with children to provide emergency shelter and essential services need to follow these children to their permanent housing. Nurses need to be skillful in conducting comprehensive assessment, screening for depression and child development screening. Nurses can advocate for programs allowing single parent mothers to receive job training and workplace skills. These mothers will need help finding safe childcare for their children. Most importantly, family nurses need to help these families learning parenting skills so they can build strong healthy relationships with their children.

In the United States today, as well as in Canada, the concern about the gender gap between men and women and younger/older workers is narrowing, but remains consistent (PEW Research Center, 2017). In 2015 women earned 83% of what men earned for both full-time and part-time work. For example, for women in the 25–34 year age group the gap is smaller as these women earned 90% of what men earned. A few women find higher paying jobs that were traditionally held by men. However, women mostly have jobs in the lower-paying occupations. This finding is specifically difficult given the number of single mothers.

The Pew Research Center (2016) explored the shrinking middle class in the United States. The following five trends were noted:

1. With fewer Americans in the middle-income tier, the economic tiers above and below have grown in significance over time.
2. The share of adults in the upper-income tier increased more than the lower-income share in about half of the metropolitan areas analyzed.
3. Nationally, the share of adults in the middle class has fallen since 2000 and the shares in the lower- and upper-income tiers have increased.

4. The 10 metropolitan areas with the greatest shares of middle income adults are mostly located in the Midwest.
5. There is notable variation in the median income of middle-class households across U.S. metropolitan areas. For example, the range was from $70,000 in most households, but the highest reported was $81,283 and lowest was $64,549.

Today, more than 43.1 million Americans, including 14.5 million children, live in poverty in the United States (U.S. Census Bureau, 2015b). As explored further in the following sections on race and gender, African American families and those with female heads of households disproportionately account for those living at or below the poverty level. African Americans earn 61% ($31,969) of what non-Hispanic white individuals earn ($52,423). Women continue to earn 80% of what men earn overall (American Association of University Women, 2017; DeNavas-Walt, Proctor, & Smith, 2007).

Canada fares only slightly better, as a widening income disparity also exists there. Whereas the top 10% of incomes represents more than a quarter of total incomes, the bottom 10% only represents 1/40th of total incomes. The 80% in between earn the remaining 75% (Canadian Centre for Policy Alternatives, 2017). The Canadian Index of Wellbeing [CIW] (2012, p. 2) reported that Canada, since 2008, is experiencing an economic backslide. From 1994 to 2010, even though Canada's GDP grew by an impressive 28.9%, improvements in Canadians' well-being grew by a significantly smaller 5.7%. The key message is that despite years of steady economic growth in Canada, this prosperity has not been fairly distributed among the Canadian population (CIW, 2012) because income disparities continue to rise. CIW further pointed out that income inequality, measured as the difference between the richest 20% and the poorest 20% of Canadian families, is particularly problematic because this gap has grown by over 40% since 1994.

In the United States availability of employment-based health coverage has declined from 64.4% in 1997 to 56.5% in 2010. By 2015 the rate had climbed to 90.9% owing to the Affordable Care Act (Barnett & Vornovitsky, 2016). This increase has provided many more citizens and their dependents with health coverage, but many are faced with high deductible plans and high monthly premiums. The highest number of families covered by health insurance remains those with employer-covered care, at 56% of the population. Yet, many employers are requiring higher shared costs of health insurance from their employees.

The number of families living in poverty covered by government-funded programs has steadily grown to 37% of the population. With this continued growth in health care coverage for families in the United States, we are still faced with 29 million children not covered by health insurance, with a majority of those children being African American or Hispanic (Barnett & Vornovitsky, 2016). The cost of health coverage is well beyond the means of those living in or close to the poverty level. Meanwhile, the public debate on an appropriate level of support for families who lack basic housing, food, health services, or social stability continues.

Another important factor that affects poor families is a lack of affordable day care. To relieve stress on the families and to escape poverty, families need reliable and quality day care allowing both parents to work. Child-care costs are estimated at 7% of the income of working families, with higher percentages paid by single working mothers. Working mothers with children under age 18 years pay an average of $143 per week for child care, an increase of $59 per week over the past two decades in spite of no increase in the average mother's annual income ($19,680 in 1990 compared with $19,098 in 2011) (U.S. Census Bureau, 2015b). Although the quality of child care can have a profound effect on the well-being of children, families living in poverty struggle to find and afford this care. Therefore, many families living in poverty rely on older siblings or other family members to care for children during working hours, often placing these children at risk for developmental delays and injuries from accidents.

Multiple other factors worsen the influence of poverty on health outcomes (Woolf, Johnson, Phillips, & Philipsen, 2007), including access to resources, health literacy, gender, ethnicity, and education. All these factors are considered major contributors to poor health, particularly cardiovascular disease (Shikatani et al., 2012), type 2 diabetes (Chaufan, Constantino, & Davis, 2011; Pilkington et al., 2011), higher blood pressure, mental illness (Mental Health Commission of Canada, 2012), and poorer adherence to medications. Children who live in poverty, especially during the early years or for an extended period of time, are at significant risk of poor

health outcomes and developmental delays (American Academy of Pediatrics, 2016). Americans who live in poverty are at higher risk of developing chronic illness, especially depression (Brown, 2012). Even a nominal copay of $2 has been shown to decrease the number of visits to a physician for those living in poverty (USDHHS, 2015a, p. 6). This results in poorer health outcomes. It is important that nurses and other health care providers support policies that help to eradicate poverty and the resulting health disparities (Kirkpatrick & Tarasuk, 2009).

Gender

Gender is a social determinant everywhere, with women and sexual minorities experiencing disparities in access to resources and well-paying jobs (Mikkonen & Raphael, 2010). Women earn less than men when performing the same job, approximately 80% of men's wages (American Association of University Women, 2017; DeNavas-Walt, Proctor, & Smith, 2007), yet they are more likely than men to be heads of single-parent households. In fact, gender is one of the factors that further exacerbates poverty and, in turn, contributes to even greater health disparities. Gender affects health care in other ways as well. For example, women who are at risk of heart disease are 11% less likely than men to have been told they are at risk and receive counseling about risk modification (Leifheit-Limson et al., 2015). Women with ischemic heart disease are more likely to be under-recognized and treated than men (Graham, 2016). Women are also less likely to receive adequate pain management (Gravely & Bair, 2016).

Health Disparities in the Lesbian, Gay, Bisexual, and Transgender (LGBT) Population

Arguably one of the most significant areas of current relevance to family health in North America relates to families with nonheterosexual or non-gender-conforming identities. LGBT families characterize a growing number of households in the United States (U.S. Census Bureau, 2015c). Some estimates from these data suggest that there has been as much as a 51.8% increase in the number of formal same-sex households from the previous decade, although the prevalence in the overall population is still quite small at approximately 1.5% of U.S. households. Approximately 17% of these households have children, with a majority being biological children (U.S. Census Bureau,

2015c). This prevalence is significant because with the federal definition of family currently changing, these couples and parents face several challenges with insurance access, financial benefits and death planning, decision-making abilities, and other key policy-related family health challenges. In Canada, where same-sex marriages are legalized, same-sex marriages have all the rights, duties, and privileges that come with being a married couple. Nevertheless, the stigma associated with homosexuality remains in varying degrees, so the issues cited in the text that follows are similar in both countries.

According to data presented by the *Healthy People 2020* initiative, LGBT individuals face several specific health disparities such as stigma, discrimination-related mental health disorders, and increased rates of suicide and substance abuse (USDHHS, 2013b). Because of systemic and policy-related stigma and barriers, these individuals experience significant differences in health-seeking and health-promoting behaviors: They are far more likely to delay accessing health care; they are less likely to receive preventive screens such as mammograms; and they experience greater alcohol and tobacco use, as well as physical violence, than their heterosexual counterparts (Krehely, 2009). Families with LGBT youth are particularly vulnerable and experience significant family life challenges related to stigma and acceptance. As such, LGBT adolescents experience much higher rates of homelessness, prostitution, and substance use, and they are at increased risk of infectious diseases such as human immunodeficiency virus (HIV), hepatitis, and a host of sexually transmitted infections (Ryan, Huebner, Diaz, & Sanchez, 2009). Additional family policies are needed to decrease these disparities.

To combat these individual and family health problems, San Francisco State University completed a significant family-based intervention project to assist families to develop skills and attributes of acceptance, particularly among families with high degrees of religiosity (Ryan, Russell, Huebner, Diaz, & Sanchez, 2010). Their Family Acceptance Project provided an entire evidence-based family intervention plan and resources available to the general public, along with links to peer-reviewed research aimed to assist families, that can be accessed at http://familyproject.sfsu.edu. Efforts such as these, aimed at assisting families at the individual and community levels, in combination with systems of health research provide an important link between family policy development and LGBT individual and family health issues.

Race and Ethnicity

Racial and ethnic minority groups, or people of First Nation status, tend to have lower incomes and lower-quality jobs (Mikkonen & Raphael, 2010), factors that contribute directly to health disparities. Recent Canadian data show that the health of non-European immigrants of color deteriorates over time whereas the health of European immigrants is actually superior to that of Canadian-born residents. Hispanic and Latino men are three times as likely to contract HIV as white men and Latino populations are disproportionately affected by HIV, accounting for nearly 20% of new infections in the United States (Centers for Disease Control and Prevention [CDC], 2015). Other examples of disparities based on race and ethnicity are as follows: African American, American Indian, and Puerto Rican infants have higher death rates than white infants; African Americans, Hispanics, American Indians, and Alaska Natives are twice as likely to have diabetes than non-Hispanic whites; and Hispanic and African American older adults are less likely than non-Hispanic whites to receive influenza and pneumococcal vaccines (CDC, 2013a; Rodriguez, Chen, & Rodriguez, 2010).

Additionally, members of these groups may experience overt or subtle differences in treatment in the health care system because of discrimination against minority populations. Self-reported racial or ethnic discrimination encountered by health care providers is significantly associated with lower quality of care indicators, such as development of foot disorders and regulation of HbA1c in individuals with diabetes (Peek, Wagner, Tang, Baker, & Chin, 2011). Other recent studies indicate that although minority populations are more likely to require health care, they are less likely to receive health services. Further, even when access is equal, minority populations are far less likely to receive surgical or other therapies. Nurses have the moral obligation to advocate for clients who are faced with discrimination in the system and ensure that they receive the same care and treatment as everyone else.

Presence of Chronic Illness

The presence of chronic illness is a determinant that leads to health disparities beyond the mere presence of the chronic illness. Chronic illness, especially in the face of poverty, often results in poor quality of life and increased financial strain, especially for those who have no or limited access to health care and resources. In severe cases chronic illness also leads to the inability to work and, therefore, forces those who are ill to rely on the social safety net, which has been increasingly cut back over the last 20 years (Mikkonen & Raphael, 2010). Despite improvements in treatment and management strategies for chronic illness improving both quantity and quality of life, social determinants continue to place disadvantaged populations at risk of poor outcomes from chronic illness. Likewise, the presence of chronic illness itself is a determinant that leads to health disparities for and between families. If one family member is ill, then the whole family is affected and often has to pick up the financial and care burden. This is true for the United States and Canada where many medications and access to home care, for example, are not covered by universal health care. The following section explores several common chronic illnesses and the ways that they contribute to health disparities.

Type 2 Diabetes

Type 2 diabetes is on the increase and is four times more likely in low-income communities than in their higher-income counterparts. Lower-income communities often also coincide with high proportions of immigrant populations and people on social assistance (Mikkonen & Raphael, 2010). Health promotion efforts involving diet and exercise to ward off obesity have a significant influence on disease rates; however, they require sufficient resources (Webster, Sullivan-Taylor, & Terner, 2011). Because of a lack of resources, preventive measures, such as keeping a healthy weight, are much less likely in lower-income groups (Chaufan et al., 2011; Dinca-Panaitescu et al., 2012; Raphael et al., 2011). Aboriginal peoples, for example, only developed diabetes when they started to eat Western foods instead of their traditional diets. Before the 1940s, this disease was virtually unknown in that group (Health Canada, 2015).

Dinca-Panaitescu et al. (2012) presented research showing that even with obesity levels the same, diabetes rates were four times higher among those persons who lived in lower-income neighborhoods, confirming that the reasons for this disparity are complex and multilayered. These layers include lack of needed resources for a healthy lifestyle, such as healthy diets; lack of exercise; inability to pay for prescription drugs; lower incomes; unhealthy environments; racial or ethnic discrimination; and stress. Researchers have found evidence that worry

and chronic stress, which lead to high cortisol levels, play a role in chronic disease (Brunner & Marmot, 2006). Chronic stress disproportionately affects most minority ethnic groups who are often subject to discrimination and the constant worries attached to low incomes. When people have to cope with the added expenses of the illness it increases stress further, creating a cycle and exacerbating chronic illness. As stated earlier, the social determinants that create health disparities are multilayered, complex, and mutually reinforcing.

Asthma and Other Lung Diseases

According to the American Lung Association (2017), approximately 9% of adults and children in the United States report a diagnosis of asthma, and the incidence of asthma is increasing with similar reports from Canada (Public Health Agency of Canada, 2012). Direct health costs for treating asthma are estimated to be $10 billion annually. Asthma is the leading chronic illness among children and is the third leading cause of hospitalization for children younger than 15 (American Lung Association, 2017). It is associated with poor-quality physical environments such as regions with increased air pollution and substandard housing. Major asthma attack triggers include secondhand tobacco smoke, dust, pollution, cockroaches, pets, and mold. Less common triggers include exercise, extremes of weather, food, and hyperventilation (National Center for Environmental Health, 2017).

In adults chronic obstructive pulmonary disease (COPD) and lung cancer are serious chronic diseases that shorten life and decrease its quality. Lung diseases, similar to all other diseases, are associated with social determinants such as poverty, as well as with considerable health care costs.

HIV/AIDS

The incidence of HIV infection, although decreasing in many age groups, continues to climb in 25- to 29-year-olds. During 2010 to 2014, 33.4 individuals age 25 to 29 years per 100,000 in the United States were diagnosed with HIV infection. Those individuals of color continue to have a higher infection rate, with African Americans of all age groups being diagnosed at a rate of 44.3 individuals per 100,000 compared with Whites at 5.3 individuals per 100,000 (CDC, 2015a). Although this infection is more successfully treated with antiviral medications, those living in poverty and of color continue to struggle with access to care to delay the onset of AIDS.

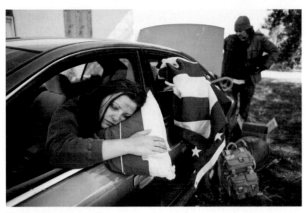

© *iStock.com/powerofforever*

Mental Illness

Mental illness is widespread and very debilitating, particularly because of the stigma attached. It is estimated that one in five persons in North America will have a mental illness at some point in his or her life. Mental illness can strike at any age, including childhood. Those with mental illness who are poor are more likely to end up homeless and destitute (Canadian Mental Health Association [CMHA], 2009).

Cancer and Heart Disease

In North America it is estimated that four persons out of ten will develop cancer in their lifetime. In recent years, with improved detection and treatments, many cancers are now cured or, similar to HIV infection, can become chronic diseases that people live with for many years. In Canada the top three causes of deaths are cancer, cardiovascular diseases, and cerebrovascular disease. Twenty-nine percent of all deaths in Canada are from heart disease (Statistics Canada, 2017). As persons with chronic illnesses live and work within their communities, they need to learn how to self-manage their conditions (see Chapter 9 for more about self-management in chronic illness). (Nurses have a large role to play here as advocates and coaches when they care for individuals and families within the context of their physical and social environments. One of the roles of nurses to help clients with chronic diseases is teaching health literacy.

Health Literacy

Health literacy, first noted in the *Healthy People 2010* objectives and more recently identified in the *Healthy People 2020* objectives, is defined as "the degree to which individuals have the capacity to obtain, process, and understand basic health information and services needed to make appropriate health decisions" (USDHHS, 2010, p. 1). Health literacy is one of the social determinants that contributes to health disparities; however, although a relationship between health disparities and health literacy has been established, it is complex. The IOM found that approximately 9 out of 10 adults have difficulty understanding health information (IOM, 2011), and the Canadian Council on Learning (2007) found 60% of Canadians are health illiterate. Individuals with low health literacy do not understand health information; this affects their health outcomes disproportionately because they seek fewer health screenings, they use urgent or emergency care, they experience errors in medication dosing and scheduling, they lack alternatives in treatment regimens, and they are unable to access accurate health-related information.

As educators and advocates, nurses must consider the health literacy of the patients and families that they serve (Office of Disease Prevention and Health Promotion, 2017). Explaining health-related concepts in plain language will help to ensure that patients understand the information correctly. Nurses may also assist families by filling out complicated forms when applying for social support or filing insurance claims (Street Health Report, 2007).

Risks and Behaviors That Contribute to Health Disparities

This section focuses on the behavioral health determinants that contribute to health disparities. In popular discussions, and sometimes among health care providers, health-related behaviors are treated as resulting solely from conscious choice by individuals who are to blame if their risky behavior leads to poor health outcomes. Many health activists, by contrast, seek to place blame on commercial interests that profit from these behaviors or on government policies that protect them. Research on the causes of risky behaviors is much less developed than is research on the consequences of such behaviors. Even so, it is clear that these risky behaviors are the result of multiple causes and can be influenced by health policy in multiple ways (Braveman & Gottlieb, 2014). This section explores obesity, alcohol use, smoking, and other risk factors specifically pertinent to adolescents.

Obesity

In North America, one of the most disturbing trends in health over the past decade has been the increase in the proportion of the population that is overweight or obese. Obesity is defined as body mass index (BMI) at or above the 95th percentile of the sex-specific BMI, according to the CDC's BMI-for-age growth charts (CDC, 2010). BMI is calculated as weight in kilograms divided by the square of height in meters. Obese people are more likely than are those of normal weight to suffer from heart disease, stroke, diabetes, gallstones, sleep apnea, and some types of cancer (CDC, 2017a). Hypertension, musculoskeletal problems, and arthritis tend to be more severe in people who are obese. Obesity increased little in the U.S. population between the early 1960s and 1980. Since 1980, however, obesity has increased dramatically in the United States. Fifteen percent of American adults were obese in the mid-to-late 1970s. The prevalence of obesity doubled in the two subsequent decades to 31% by 2000; by 2010, nearly 36% of adults were obese (CDC, 2012). Women (36.2%) are more likely than men (32.6%) to be obese (Shields, Carroll, & Ogden, 2011).

Obesity rates are lower in Canada than in the United States, but Canadian rates have also increased rapidly in recent years. Approximately 24% of Canadian adults were obese in the period from 2007 to 2009 (Shields et al., 2011). In contrast with the United States, men in Canada were more likely to be obese than women; trends in the incidence of obesity are now similar for both: Between 2007 and 2009, 24.3% of men and 23.9% of women were obese in Canada (Shields et al., 2011).

Between 2009 and 2010, more than one third of adults age 65 and older in the United States were obese (CDC, 2012). Since 1999 the incidence of obesity among older adults has increased, especially among men. With projections for the number of older adults to more than double from 44.2 to 88.5 million by 2050, obesity in this group will contribute significantly to health care costs (Fakhouri, Ogden, Carroll, Kit, & Flegal, 2012).

The percentage of children and teenagers who are obese has been increasing dramatically since the 1980s. In the mid 1980s in the United States, only 5% of children were obese, yet by the early 2000s obesity increased to 18% among children and adolescents (Federal Interagency Forum on Child and Family Statistics, 2014). The CDC (2016) revealed for the first time in decades that there is a slight improvement in obesity rates in the United States among preschool children who live in low poverty and receive Women, Infant, and Children (WIC) services. From 2008 through 2011, data were collected in 43 states and territories for preschool children who participate in the Women, Infants, and Children (WIC) federally funded program. There was a slight decrease in the obesity rates in 19 of these states, with the largest decrease of 1% in Florida, Georgia, Missouri, New Jersey, and South Dakota. One factor that could contribute to this new trend is changes in the WIC program, which include eliminating juice from food packets, including fewer foods with saturated fats, and providing easier access to fruits and vegetables. Along with these changes, the breastfeeding rates in the United States continue to increase. Although this is an excellent trend, childhood obesity remains of deep concern as one in eight children are obese, with one in five African American children and one in six Hispanic children still obese. Boys and girls have been historically about equal in their likelihood to be overweight, but between 2007 and 2008 a higher percentage of boys (21.2%) were obese than girls (17.3%). Mexican American and African American teenagers are more likely to be overweight than are non-Hispanic white teenagers. Between 2007 and 2008, the percentage of overweight Mexican American teenagers was 24.2% compared with 22.4% for African Americans and 17.4% for whites (Federal Interagency Forum on Child and Family Statistics, 2014).

Obesity in Canadian children has nearly tripled in the last 3 decades (Government of Canada, 2016). In 2014, 6.3% (125,000) of 12- to 17-year-old Canadian youth were obese and 16.9% (343,000) were considered as overweight (Statistics Canada, 2014). Of these children who had excess weight, 28.5% were boys and 16.9% were girls. Similarly the obesity rates have increased in children from the United States, which has more than tripled since 1970 (CDC, 2017b).

Children who are overweight experience many physical health conditions. They are at risk for having other chronic illnesses, such as asthma (Lang, 2014), bone and joint problems (Widhalm et al., 2014), type 2 diabetes (Hagman, Danielsson, Brandt, Ekbom, & Marcus, 2016), and increased risk for heart disease (Ajala, Mold, Boughton, Cooke, & Whyte, 2017). In addition, these children are bullied and teased more than other children and often suffer from isolation, depression and lower self-esteem (Puhl, Latner, O'Brien, Luedicke, & Forhan, 2016). Obesity in childhood is a known precursor to obesity in adulthood (Faienza, Wang, Fruhbeck, Garruti, & Portincasa, 2016).

The costs of obesity and related medical conditions for children through adulthood in the U.S. is estimated to be as high as $141 billion annually in outpatient visits, prescription medications, and emergency room visits (Finkelstein et al., 2012). The most common recommendations for the treatment of overweight and obesity include participating in physical exercise and following dietary guidelines for healthy eating. Although healthy diets and exercise are part of the solution to the obesity epidemic, nurses must consider constraining social and policy factors determining health, including lack of access to healthy foods, unsafe neighborhoods with limited facilities for physical exercise, and cultural beliefs and attitudes about weight and health. Overall, we know that losing weight reduces and sometimes corrects type 2 diabetes. Obesity plays a major role in cardiovascular diseases and puts unnecessary stress on joints, which causes them to become deteriorated with painful arthritic symptoms. In general this condition leads to debilitating health problems and may also lead to self-esteem issues, particularly in younger people.

Tobacco

Smoking and substance abuse are critical behavioral health determinants that lead to multiple health disparities among families in the United States and Canada. Although smoking is still prevalent, it has declined steadily among adults in the United States. In 1965 more than half of adult men smoked, as did a third of adult women (USDHHS, 2015b). Smoking has declined more rapidly for men than for women, and the gap between sexes has narrowed. By 2011, approximately 21.5% of adult men and 17.3% of adult women were current smokers. Prevalence of cigarette smoking is highest among American Indians/Alaska Natives (31.4%), followed by whites (21.0%), African Americans (20.6%), Hispanics (12.5%), and Asians (excluding Native Hawaiians and other Pacific Islanders) (9.2%) (USDHHS, 2015b). In Canada, just under 4 million or just over 1 in 10 Canadians reported smoking regularly or occasionally (Government of Canada, 2016b). As in the United States, more men (24.2%) were smokers than women (17.4%) (Statistics Canada,

2016). More Canadians are trying e-cigarettes. In 2015 3.9 million or 13% of Canadians 15 years or older reported trying e-cigarettes compared to 2.5 million or 9% in 2013 (Government of Canada, 2016b).

Smoking is a significant behavioral health determinant. It harms most body organs, reduces circulation, and causes several diseases, including coronary heart disease, chronic obstructive lung diseases, lung cancer, leukemia, and other types of cancer. Smoking also has adverse reproductive effects and is associated with infertility problems, low birth weight, and stillbirth. Smokers are at higher risk than nonsmokers of developing many other diseases and chronic health conditions (USDHHS, 2015a). The myriad of health implications from smoking are of critical importance for nurses to consider when planning care for families with members who smoke. The impact of the behavior on the entire family should be included in all health teaching, with realistic goals set by the nurse and family in collaboration with one another.

Alcohol

Use of alcohol is a risk factor and determinant for a wide range of poor physical and mental health outcomes. Alcohol use is legal for adults, although impaired driving (DUI) and, to a lesser extent, public drunkenness are banned. Alcohol use is illegal for minors, although widely tolerated in both the United States and Canada. In 2011, 62.6% of American adult men (age 21 or older) and 50.9% of American adult women reported that they currently drank alcohol. Almost one third of men and 16% of women reported "binge drinking" (defined as the consumption of five or more drinks on one occasion for men and four or more drinks for women) during the preceding month. In the United States, non-Hispanic whites were statistically more likely than other race groups to be current drinkers, whereas Native Americans were statistically more likely than other race groups to be binge drinkers (CDC, 2013b). In Canada in 2011, 18.7% of those who consumed alcohol engaged in chronic drinking, defined as 10 or more drinks per week for women and 15 or more for men; and 13.1% engaged in acute drinking, defined as three or more drinks during a single occasion for women and four or more drinks for men (Health Canada, 2015).

The prevalence of illegal drug use, the particular drugs used, and the methods in which they are taken vary considerably over time among racial and ethnic groups, across social and economic classes, and among regions of the country or even neighborhoods. The following statistics are all from the Substance Abuse and Mental Health Services Administration National Survey on Drug Use and Health from 2013 (National Institute on Drug Abuse, 2015). In 2013 an estimated 24.6 million Americans or 9.4% of the population over the age of 12 reported using an illicit drug in the last month (National Institute on Drug Abuse, 2015). The use of marijuana has increased from 14.5 million (5.8% of those over the age of 12) to 19.8 million (7.5% of those over the age of 12). Methamphetamine use is on the rise with an increase from 353,000 in 2010 to 595,000 in 2013. Most new people who use drugs are in their teens with about 7800 new users a day in the United States. More than half of the 7800 new drug users start with marijuana. Drug use is highest in people between 18–20 years of age with 22.6% of the population reporting drug use. However, drug use is increasing in those who are in their fifties and sixties, which is thought to be related to the aging baby boomer population.

Although drinking by underage persons from 12–20 has declined between 2002 and 2013 from 28.8% to 22.7% (National Institute on Drug Abuse, 2015). Binge drinking is more common among men (30.2%) compared to women (16.0%). Alcohol and substance abuse have serious consequences for individual health. Individuals who engage in excessive drinking are more likely to suffer from high blood pressure and to develop chronic diseases such as liver cirrhosis, pancreatitis, and different types of cancers (Dasgupta, 2011). Excessive drinking also affects psychological health. In addition, substance abuse causes unintentional injuries produced by car accidents, drowning, falls, and other types of incidents.

Adolescent Health Practices and High Risk Behaviors

Once children survive the first year of life, the risk of death decreases dramatically (Federal Interagency Forum on Child and Family Statistics, 2014). The risk of death increases again in the teen years as youths, especially male and minority youths, are subject to heightened threat of fatal motor vehicle accidents and homicides. In the United States, African American teenage males are more often victims of homicide than teens in other racial and ethnic groups (Federal Interagency Forum on Child and Family Statistics, 2014). For young Americans ages 10 to 24 years, the most common cause of death

in 2014 was unintentional injuries, accounting for 40% of deaths in this age group. The second most common cause of death was suicide, accounting for 17% of deaths, followed by homicides at 15% among this age group (Heron, 2016). Additionally, the risk of dying for those between 10 and 24 years of age was more than twice as high for boys as for girls. Asian or Pacific Islander teenage girls have the lowest mortality rates and African American teenage boys have the highest, at 99 per 1000 youth (Federal Interagency Forum on Child and Family Statistics, 2014). These distressing statistics can be attributed to the fact that adolescents are engaging in many high risk adult behaviors such as driving, using alcohol and drugs, and increasing their independence—all without the experience of adults.

Still, in the United States, from 1991 to 2014, adolescent smoking and alcohol consumption significantly declined (Federal Interagency Forum on Child and Family Statistics, 2014). And although the use of illicit drugs increased substantially in the mid 1990s, these rates likewise decreased during the 2000s. Despite some historical fluctuations in the rate of smoking over the last several decades, by 2014 only 11% of high school seniors reported regular cigarette use in the last month (Federal Interagency Forum on Child and Family Statistics, 2014; Kann et al., 2016). Smoking is more likely among white adolescents than among youths in minority populations, and more common among males than females in all ethnic and racial groups. African Americans were the least likely to report engaging in most of these behaviors (Kann et al., 2016). The rates of alcohol use for Canadian adolescents remained relatively stable during the 1990s but decreased in the 2000s. During 2013 the rates of alcohol use were 60% for both boys and girls ages 15 to 19 years, with 20% drinking to excess (Government of Canada, 2013). Fewer Canadian adolescents smoke today than was the case a decade ago. In 2013 slightly more than 11% of adolescents ages 15 to 19 smoked daily or occasionally compared with nearly 30% in 1994 (Government of Canada, 2013).

Researchers evaluating large data sets of representative samples of young people over time, such as the National Study of Adolescent Health, are beginning to untangle the effects of peer influences, family factors, school climate, and neighborhood contexts on youth risk-taking behavior (CDC, 2016). As this section reflects, multiple, complex, and challenging factors contribute to the nurse's ability to evaluate risks and behaviors that lead to health disparities. Families comprised of members demonstrating one or more of these risks or behaviors may present challenges to the nurse as he or she develops a comprehensive plan of care that meets the needs of all family members. Nevertheless, it is important that each family member be assessed and evaluated for high risk behaviors and risks for health disparities when creating a family plan of care.

HEALTH CARE POLICIES

Health Care Policies in the United States

The Emergence of Universal Health Care

Providing health care to families based on a human rights and legal perspective may promote health equity by transforming and developing policies, programs, and laws that inhibit the limited or restricted access to health care services to families. Ethical issues emerge with the definition of family and how social determinants shape health in the United States. Social insurance and universal programs funded through taxes protect citizens who are facing economic hardships resulting from a loss of wages, retirement, illness and disability, or the death of the primary wage earner (Karger & Stoesz, 2002).

President Theodore Roosevelt attempted to enact a national health care policy in the early 1900s (Physicians for a National Health Program, 2016). Mimicking insurance plans that protect against adversity, the first social insurance policy was the Old-Age, Survivors, and Disability Insurance (OASDI), signed into law by President Franklin D. Roosevelt and commonly called the Social Security Act of 1935. The Social Security Act was the government's direct response to the Great Depression and offered minimum income to unemployed and retired workers. The federal government also provided survivor benefits to widows and children and services for older adults, persons who were blind, and children with disabilities. Other money was set aside for vocational therapy, public health care in rural areas, and educating public professionals.

Later in 1939, President Roosevelt attempted to pass the Wagner National Health Act, which was taken out of the Social Security Bill. Despite the collapse of the Wagner National Health Act, the study of health care remained in the Social Security Act. The passage of this New Deal policy marked one of the greatest contributions to a universal health care program in the United States. Following the enactment of the Social Security Act of 1935, the Truman administration added the Old-Age and Survivors Insurance section of this act, which provided 60 days of hospital insurance per year for retired adults ages 60 and older (Oberlander & Laugesen, 2015). It took the country until the 1960s to reexamine health care concerns at the national level. The Medicare and Medicaid Services enacted in 1966 were similar to national health care services provided to citizens in other Westernized countries (Kaiser Family Foundation, 2015).

Contemporary Medicare and Medicaid Services

The U.S. Centers for Medicare (2017a) and Medicaid Services (2017b) is a current government agency in the United States with responsibility for Medicare, Medicaid, the State Health Insurance Children's Program (SCHIP, now known more commonly as CHIP), the Health Insurance Portability and Accountability Act (HIPAA), and the Clinical Laboratories Improvement Amendment (CLIA). Medicare is a health insurance program for people 65 years and older, certain younger people with disabilities, and those with end-stage renal disease (ESRD). Medicare covers more than 55 million persons on an annual basis (Kaiser Family Foundation, 2015), with a growth from 19 million in 1966 to 52 million in 2012. The recent increase in the growth of Medicare recipients can be explained in large part by the number of baby boomers now aging into Medicare benefits (Kaiser Family Foundation, 2015).

There are four parts to Medicare:

- *Part A* provides inpatient hospital care, care in nursing facilities, hospice care, and a limited amount of home care services (U.S. Centers for Medicare & Medicaid Services, 2017c).
- *Part B* of the Medicare program covers some of the costs associated with physician and outpatient care, medical supplies, and preventive services.
- Known as Medicare Advantage Plans, *Part C* is a nongovernmental plan. Private companies hold contracts with Medicare, offering Parts A and B services. Humana Medicare Advantage is an example of a health maintenance organization that contracts health insurance to Medicare recipients.

Other Advantage Plans may be organized as preferred provider organizations, private fee-for-service plans, special needs plans, and Medicare medical savings account plans.

■ *Part D*, Prescription Drug Coverage, is another feature of Medicare. Medicare.gov at https://www.medicare.gov/part-d/ outlines some of the plans used to cover prescription drug costs, such as Medicare private-fee-for-services and Medicare medical savings account plans. To put prescription drug costs in context, Schondelmeyer and Purvis (2016) report that brand name drugs used for a prolonged period of time may cost an average of $5800 per year. For the average older adult who takes 4.5 prescription drugs on a monthly basis, the annual cost of pre-scription drugs may be as high as $26,000 per year. Medicare beneficiaries are allocated $24,150.00 for prescription drugs.

The enactment of Medicaid moved health care for vulnerable populations from the responsibility of state and local governments and charitable orga-nizations to the federal government. Medicaid is a federal–state partnership health insurance program for eligible groups with lower income. In contrast with Medicare, which is managed by the federal government, Medicaid is managed by individual states. Unlike Medicare, Medicaid is a means-test public assistance program, or only offered to those who meet specific criteria, rather than a universal plan (Karger & Stoesz, 2002). Further, Medicaid is not a social insurance program. Medicaid offers health care to persons living in poverty by physicians who accept patients who rely on Medicaid. Discussed later in this chapter, an expansion of Medicaid was a feature of the Patient Protection and Affordable Care Act of 2010 (Affordable Health Care Act or PPACA). The federal government outlined a provision to assist citizens whose incomes fell underneath 138% of the federal poverty level. This would equate to $12,060 for individuals to $24,600 for a family with four members (U.S. Centers for Medicare & Medicaid Services, 2016). Looking at the influence of the expansion of Medicaid, McMorrow, Kenny, Long, and Gates (2017) reported a decline in the uninsured rate for people who are poor and childless from 45.4% in 2013 to 16.5% in 2015.

In addition to Medicare and Medicaid, CHIP was enacted in 1997 to address the lack of health insurance coverage for children who did not qualify for Medicaid (U.S. Centers for Medicare & Medicaid Services 2017c). Similar to Medicaid, this program represents a federal–state government partnership. States have three options for implementing CHIP: (1) creating a new health care program for children; (2) building on the current Medicaid program; or (3) using some combination of these two options. For example, more than 28 million children were covered by Medicaid with an additional 5.7 million receiving health care via the CHIP program (Rudowitz, Artiga, & Arguello, 2014). The disparities in health care coverage for children varies across states. For example, approximately 50% of children receive Medicaid coverage in Mississippi, New Mexico, and West Virginia compared with fewer than 30% in Maryland, Rhode Island, and Utah (Kaiser Family Foundation, 2015). Ten percent of children remain with no health coverage in Alaska and Oklahoma compared with fewer than 5% of children without health care coverage in California, Alabama, and Tennessee. Overall, 39% of children in the United States are covered by Medicaid and 48% are covered through an employer's insurance program. Given the health disparities in adults, it is not surprising that a greater number of poor children and children of color are more likely to be covered by CHIP and Medicaid than family or parental health care plans compared with children from white families.

To continue to promote the well-being of children, the federal government expanded the CHIP program. In 2009, President Obama signed the Children's Health Insurance Program Reauthorization Act (CHIPRA) into law, which has been extended through September 2017, providing new financial resources and options to expand and improve health coverage for children through both Medicaid and CHIP (National Conference of State Legislatures, 2017). Hopefully, the CHIP program will be reauthorized beyond 2017 even though services are financed until 2019. This restructuring of the program allocated over $25.5 billion to help states insure low income children. During 2016, 8.9 million children were enrolled in CHIP (Center for Children and Fam-ilies, 2017).

Also worth noting is the Prenatal Care Assistance Program (PCAP), which targets pregnant women who meet certain income requirements and are eligible for part of the Medicaid system. The PCAP program includes prenatal care, delivery services, postpartum care up to 2 months after the birth of the baby, referral to the Women, Infants, and Children

(WIC) program, and infant care for 1 year (United States Department of Agriculture, 2015).

Because in the United States the majority of government health care programs are managed and delivered by individual states with only partial monetary support by the federal program, the burden to state budgets is enormous. Some unique programs have been implemented to help individual states bridge this gap in costs of health care coverage.

Patient Protection and Affordable Care Act

The United States is in the midst of a transition to a more affordable and accessible health care system. The Patient Protections and Affordable Care Act (PPACA) of 2010 (2010) had the goal of universal health care for every citizen. The objectives of this act included:

1. To decrease the number of uninsured U.S. citizens
2. To decrease the health costs in the United States
3. To improve the efficiency of health care
4. To decrease discrimination by insurance companies based on preexisting conditions
5. To improve health care outcomes (Levitsky, 2013)

The intent of this act was to assure that every American citizen be covered by health insurance through the workplace, through the federal or state government (i.e., Medicare and Medicaid Services), or through private purchase of insurance. The PPACA also assured a *Patient Bill of Rights* that placed restrictions on denying insurance based on preexisting conditions, and that no insurance company could increase annual rates above 10%. The act also provided free services for expectant mothers, contraceptive care, domestic violence screening and treatment, and well-women's health care. Finally, the CHIP program was expanded to every state and included free well-child checks, vaccinations, vision examinations, behavioral assessment and care, and screening for autism for low-income children. Beginning in 2013, the approximately 40 million uninsured U.S. citizens were able to access health coverage through the Health Insurance Marketplace, a set of government-regulated and standardized health care plans that allowed those without insurance to submit one application to choose from multiple private-sector policies. The selection was based on their individual eligibility and ability to pay the set monthly premiums (Levitsky, 2013).

Despite much legislative and legal wrangling, the PPACA was upheld by the U.S. Supreme Court in 2012 and implementation efforts began in 2013 (Kaiser Family Foundation, 2012). Although the PPACA achieved its intended goals, it did not specifically intend to, nor succeed at, decreasing health disparities as many hoped it would. Rather, the goal of U.S. citizens having access to health care insurance was achieved. The outcome still left many without the ability to pay for needed services beyond limited preventative care and without affordable health care to treat acute and chronic conditions unless they qualified for Medicaid. Further, even those who qualified for Medicaid or Medicare often could not find a provider willing to take state or federally funded insurance, and high deductible rates set by the insurance companies were a burden to most outside the Medicare and Medicaid Services. A clear distinction to consider is that access to health insurance does not guarantee access to quality, affordable, and equitable health care.

Despite the progress brought by these recent changes to the health care system, the United States continues to face health disparity. The long-standing lack of universally available health care has resulted in a return to trying to establish a health care system that meets the needs of the citizens, the insurance companies, and the providers. The basic question continues to be debated: "Do the citizens of the U.S. have a right to health care?" (Levitsky, 2013). An often cited conservative view is that health and health care is an individual responsibility reliant on individual choices (Stahl, 2016). Because of the liberal view that the PPACA did not decrease health disparities and the conservative view that the act encouraged health care as an unattainable and inappropriate right, the PPACA is being threatened by the current administration of the United States. To date, however, a new replacement system has not yet been approved. Seven different programs have been considered for review, with recommended changes centering around allowing individuals to purchase insurance across state lines, increasing Medicare age eligibility to 67 years old, decreasing eligibility for Medicaid services, changing tax liabilities and benefits for employers and citizens, and changing policies for how individual states can use federal dollars (Kaiser Family Foundation, 2015).

Currently, there are no policies that guarantee the right to health care in the United States with the exception of the social insurance program of Medicare and need-based programs and policies. These include Medicaid services laws prohibiting denial of health care based on discriminatory grounds. An example of this is the Emergency Medical Treatment and Active Labor Act (EMTALA), which assures that hospitals cannot refuse to treat anyone who comes to the emergency room for care regardless if they can pay or not or have insurance coverage, however this act has remained an unfunded mandate since created in 1986 (American College of Emergency Physicians, 2016). This act, however, does not guarantee diagnosis and ongoing treatment, but rather stabilization of symptoms with the assumption that the individual will receive comprehensive care from a primary care provider or outpatient specialist (Levitsky, 2013).

In 2015 the National Health Interview Survey (CDC, 2015b) found that 83.6% of adults aged 18 or older reported having contact with a primary care provider. The majority of the people reporting seeing a primary care provider within 6 months were those over 75 years of age. The percent of children who had contact with a primary care provider in the past year was 93.0%. Children 0–4 years had the most contact, followed by 5–11 years, then 12–17 years of age. In 2011, National Hospital Ambulatory Medical Care Survey (CDC, 2011), the number of hospital outpatient visits totaled 125.7 million with those in the 45–64 age range having the most visits. In 2013, the number of visits to a physician's office was 922.6 million (CDC, 2013c), with those in the 45–64 age range having the most visits. The number of emergency room visits in 2013 totaled 130.4 million, of which 37.2 million being injury-related visits, 12.2 million resulting in hospital admission of which 1.5 million were to critical care units (CDC, 2013d).

For family nurses, another important model of care to consider is family-focused care. This model of primary care includes the family as the client and recognizes the importance of addressing all family members when caring for an individual with health care needs. This is especially important for children with special health care needs (CSHCN) because family-focused care has shown to improve health outcomes across time. A recent study using the 2005 to 2006 National Survey of Children with Special Health Care Needs found that only 66% of families with CSHCN received family-focused care. Of further concern is that the biggest predictor of not receiving family-focused care was those families of color or those with English as a second language (ESL). These variables were stronger in predicting lack of family-focused care above socioeconomic levels, education levels, family structure, and urban-versus-rural geographic areas (Coker, Rodriguez, & Flores, 2010). The importance of primary care, especially family-focused primary care, cannot be overstated. Yet, similar to many other areas of health disparity, specific groups continue to struggle to obtain primary care, leading to continued negative health outcomes. Health policies can make a difference and have done so in other countries.

Health Care Policies in Other Countries

Other countries, including countries in South America, South Africa, Europe, and Asia, support laws and national policies with funding to protect civil rights, political rights, and social welfare rights. Social welfare rights include security, housing, education, clean water, food, and *health care*. In spite of programs that not only cover universal health care but also face challenges such as access and treatment of HIV/AIDS, prescription medications, reproductive health care, and comprehensive preventive health care, national health care costs in these nations are consistently lower than that in the United States. The United States is unique in its struggle with the ongoing debate on whether health care should be governed by citizens' social rights versus market value and fiscal profits for those administering or providing health care. In spite of the majority of the public consistently stating that health care should be a right, there have not been any policies that reflect this opinion. Another fear that prevents universal health care policies from being passed in the United States is a fear that, because of the expense of universal health care, health care would be rationed. This is because of the outcome of other rationing programs across history, including rationing of food and gas during World War II and rationing of gas with long gas lines during the oil crisis of 1976. Health care, however, is currently already rationed through pricing, employment, and access (Hoffman, 2012).

Health Care Policies in Canada

By way of contrast, Canada has boasted universal, federally funded health care access for physicians' services, hospital care, and diagnostics since the 1966

Medical Care Act (Canadian Museum of History, 2010). The Medical Care Act Canada 1966 has had a major influence on family policy affecting health care. It ensures that on a national level hospital care, doctor's visits, and diagnostic services are accessible to everyone without charge. Many people also have additional extended benefit plans through their employers for medication coverage, dental care, and other therapies. Persons who are on social assistance programs, such as welfare or disability pensions, as well as those receiving old-age pensions have additional publicly funded coverage for essential medications and basic dental care. However, these additional benefits do not extend to those working for low wages with no additional benefits and who often cannot afford their medications (Pilkington et al., 2010). Although some provincially funded coverage is available for this group, obtaining it is very difficult; it is only meant for dire situations of need and disqualifies most of those working for low wages. Therefore, many prescriptions remain unfilled because choices have to be made between paying the rent, feeding the family, and buying medications (Pilkington et al., 2010). Although universal health care exists, it does not cover all aspects of health. Similar to other Westernized countries with universal health care, there remains a gap in the health care delivery for those who lack private insurance. Provinces and municipalities in Canada provide long-term care for persons in need, but access to care is a challenge because of an insufficient number of facilities and providers. At times, some provinces have attempted to implement user fees for doctor and emergency department visits. Because of immense public pressure, the federal government has thus far stepped in to stop this practice. One policy severely curtailing federal health care funding for refugees was implemented in 2012 by the federal government, leaving this vulnerable and often traumatized group unprotected (Canadian Association of Community Health Centres, 2012; Service Canada, 2012). This move was seen as a major injustice by the public as well as physicians' and nurses' associations. This act was also criticized by hospital groups and community health centers who have voiced a strong and unified opposition to this policy. In the meantime, much-needed care for refugees is provided by free volunteer health care providers, whereas individual hospitals and provinces are absorbing the costs for emergency treatments within their general budgets (CACHC, 2012).

HEALTH PROMOTION POLICIES

Health promotion generates health improvements through multiple approaches of research, public education, changes in the physical and social environment, regulation of disease- and injury-promoting activities or behaviors, and improved access to high-quality health care through policies that mitigate disparities and promote equity. For effective outcomes, these policies must consider the social determinants of health as the foundational concepts influencing health (Marmot, 1993; Mikkonen & Raphael, 2010). In 1990, at the urging of the U.S. Surgeon General, the U.S. federal government published a national agenda for health promotion titled *Healthy People 2000* that identified 319 objectives for health promotion and set measurable goals for achieving them. Many of the objectives for the decade dealt with health behaviors such as physical activity and exercise; tobacco, alcohol, and drug use; violent and abusive behaviors; safer sexual practices; and behaviors designed to prevent or mitigate injuries. These objectives were set as national goals to be realized through a combination of public sector, private sector, community, and individual efforts (see National Center for Health Statistics (2011) for a complete list of objectives and an assessment of progress toward their achievement). The outcomes to date appear to be mixed with considerable success in some areas, including increases in moderate physical activity; moderate improvements in some others, including decreases in "binge drinking" and increases in safer sexual practices; and little progress in some other behavioral objectives, including marijuana use and tobacco use during pregnancy (National Center for Health Statistics, 2011). A new set of objectives and measurable goals were established in *Healthy People 2010* and revised again in *Healthy People 2020*. The relevant *Healthy People* goals provide a standardized approach to assess changes in behaviors that determine health outcomes. Numerous tables in the statistical yearbooks published by the National Center for Health Statistics form a scorecard for this national health promotion effort.

Ensuring access to health and illness care services is one way to improve the health of individuals and families. Health promotion efforts aimed at the first five years of life are known to reduce the population level burden of disease (Mistry et al., 2012). Using upstream approaches, children should receive necessary immunizations and should be evaluated on a regular basis for normal growth and development. Likewise, it is important that adults be adequately immunized and screened for hypertension, diabetes, and cancer at appropriate ages and intervals. The Canadian government introduced the Healthy Kids Strategy (Webb, 2013) with the focus on health promotion of children including support before and during pregnancy, early years, initiatives to promote healthy eating and building healthy environments for children in their communities. The approach is to address health in young children to improve the longer term health outcomes.

Although much emphasis has been on the roles parents have in ensuring that their children receive needed services, many adults also have responsibilities for the health care of aging parents. Adults with both children and aging parents dependent for support struggle with access to health care and management of illnesses and therefore experience a particularly difficult burden in today's world. They are referred to as the "sandwich generation" and are in danger of caregiver burnout (Boyczuk & Fletcher, 2016). Adequate supports for families are needed so they do not have to shoulder the burden of care alone. Suggestions for promising approaches are health coaches, particularly registered nurses (RNs), who develop a trusting relationship with their clients and act as advisors and resources for the clients. The RN-Health Coach was recently introduced in the United States with good results and is currently piloted in Canada as well (Change Foundation, 2013).

Avoiding Growing Health Care Disparities

There are several areas in particular need of additional family policy to help stem growing disparities.

Elder Care

In 2012 the population of people aged 65 or over in the United States was 43.1 million (USDHHS, 2013c). The Administration on Aging (USDHHS, 2013c) predicts that by 2040 there will be about 79.7 million and by 2060 that number will increase to 92 million. The number of the population of those 85 years and over was 5.9 million and is expected to triple to 14.1 million by 2040.

About half of the people over 65 years (57%) in 2012 lived with their spouse (USDHHS, 2013c). Of those 71% (13.8 million) were older men and 45% (10.7 million) were women. About 8.4 million women and 3.7 million men lived alone. Among the women 75 and older almost half lived alone.

The provision of care to the elderly is growing both as a family responsibility and as a profession. More women are caregivers than men. Policies such as the Family and Medical Leave Act are written as gender neutral, but women experience a general expectation that they will be the caregivers regardless of the burden that places on them. Lay caregivers are unpaid, which benefits social programs, especially Medicare and Medicaid. Home care in Canada is also poorly funded and benefits enormously from free labor by family members. Women who provide lay home health care experience much greater levels of stress than their other family members, as well as more alienation from those outside of the home (Revenson et al., 2016). Respite care and increased home health nursing and other supports are needed here to ease the burden (Bookman, Harrington, Pass, & Reisner, 2007; Change Foundation, 2013). Recently, some parts of Canada introduced compassionate care benefits, which apply when the death of a family member is expected within the next 6 months. A family caregiver can be granted up to 6 weeks leave from work, during which time she receives Employment Insurance benefits (Employment Insurance Compassionate Care Benefits, 2013). Day care for older adults and increasing funding for community-based care in the home would make it easier for older people to stay out of costly institutional care and increase their quality of life. This type of care needs to include house calls by doctors, nurses, physical therapists, and other health care providers if clients are unable to go to appointments. It also needs to focus on home safety (Change Foundation, 2013). It could go a long way toward reducing health disparities imposed by chronic illness by providing access to optimal care for vulnerable older persons.

Women's Reproductive Rights

Women's reproduction is another area where family policy could help stem health disparities. In the United States Medicaid policies and procedures relative to women requesting publically-funded tubal ligations for sterilization have not changed since 1978 (Borrero, Nikki, Potter, & Trussell, 2014). Women who qualify for Medicaid must complete the "Consent to Sterilization" section of the Medicaid Title XIX form at least 30 days and no more than 180 days before undergoing the procedure. It is possible to waive the 30-day requirement, but at minimum 72 hours are required between the request and procedure. Women who desire a tubal ligation immediately after birth are significantly affected by this ruling. Other groups at a disadvantage are low income and women from minority racial and ethnic groups.

In 2014, approximately 30% of women in the United States had an abortion before the age of 45 (Jones & Jerman, 2017). The total number of abortion providers declined 4% from 2008 to 2011. Forty-four laws to limit access to abortions were implemented in 2008–2010 in 18 states. And in 2011 there were 62 additional laws restricting access in 21 states. Even though these laws were passed the national rates of abortion remained constant. However these laws stigmatize abortion and may create fear in women.

On a similar note, some pharmacists across both countries have refused to fill prescriptions for contraceptives, including emergency contraception, stating that doing so is in direct conflict with their moral and personal beliefs (Card, 2017). Women, who are often unaware of these reproductive health issues until they are directly affected, are outraged when pharmacists' beliefs override their right to services. Women have a legal right to access prescription medications. The question is, whose rights prevail? In Canada, religious-based health care institutions, as well as individuals, can also refuse abortions and birth control counseling, although women have the right to these services under the Canadian Charter of Rights and Freedoms. Those who are refusing to provide the services are legally required to refer the women to another practitioner who is willing to perform the service. In underserviced areas, this might mean traveling long distances, which not all women can afford.

In the United States, according to the Guttmacher Institute (2017), 45 states have a policy that allows health care providers, including nurses and pharmacists, to refuse to participate in the delivery of reproductive health services, which could leave many women with no choice regarding their reproductive health. Once again, gender, socioeconomic position, and geography seem to be determinants of health that disproportionately disadvantage women by denying them access to care. Both countries are in need of family policy to help mitigate these disparities.

THE NURSE'S ROLE IN ADVOCACY FOR FAMILY POLICY

An important role of the nurse historically and today is to advocate for family policies to promote the health of clients and families, particularly those who are disadvantaged. As holistic care providers, nurses are in an excellent position to inform the public, including politicians, about what policies are needed and why, and to negotiate for, and help clients and families obtain, the best possible resources established by family policies.

Historical Involvement in Family Policy

Historically, nurses have worked closely with vulnerable populations and developed unique solutions to challenging health care problems. Many of these interventions took place in the community setting and focused on the family, not just the individual. The profession of nursing historically has been involved in social issues and has worked tirelessly to advocate and provide a voice to many vulnerable populations. For example, in 1737 Marguerite Dufrost de Lajemmerais began a now internationally known campaign to serve vulnerable populations. She and her supporters were the first to offer care to vulnerable women in Canada at a time that only men were provided health care in hospitals. Because of her dedication to vulnerable populations, women and native citizens received health care, food, and shelter (The History of the Grey Nuns, n.d.). The Grey Nuns were Catholic, religious sisters who established themselves in the city of Montreal, Canada, and spread to multiple countries across the world (Hardill, 2006). In England, in the mid 19th century, Florence Nightingale began to reform the Poor Houses of London and stressed the importance of the environment in health care (Hardill, 2006; Monteiro, 1985). The Henry Street Settlement (HSS) in New York City, founded by Lillian Wald, likewise demonstrated nursing's role as an advocate for vulnerable populations. Founded in the late 19th century, the mission of the HSS was to provide health care for poor immigrants (Henry Street Settlement, 2017). Today, the HSS continues to function as a community center for families in New York through its midwifery and nurse practitioner program. Mary Breckinridge established the Frontier Nursing

Service (FNS) in Hyden, Kentucky, in 1925. The FNS introduced community-based midwifery care to the women of Appalachia, a vulnerable population with distinct health care needs. These nurses were serving the needs of women and vulnerable minority populations who, at the time, had no human rights, such as voting or owning property.

In the early 20th century, as nursing care moved into the hospital setting, the role of the nurse changed. Nurses lost their autonomous practice as healers and became subordinated to physicians. Care became increasingly centered on the medical model and focused on curing the sick individual as opposed to caring for the human response to illness in the context of the physical and social environments. Assessing the influence of the determinants of health and evaluating their effects on the overall health of the individual and family lost much of its importance because care delivery became focused on the individual's medical diagnosis. Family-focused care increased in awareness in the 1990s, largely because of work by scholars Hanson, Wright, Leahey, Feetham, and Bell. Family nursing grew to an international awareness with the start of the International Family Nursing Association, building a strong foundation for nurses' role in recognizing families and in advocating for family-focused care.

Nursing Today

Numbering more than four million in the United States and 406,817 nurses in Canada with 293,205 RNs, 107,923 LPNs, 5,689 RPNs and 3,966 nurse practitioners (Canadian Institute for Health Information, 2014), nurses comprise the largest segment of the United States and Canadian health care workforce and must be active leaders in improving the access to and quality of health care. Today most front-line nurses in the United States and Canada function primarily in the acute care setting, a practice that supports an inadequate perspective and understanding of the social determinants of health and an associated limitation in advocacy. This limited involvement, however, is changing as the transformation of health care through the Patient Protection and Affordable Care Act (PPACA) in the United States has taken place, and talk in both countries has moved care from institutions into the community.

In 2010 the IOM released a report outlining key recommendations for preparing the nursing workforce to meet the needs of the population: *The*

Future of Nursing: Leading Change, Advancing Health. This landmark report described the need to harness the power of nurses to realize the objectives set forth in the PPACA by transforming the health care system from one that focuses on the provision of acute care services to one that delivers health care where and when it is needed, ensuring access to high-quality preventive care in the community. The IOM committee explained that nurses will need to be full partners in redesigning efforts, to be accountable for their own contributions to delivering high-quality care, and to work collaboratively with leaders from other health care professions by taking responsibility for identifying problems, devising and implementing solutions to those problems, and tracking improvements over time to ensure the health of the population (IOM, 2011).

It is estimated that in the United States one in every 45 voters is a nurse (American Nurses Association, 2014). The Canadian Nurses Association (2013) took a bold step in the role of nurses to address health and social disparities. The Canadian National Expert Commission report, *A Nursing Call to Action: The Health of our Nation, the Future of our Health System* (Canadian Nurses Association, 2012) "recommends that the use of a cost-effective, wellness-based model that places greater emphasis on primary care, health promotion and the prevention and management of chronic diseases" (Canadian Nurses Association, 2013, p. 6). In addition, it suggests that care be moved as much as possible from acute care facilities to community sites. Nurses are designing new nurse-led programs in multiple areas of health care with a specific focus on improving access to care, reducing pain, management of care for chronic conditions and health promotion/prevention.

Advancing health care will require a cultural shift in the expectations of the nursing profession regarding education, practice, and advocacy for vulnerable populations. In Canada, Pilkington et al. (2011) found that, even in community-based health care centers, many nurses failed to take into account the clients' social and housing conditions when planning health education and care because these concepts were not included in the standard nursing assessment forms. The allotted time spent with clients was mostly focused on traditional health teaching about lifestyle changes despite the fact that these same nurses indicated that assessment of access to necessary resources was a critically important component for success in meeting clients' needs to promote their health. This trend emphasizes the need for nursing educators to reexamine how nurses can better understand social and family policy in order to effectively improve the health care of their clients.

Nurses have to look beyond health behaviors and medications as primary interventions and instead look at and treat underlying social issues, including:

- Poverty and the lack of employment security
- Unequal access to health care
- Lack of education and health literacy
- Stigma of mental illness, obesity, and HIV infection
- Racism and social exclusion
- Individual, family, and community stress
- Lack of social support and isolation
- Food insecurity and lack of quality nutrition

The PPACA (2010) made many stipulations that directly affect nurses' role in care and the salient need for nurses to become actively involved in family policy. For example, the PPACA required all adults to have a primary care provider by 2014. This requirement put a strain on an already dearth of family practice physicians. Nursing leaders stepped up and advocated to increase investment in funding education for advanced nurses with the goal of nurses being able to meet the need of primary care access. Likewise, the PPACA increased funding to those who provided care to underserved populations. Nurses increased their efforts to document their care of underserved populations, thereby increasing funding for nursing care across both urban and rural populations (Mahoney & Jones, 2013).

Brewah (2009) recommended integrating advocacy into nursing curricula and staff education. Primomo (2007) studied the influence of an educational intervention on political awareness in a group of graduate nursing students and found that perceived competence among the students increased after the intervention. Hewison (2007) described an organized method for policy analysis to be used by nurse managers. The method involves a process by which a summary of the policy is developed, including its origin and status, a history and link to other policy initiatives, and, finally, themes and elements of nursing practice affected by the policy. Once the analysis is concluded, the nurse can take a position on whether this policy will meet the needs of the constituency. Nurses with strong policy analysis skills

are critical to improving health for all citizens and to closing the health disparities gap.

Professional nurses with an interest in learning more about their role in the family policy arena can find resources through professional associations or can extend their knowledge by taking continuing education courses in a health care policy. One example is the Washington Health Policy Institute conducted by George Mason University in Arlington, Virginia. Nurses and other health care providers spend one week learning about health and family policy, strategies to advocate for at-risk populations, and how to influence policy makers. Similarly, in Canada, the Canadian Nurses Association (CAN) and provincial associations such as the Registered Nurses' Association of Ontario (RNAO) also offer information, workshops, and training for nurses to gain skill in health care policy development. Family policies are a major contributing factor to the mitigation of health disparities. Nurses have the ability to influence policy on many levels and thereby improve the health outcomes of the most vulnerable populations.

Nursing Policy, Research, and Education

Many important policies are at the institutional level where nurses work; nursing practice, research, and education should reflect this orientation.

Nurses Influencing Family Policy

The implications of becoming involved in the influence of family policy as a context for nursing care of families are limitless, especially in community and institutional settings. Nurse involvement in policy development can constitute a wide range of activities, from the micro-level by asking open-ended questions about sexual orientation to the meso-level by asking about housing and food security or environmental safety in the community, to the macro-level where nurses can inform institutional policies in the workplace, to the exo-level where nurses may petition government representatives regarding development of needed policies or modification of harmful or absent policies.

Nurses can influence policy from the initial assessment of families in clinics and hospitals to discharge planning for return to the community including open exploration of potential support and resources, avoiding the omission and assumption that any resources are automatically available. Specific strategies for nurses to get involved in influencing policy from micro- to exo-levels include:

- Join committees in your institution to change relevant policies (e.g., include questions regarding available resources in assessment forms; make sure needed resources are available before discharge; ensure follow-up after discharge or referrals).
- Join professional associations and advocate for needed family policies.
- Write to or phone elected representatives regarding needed policies or changes to those that are harmful.
- Join community advocacy groups, such as those requesting affordable day care.
- Join boards of directors for agencies, such as social housing and community health centers (CHCs).

Nursing Research

Nursing research has already developed useful tools and frameworks for providing nursing care across cultural barriers and under difficult circumstances. The recent development of community-based participatory research models (Minkler & Wallerstein, 2008) provides a methodology for studies more respectful of the potentially diverse views of family in a community. This approach requires the nurse researcher to establish a relationship with the community in which the study is to occur *before* the development of the research question. By sharing all stages of the research process with the members of the community, nurse scientists can use this collaborative approach to examine health disparities directly affected by community improvement based on the results of the study. Adopting this level of respect for reshaping nursing studies of "family" helps nurses gain a more complete understanding of health care for all types of families. This approach is particularly important as trends in care move away from acute care institutions toward community-based care delivery in both the United States and Canada. Nurses are particularly well positioned to participate in policy changes and program development in collaboration with an interdisciplinary team, including their clients and families (Hankivsky & Christoffersen, 2008).

Nursing Education

As discussed previously, there is currently very little inclusion of family policy development and advocacy work in nursing curricula. Opportunities for learning experiences in settings that have established services for vulnerable populations provide the nursing student with clinical situations in which to practice assumption-free assessment skills and learn about diverse life situations and needs. Homeless shelters, services for gay and lesbian adolescents, shelters for victims of intimate partner abuse, outreach centers for sex workers, and street syringe and needle exchange programs all reach a disproportionate share of individuals whose family experiences are not the idealized norm (Hunt, 2007). Working in coalition with clients and other health care providers, nurses can ensure the maximum beneficial influence of such policies on the needs of families, communities, and society (Bergan & While, 2012; Brewah, 2009).

The inclusion of health policy in nursing education has the potential to increase the sensitivity of nurses to social and health policy issues. Policy involvement is about empowering others through leadership, not exerting power over others (Brewah, 2009). Nurses must understand that it is not sufficient to provide care in isolation from the forces that increase risk for disease or limit access to medical services. Electives in history, economics, and political science further inform nurses' understanding of policy. The IOM recommends that nurses engage in lifelong learning, thereby speaking to the need for nurses to engage in professional practice that strives to stay current on the state of the science in health care and the influences of public policy on the delivery of that health care (IOM, 2011). Nurses at all levels must be able to understand current affairs, join nursing and other advocacy organizations, and participate in local, state and provincial, or national political processes. Nurses should be educated to take on responsibility of advocating for equity and social justice to help develop family-friendly policies.

Clearly, nurses can be instrumental in having an impact on family policies that affect the health of citizens they serve. The American Nurses Association Code of Ethics (2015) addresses social policy in Provision 8: "The nurse collaborates with other health professionals and the public to protect human rights, promote health diplomacy, and reduce health disparities" (Lachman, Swanson, & Winland-Brown, 2015). . . ." This provision recommends that nurses work in conjunction with community organizations and legislative policy at the state and national level.

Case Study: Smith Family

Heather is a 19-year-old female diagnosed with bipolar disorder. She was recently hospitalized for 10 days because of experiencing a manic episode with psychotic symptoms. During her hospitalization she admitted stopping her medications because she could no longer afford the high cost and her parents' insurance had a high deductible that would not cover her medications until that deductible was met. Since her hospitalization, however, the deductible was met and she was now interested in returning to medications and to stabilizing her mood. During the discharge planning, Heather met with her psychiatrist, mental health nurse, and her parents.

Heather's history includes being diagnosed with depression at age 13 years with a trial on sertraline (Zoloft) for 2 years. Although her depression symptoms went into remission, her parents noted that she became increasingly agitated and argumentative. During her sophomore year in high school, she became involved with a "rough crowd" and started using marijuana daily, with periods of depression lasting months, followed by weeks of argumentative behavior, poor sleep, and rapid mood shifts. She also started failing her classes, which her parents noted was unusual as she had been identified as a talented and gifted child in elementary school. Her parents sought treatment from a new psychiatrist at that point, and she was diagnosed with bipolar I disorder. She was tried on several mood stabilizers and finally stabilized on paliperidone (Invega) titrated to 6 mg per day. During her senior year in high school she stopped taking her medications because she believed she was stable and no longer needed medication. She quickly became agitated and started believing she was directly talking to characters on the television. She also stole her parents' credit card and purchased more than $2000.00 of items that she later admitted she did not want or need. She agreed to go back on her medication and her symptoms stabilized over the course of 3 weeks. Heather did well upon her return to school and through credit recovery graduated successfully from high school. She attended the local community college for 1 year and was starting her second year when she decided to stop her medications again because of the high cost. Her parents both complained monthly about having to pay $880.83 per month to cover her medications (GoodRx, 2017). They noted that their current insurance, offered by Heather's father's employer, cost the family $600.00 per month and had a $10,000.00 deductible. Heather noted that she had applied for disability services and Medicare health coverage owing to her diagnosis of bipolar I disorder, but was denied because of her successful functioning in school when stable. She also tried to apply for Medicaid services in light of her low income as a student and her bipolar diagnosis but was denied because she had creditable insurance through her father's employer (U.S. Centers for Medicare & Medicaid Services, 2017b). She stated that she did not want to be a burden on her parents, already felt guilty asking them to help her with her tuition and living costs, and did not want to also ask for money to cover her medication costs. Heather's parents asked what could be done to help them afford the high cost of keeping Heather stable. Heather's father anxiously pointed out that the hospital bill thus far was $7595.00 and only covered 9 days, that amount did not include the cost of medications during the hospital stay (Stensland, Watson, & Grazier, 2012). He lamented that his high deductible insurance plan was the best they could afford at this time.

The nurse asked this family what their goals were, both individually for Heather and as a family. Heather stated that she wanted to complete her college degree in old English literature and eventually teach at a university. She was hoping to eventually obtain her doctorate degree in Victorian literature. She said she worried that her diagnosis of bipolar disorder would interfere with that plan because she could not imagine being able to pay for her medications. She now understood how critical it was to take her medications; otherwise, she would be disabled and unable to complete school or be successful at any job. Heather's parents agreed with Heather's goals and stated that they too were worried that successful treatment of her disorder was not affordable.

Heather's psychiatrist stated she believed the paliperidone (Invega) was the best option for successful treatment of Heather's bipolar disorder because of her psychotic symptoms with mania. She also noted that Heather's previous psychiatrist had appropriately tried less expensive mood stabilizers (i.e., risperidone and lithium) but because of intolerable side effects (i.e., tremors, weight gain, and abnormal thyroid function) and break-through manic symptoms, these medications were discontinued and Heather was given paliperidone with good results. Up until she stopped taking her medication she was stable and doing well in school, with relationships, and was getting along well with her parents.

Heather's family history included being the only child of her biological parents. Her parents denied any history of depression, anxiety, or bipolar disorder, but her father noted that his brother was also diagnosed with bipolar disorder and spent most of his life in and out of inpatient care. Heather's mother noted that her mother suffered from depression and anxiety but was stable on an antidepressant medication. Heather was close to her biological grandparents but did not have any contact with her

(continued)

Case Study: Smith Family *(cont.)*

paternal uncle. She noted that her mother was also an only child. Heather stated she had a boyfriend that she had been dating for the past 2 years. He was also a student, studying biology at the community college. She stated that she had a stable group of friends and spent time several days per week with these friends. She said that she no longer used drugs or alcohol because she recognized the negative effects of drugs and alcohol on her mood stability. Heather stated that she was also seeing the counselor at the community college weekly to help her learn strategies for mood regulation. See Figure 4-1, the Smith family genogram, and Figure 4-2, the Smith family ecomap.

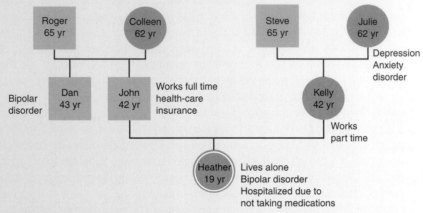

FIGURE 4-1 Smith Family Genogram

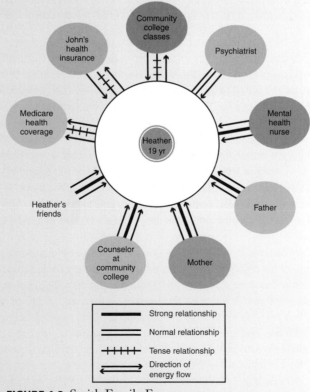

FIGURE 4-2 Smith Family Ecomap

Case Study: Smith Family *(cont.)*

The nurse helped the family prioritize steps to assure that Heather's goals and the family's goals would be supported. The policies that affected this family the most included:

- *Medicare eligibility mandates coverage for disabled individuals.* Heather, unfortunately, did not meet the criteria for being disabled as she functioned well when she was on her medication. She could stop medication; if her functionality declined she would then qualify for Medicare. This option, however, would not support her goals of striving for a successful career. Heather stated that she would rather look for other options to fund her medication.
- *Medicaid eligibility mandates coverage for certain groups of vulnerable populations, including those living in the federally accepted poverty range.* Although the PPACA increased the numbers of individuals eligible for Medicaid coverage, those with creditable insurance through an employer are not eligible. As long as Heather was covered under her parents' insurance plan she would not qualify for Medicaid benefits. The family analyzed whether it would be more cost effective not to take Heather as a tax deduction as a dependent and cancel her insurance versus continuing her coverage but having to pay for her mental health care, including medications. They decided to visit their accountant to discuss these two options. Heather stated that she would feel more comfortable if she qualified for Medicaid and that she had researched that Medicaid does cover the cost of paliperidone (Invega) (GoodRx, 2017). She also learned that Medicaid would cover the cost of counseling should she decide to transfer her counseling services to the county mental health clinic.
- *Employer-supported insurance programs offer employees a discount on their monthly premiums.* Even with this discount, however, families are spending an average of $6422.00 per year on health care costs, including insurance premiums and high deductible expenditures (The Common Wealth Fund, 2016). Although each state is different, the percentage of health care costs on the family income ranges from a low of 6.8% in Massachusetts to a high of 14.7% in Mississippi (The Common Wealth Fund, 2016). The PPACA allowed children to remain on their parents' plans until age 26 years. Although this allows young adults the opportunity to have health insurance, the high deductibles associated with most employer-based programs continue to place a burden on most families, including those with young adult children.
- *Many community and national programs attempt to ease the burden of high cost prescriptions for most individuals.* These programs are often offered through community agencies or pharmaceutical companies. Of interest is that many of these medication discount programs are only given to those with private insurance. Heather's nurse found out that Heather qualified for a discount program, reducing her medication costs by 50% (GoodRx, 2017).

Heather is one of many individuals with a chronic condition that face the dilemma of how to treat symptoms given the continued high cost of health care. Although hospitalization is significantly more expensive than outpatient care and stabilizing medications, many, such as Heather, end up in the emergency department or inpatient care because of not being able to pay for outpatient care and medications. Family policies provide health care coverage for many, but not all. Further, many chronic conditions place individuals in a stigmatized group, further blocking their access to care. Mental health disorders are a large group of chronic conditions commonly stigmatized. Heather was lucky to have a mental health nurse interested in family policies that would help better stabilize Heather's symptoms and help her reach her goals. Future efforts are needed to assure all individuals and families, including young adults, are not burdened with high cost health care that in the end may cause an increase in chronic disabilities rather than supporting successful functioning in the community.

SUMMARY

This chapter has focused on family health policies and how continued health disparities continue to leave many vulnerable populations with inadequate and unequal health care. As nursing care shifts from institutions into the community, nurses who want to deliver the most effective family-focused care need to return to historical role models in nursing, with leaders working hard to provide health care to those in need. They need to become knowledgeable about the influence of the political social structures that are facilitating or hindering health promotion and particularly affect those vulnerable families impacted by racism and exclusion. Promoting health and mitigating disparities, nurses have to be aware of and keep in mind the following:

- Health disparities arise from complex, deeply rooted social issues including racism and stigma.

- Health disparities are directly related to the social and political structure of a society, which gives rise to the determinants of health.
- The social determinants of health include poverty, housing, education, employment and food security, accessibility to health care, presence of chronic illness, gender, and being of an ethnic, racial, or sexual minority.
- The three levels of racism—institutional racism, personally mediated racism, and internalized racism—provide a foundation for understanding the causes and potential solutions of health disparities.
- Interventions at the micro-, meso-, macro-, and exo-levels are important to realize in addressing changes to family policies.
- All social determinants of health intersect and mutually reinforce each other.
- The social determinants are the root causes of illness and health because they affect lifestyle possibilities and limitations and access to health care resources.
- The policy decisions made by a society or government about families and what constitutes a legal relationship, and how health care is delivered, have a profound effect on families and their health.
- In the past, the profession of nursing had a well-defined role in advocating for vulnerable populations. In the last century, nursing involvement in the development of health policy has declined because of a focus on medical diagnosis rather than whole individuals and families in their environmental and social contexts.
- Nurses today need to get involved in policy development at institutional and societal levels to promote health and well-being for families.
- Nursing professionals can benefit from theoretical and practical education about family policy issues that are broad and complex, and that result in resounding effects on the health of the family.
- Family nursing practice has the potential to improve the health of all families regardless of definition and composition by closely collaborating with clients and interdisciplinary health care teams.
- Nursing education needs to include teaching policy development and advocacy.
- Nursing research should include collaborative, community-based participatory research with families for best meeting their needs because they are the experts of their own lives.
- Nurses are in a unique and key position to make a difference in the health of families.

DavisPlus | For additional resources and information, visit **http://davisplus.fadavis.com**. References can be found on *DavisPlus*.

Chapter 5

Family Nursing Assessment and Intervention

Joanna Rowe Kaakinen, PhD, RN

Critical Concepts

- Families are complex social systems with which nurses interact in many ways and in many different contexts; the use of a logical systematic family nursing assessment approach is important.

- In the context of family nursing, the creative nurse thinker must be aware of possibilities, be able to recognize the new and the unusual, be able to decipher unique and complex situations, and be inventive in designing an approach to family care.

- Nurses determine the theoretical and practice lens(es) through which to analyze the family event.

- Knowledge about family structures, functions, and processes informs nurses in their efforts to optimize and provide individualized nursing care, tailored to the uniqueness of every family system.

- Nurses begin family assessment from the moment of contact or referral.

- Family stories are narratives that nurses construct in framing, contextualizing, communicating, and providing interpretations of their family clients' needs as they exercise clinical judgment in their work.

- Interacting with families as clients requires knowledge of family assessment and intervention models, as well as skilled communication techniques so that the interaction will be effective and efficient for all parties.

- The family genogram and ecomap are both assessment data-gathering instruments. The therapeutic interaction that occurs with the family while diagramming a genogram or ecomap is itself a powerful intervention.

- Families' beliefs about health and illness, about nurses and other health care providers, and about themselves are essential for nurses to explore in order to craft effective approaches to family interventions and to promote health literacy.

- Families determine the level of nurses' involvement in their health and illness journeys, and nurses seek to tailor their work and approach accordingly.

- Nurses and families who work together and build on family strengths are in the best position to determine and prioritize specific family needs; develop realistic outcomes; and design, evaluate, and modify a plan of action that has a high probability of being implemented by the family.

- The final step in working with families should always be for nurses to engage in critical, creative, and concurrent reflection about the family, their work with the family, and their own professional practice.

One of the most difficult and challenging aspects of working with families that nurses will encounter is how not to compare, judge, or assume what is the best action for the family or client based on nurses' personal experience with their own families. The way in which a nurse interacts with another person sets in motion a multitude of possibilities. The nurse who stops to mentally prepare becomes fully present for the patient and family before entering the room, which brings the best of self to that interaction. Using therapeutic self in interactions places the other's illness story at the focal point of care. Being always curious about the other's experience, thoughts, life, and needs explores varied possible outcomes. The nurse who is open to diversity welcomes the other as a partner in care. This way of practicing family nursing is known as relational inquiry (Doane & Varcoe, 2015; Varcoe & Doane, 2015).

RELATIONAL INQUIRY FAMILY NURSING PRACTICE

Relational inquiry family nursing practice is oriented toward enhancing the capacity and power of people/families to live a life that is meaningful from their own perspective. Although this may involve treating and preventing disease or modifying lifestyle factors, the primary focus is to enhance peoples' well-being, as well as their capacity and resources for meaningful life experiences. Thus, relational inquiry focuses very specifically on how *health is a socio-relational experience* that is strongly shaped by contextual factors.

> *Like a scientific inquiry, inquiry-based nursing practice involves being in that in-between relational space of knowing/not knowing, being curious, looking for what seems significant, examining the interrelatedness between the elements as well as the relevance of those interrelationships in the experiential moment and also acting toward them.* (Doane & Varcoe, 2015, p. 6)

Families, health, and family nursing are understood to be shaped by the historical, geographical, economic, political, and social diversity of the particular person's/family's context. By purposefully working with this diversity, nurses are prepared to take into account the contextual nature of people's/families' health and illness experiences and how their lives are shaped by their intrapersonal, interpersonal, and contextual circumstances in order to provide the most appropriate care.

Understanding and working directly with context provides a key resource and strategy for responsive, health-promoting family nursing practice. "Context" is not something outside or separate from people; rather, contextual elements (e.g., socioeconomic circumstances, family and cultural histories) are literally embodied in people and within their actions and responses to particular situations (Varcoe & Doane, 2015). Having an appreciation for the range of diverse experiences and how the dynamics of geography, history, politics, and economics shape those experiences allows nurses to provide more effective care to particular families, better understand the stresses and challenges families face, and better support families to draw on their own capacities.

Context is considered something that is integral to the lives of people, as something that shapes not only people's external circumstances and opportunities but also their physiology at the cellular level (Varcoe & Doane, 2015). In other words, context is embodied. For example, if a person is born into a middle-class, English-speaking, Euro-Canadian family, the very way that person speaks—accent, intonation, vocabulary—is shaped by that context. The way that a person's body grows is influenced by the nutritional value of the food and quality of water available, the level of stress in the family, the quality of housing the family has, and the opportunities for rest and physical activity. Similarly, the person's sense of self and expectations for his or her life are shaped by the circumstances into which the person is born. The individual's success in education will depend not only on what educational opportunities are available, but also on how the person comes to that education—for example, how well fed or hungry, well rested or tired, or confident and content he or she is—and the economic resources available that shape which school the person attends. It will also be affected by how education is valued within the person's family or community. Thus, a person's/family's multiple contexts cannot be understood as being outside or separate from one's self, or even as necessarily under one's control. Rather, people/families embody their circumstances, and their circumstances embody them. Although people have some influence over their circumstances, such influence generally is more limited than we would like to imagine. Moreover, the contextual elements, and the experiences to which those elements give rise, live on in people. That is, past contexts go forward within people, shaping how they experience present and future situations.

People are both influenced *by* their context and live *within* contexts (Varcoe & Doane, 2015). Throughout nursing careers, nurses provide care in specific contexts, and families will live in their own diverse contexts. Consciously considering the interface of these differing contexts and how they are shaping families' health and illness experiences is vital to providing responsive, health-promoting care. Also foundational to this process is the need to inquire into how context shapes the life of a nurse and his or her practice. This self-reflection enables nurses to more intentionally choose how to draw on those influences to enhance responsiveness to the needs of families. For example, many nurses practice in health care settings where they are surrounded by well-educated and financially stable professionals. This context contrasts with many clients who may lack education and live in low-income and unstable housing because of financial instability. When a nurse recognizes this difference, care can then include sensitivity to the disparity between these two contexts.

Through a relational inquiry lens of family nursing, nurses look for how people, situations, contexts, environments, and processes are integrally connecting with and shaping each other. Nurses step outside their personal experience of family and actively engage in conversations to uncover the family illness story (Wright & Leahey, 2013). The illness story differs from the medical story. The medical story is about the patient who has the disease or health problem and includes signs and symptoms, medications, treatment regimen, and prognosis or trajectory of illness. The family illness story is how the family and each member live through the experience of the illness or health event. "Relational practice is a humanely involved process of respectful, compassionate, and authentically interested inquiry into another" (Doane & Varcoe, 2015, p. 200).

Without a careful consideration of context and its influence on families' health and illness experiences, nurses typically draw uncritically on stereotypes in ways that limit possibilities for the families they serve. By inquiring into the context of families, nurses are able to provide optimal responsive, ethical, and appropriate care. It is through relational inquiry that nurses connect across differences and work with the family by providing options and choice to help them determine the best decisions for them and

their family in this situation at this point in time. Relational inquiry is the foundational value inherent in all aspects of family nursing, but especially for assessment and specific, tailored family interventions.

Family-centered care (FCC) principles should be applied in all interactions between nurses and families or other health care providers. According to the Institute for Patient- and Family-Centered Care (IPFCC, n.d.), the core principles of FCC are respect and dignity, information sharing, participation, and collaboration. The goal of FCC is to increase the mutual benefit of health care provision for all parties, with a focus on improving the satisfaction and outcomes of health care for families (IPFCC, n.d.). By utilizing these principles in all aspects of the family nursing approach, from assessment through intervention and evaluation, nurses can facilitate exchanges of shared expertise, which lead to better holistic health outcomes.

THERAPEUTIC APPROACH TO WORKING WITH FAMILIES

During the initial interaction with families, it is critical for nurses to introduce themselves to the family, meet all the family members present, learn about the family members not present, clearly state the purpose for working with the family, outline what will happen during this session, and indicate the length of time the meeting will last. Taking these actions demonstrates respect for family members and their unique story. To continue with this precedent, the nurse needs to develop a systematic plan for the first and all following family meetings. This focus on respect, dignity, and collaboration in initial meetings helps to establish relationships that are therapeutic; effective, satisfying partnerships between nurses and families are critical as they work together toward health-related goals.

Nurses who use a therapeutic approach to family meetings have found that their focus on FCC increases, and that their communication skills with families becomes more fluid with experience (Harrison, 2010; Martinez, D'Artois, & Rennick, 2007). When nurses use therapeutic communication skills with families, the families report feeling a stronger rapport with the nurse, an increased frequency of communication between families and the nurse occurs, and families perceive these nurses to be more competent (Harrison, 2010; Martinez et al., 2007).

Conducting family meetings requires not only skilled communication strategies but also knowledge of family assessment and intervention models. Nurses use a variety of data collection and assessment instruments to help gather information in a systematic and efficient manner. Therefore, it is important that the instruments be carefully selected so they are family friendly and render information pertinent to the purpose of working with the family.

FAMILY NURSING ASSESSMENT

Central to the delivery of safe and effective family nursing care is the nurse's ability to make accurate assessments, identify health problems, and tailor plans of care. Each step of working with families, whether applied to individuals within the family or the family as a whole, requires a thoughtful, deliberate reasoning process. Nurses decide what data to collect and how, when, and where those data are collected. Nurses determine the relevance of each new piece of information and how it fits into the emerging family story. Before moving forward, nurses decide whether they have obtained sufficient information on problem and strength identification, or whether gaps exist that require additional data gathering.

Nurses must always be aware that "common" interpretations of data may not be the "correct" interpretations in any given situation, and that commonly expected signs and symptoms may not appear in every case or in the same data pattern presentation. The ability of nurses to be open to the unexpected and to be alert to unusual or different responses is critical to determining the primary needs confronting the family. Nurses should be able to perceive what is not obvious and to understand how this family story is similar to or different from other family stories.

The family nursing assessment includes the following steps:

- *Assessment of the family story*: The nurse gathers data from a variety of sources to see the whole picture of the family experience.
- *Analysis of the family story*: The nurse clusters the data into meaningful patterns to see how the family is managing the health event. The family needs are prioritized using a Family Reasoning Web.

- *Design of a family plan of care*: Together, the nurse and family determine the best plan of care for the family to manage the situation.
- *Family intervention*: Together, the nurse and family implement the plan of care incorporating the most family-focused, cost-effective, and efficient interventions that assist the family to achieve the best possible outcomes.
- *Family evaluation*: Together, the nurse and family determine whether the outcomes are being reached, are being partially reached, or need to be redesigned. Is the care plan working well, does a new care plan need to be put into place, or does the nurse/family relationship need to end?
- *Nurse reflection*: Nurses engage in critical, creative, and concurrent reflection about themselves and their own family experiences, the family client, and their work with the family.

Engaging Families in Care

Background and First Contact

Nurses encounter families in diverse health care settings for many different kinds of problems and circumstances. Every family has a story about how the potential or actual health event influences its individual members, family functioning, and management of the health event. Nurses are charged with gathering, sifting, organizing, and analyzing the data to craft a clear view of the family's story. Nurses filter data gathered in the story through different views or approaches, which affects how they think about the family as a whole and about each individual family member. For example, a family who is faced with a new diagnosis of a chronic illness would have different needs than a family who is faced with a member dying of an end-stage chronic illness. Nurses might use different strategies if the patient is in the acute hospital setting, or an assisted living center, or living at home.

The underlying theoretical approach used by the nurses working with families influences how they ask questions and collect family data. For example, if the family is worried about how its 2-year-old child will react to a new baby, such as in the Bono family case study presented later in this chapter, the nurse may elect to base the assessment and interventions on a family systems theoretical view or the developmental family life cycle theoretical view. Refer to Chapter 2 for a detailed discussion of working with families from different theoretical perspectives.

Data collection, which is the first part of assessment, involves both subjective and objective family information that is obtained through direct observation, examination, or in consultation with other health care providers. In all cases, family assessment begins from the first moment that the family is referred to the nurse. Following are some circumstances in which a family is referred to a nurse:

- A family is referred by the hospital to a home health agency for wound care on the feet of a client with diabetes.
- A couple seeks advice for managing their busy life with three children as the mother returns home from the hospital following an unplanned cesarean section.
- A family calls the Visiting Nurse Association to request assistance in providing care to a family member with increasing dementia.
- A school nurse is asked by the school psychologist to conduct a family assessment with a family who is suspected of child neglect.
- A physician requests a family assessment for a child who has nonorganic failure to thrive.
- A family with a member with critical care needs is asked to make decisions about life-sustaining treatments in the intensive care unit.

Making Community-Based Appointments

As soon as a family is identified, the nurse begins to collect data about the family's story. Sources of data that can be collected before contacting a family for a home or clinic appointment are listed in Box 5-1. Specifically, the nurse needs to know the following information:

- The reason for the referral or requested visit
- The family knowledge of the visit or referral

- Specific medical information about the family member with the health problem
- Strategies that have been used previously
- Insurance sources for the family
- Family problems identified by other health providers
- Family demographic data, when available, such as the number of people and ages of family members or basic cultural background information
- The need for an interpreter

Before contacting the family to arrange for the initial appointment, the nurse needs to decide whether the most appropriate place to conduct the appointment is in the family's home or the clinic/office. The type of agency where the nurse works may dictate this decision. Advantages and disadvantages of a home setting and a clinic setting are listed in Table 5-1.

Contacting the family for the appointment provides valuable information about the family. It is imperative that the nurse be confident and organized when making the initial contact. Information that is important for the nurse to note is whether the family acts surprised that the referral was made, shows reluctance in setting up a meeting, or expresses openness about working together. The family also gathers important information about the nurse during the initial interaction. For example, family members will notice whether the nurse takes time to talk with them, uses a lot of words they do not understand, or appears organized and open to working with the family. To facilitate the best possible outcomes in engaging families for the first time to learn about their health and illness story, effective nurses consider the family and its needs as central to starting a successful collaboration. This relationship of trust begins from the moment of first contact with families. As a guide, Box 5-2 outlines steps to follow when making an appointment with a family.

BOX 5-1

Sources of Preencounter Family Data

- *Referral source*: includes data that indicated a problem for this family, as well as demographic information.
- *Family*: includes family members' views of the problem, surprise that the referral was made, reluctance to set up the meeting, and avoidance in setting up the appointment.

- *Previous records*: records in the health care system or that are sent by having the client sign a release for information form, such as process logs, charts, phone logs, or school records.

Table 5-1 Advantages and Disadvantages of Home Visits Versus Clinic Visits	
Home Visit	**Clinic Visit**
Advantages	
• Opportunity to see the everyday family environment.	• Conducting the family appointment in the office or clinic allows for easier access to consultants.
• Observe typical family interactions because the family members are likely to feel more relaxed in their physical space.	• The family situation may be so strained that a more formal, less personal setting will facilitate discussions of emotionally charged issues.
• More family members may be able to attend the meeting.	
• Emphasizes that the problem is the responsibility of the whole family and not one family member.	
Disadvantages	
• Home may be the only sanctuary or safe place for the family or its members to be away from the scrutiny of others. Therefore, conducting the meeting in the home would invade or violate this sanctuary and bring the clinical perspective into this safe world.	• May reinforce a possible culture gap between the family and the nurse.
• The nurse must be highly skilled in communication, specifically setting limits and guiding the interaction, or the visit may have a more social tone and not be efficient or productive.	

BOX 5-2

Setting Up Family Appointments

When organizing family appointments:

■ Introduce yourself.
■ State the purpose of the requested meeting, including who referred the family to the agency.
■ Do not apologize for the meeting.
■ Be factual about the need for the meeting but do not provide details.

■ Offer several possible times for the meeting, including late afternoon or evening.
■ Let the family select the most convenient time that allows the majority of family members to attend.
■ Offer services of an interpreter, if required.
■ Confirm the date, time, place, and directions.

Family Assessments in Acute Care Settings

Nurses in acute care settings encounter the families of their individual patients on a daily basis. The degree to which nurses feel comfortable and to which they demonstrate clinical competence engaging families varies widely. Because of the short length of stay in acute hospitals and the increasing population of people with chronic illnesses who need help with symptom management of both their acute health problem and their chronic illness, nurses in acute care settings often feel there is little time to engage families effectively. Lack of time, in fact, has been identified by nurses as the primary barrier to engaging families, though there are many other barriers as well, including nurse bias, safety concerns, and negative nurse attitudes about working with families (Duhamel, Dupuis, Turcotte, Martinez, & Goudreau, 2015; Segaric & Hall, 2015). It is critical that nurses gain skill and comfort with families in acute care settings as families are the primary caregivers following the discharge of their family members. Families need the help of nurses in order to learn how to provide effective post-discharge care tasks; engage in shared decision making with health care providers; understand the current health status of their ill family member; balance admission and post-discharge family life demands; assist families during critical events such as resuscitation; and solve ethical dilemmas that arise in the care of their loved one. With this extensive list of needs, it is essential that nurses in acute care settings intentionally and effectively engage families (Al-Mutair, Plummer, O'Brien, & Clerehan, 2013).

Nurses in acute care settings encounter several challenges, including caring for several acutely ill persons simultaneously, managing the informational needs of interdisciplinary providers, and coping with a host of distractions that often keep nurses away from the bedside. Older adult patients, especially those with dementia, and their families have specific needs (Moyle, Bramble, Bauer, Smyth, & Beattie, 2016) that nurses need to be aware of in order to achieve the best outcomes (Palmer & Kresevic, 2014). Therefore, nurses who seek to engage families, complete family assessments, and implement family interventions must be highly efficient and creative. Several specific strategies and tools must be used to accomplish a meaningful and effective experience. Refer to Chapter 14 for an in-depth discussion of acute care family nursing needs, and for families where patients are older adults refer to Chapter 15.

Using Interpreters With Families

It is critical for the nurse to determine whether an interpreter is needed during the family meeting, because the number of families for whom English is a second language is increasing. With the growing immigrant population in the United States that needs health care, hospitals are struggling to meet the needs of families who are limited in English proficiency (Tienda & Haskins, 2011). Language barriers have been found to complicate many aspects of patient care, including comprehension and adherence to plans of care, and may result in poor health outcomes (Palmer & Kresevic, 2014). Furthermore, language barriers have been found to contribute to adverse health outcomes, compromised quality of care, avoidable expenses, dissatisfied families, and increased potential for medical mistakes (Flores, Abreu, Barone, Bachur, & Lin, 2012; Palmer & Kresevic, 2014). Thus, it is essential that nurses who are not bilingual use interpreters when working with non–English-speaking families. Even though health care providers may know the benefits of using an official interpreter, many choose not to use them (Vidaeff, Kerrigan, & Monga, 2015). One of the main reasons reported for not using official interpreters is that it takes more time (Parsons, Baker, Smith-Gorvie, & Hudak, 2014).

The types of interpreters that nurses solicit to help work with families have the potential to influence the quality of the information exchanged and the family's ability to follow the suggested plan of action. One of the most common types of interpreters used is bilingual family members or friends, called *ad hoc family interpreters* or *child language brokers* when using children. The problems with using family members as interpreters are that they have been found to buffer information, alter the meaning of the content, or make the decision for the person for whom they are interpreting (Flores et al., 2012; Palmer & Kresevic, 2014). The ad hoc family member interpreter also has been found to lack important language skills, especially when it comes to medical interpretation (Flores et al., 2012; Palmer & Kresevic, 2014) and when children are used as interpreters (Anguiano, 2012). If the ad hoc family member interpreter is a child, the information that is being discussed may be frightening or the topic may be too personal and sensitive (Anguiano, 2012; Palmer & Kresevic, 2014; Russell, Morales, & Ravert, 2015). Using ad hoc family interpreters also raises confidentially issues (Gray, Hilder, & Donaldson, 2011). Therefore, it is not ideal for nurses to use a family member for interpretation, especially if another choice is available.

The use of a qualified medical interpreter is the preferred approach for interpretation. However, it is not sufficient that a person speaks a specific language; it is also important to consider the interpreter's ethnic origin, religious background, gender, language or dialect, social group, clothes, appearance, and attitude (Hadziabdic, Albin, Heikkilä, & Hjelm, 2014). If a qualified medical interpreter cannot come to the meeting in the family home, the nurse should plan to use a speaker phone so that the professional interpreter can be involved in the conversation with the family. One of the problems with using an interpreter on the phone is that interpreters do not have the advantage of seeing the family members in person and cannot observe nonverbal communication (Gray et al., 2011; Hadziabdic, Heikkilä, Albin, & Hjelm, 2011). Also, the nurse should be aware that using a telephone interpreter introduces another outside person into the family setting, which may be perceived as impersonal by the family (Hadziabdic et al., 2014; Hadziabdic et al., 2011).

FAMILY NURSING ASSESSMENT MODELS AND INSTRUMENTS

Nurses practice family nursing using a variety of tools. The following three family assessment models have been developed by family nurses. The Family Assessment and Intervention Model and the FS³I were developed by Berkey and Hanson (1991). Friedman developed the Friedman Family Assessment Model (Friedman, Bowden, & Jones, 2003). The Calgary Family Assessment Model (CFAM) and Calgary Family Intervention Model (CFIM) were developed by Wright and Leahey (2013). These three approaches vary in purpose, unit of analysis, and level of data collected. Table 5-2 has a detailed comparison of the essential components of these three family assessment models.

Table 5-2	**Comparison of Family Assessment Models Developed by Family Nurses**		
Name of model	Family Assessment and Intervention Model and the Family System Stressor-Strength Inventory (FS³I)	Friedman Family Assessment Model	Calgary Family Assessment and Intervention Model
Citation	Berkey & Hanson (1991)	Friedman, Bowden, & Jones (2003)	Wright & Leahey (2013)
Purpose	Concrete, focused measurement instrument that helps families identify current family stressors and builds interventions based on family strengths	Concrete, global family assessment interview guide that looks primarily at families in the larger community in which they are embedded	Conceptual model and multidimensional approach to families that looks at the fit among family functioning, as well as effective and behavioral aspects
Theoretical underpinnings	Systems:	Developmental	Systems:
	Family systems	Structural-functional	Cybernetics Communication Change Theory
	Neuman systems	Family stress-coping	
	Model:	Environmental	
	Stress-coping theory		
Level of data collected	Quantitative:	Qualitative:	Qualitative:
	Ordinal and interval	Nominal	Nominal
	Qualitative:		
	Nominal		
Settings in which primarily used	Inpatient	Outpatient	Outpatient
	Outpatient	Community	Community
	Community		
Units of analysis	Family as context	Family as client	Family as system
	Family as client	Family as component of society	
	Family as system		
	Family as component of society		
Strengths	Short	Comprehensive list of areas to assess family	Conceptually sound
	Easy to administer		
	Yields data to compare one family member with another family member		
	Assess and measure focused presenting problem		
Weaknesses	Narrow variable	Large quantities of data that may not relate to the problem	Not concrete enough to be useful as a guideline unless the provider has studied this model and approach in detail
		No quantitative data	

Family Assessment and Intervention Model

The Family Assessment and Intervention Model, originally developed by Berkey and Hanson (1991), is presented in greater detail in Chapter 2, but is worth exploring in this context as well. The Family Assessment and Intervention Model is based on Neuman's health care systems model (Kaakinen & Tabacco, 2015).

According to the Family Assessment and Intervention Model, families are subject to tensions when stressed. The family's reaction depends on how deeply the stressor penetrates the family unit and how capable the family is of adapting to maintain its stability. The lines of resistance protect the family's basic structure, which includes the family's functions and energy resources. The family core contains the patterns of family interactions and strengths. The basic family structure must be protected at all costs or the family ceases to exist. Reconstitution or adaptation is the work the family undertakes to preserve or restore family stability. This model addresses three areas: (1) health promotion, wellness activities, problem identification, and family factors at lines of defense and resistance; (2) family reaction and instability at lines of defense and resistance; and (3) restoration of family stability and family functioning at levels of prevention and intervention.

The FS³I is the assessment and intervention tool that accompanies the Family Assessment and Intervention Model. The FS³I is divided into three sections: (1) family systems stressors—general; (2) family stressors—specific; and (3) family system strengths.

Nurses can assess family stability by gathering information on family stressors and strengths. The nurse and family work together to first assess the family's general, overall stressors, and then specific family problems. Identified family strengths give an indication of the potential and actual problem-solving abilities of the family system. A plus to the FS³I approach is that both quantitative and qualitative data are used to determine the level of prevention and intervention needed. The family is actively involved in the discussions and decisions. Moreover, this assessment and intervention approach focuses on both family stressors and strengths, and provides a theoretical structure for family nursing.

Friedman Family Assessment Model

The Friedman Family Assessment Model (Friedman et al., 2003) is based on the structural-functional framework and developmental and systems theory. This assessment model takes a macroscopic approach to family assessment by viewing families as subsystems of the wider society, which includes institutions devoted to religion, education, and health. Family is considered an open social system and this model focuses on family's structure, functions (activities and purposes), and relationships with other social systems. The Friedman Family Assessment Model is commonly used when the family-in-community is the setting for care (e.g., in community and public health nursing). This approach enables family nurses to assess the family system as a whole, as a subunit of the society, and as an interactional system. Box 5-3 delineates the general assumptions of this model (Friedman et al., 2003, p. 100).

Structure refers to how a family is organized and how the parts relate to each other and to the whole.

BOX 5-3

Underlying Assumptions of Friedman's Family Assessment Model

The Friedman's Family Assessment Model includes the following underlying assumptions:

- A family is a social system with functional requirements.
- A family is a small group possessing certain generic features common to all small groups.

- The family as a social system accomplishes functions that serve the individual and society.
- Individuals act in accordance with a set of internalized norms and values that are learned primarily through socialization.

Source: Friedman, M. M., Bowden, V. R., & Jones, E. G. (2003). *Family nursing: Research, theory & practice* (5th ed.). Upper Saddle River, NJ: Prentice Hall/Pearson Education.

The four basic structural dimensions are role systems, value systems, communication networks, and power structure. These dimensions are interrelated and interactive, and they may differ in single-parent and two-parent families. For example, a single mother may be the head of the family, but she may not necessarily take on the authoritarian role that a traditional man might in a two-parent family. In turn, the value systems, communication networks, and power structures may be quite different in the single-parent and two-parent families because of these structural differences.

Function refers to how families go about meeting the needs of individuals and meeting the purposes of the broader society. In other words, family functions are what a family does. The functions of the family historically are discussed in Chapter 1, but the following specific family functions are considered in this approach:

- Pass on culture, religion, and ethnicity
- Socialize young people for the next generation (e.g., to be good citizens, to be able to cope in society through education)
- Exist for sexual satisfaction and reproduction
- Provide economic security
- Serve as a protective mechanism for family members against outside forces
- Provide closer human contact and relations

The Friedman Family Assessment Model form consists of six broad categories of interview questions: (1) identification data, (2) developmental stage and history of the family, (3) environmental data, (4) family structure (i.e., role structure, family values, communication patterns, power structure), (5) family functions (i.e., affective functions, socialization functions, health care functions), and (6) family stress and coping. Each category has several subcategories (Friedman et al., 2003).

Friedman's assessment was developed to provide guidelines for family nurses who are interviewing a family. The guidelines categorize family information according to structure and function. Friedman's Family Assessment Model Form exists in both a long form and a short form. The long form is quite extensive (13 pages), and it may not be possible to collect all the data in one visit. Moreover, all the categories of information listed in the guidelines may not be pertinent for every family. Similar to other approaches, this model has its strengths and weaknesses. One problem with this approach is that it can generate large quantities of data with no clear direction as to how to use all the information in diagnosis, planning, and intervention. The strength of this approach is that it addresses a comprehensive list of areas to assess the family. Further, a short assessment form has been developed to highlight critical areas of family functioning. The short form, which is included in Appendix found on Davis*Plus*, outlines the types of questions the nurse can ask.

Calgary Family Assessment Model

The CFAM by Wright and Leahey (2013) blends nursing and family therapy concepts that are grounded in systems theory, cybernetics, communication theory, change theory, and a biology of recognition. The following concepts from general systems theory and family systems theory make up the theoretical framework for this model (Wright & Leahy, 2013, pp. 21–44):

- A family system is part of a larger suprasystem and is also composed of many subsystems.
- The family as a whole is greater than the sum of its parts.
- A change in one family member affects all family members.
- The family is able to create a balance between change and stability.
- Family members' behaviors are best understood from a perspective of circular rather than linear causality.

Cybernetics is the science of communication and control theory; therefore, it differs from systems theory. Systems theory helps change the focus of one's conceptual lens from parts to wholes. By contrast, cybernetics changes the focus from substance to form. Wright and Leahey (2013) drew two useful concepts from cybernetics theory:

- Families possess self-regulating ability.
- Feedback processes can simultaneously occur at several system levels with families.

Communication theory in this model is based on the work of Watzlawick and colleagues (Watzlawick, Weakland, & Fisch, 1967, 1974). Communication represents the way that individuals interact with one another. Concepts derived from communication theory used in the CFAM are as follows (Wright & Leahey, 2013):

- All nonverbal communication is meaningful.
- All communication has two major channels for transmission: digital (verbal) and analogical (nonverbal).
- A dyadic relationship has varying degrees of symmetry (similarity) and complementarity (divergence, contrast, or complementary characteristics).
- All communication has two levels: content and relationship.

Helping families to change is at the very core of family nursing interventions. Families need a balance between change and stability. Change is required to make things better, and stability is required to maintain some semblance of order. Several concepts from change theory are important to this family nursing approach (Wright & Leahey, 2013):

- Change is dependent on the perception of the problem.
- Change is determined by structure.
- Change is dependent on context.
- Change is dependent on co-evolving goals for treatment.
- Understanding alone does not lead to change.
- Change does not necessarily occur equally in all family members.
- Facilitating change is the nurse's responsibility.
- Change occurs by means of a "fit" or meshing between the therapeutic offerings (interventions of the nurse) and the bio-psycho-social-spiritual structures of family members.
- Change can be the result of a myriad of causes.

Figure 5-1 shows the branching diagram of the CFAM (Wright & Leahey, 2013, p. 48). The assessment questions that accompany the model are organized into three major categories: (1) structural, (2) developmental, and (3) functional. Nurses examine a family's structural components to answer these questions: Who is in the family? What is the connection between family members? What is the family's context? Structure includes family composition, sex, sexual orientation, rank order, subsystems,

and the boundaries of the family system. Aside from interview and observation, strategies recommended to assess structure include the genogram and the ecomap.

The second major assessment category in the Calgary approach is family development, which includes assessment of family stages, tasks, and attachments. For example, nurses may ask, "Where is the family in the family life cycle?" Understanding the stage of the family enables nurses to assess and intervene in a more purposeful, specific, and meaningful way. There are no actual instruments for assessing development, but nurses can use developmental tasks as guidelines.

The third area for assessment in the CFAM is family functioning. Family functioning reflects how individuals actually behave in relation to one another, or the "here-and-now aspect of a family's life" (Wright & Leahey, 2013, p. 116). Aspects of family functioning include activities of daily life, such as eating, sleeping, meal preparation, and health care, as well as emotional communication, verbal and nonverbal communication, communication patterns (the way communication and responses are passed back and forth between members), problem solving, roles, influence and power, beliefs, and alliances and coalitions. Wright and Leahey indicate that nurses may assess in all three areas for a macroview of the family, or they can use any part of the approach for a microassessment. Wright and Leahey developed a companion model to the CFAM called the CFIM. This intervention model provides concrete strategies by which nurses can promote, improve, and sustain effective family functioning in the cognitive, affective, and behavioral domains. The strength of the Calgary Assessment and Intervention Model is that it is a conceptually sound model that incorporates multiple theoretical aspects into working with families. The strength of this approach is also its weakness in that unless you are intimately knowledgeable with the model and the interventions, it is difficult to implement in acute care settings.

Family Assessment Instruments

There are approximately 1000 family-focused instruments that have been developed and used in assessing family-related variables (Touliatos, Perlmutter, & Straus, 2001; Westmoreland, Bouffard, O'Carroll, &

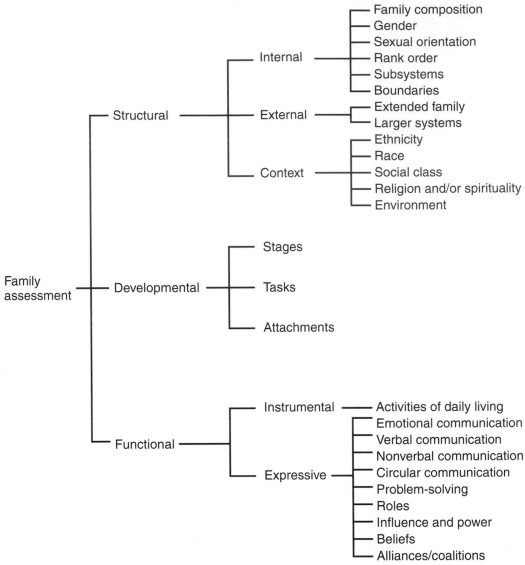

FIGURE 5-1 Calgary Assessment Model Diagram (*Wright L. M., & Leahey, M. (2013). Nurses and families: A guide to family assessment and intervention (6th ed.). Philadelphia, PA: F. A. Davis, with permission.*)

Rosenberg, 2009). Box 5-4 lists family nursing instruments that have been developed by family nursing scholars. The selection of the appropriate instrument to use can be complex. Sometimes, a simple questionnaire or instrument can be completed in just a few minutes. No one instrument for data collection on family history or experience is relevant in all contexts for all purposes (Wilson et al., 2012). To select the most appropriate assessment instrument, be sure the instrument has the following characteristics:

- Written in uncomplicated language at a fifth-grade level
- Only 10 to 15 minutes in length
- Relatively easy to score
- Offers valid data on which to base decisions
- Sensitive to sex, race, social class, and ethnic background

Regardless of which assessment/measurement instrument is used, families should always be informed of how the information gathered through the instruments will be used by the health care providers.

BOX 5-4
Family Nursing Instruments Developed by Family Nurse Scholars

Family Functioning Variables

Feetham Family Functioning Survey (FFFS)	• Suzanne Feetham, **USA** (E-mail: stfeetham@gmail.com) • Hohashi, N., Honda, J., & Kong, S. K. (2008). Validity and reliability of the Chinese version of the Feetham Family Functioning Survey (FFFS). *Journal of Family Nursing, 14*(2), 201–223. • Hohashi, N., Maeda, M., & Sugishita, C. (2000). Development of the Japanese-language Feetham Family Functioning Survey (FFFS) and evaluation of its effectiveness. *Japanese Journal of Research in Family Nursing, 6*(1), 2–10. [in Japanese] • Roberts, C. S., & Feetham, S. L. (1982). Assessing family functioning across three areas of relationships. *Nursing Research, 31*(4), 231–235. • Sawin, K. J., & Harrigan, M. P. (1995). Well-established self-report instruments: Feetham Family Functioning Survey (FFFS). In K. J. Sawin & M. P. Harrigan (Eds.), *Measures of family functioning for research and practice* (pp. 42–49). New York, NY: Springer.
Family Management Measure (FaMM)	• Kathleen Knafl, Janet Deatrick, Agatha Gallo, **USA** (Web site: http://nursing.unc.edu/research/office-of-research-support-and-consultation/family-management-measure/) • Knafl, K., Deatrick, J. A., Gallo, A., Dixon, J., Grey, M., Knafl, G., & O'Malley, J. (2011). Assessment of the psychometric properties of the Family Management Measure. *Journal of Pediatric Psychology, 36*(5), 494–505.
Family Functioning, Health, and Social Support Instrument (FAFHES)	• Paivi Åstedt-Kurki, Marja-Terttu Tarkka, Eija Paavilainen, Kristiina Lehti, **FINLAND** (E-mail: paivi.astedt-kurki@uta.fi) • Åstedt-Kurki, P., Tarkka, M.-T., Paavilainen, E., & Lehti, K. (2002). Development and testing of a family nursing scale. *Western Journal of Nursing Research, 24*(5), 567–579. • Åstedt-Kurki, P., Tarkka, M.-T., Rikala, M.-R., Lehti, K., & Paavilainen, E. (2009). Further testing of a family nursing instrument (FAFHES). *International Journal of Nursing Studies, 46*(3), 350–359.
Family Health Routines (FHR)	• Sharon Denham, **USA** (E-mail: sdenham@mail.twu.edu) • Kanjanawetang, J., Yunlbhand, J., Chaiyawat, W., Wu, Y.-W. B., & Denham, S. A. (2009). Thai family health routines: Scale development and psychometric testing. *Southeast Asian Journal of Tropical Medicine and Public Health, 40*(3), 629–643.
Assessment of Strategies in Families–Effectiveness (ASF–E)	• Maire-Luise Friedemann, **USA** (Web site: http://www2.fiu.edu/~friedemm/asfdevelopment.htm) • Friedemann, M.-L. (1991). An instrument to evaluate effectiveness in family functioning. *Western Journal of Nursing Research, 13*(2), 220–236; Cardea, J. M., Harrison, M., & Lenz, E.R., discussion pp. 236–241. • Friedemann, M.-L., & Smith, A. A. (1997). A triangulation approach to testing a family instrument. *Western Journal of Nursing Research, 19*(3), 364–378.
Iceland-Expressive Family Functioning Questionnaire (ICE-EFFQ)	• Eydis Sveinbjarnardottir, Erla Kolbrun Svavarsdottir, & Birgir Hrafnkelsson, **ICELAND** (E-mail: eks@hi.is) • Sveinbjarnardottir, E. K., Svavarsdottir, E. K., & Hrafnkelsson, B. (2012a). Psychometric development of the Iceland-Expressive Family Functioning Questionnaire (ICE-EFFQ). *Journal of Family Nursing, 18*(3), 353–377.
Iceland-Expressive Family Functioning Questionnaire (ICE-EFFQ)	• Margrét Gisladottir, Erla Kolbrun Svavarsdottir, **ICELAND** (E-mail: eks@hi.is) • Gisladottir, M., & Svavarsdottir, E. K. (2016). Development and psychometric testing of the Iceland-Family Illness Beliefs Questionnaire. *Journal of Family Nursing, 22*(3), 321–338.

(continued)

BOX 5-4

Family Nursing Instruments Developed by Family Nurse Scholars *(cont.)*

Family Functioning Variables

F-COPES	• McCubbin, H. I., Thompson, A., & McCubbin, M. A. (1996). *Family assessment: Resiliency, coping and adaptation-inventories for research and practice.* Madison, WI: University of Wisconsin.
Survey of Family Environment (SFE)	• Naohiro Hohashi & Junko Honda, **JAPAN** (E-mail: naohiro@hohashi.org)
	• Hohashi, N., & Honda, J. (2012). Development and testing of the Survey of Family Environment (SFE): A novel instrument to measure family functioning and needs for family support. *Journal of Nursing Measurement, 20*(3), 212–229.

FAMILY NURSE/FAMILY CARE VARIABLES

Family Nursing Practice Scale (FNPS)	• Peggy Simpson, **CANADA**; Marie Tarrant, **HONG KONG** (E-mail: peggysimpson01 @gmail.com)
	• Simpson, P., & Tarrant, M. (2006). Development of the Family Nursing Practice Scale. *Journal of Family Nursing, 12*(4), 413–425.
Family Nurse Caring Beliefs Scale (FNCBS)	• Sonja Meiers, Patricia Tomlinson, Cynthia Peden-McAlpine, **USA** (E-mail: smeiers @winona.edu)
	• Meiers, S. J., Tomlinson, P., & Peden-McAlpine, C. (2007). Development of the Family Nurse Caring Belief Scale (FNCBS). *Journal of Family Nursing, 13*(4), 484–502.
Families' Importance in Nursing Care: Nurses' Attitudes (FINC-NA)	• Eva Benzein, Pauline Johansson, Kristofer Arestedt, Agneta Berg, Britt-Inger Saveman, **SWEDEN** (E-mail: eva.benzein@lnu.se; britt-inger.saveman@nurs.umu.se)
	• Benzein, E., Johansson, P., Årestedt, K. F., Berg, A., & Saveman, B.-I. (2008). Families' importance in nursing care: Nurses' attitudes—An instrument development. *Journal of Family Nursing, 14*(1), 97–117.
	• Saveman, B.-I., Benzein, E. G., Engström, A. H., & Årestedt, K. (2011). Refinement and psychometric re-evaluation of the instrument: Families' Importance in Nursing Care–Nurses' Attitudes. *Journal of Family Nursing, 17*(3), 312–329.
Parents' Perceptions of Care (PPC)	• Hanna Maijala, Tiina Luukkaala, Paivi Åstedt-Kurki, **FINLAND** (E-mail: paivi.astedt -kurki@uta.fi)
	• Maijala, H., Luukkaala, T., & Åstedt-Kurki, P. (2009). Measuring parents' perceptions of care. Psychometric development of a research instrument. *Journal of Family Nursing, 15*(3), 343–359.
Family Nurse Presence Scale (FNP)	• Sandra Eggenberger, **USA** (E-mail: sandra.eggenberger@mnsu.edu)
Iceland-Family Perceived Support Questionnaire (ICE-FPSQ)	• Eydis Sveinbjarnardottir, Erla Kolbrun Svavarsdottir, & Birgir Hrafnkelsson, **ICELAND** (E-mail: eks@hi.is)
	• Bruce, E., Dorell, A., Lindh, V., Erlingsson, C., Lindkvist, M., & Sundin, K. (2016). Translation and testing of the Swedish version of the Iceland-Family Perceived Support Questionnaire with parents of children with congenital heart defects. *Journal of Family Nursing, 22*(3), 298–320.
	• Sveinbjarnardottir, E. K., Svavarsdottir, E. K., & Hrafnkelsson, B. (2012b). Psychometric development of the Iceland-Family Perceived Support Questionnaire (ICE-FPSQ). *Journal of Family Nursing, 18*(3), 328–352.

Sources: Bell, J. (2016a). *Family nursing research instruments developed by family nurses* (Web log Post). Retrieved from janicembell .com/2015/08/family-nursing-research-instruments-developed-by-family-nurses/; and Sawin, K. J. (2016). Measurement in family nursing: Established instruments and new directions [Guest editorial]. *Journal of Family Nursing, 22*(3), 287–297.

Two family data-gathering instruments that should be used in working with families are the family genogram and the family ecomap. Both are short, easy instruments and processes that supply essential family data and engage the family in therapeutic conversation.

Family Genogram and Family Ecomap

Genograms and ecomaps provide health care providers with visual diagrams of the current family story and situation (Harrison & Neufeld, 2009; Kaakinen & Tabacco, 2015). The information gathered from both the genogram and ecomap help guide the family plan of action and the selection of intervention strategies (Ray & Street, 2005). One of the major benefits of working with families using these two instruments is that family members can feel and visualize the amount of energy they are expending to manage the situation, which in itself is therapeutic for the family (Harrison & Neufeld, 2009; Holtslander, 2005; Rempel, Neufeld, & Kushner, 2007).

The use of genograms and ecomaps among nurses and other health care providers is growing and these useful tools are being applied in several practice and research contexts. Genograms, used historically in the context of genetic prediction and counseling, have been applied alongside ecomaps as primary assessment and decision-making tools in acute centers (Leahey & Svavarsdottir, 2009; Svavarsdottir, 2008). Examples of how other health care providers have applied the use of these tools include enhancing health promotion (Kehoe & Kehoe, 2008); increasing provider cultural competence and spiritual assessment of families (Hodge & Limb, 2010); and assessment of child social support systems (Baumgartner, Burnett, DiCarlo, & Buchanan, 2012). It is clear that generating and annotating visual data in these diagrammatic forms will be increasingly useful to nurses caring for families in many settings and contexts.

Family Genogram

The *family genogram* is a format for drawing a family tree that records information about family members and their relationships during at least three generations (McGoldrick, 2016; McGoldrick, Gerson, & Petry, 2008). In addition, the genogram captures significant non-blood kin who are considered family, as well as pets. This diagram offers a rich source of information for planning intervention strategies because it displays the complexity of a family visually and graphically in a way that provides a quick overview. Family genograms help both nurses and families to see and think systematically about families and the impact of the health event on family structure, function, and processes.

The three-generational family genogram had its origin in Family Systems Theory (Bowen, 1985; Bowen & Kerr, 1988). According to family systems, people are organized into family systems by generation, age, sex, or other similar features. How a person fits into his or her family structure influences its functioning, relational patterns, and what type of family he or she will carry forward into the next generation. Bowen (1985) incorporated Toman's (1976) ideas about the importance of sex and birth order in shaping sibling relationships and characteristics. Furthermore, families repeat themselves throughout generations in a phenomenon called the *transmission of family patterns* (Bowen, 1985). What happens in one generation repeats itself in the next generation; thus, many of the same strengths and problems get played out from generation to generation. These include psychosocial, physical, and mental health issues.

Nurses establish therapeutic relationships with families through the process of asking questions while collecting family data. Families become more engaged in their current situation during this interaction as their family story unfolds. Both the nurse and the family can see the "big picture" historically on the vertical axis of the genogram and horizontally across the family (McGoldrick, 2016; McGoldrick et al., 2008). This approach can help families see connectedness, and help identify potential and missing support people.

The diagramming of family genograms must adhere to specific rules and symbols to ensure that all parties involved have the same understanding and interpretations. It is important not to confuse family genograms with a family genetic pedigree. A family pedigree is specific to genetic assessments (see Chapter 8), whereas a genogram has broader uses for family health care practitioners. Genograms may assist nurses to offer a more comprehensive, holistic nursing care perspective (Charnock, 2016; Gallagher, 2013). Creative blended models built upon these ideas are emerging in practice with innovative applications such as the use of color coding for enhancing multimodal understanding of children and families (Driessnack, 2009).

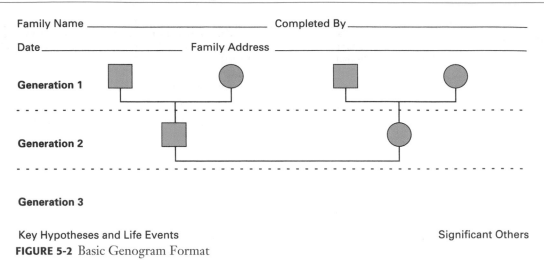

Key Hypotheses and Life Events   Significant Others

FIGURE 5-2 Basic Genogram Format

Figure 5-2 provides a basic genogram from which a nurse can start diagramming family members during the first, second, and third generations (McGoldrick, Gerson, & Schellenberger, 1999). Figure 5-3 depicts the genogram symbols used to describe basic family membership and structure, family interaction patterns, and other family information of particular importance, such as health status, substance abuse, obesity, smoking, and mental health comorbidities (McGoldrick et al., 2008). The health history of all family members (e.g., morbidity, mortality, and onset of illness) is important information for family nurses and can be the focus of analysis of the family genogram. An example of a family genogram developed from one interview is contained in the Bono family case study that follows.

The structure of the interview for gathering the genogram information is based on the reasons why the nurse is working with the family. For example, if the context of creating a genogram is that of obtaining a health history aimed at uncovering family patterns of illness, the nurse may wish to explore more fully the health history of each generational family member. If, on the other hand, the context of the nursing care is determining the nature of social relationships and roles among family members to craft an acute care plan of discharge, the nurse may wish to focus the interview more closely on determining who is directly in the home and how their relationships function to aid in the recovery of the ill family member. A suggested format for conducting a concise, focused family genogram interview is outlined in Box 5-5. Most families are cooperative and interested in completing their genogram, which becomes a part

of their ongoing health care record. The genogram does not have to be completed at one sitting. As the same or a different nurse continues to work with a family, data can be added to the genogram over time in a continuing process. Families should be given a copy of their own genogram.

Family Ecomap

A *family ecomap* provides information about systems outside of the immediate nuclear family that are sources of social support or that are stressors to the family. The ecomap is a visual representation of the family unit in relation to the larger community in which it is embedded (Kaakinen & Tabacco, 2015). It is a visual representation of the relationship between an individual family and the world around it (McGoldrick et al., 2008). The ecomap is thus an overview of the family in its current context, picturing the important connections among the nuclear family, the extended family, and the community around it.

The blank ecomap form consists of a large circle with smaller circles around it (Figure 5-4). A simplified version of the family is placed in the center of the larger circle to complete the ecomap. This circle marks the boundary between the family and its extended external environment. The smaller outer circles represent significant people, agencies, or institutions with which the family interacts. Lines are drawn between the circles and the family members to depict the nature and quality of the relationships, and to show what kinds of energy and resources are moving in and out of the immediate family. Straight lines show strong or close relationships; the more pronounced the line

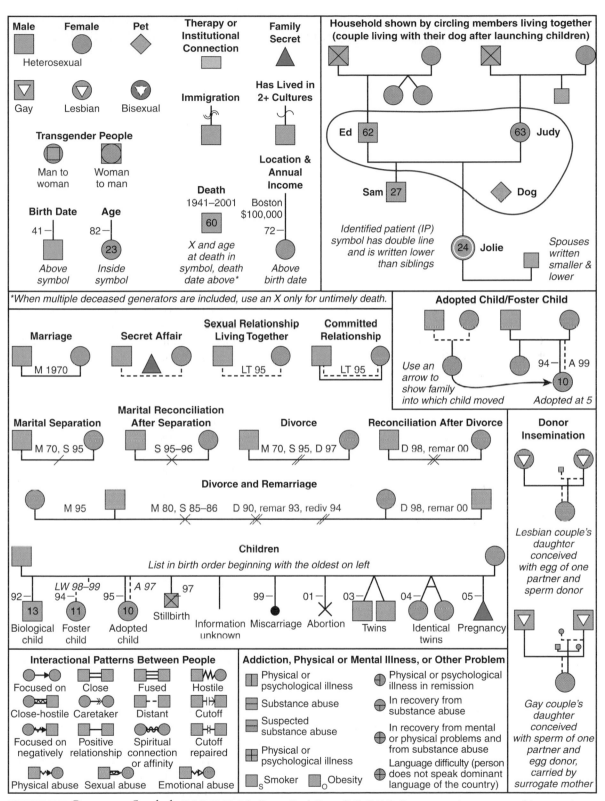

FIGURE 5-3 Genogram Symbols (*McGoldrick, M., Gerson, R., & Petry, S. S. (2008).* Genograms: Assessment and intervention *(3rd ed.); and McGoldrick, M., Gerson, R., & Schellenberger, S. (1999).* Genograms in family assessment *(2nd ed.); with permission from W.W. Norton).*

BOX 5-5

Family Genogram Interview Data Collection

During a family genogram interview, do the following:

- Identify who is in the immediate family.
- Identify the person who has the health problem.
- Identify all the people who live with the immediate family.
- Determine how all the people are related.
- Gather the following information on each family member.
  - Age
  - Sex

- Correct spelling of name
- Health problems
- Occupation
- Dates of relationships: marriage, separation, divorce, living together, living together/committed
- Dates and age of death
- Seek the same information for all family members across each generation for consistency and to reveal patterns of health and illness.
- Add any information relative to the situation, such as geographical location and interaction patterns.

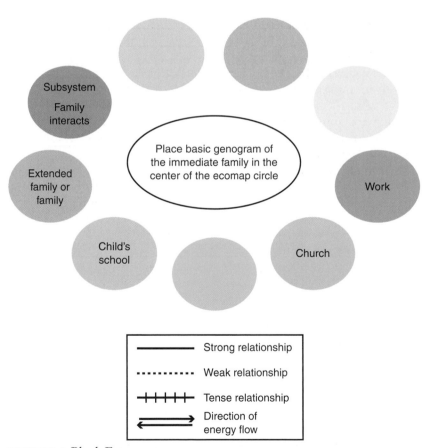

FIGURE 5-4 Blank Ecomap

or the greater the number of lines, the stronger the relationship. Straight lines with slashes denote stressful relationships, and broken lines show tenuous or distant relationships. Arrows reveal the direction of the flow of energy and resources between individuals, and between the family and the environment. Ecomaps not only portray the present situation but also can be used to set goals; for example, to increase connections and exchanges with individuals and agencies in the community.

See the Bono family case study later in this chapter for an example of a completed ecomap.

The value of using a genogram and ecomap in family nursing practice is extensive. By creating a visual picture of the system in which the family exists, families are more able to envision alternative solutions and possible social support networks (Rempel et al., 2007). Ecomaps help patients in palliative care identify who is important and who they desire to have involved in their lives (Gallagher, 2013). Family genograms have been used by nurses in diverse cultures: for example, in Brazil to work with children who have special needs (Neves, Cabral, & da Silveira, 2013); in Brazil, as identified in a systematic review of Brazilian use of family genograms and ecomaps (Nascimento, Dantas, Andrade, & de Mello, 2014); in Iceland working with families, children, and adolescents in active cancer treatment (Svavarsdottir & Sigurdardottir, 2013); and in Sweden for using spiritual ecomaps as a component of care (Hodge, 2015). In addition, the process of this data collection itself helps to expose a clearer picture of the supportive or unsupportive family relationships that are going on in a family system (Neufeld, Harrison, Hughes, & Stewart, 2007). This information will enhance understanding of the family's social network with their caregivers (Rempel et al., 2007).

Family Health Literacy

The definition of health literacy has evolved. The following definition is the most comprehensive and explanatory:

Health literacy is linked to literacy and entails people's knowledge, motivation and competence to access, understand, appraise, and apply health information in order to make judgments and decisions in everyday life concerning healthcare, disease prevention and health promotion to maintain or improve quality of life during the life course. (Sorensen et al., 2012, p. 3)

Concepts of health literacy include the comprehension of medical words, the ability to follow medical instructions, and the understanding of the consequences when instructions are not followed (Rutherford et al., 2016). As many health care providers have limited ability to identify patients with low health literacy, the Agency for Healthcare Research and Quality (AHRQ) suggests that health care providers should use health literacy guidelines for low literacy with all patients (Brega et al., 2015). The AHRQ has an online toolkit (see www.ahrq.gov/professionals/quality-patient-safety/quality-resources/tools/literacy-toolkit/index.html) that is an excellent resource for all health care providers. Nurses who understand the concept of health literacy will provide education, materials, and other supports, such as videos or Web sites that are accessible to the family.

Health literacy is an important measure for health care providers because lower health literacy is strongly associated with poor health outcomes (Berkman, Sheridan, Donahue, Halpern, & Crotty, 2011; Dickens, & Piano, 2013; Federman et al., 2014; French, 2015; Parnell, 2014; Watts, Stevenson, & Adams, 2017). Health literacy plays a primary role in people's ability to gain knowledge, make decisions, and take actions that result in positive health outcomes (Dickens & Piano, 2013; Sorensen et al., 2012), especially when managing a chronic illness (Dickens & Piano, 2013; Watts et al., 2017).

Multiple approaches to helping patients understand their health and health care needs have been designed. Table 5-3 includes tips for successful oral education and Box 5-6 outlines guidelines for improving readability and visualization of written material.

Nurses need to approach assessment of a family's health literacy with sensitivity and understanding. It is a crucial element to take into consideration during the analysis of the family story and in the development of the family action plan.

ANALYSIS OF THE FAMILY STORY

One of the challenges of data collection is organizing the individual pieces of information so that the "big picture" or whole family story can be understood and analyzed. To understand the family picture, the nurse must consolidate the data that were collected into meaningful patterns or categories. This process helps the nurse visualize the relationships between and among the patterns to uncover how the family is managing the situation. Diagramming the family and the relationships between the data groups assists in identifying the most pressing issues or problems for the family. If the family and nurse focus on solving these major family problems, the outcome will have a ripple effect by positively influencing the other areas of family functioning.

Table 5-3	**Tips for Successful Oral Education**	
Language Elements	**Recommendations**	**Example**
Use the active voice.	• The subject of the sentence is performing the action.	• You will take your medications with breakfast. **NOT** The medications are taken at breakfast.
Converse: be interactive.	• Limit long monologues.	• What questions do you have for me? (Ask this several times in the teaching session.)
Be considerate toward listeners.	• Announce topics.	• Aspirin. Aspirin helps stop heart attacks.
	• Periodically call the learner by name.	• Rosie, could you tell me what you ate yesterday?
	• Convey information in little stories.	• I know a woman named Charisse who forgot to take her Plavix for 3 days, and then WHAM, she got chest pain and came back to the emergency room. And guess what? The metal coil they just put in her heart had blocked off and caused another heart attack!
Give "need to know" rather than "nice to know" information.	• Reinforce important information (such as the prescription regimen).	• Take your water pill every morning, right after breakfast. **NOT** Your diuretic works on the distal loop of Henle.
	• Limit information on pathophysiology.	• When you leave the hospital today, I want you to remember to make your follow-up appointment, take your Plavix every day, and call us if you have any chest pain.
	• Provide information in three to five chunks in each session.	
Focus on the patient.	• Contextualize the information being taught.	• In the morning, get out of bed, go to the bathroom, and then weigh yourself. Do this every day, before you eat or drink anything for breakfast.
	• Use everyday language familiar to the patient.	• Fast food is really bad for your health.
Be mindful of language complexity.	• Speak in short sentences (fewer than 15 words).	• If you have chest pain, go to the emergency room.
	• Use words with fewer than three syllables.	• Drink a lot of water with these pills.
	• Decrease medical jargon.	• Your water pill will make you pee a lot.

Source: Dickens, C., & Piano, M. R. (2013). Health literacy and nursing: An update. *American Journal of Nursing, 113*(6), 52–57, Wolters Kluwer Health, Inc. with permission.

BOX 5-6

Guidelines for Improving Readability and Visuals of Written Materials

Criteria	Specifications
Typography	• Use bold or underlined headers.
	• Use sans serif or serif 12- to 14-point fonts.
	• Do not use all caps for headers.
	• Use white space around your main content area.
	• Use high-contrast colors (black on white).
Layout	• Put the most important information first.
	• Limit bullet points to 3 to 7 items at a time.
	• Turn sentences into lists.
	• Create headings with subheadings.

(continued)

BOX 5-6

Guidelines for Improving Readability and Visuals of Written Materials (cont.)

Criteria	Specifications
Language	• Explain how to perform the action, **NOT** the mechanism of action.
	• Limit use of "not," "don't," or "unless."
	• Select familiar words and use them frequently.
	• Provide specific action steps.
	• Keep paragraphs short.
	• Use active, **NOT** passive, voice.
	• Use words with one or two syllables when possible.
	• Limit the use of jargon or scientific language.
	• If you have to use medical jargon, define the word.
	• Provide text at the fifth grade or lower reading level.
Graphics	• Use captions that explain each graphic.
	• Place illustrations adjacent to text on the page.
	• Do not use shading or graying.
	• Do not use cues, such as circles or arrows.
	• Use photographs to portray real-life events and emotions.
	• Use culturally relevant images.
	• When showing a sequence, number the images.

Source: Dickens, C., & Piano, M. R. (2013). Health literacy and nursing: An update. *American Journal of Nursing, 113*(6), 52–57, Wolters Kluwer Health, Inc. with permission.

The Family Reasoning Web (Figure 5-5) is an organizational tool to help analyze the family story by clustering individual pieces of data into meaningful family categories. The components of the Family Reasoning Web have been drawn from various theoretical concepts, such as Family Structure and Function Theory, Family Developmental Theory, Family Stress Theory, and family health promotion models. This systematic approach to collecting and analyzing information helps structure the information collection process to ensure the inclusion of important pieces of information. The categories of the Family Reasoning Web are as follows:

1. Family routines of daily living (i.e., sleeping, meals, child care, exercise)
2. Family communication
3. Family supports and resources
4. Family roles
5. Family beliefs
6. Family developmental stage
7. Family health knowledge
8. Family environment
9. Family stress management
10. Family culture
11. Family spirituality

Once the data have been placed into the categories of the Family Reasoning Web template, the nurse assigns a family nursing diagnosis to each category. "A nursing diagnosis is defined as a clinical judgment about individuals, families, or community responses to actual or potential health problems/life processes. Nursing diagnoses link information to care planning. Nursing diagnoses provide the basis for selecting nursing interventions to help achieve outcomes for which nurses are accountable" (Doenges, Moorhouse, & Murr, 2016, p. 10). The following case study presents more information on nursing diagnoses.

NANDA International Inc. (NANDA-I) has approved more than 200 nursing diagnoses that are used in multiple member countries. NANDA-I nursing

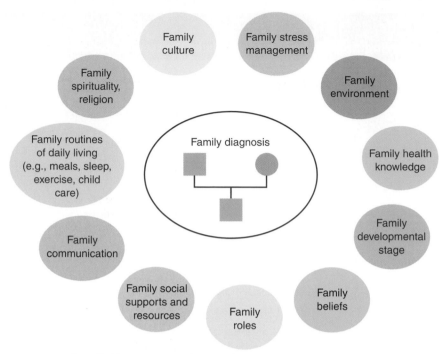

FIGURE 5-5 Family Reasoning Web Template

diagnoses that are specific to families are listed in Box 5-7. If the pattern of family data in the specific category in the Family Reasoning Web does not match one of the NANDA-I nursing diagnoses, nurses are encouraged to create a family nursing diagnosis that captures the family problem. Nursing diagnosis manuals are extremely important resources for nurses because family nursing diagnoses are readily linked with both the Nursing Intervention Classification (NIC) (Bulechek, Butcher, Dochterman, & Wagner, 2013) and the Nursing Outcomes Classification (NOC) (Moorhead, Johnson, Maas, & Swanson, 2012) data sets. These resources provide many new ideas for family interventions and suggest focused family outcomes that can be explored with families.

Other diagnostic classification systems that can be used to identify problems include the Omaha System–Community Health Classification System (Martin, 2005; The Omaha System, 2016), the *Diagnostic and Statistical Manual of Mental Disorders, Fifth Edition* (*DSM-5*; American Psychiatric Association, 2013), and the *International Classification of Diseases, Tenth Revision, Clinical Modification* (*ICD-10-CM*; Centers for Disease and Control Prevention, 2016). See Boxes 5-8 and 5-9, respectively, for examples of selected family diagnoses from the *DSM* and *ICD-10-CM* sources.

A rapidly growing system of diagnostic language relevant to nursing in North America is that of the World Health Organization *ICD* companions, the *International Classification of Functioning (ICF)*, and its related child and youth version *(ICF-CY)* (World Health Organization, 2016). This broad schema of classification focuses on making diagnostic statements of health impact in four domains: body structure, body function, activity and participation, and environment (World Health Organization, 2016). Family nursing practice greatly involves the focus on the domains of activity and participation and the environmental context of family life. Given that nurses' primary focus with individuals and families is the functional aspect of health in daily life, this system of categorizing and coding functional outcomes of health is compelling. The *ICF* and *ICF-CY* approaches are being used with expanded focus in Europe and Canada particularly (Florin, Ehrenberg, Ehnfors, & Björvell, 2013; Raggi, Leonardi, Cabello, & Bickenbach, 2010).

After the categories have been assigned and a family nursing diagnosis determined, the next step in analyzing the family story is for the nurse and family to work together to determine the relationships between the categories. Arrows are drawn between the family categories to show the direction of influence if the data in one category influence the data in another

BOX 5-7

NANDA-I Nursing Diagnoses Relevant to Family Nursing

Following are nursing diagnoses relevant to family nursing:

- Ineffective childbearing process
- Risk for ineffective childbearing process
- Risk for impaired parent/infant/child attachment
- Caregiver role strain
- Risk for caregiver role strain
- Ineffective role performance
- Parental role conflict
- Compromised family coping

- Disabled family coping
- Readiness for enhanced family coping
- Dysfunctional family processes: alcoholism
- Readiness for enhanced family processes
- Interrupted family processes
- Readiness for enhanced parenting
- Impaired parenting
- Risk for impaired parenting
- Relocation stress syndrome
- Ineffective role performance
- Ineffective family therapeutic regimen management

Source: Doenges, M. E., Moorhouse, M. F., & Murr, A. C. (2016). *Nursing diagnosis manual: Planning, individualizing, and documenting client care* (5th ed.). Philadelphia, PA: F. A. Davis, with permission.

BOX 5-8

Selected Family-Centered Diagnoses From *Diagnostic and Statistical Manual of Mental Disorders, Fifth Edition*

V61.9	Relational problem related to a mental disorder or general medical condition
V61.20	Parent-child relational problem
V61.10	Partner relational problem
V61.8	Sibling relational problem
V71.02	Child or adolescent antisocial behavior
V62.82	Bereavement
V62.3	Academic problem
V62.4	Acculturation problem
V62.89	Phase-of-life problem

Source: American Psychiatric Association. (2013). *Diagnostic and statistical manual of mental disorders (DSM-5)* (5th ed.). Arlington, VA: American Psychiatric Association Publishing.

BOX 5-9

Selected Family-Centered Diagnoses From *ICD-9-CM*

313.3	Relationship problems
313.8	Emotional disturbances of childhood or adolescence
V61.0	Family disruption
V25.09	Family planning advice
V61.9	Family problem
94.41	Group therapy
94.42	Family therapy

Source: Centers for Disease Control and Prevention. (2016). *International classification of diseases, tenth revision, clinical modification (ICD-10-CM)*. Retrieved from www.cdc.gov/nchs/icd/icd10cm.htm

category. The important family problems or issues surface by systematically working through all the relationships because they are the ones that have the most arrows indicating the strongest relationships to all other areas of family functioning. This step reveals the primary family problems.

Another dimension of the family story that is of importance to nurses is the dimension of beliefs. Family and family member beliefs about health, illness, health care providers, and even their own roles and processes are of great importance for nurses to assess in planning to provide optimal care. The Beliefs and Illness Model by Wright and Bell (2009) suggests that nurses should assess families' beliefs in several areas, specifically, family structure, roles, communication, and decision-making authority; beliefs about health and illness (how they are defined, why they occur, how they are managed); and beliefs about health care providers (their intentions, motivations, and knowledge and the meaning of their presence and actions to the families and their health or illness experience). Individuals and families often behave based upon their beliefs and, thus, any attempt for nurses to engage families in health promotion, health literacy, or health intervention in any setting requires an exploration of these key areas. After verifying all these findings with the family, the next step is to work with the family to understand their preferences for decision making and design a family plan of care accordingly.

Shared Decision Making

Family nurses should explore how involved the family would like to be in the decision-making processes. Universal needs of families include consistency, clarity, comprehensive information, and involvement in shared decision making with the health care provider (Elwyn et al., 2013; Légaré & Thompson-Leduc, 2014). One of the problems with the implementation of shared decision making is that individual health care providers may have a different definition and understanding of the components of this concept, as well as personal biases and beliefs about how individuals and families may or may not wish to participate (Elwyn et al., 2013). Shared decision making is not just informing the family of the decisions and keeping the lines of communication open, nor is it the health care providers determining what decisions the family can make. Shared decision making is defined as "a collaborative

process that allows patients and their providers to make health care decisions together, taking into account the best scientific evidence available as well as the patient's values and preferences" (Informed Medical Decisions Foundation, 2017). Patients and families vary in the process and degree to which they would like to be involved in decision making (Dy & Purnell, 2012; Légaré & Thompson-Leduc, 2014; Stiggelbout, Pieterse, & De Haes, 2015). Nurses should not assume that patients' or families' reluctance to engage in the decision-making process means that they do not want to be involved, as reluctance could be related to several factors, such as a lack of self-efficacy (Légaré & Thompson-Leduc, 2014), health statistics being poorly understood by patients (McCaffery, Smith, & Wolf, 2010), some patients having difficulty imagining their future health state or events (McCaffery et al., 2010), and some patients believing that the physicians are supposed to make these decisions (Hawley & Morris, 2017).

The amount of information families seek or need changes during the course of the health event, the stage of the illness, and the likelihood of a cure (Stiggelbout et al., 2015). Supporting the hypothesis that not all families and family members want full involvement in making health care decisions, Makoul and Clayman (2006) outlined the following nine options for shared decision making (p. 307):

- Doctor alone
- Doctor led and patient acknowledgment sought or offered
- Doctor led and patient agreement sought or offered
- Doctor led and patient views/option sought or offered
- Shared equally
- Patient led and doctor views/opinions sought or offered
- Patient led and doctor agreement sought or offered
- Patient led and doctor acknowledgment sought or offered
- Patient alone

Studies have shown that some patients who elected to defer decisions to their health care provider want more involvement in making decisions after knowing more about their health situation (Stiggelbout et al., 2015). At the beginning of a health event that requires shared decision making, many patients and their family members do not have clearly defined preferences

(Pieterse, de Vries, Kunneman, Stiggelbout, & Feldman-Stewart, 2013).

Several instruments have been designed to assist providers and patients/families to work through their preferences and participate in decision making. One of the major concerns about use of these instruments is that they are not well-tested when working with patients/family of minority race/ethnic backgrounds (Hawley & Morris, 2017) or with patients with lower health literacy (McCaffery et al., 2010). An option grid is one strategy for implementation of shared decision making (Elwyn et al., 2013). An option grid is developed by the family nurse and keeps health literacy principles at the fifth-grade level. Elwyn et al. specifically developed the grid format as a decision-making paper worksheet addressing common therapeutic approaches to specific health conditions where patients and families could view the benefits or drawbacks associated with different possible treatment decisions. On the worksheet, the most relevant, frequently asked questions about a specific condition make up the rows of the grid, and the specific options available for the decision make up the columns. Patients are given the paper grid and talked through the options available to them with their provider. For example, see Table 5-4 for an option grid that a nurse could design to help parents determine respite placement for their 12-year-old daughter who is medically fragile with severe cerebral palsy. This specific tool shows promise for nurses working with families because not only does it represent the principles of FCC in practice, but it is also useful because families often have difficulties understanding their options and the potential benefits or consequences associated with their choices.

Another approach to shared decision making is to use the Patient/Parent Involvement Information Assessment Tool (PINT) developed by Sobo (2004). The PINT is a self-administered survey that can be kept in the medical record to facilitate and target information for communication between the health care team and the family. In the challenge to collaborate in the care and meet the needs of individuals and family members, nurses may ask the following two sample questions from the PINT tool (Sobo, 2004, p. 258):

1. When possible, what level of information would you prefer to receive?
   - The simplest information possible
   - More than the simplest, but want to keep it on everyday terms
   - In-depth information that you can help me understand

Table 5-4	Example of Option Grid

The following is an example of an option grid for helping a family to decide about 1-week respite placement for their 12-year-old medically fragile child

Option 1: Home	Option 2: Grandmother's Home	Option 3: Nursing Home
Child knows own home and is around familiar surroundings.	Child has been to grandmother's home only a couple of times because it is in a different city.	New setting for child.
Home is adapted to the child's needs and wheelchair.	Home is not adapted to the physical care needs of the child, such as wheelchair and bathing.	Setting can accommodate the child's special needs and wheelchair.
Caregiver would be the skills trainer who knows the child.	Caregiver is grandmother, who the child knows well and has spent considerable time with.	No personal relationship with caregivers in this setting. Grandmother could visit during the day.
Parents are comfortable with the child being with the skills worker during the day, but do not have experience with this person at night.	Parents are comfortable with the child being with the grandmother. Grandmother has helped take care of the child for short times before, such as a weekend.	Parents do not have a relationship with the caregivers in this setting.
Cost: $250 a day for 7 days for a total of $1,750. This would come out of the parents' pocket because insurance does not cover this care.	Cost: Nothing.	Cost: Covered by insurance.

- As much in-depth and detailed information as can be provided

2. When possible, what decision-making role do you want to assume?
   - Leave all decisions to the health care team
   - Have the care team make the decisions about care with serious consideration of our views
   - Share in the making of the decisions with the health care team
   - Make all the decisions about care with serious consideration of the health care team advice

Shared decision making requires that health care providers tailor their communication, accommodate their talk to the level of the family, and present information in a way that allows the family to make informed choices.

FAMILY NURSING INTERVENTION

The family plan of action (or care) is designed by the nurse and the family to focus on the concerns that were identified in the Family Reasoning Web as the most pressing or as causing the family the most stress. The plan should account for the family's preferences for decision making and should meet the family members' health literacy needs. The more specific the family plan of action and the interventions, the more positive the outcomes. The role of the nurse is to offer guidance to the family, provide information, and assist in the planning interventions. Working with families from an outcome perspective helps to clarify what information and resources are necessary to address the family need. The following four points will help the family break the plan into action steps:

1. We need the following type of help.
2. We need the following information.
3. We need the following supplies or resources.
4. We need to involve or tell the following people about our family action plan.

For the purposes of clarity and evaluation, this plan should be a written document. The action steps or interventions should be clear and concise. The plan should outline specifically who needs to do what by when and also articulate the time frame in which the nurse will follow up. The last step of any family action plan should entail evaluation that involves the nurse and family reflecting and sharing ideas about what

worked well, what needs to continue to be addressed by the family, and avenues for seeking help in the future.

Working with families to improve health and adapt to illness is the primary goal of family health care nursing. Nevertheless, although there is direct evidence of the potential outcomes and effects associated with family nursing intervention, few studies have been conducted longitudinally or across multiple populations. What has been distilled from the bodies of literature on family health care intervention is that family intervention does seem to produce better effects than usual, individual-focused medical care; greater effects have been shown in improving child health than adult health in some chronic conditions; and family-focused intervention examples found in childhood obesity efforts reveal the most compelling effects (Chesla, 2010).

Chesla (2010) also articulated that the means of interventions varied and ranged from simple home visits to coach families to much more complex educational and skill-developing strategies. Nurses were involved in relationship-based interventions to improve family communication, problem solving, and skill building as they related to illness or health management. The more tools nurses tended to use to assist families (multimodal) as part of their care plans, the better the outcomes seemed to be, particularly in managing complex health conditions that required numerous lifestyle changes. Family members were sometimes noted to be beneficiaries of interventions, experiencing unique and improved outcomes that were separate from the health of the patient (Chesla, 2010). The field requires additional intervention strategies and resulting evidence of outcomes, though more frequent examples are beginning to emerge in practice (Svavarsdottir & Jonsdottir, 2011).

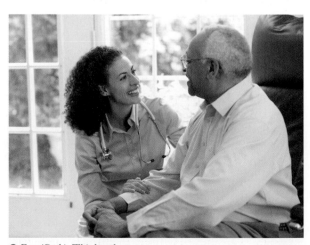

© Fuse/Corbis/Thinkstock

Nurses help by (1) providing direct care, (2) removing barriers to needed services, and (3) improving the capacity of the family to act on its own behalf and assume responsibility. Family nursing interventions can be directed toward improving the health outcomes of the member with the illness or condition, the family members' health-related outcomes of caregiving, or a combination of both. One of the important aspects of working with the family is the nurse-family relationship, which is an intervention in and of itself as families can experience a sense of strength, comfort, and confidence that can be therapeutic and useful (Friedman et al., 2003).

The nurse is responsible for helping the family implement the plan of care. The nurse can assume the role of teacher, role model, coach, counselor, advocate, coordinator, consultant, and evaluator in helping the family to implement the plan of care they jointly create. The types of interventions are limitless because they are designed with the family to meet its needs in the context of its family story. The three examples that follow illustrate different family nursing interventions in various contexts.

Brief Therapeutic Conversations in Acute Care

Brief therapeutic family conversations or interviews are an important family intervention (Bell, 2016b) and have been linked to improved health outcomes (Street Jr., Makoul, Arora, & Epstein, 2009). These brief interviews could include nurses making introductions to family members, collecting focused data to complete simple genograms and ecomaps, and opening pathways of knowing about a family's self-defined needs and priorities (Wright & Leahey, 2013). Svavarsdottir, Tryggvadottir, and Sigurdardottir (2012) conducted a study measuring families' perceptions of nurse support and family members' own reports of family functioning. The study compared families who received brief family intervention interviews with nurses and those who did not. Predictably, families who received the nursing intervention interview reported feeling more supported than those who did not. Surprisingly, this finding was true for families with a child with an acute health crisis but was not true for those coping with chronic conditions. Expressive family functioning did not seem to change in the latter situation. Families of acutely ill children, however, may experience significant benefits when nurses take

small amounts of time to enact simple family health care strategies (Svavarsdottir et al., 2012).

Home Visits and Telephone Support

Nursing visits to family homes are part of the early historical tradition of nursing and are appropriate to use today in family nursing. Northouse et al. (2007) utilized a clinical trial design to provide three in-home support visits along with two follow-up telephone calls to partnered couples where men were living through prostate cancer treatment. In the study, both patients and partners who received the in-home visits and phone calls reported that their communication and relationship with one another improved. Nurses offered these families coaching in communication, facilitated discussions that identified the beliefs and needs of both partners, and helped the families make decisions about care tasks and life balance. The partners seemed to benefit by demonstrating improved quality of life, increased self-efficacy, and less overall caregiving negativity than partners who did not receive the intervention. Additionally, some spouses continued to report these effects for up to 8 months following the intervention, suggesting that the act of providing access to nurses in the home and via telephone helped spouses long after the contact ended (Northouse et al., 2007).

Self-Care Talk for Family Caregivers

Nurses caring for families can intervene to promote health by helping families to identify potential health risks that stress the health of the family, such as when a 45-year-old father and husband with metabolic syndrome refuses to adhere to diet and exercise interventions. Parker, Teel, Leenerts, and Macan (2011) proposed a unique family nursing intervention for developing self-care motivation and implementation in family caregivers of people with high-acuity health needs; it is widely known that intensive periods of caregiving can result in worsening health of caregivers. In this intervention, family nurses made a series of six extended telephone calls that helped the family caregivers identify the barriers they faced in taking care of themselves. Using a theory-based framework, the nurses then assisted the caregivers to remove those barriers and implement self-care strategies to improve the caregivers' health. Clinical trial research is needed to demonstrate the efficacy and effectiveness of this intervention, but early evidence from similar approaches indicates that the ideas have promise for improving caregiver health. Moreover, the relational nature of the intervention, supplied entirely by telephone, is creative and has implications for nurses serving families in a variety of settings, including those in rural locations.

FAMILY NURSING EVALUATION

In making clinical judgments, nurses employ critical thinking to determine whether and to what extent they have met an outcome. The means of measuring desired changes in outcomes varies with the specific problem upon which the action plan is focused. For example, if the family has identified that a primary focus problem is disrupted sleep routines for their young child with attention deficit-hyperactivity disorder, the nurse may propose that the family create a simple chart to measure its new routine of sleep hygiene practices on a daily basis. The family determines that, at present, the child is not able to fall asleep with ease on any given night and sets a goal to have the child fall asleep with ease three nights a week initially. Using the simple daily charting concept, the nurse and family can easily look to the collected data at a specified time to determine if the goal has been met. The team makes the decision about whether to proceed as originally planned, to modify the family action plan, or to revisit the family story in total. As indicated previously, the critical reasoning approach of thinking about families and their needs is not linear. In practice, a constant flow occurs between the components of the family assessment and intervention strategy with plans being continually evaluated and modified through reflection.

There can be many reasons underlying a lack of success in meeting desired outcomes when working with families, some of which may be related to family factors, others to nurse factors, and even others to additional environmental factors. Apathy and indecision are examples of potential family barriers. Family apathy may occur because of value differences between the nurse and the family. The family may be overcome with a sense of hopelessness, may view the problems or bureaucracy as too overwhelming, or may have a fear of failure. Nurses also should consider whether they themselves impose barriers. Examples of nurse barriers to achieving desired family outcomes could include discrepant values or beliefs from the family, resulting in a lack of follow-through on the part of the nurse; not listening to family concerns about the problems of importance, leading to two separate, rather than one unified, outcome goal; or even lack of time and resources needed for the nurse to address the family needs in a timely fashion. Examples of additional environmental factors that act as barriers to desired outcomes can be things such as a change in the prescription formulary that limits access to the effective drug of choice on a family's insurance plan, lack of access to an appropriate specialty care provider because of rural geography, or the loss of a job by the primary wage earner in the family. A more detailed list of possible barriers to family outcomes can be found in Box 5-10.

Aside from evaluating outcomes, another important part of the family evaluation is the decision when to end the relationship with the family. Sometimes care with a family ends suddenly. In this case, it is important for nurses to determine the forces that brought about the closure. The family may seek to end the relationship prematurely, which may require a renegotiating process. The insurance or agency requirements may place a financial constraint on the amount of time nurses can work with a family. Other times, the family-nurse relationship comes to an end more naturally, such as when the nurse

---

BOX 5-10

Barriers to Family Outcomes

The following are barriers to family outcomes:

- Family apathy
- Family indecision about the outcome or actions
- Nurse-imposed ideas
- Negative labeling
- Overlooking family strengths

- Neglecting cultural or gender implications
- Family perception of hopelessness
- Fear of failure
- Limited access to resources and support
- Limited finances
- Fear and distrust of health care system

and family together determine that the family has achieved the intended outcomes. Whatever the reason for the end of the nurse-family relationship, it is crucial that closure be achieved between the parties.

Building closure into the family action plan will benefit the family by providing for a smooth transition process. Strategies often used in this transition include decreasing contact with the nurse, extending invitations to the family for follow-up, and making referrals when appropriate. If possible, this process should include a summary evaluation meeting where the nurse and family put formal closure to their relationship. Following up with a therapeutic letter can encourage families to continue positive adaptation. The therapeutic letter should include recognition of the family achievement, a summary of the actions, commendations to each

family member, and an insightful question for the family to think about in the future that may provide the family with a future direction (Wright & Bell, 2009). An example of a therapeutic family letter is found in Box 5-11.

NURSE AND FAMILY REFLECTION

The final step in critically thinking about family nursing is for nurses and families to engage in vital, creative, and concurrent reflection about their work together. There are two purposes of engaging in individual and collaborative reflection: to facilitate evaluation of progress toward the desired family outcomes and to increase expertise of the nurse.

BOX 5-11
Example of Therapeutic Family Letter

Dear W., H., and T.,

First, I want to thank all of you for allowing me the opportunity to get acquainted with your family. I appreciated your openness and willingness to talk with me.

During our time together, we discussed several issues that were important to your family. One of these issues was the ongoing possibility of H., losing his job because of the seasonal nature of his work. We explored the effects of potential job loss on a personal and family level.

H., you expressed some concern about your ability to provide adequately for your family. You indicated a personal constraining belief that a lack of steady employment meant that you were letting your family down and not providing for them. We discussed the idea that a paying job is only one part of the entire family support system that you provide. We explored some examples of noneconomic means of support, such as specific tasks related to farm chores, household management, and child care. If your job situation changes again, I hope you will find some of these suggestions helpful.

W., I was so impressed with your ability to juggle your caregiving job with home, farm, kids, and spouse. I can't think of many women who could handle all that with such strength and grace. With all that you do, it's not surprising that there isn't much time left over for your own personal endeavors. We discussed your constraining belief that you had to be responsible for everything. You envisioned the possibility of letting go of certain tasks

and suggesting ways to share other tasks more equitably among family members. If you and your family choose to implement some task-sharing ideas, I sincerely hope this will work for all of you.

T., you have mapped out a path to higher education and a future career. You have every reason to expect success. We briefly touched upon what "success" might mean for you and whether success depends on the university attended. I hope you will consider my thoughts in this regard. Whatever the outcome, you have the love and support of your parents.

Finally, I would like to commend all of you for your deep devotion to each other and for putting family first. You value family time, and you strive to communicate in a way that sustains your close relationship with each other.

I would like to invite W. and H. to consider a suggestion regarding making time for just the two of you. "Couple time" is easy to overlook when you are focused on creating a loving, stable home for E. and helping to launch T. into higher education. Please remember that you two are the solid foundation of your family; the stronger your relationship is, the stronger your whole family can be.

Because of our time spent together, I came away with the feeling that your family is exceptionally strong, deeply committed to one another, and fully capable of adapting to any of life's challenges. Thank you again for your time.

Best wishes to you and your family,

Nursing student signature here

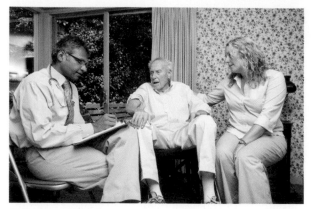

© iStock.com/jhorrocks

Evaluating Family Outcomes

The first purpose is for the nurse to reflect on the success of the family outcome in collaboration with the family as part of outcome evaluation. Reflection entails thinking about your thought process relative to this family client. Nurses can link ideas and consequences together in logical sequences by using an "if (describe a situation) . . . then (explain the outcome)" exercise, which can help the family member articulate concerns. A comparative analysis approach of the family problem can be used to analyze the strengths and weaknesses of competing alternatives. The nurse may decide to reframe the

family problem or priority need by attributing a different meaning to the content or context of the family situation based on testing, judgment, or changes in the context or content of the family story (Pesut & Herman, 1999). Although this process of reflecting with the family results in new co-created evaluation and knowledge related to the collaborative work, the nurse can also engage in this comparative reflective reasoning individually in preparation for, and as follow-up to, the discussions with the family.

Increasing Nursing Expertise

The second purpose of reflection is for nurses to build on their expertise by reflecting on client stories and their practice with each family. In essence, nurses create a library of family stories so that each time they come upon a similar family story, they can pull ideas from previous experiences. This aspect of reflection assists nurses with pattern recognition.

Yet another, more individual purpose of reflection is to engage in self-reflection and self-evaluation. By using this critical thinking strategy, nurses learn from mistakes and cement patterns of action that assist them to advance in their nursing practice from novice to expert family nurse.

A family case study follows that demonstrates critical reasoning about a family, assessment to identify concerns, and interventions to meet family needs.

Case Study: Bono Family

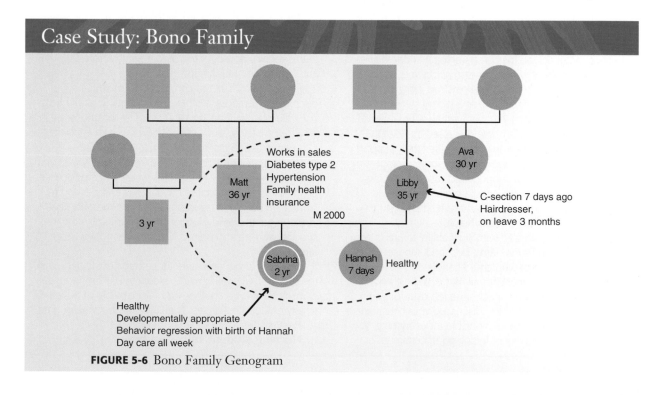

FIGURE 5-6 Bono Family Genogram

Case Study: Bono Family *(cont.)*

In preparation for her appointment with the Bono family in the mother-baby clinic, Vicki reviews the chart notes written by the nurse-midwife about the family. Vicki sees that the Bono family is coming in for a 1-week well-baby checkup of newborn infant Hannah and a follow-up for Libby, the mother, after her cesarean section (C-section) delivery 7 days ago. The note from the receptionist indicates that Libby expressed some concerns with her effectiveness in breastfeeding Hannah. The appointment book notes that the whole Bono family is coming for this visit. Vicki notes that the Bonos are a nuclear family that consists of a married couple with two biological children. Figure 5-6 shows the Bono family genogram.

Knowing that this is a nuclear family coming in for a well-baby checkup, Vicki decides to use a Developmental and Family Life Cycle theoretical approach to this family with a new member. (See Chapter 2 for details about this theoretical model.) Based on this approach, Vicki has many questions in her mind as she prepares for her appointment with the Bono family. The questions Vicki has about each family member and the whole family are presented in bulleted lists after a brief description of each family member.

Libby Bono is a 35-year-old mother recovering from a cesarean section delivery 7 days ago. She does not have any existing health problems. Libby's roles in the family are primary child-rearer, events planner, disciplinarian, and health expert. Libby is a hairdresser and is independently contracted with a hair salon. She has planned to take off 3 months for maternity leave.

- How might Libby's recovery from the cesarean section be affecting her roles in the family, especially with an active 2-year-old and a newborn?
- What are Libby's thoughts or plans for returning to work after her maternity leave?
- How is Libby adjusting to her expanded mother role? Assess Libby for postpartum depression.

Matt Bono, 36 years old, works for a snack food company in sales and distribution. His primary roles in the family are decision maker, maintenance person, pioneer, and information provider. He reports feeling little attachment to his occupation and welcomes this new birth as a change in routine and an opportunity to consider a change in his place of employment. His current medical problems include type 2 diabetes and mild hypertension; both are well managed and controlled by oral diabetic and antihypertensive medications. Currently, he is following the Weight Watchers® program to reduce his weight and to control the symptomatology experienced from his health conditions.

- How is Matt adjusting to the expanded role of father of two daughters?
- What are Matt's plans for employment, specifically about financial support for the family if he leaves his job? How would this affect health insurance for the family?

Sabrina Bono is a healthy 2-year-old girl who is developmentally appropriate. Psychologically, Sabrina is in the autonomy versus shame-and-doubt developmental stage. Her parents report that she often attempts to try new things on her own, and they frequently praise her efforts to promote independence. Her interest in potty training is developing, but still intermittent. Her immunizations are current. She normally goes to a day-care center that is close to her mother's work.

- How is Sabrina adjusting to the new baby?
- Is Sabrina showing any regression in her skills and abilities?
- Are each of the parents finding time to spend with Sabrina alone?
- How are the parents talking with Sabrina about her role as big sister?

Hannah Bono, 7 days old, was delivered after 42 weeks' gestation and was assessed as adequate for gestational age (AGA; 10th to 90th percentile), 53.75 cm and 3966 g, with American Pediatric Gross Assessment Record (APGAR) scores of 8 at 1 minute and 9 at 5 minutes.

- Is Hannah developing on target for her age and gestational age at birth?
- How often is Hannah eating, and is she gaining weight?
- How is Hannah nursing?

(continued)

Case Study: Bono Family *(cont.)*

The Bono family is a nuclear family that recently added a second child.

- What are the major concerns for the family at this time?
- Who in the family is having the most difficult adjustment to the changes brought about by the addition of a new family member?
- How is the family adjusting to these changes?
- Who or what are the support systems for this new family?

Bono Family Story:

During the appointment, Vicki confirms that family life for the Bono family has changed. Hannah was found to be healthy and developmentally appropriate. Libby is healing well from the C-section, but reported occasional discomfort when she "overdoes it." Libby's concerns about breastfeeding were easily relieved as Vicki validated her breastfeeding technique. An assessment for postpartum depression revealed that Libby is not demonstrating any signs of depression at this time. Throughout the examination of Hannah, the parents demonstrated overwhelming signs of bonding, such as talking with the infant and bragging about her beauty and temperament. During the appointment, Vicki noted that Sabrina was throwing toys and attempting to crawl onto her mother's lap while Libby was nursing Hannah. Sabrina would say "baby back" when she was upset. When Matt attempted to coddle or praise the baby, Sabrina became extremely angry with her father. They were not ignoring Sabrina but were not focused on her during the appointment. The parents' nonverbal actions showed frustration with Sabrina's behaviors. When asked, they reported that Sabrina has been very temperamental and inconsolable at day care. They reported that she had begun to show progress with toilet training before Hannah's birth but had now lost all interest.

Analysis of Bono Family Story:

To help everyone see the larger family picture, Vicki uses the Family Reasoning Web (see Figure 5-5). Based on the responses from using the Family Reasoning Web, she uncovered the following family information for analysis:

- *Family routines of daily living*: Matt and Libby are both tired from Hannah's every-3-hour breastfeeding schedule. They share some of the responsibility for comforting Hannah and seeing to her needs. Meals have been challenging as Matt has had to assume this responsibility because Libby has not recovered from her C-section. At this time, they do not have extended family support. Sabrina is still going to day care but is evidencing difficulty there.
- *Family communication*: Communication has been identified as a strength of the couple. They have a shared decision-making style. They appear nurturing with their children. Sabrina is emotionally up and down. She is clingy with her dad and ignores her mother except when she is breastfeeding Hannah. Sabrina was throwing toys when upset or frustrated. She periodically pointed to Hannah and said, "Take back."
- *Family supports and resources*: This family is fully covered under Matt's health insurance through his work. They have some family they can call on to help them. Ava, Libby's sister, volunteered to come for a visit and stay for 2 weeks. Matt's brother, his wife, and their 3-year-old child live in the same city. They have informally talked about sharing some child care. Both parents need to work to sustain their family lifestyle. Libby does not have benefits in her contracted hairdresser job. When she is off work, she does not make money. She does not have paid maternity leave. The couple planned for Libby to take 3 months off from work. The needs identified are for some immediate family support with everyday living and some financial concern at the end of the 3 months, given that the family had not planned for a longer period of reduced income.
- *Family roles*: All the family members are experiencing role ambiguity with their new roles. Matt and Libby are now parents of two daughters. Sabrina is a big sister, and Hannah is the new infant. Matt expressed some role overload because he is assuming many of the typical daily household chores of meals, laundry, food shopping, and primary care provider for Sabrina.
- *Family beliefs*: They strongly state that "family comes first." This was a planned pregnancy. They see themselves as loving parents. They express some confusion about disciplining Sabrina given her recent behaviors.
- *Family developmental stage*: This is a nuclear family in the family-with-toddler stage. They also have a new infant; therefore, they are in two developmental stages at the same time.
- *Family health knowledge*: The family expressed that it needed more help in knowing how to help Sabrina. The parents do not know how to work with Sabrina to help her adjust to being a big sister. They are confused with Sabrina's behavior of aggression, mood swings, clinging, and pointing at the baby and saying "take back." They feel that she has lost some of her skills. Health literacy does not appear to be an issue.

(continued)

Case Study: Bono Family *(cont.)*

- *Family environment*: At this time, they have enough room in their home for a family of four. They live in a safe neighborhood, but they do not know their neighbors well.
- *Family stress management*: They express feeling stressed about Sabrina's behaviors. They are both tired. Sabrina is stressed, as evidenced by her behaviors and changes in behavior. They are dealing with the current situation on their own but are open to asking for help from family for the immediate assistance with daily living routines. They are open to learning more about how to help Sabrina.
- *Family culture*: They are white with an Italian Catholic background. They are of working lower-middle-class socioeconomic status.
- *Family spiritually*: They were both raised Catholic but are not practicing their religion. They do not belong to a church. They describe themselves as spiritual.

The parents identified that both of them and Sabrina are having difficulty adjusting to the expansion of their family and the shift in their family roles. They state that they are most concerned with Sabrina's adjustment to the new baby. They state that they just do not know the best way to help her. They shared that they thought that because this was the "second time around" they believed they could be even better parents. They have been frustrated thinking about how to cope and what to do with two young children. The nursing diagnosis *Readiness for Enhanced Parenting* is related to the new role of parents of two children and is evidenced by the parents' subjective statements about parenting, Sabrina's reactions to the new baby, and parents asking for information and help on sibling rivalry.

Bono Family Intervention:

The nurse, together with Matt and Libby, review the family genogram (see Figure 5-6), which helps the couple visualize the family. The parents decide that Ava is the best person to come to help at this time. They say they will talk later with Matt's brother and family about sharing some child care. They complete a family ecomap (Figure 5-7) to help assess what is creating stress and determine what could help alleviate family stress.

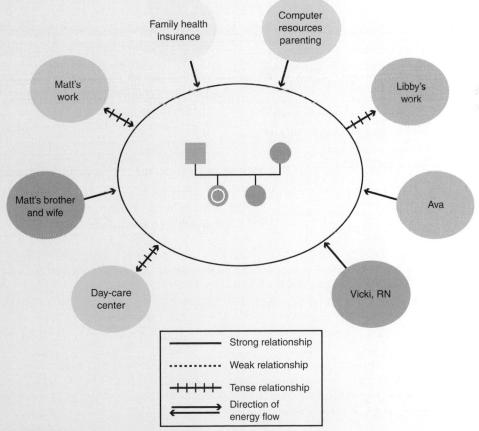

FIGURE 5-7 Bono Family Ecomap

(continued)

Case Study: Bono Family *(cont.)*

Vicki provides Matt and Libby with several educational packets about toddlers and new infants. She directs them to several online Web sites after she confirms that they have computer skills. They discuss ideas on how both parents can make personal time to spend with each daughter. They brainstorm ways to help Sabrina interact with Hannah but to keep Hannah safe from aggressive toddler behavior to a new sibling. They plan to talk with the day-care providers so they can be effective with their help for Sabrina. They will call Ava as soon as they get home to plan for her visit. Vicki makes a follow-up appointment with the Bono family for their next well-baby visit and to see how they are progressing with both children.

Bono Family Evaluation:

Vicki plans a follow-up phone call to check in with Libby and Matt. At the next visit, Vicki will revisit the family action plan with Libby and Matt to see whether their priority family concerns remain the same, or have decreased/increased or disappeared. Vicki plans to observe Sabrina's behaviors to see how she is coping and whether she is adapting in more positive ways. She will talk with the parents to assess their anxiety level. She will observe the parents and their interactions with both children.

Nurse Reflection:

Vicki reflects about her work with the Bono family. She determines that her therapeutic communication skills were excellent. She showed empathy and validated the family's concern for the added stresses that a newborn child creates for a family. The 7-day-old well-baby visit in the clinic setting presented an ideal time to observe and address parenting techniques and ease parental concerns. Learning how to shift focus from the more medical concern of the well-baby to family dynamics was the most challenging aspect, yet also the most rewarding. The interventions were appropriate and truly empowered their overall ability to cope and function as a family.

SUMMARY

- Conducting a family assessment includes the following components: assessment strategies, including how to select assessment instruments, determining the need for interpreters, assessing for family health literacy, and diagramming family genograms and ecomaps.
- Family nurses must work in partnership with families as they build from a strengths model and not a deficit model.
- Using the family assessment approach outlined in this chapter, nurses and families together identify the family priorities.
- The Family Reasoning Web is a systematic method used to ensure that families are viewed in a holistic manner, which also helps to keep the interventions oriented to family strengths.
- Family interventions need to be tailored to each individual family, with consideration of the family's structure, function, and processes.
- By subscribing to and selecting a theory-based approach to assessment, and formulating mutually derived intervention strategies, families are more likely to be committed and follow through with family plans and interventions.
- Family nurses serve as the catalyst for assessment, intervention, and evaluation that are specific to family identified needs.

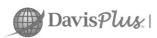 | For additional resources and information, visit **http://davisplus.fadavis.com**. References can be found on Davis*Plus*.

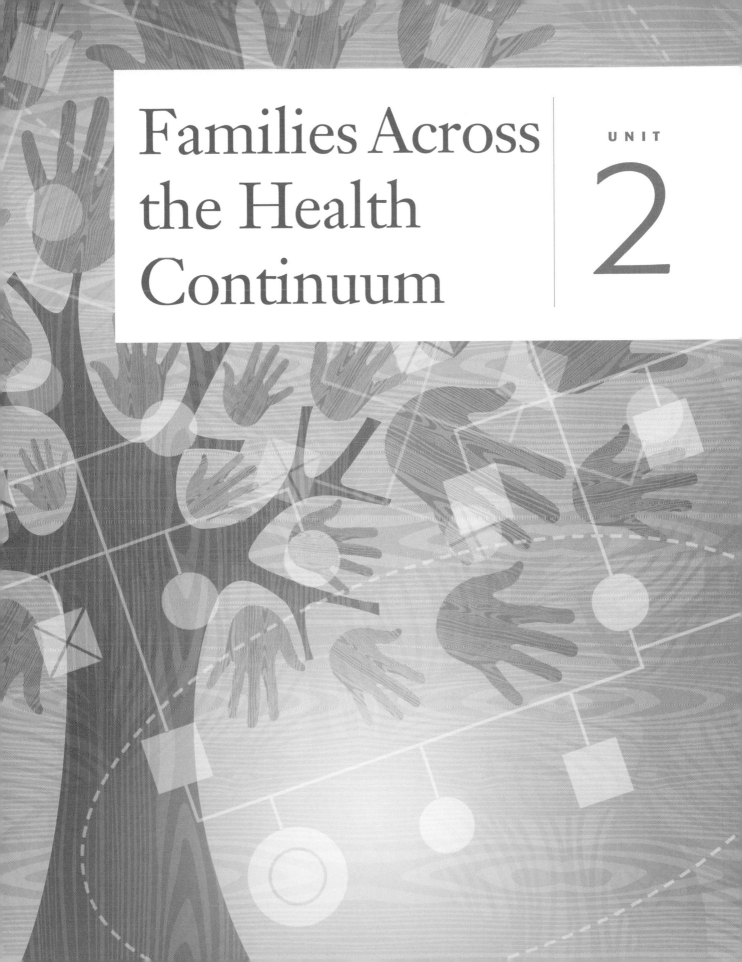

Families Across the Health Continuum

UNIT 2

Chapter 6

Family Health Promotion

YeounSoo Kim-Godwin, PhD, MPH, CNE, RN

Melissa Robinson, PhD, RN

Critical Concepts

- Family health promotion refers to activities that families engage in to strengthen the family unit and increase family unity and the quality of family life.

- Health promotion is learned within families, and patterns of health behavior are formed and passed on to the next generation.

- A major task of the family is to teach health maintenance and health promotion.

- The role of the family nurse is to help families attain, maintain, and regain the highest level of family health possible.

- Family health promotion is the byproduct of family interactions with factors outside the home and internal family processes: microsystem, mesosystem, exosystem, and macrosystem.

- Positive, reinforcing interaction between family members leads to a healthier family lifestyle.

- Different cultures define and value health, health promotion, and disease prevention differently. Clients may not understand or respond to a family nurse's suggestions for health promotion because the suggestions conflict with their health beliefs and values.

- Family health promotion should become a regular part of taking a family history and a routine aspect of nursing care.

- A primary goal of nursing care for families is empowering family members to work together to attain and maintain family health; therefore, family health promotion should focus on strengths, competencies, and resources.

Fostering the health of the family as a unit and encouraging families to value and incorporate health promotion into their lifestyles are essential components of family nursing practice. *Family health promotion* refers to the activities that families engage in to strengthen the family as a unit. Family health promotion has been defined as the process by which families work to improve or maintain the physical, social, emotional, and spiritual well-being of the family unit and its members (Loveland-Cherry, 2011). One of the major functions of the family is

to provide health care for its members, including ways to promote healthy lifestyles among the family members and to promote overall family function and well-being (Carroll & Vickers, 2014). Health promotion is learned within families, and patterns of health behavior are formed and passed on to the next generation.

Families are primarily responsible for providing health and illness care, being a role model, teaching self-care and wellness behavior, providing for care of members across their life course and during varied

149

family transitions, and supporting each other during health-promoting activities and during illness. A major task of families is to make efforts toward health maintenance and health promotion, regardless of age. For families, maintaining health and well-being is a collective effort whereby routines are established, relationships are formed that foster health in others, and quality of life is promoted when better health is experienced by multiple members of the household (Carroll & Vickers, 2014; Fiese & Everhart, 2011).

When it comes to health promotion activities, family interventions have been found to be very effective for both girls and boys, whereas youth-only programs work mostly for boys and not for girls (Kumpfer, 2014). Findings from a meta-analysis conducted by Kumpfer, Magalhães, and Kanse (2016) indicated that health promotion and disease prevention programs for youth that improve ongoing family dynamics are the most effective because they promote healthy parent–child relationships. The most relevant causal factors that emerged in the meta-analysis included improved communication, bonding, parental monitoring, supervision, discipline, and family organization and rule setting (Kumpfer et al., 2016).

The purpose of this chapter is to introduce the concepts of family health and family health promotion. The chapter presents models to represent these concepts, including the Family Health Model, the Family Resilience Framework, the McMaster Model of Family Functioning, the Family Health Promotion Model, the Developmental Model of Health and Nursing, and the Model of the Health-Promoting Family. The chapter also examines internal and external factors through a lens of the bioecological systems theory that influences family health promotion, family nursing intervention strategies for health promotion, and two family case studies demonstrating how different theoretical approaches can be used for assessing and intervening in the family for health promotion.

WHAT IS FAMILY HEALTH?

Definitions of *family health* have evolved from anthropological, biopsychosocial, developmental, family science, cultural, and nursing paradigms. The concept of family health is often used interchangeably with the terms *family functioning, healthy families,*

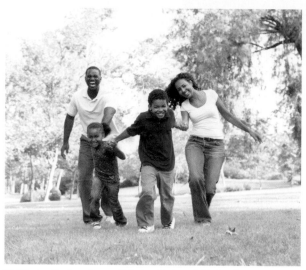

© *Monkey Business Images/Monkey Business/Thinkstock*

resilient families, and *balanced families* (Alderfer, 2011; Kaakinen & Webb, 2016; Walsh, 2012). Family scientists define healthy families as resilient (Walsh, 2016b) and as possessing a balance of cohesion and adaptability that is facilitated by good communication (Walsh, 2016b).

Family therapy definitions of family health often emphasize optimal family functioning and freedom from psychopathology (Goldenberg, Stanton, & Goldenberg, 2017). Furthermore, within the developmental framework, healthy families complete developmental tasks at appropriate times (Duval & Miller, 1985; McGoldrick, Garcia-Preto, & Carter, 2016).

Other definitions of family health focus on the totality, or *gestalt,* of the family's existence, and include the internal and external environment of the family. This perspective is rooted in general systems theory and the ecological systems theory (Novilla, 2011).

A holistic definition of family health encompasses all aspects of family life, including interaction and health care function. Different aspects of family functioning that nurses can assess or help promote to encourage overall family health care functions include family nutrition, recreation, communication, sleep and rest patterns, problem solving, sexuality, use of time and space, coping with stress, hygiene and safety, spirituality, illness care, health promotion and protection, and emotional health of family members (Alderfer, 2011; Novilla, 2011).

For the purposes of this chapter, *family health* is a holistic, dynamic, and complex state. Family health

Table 6-1	Characteristics of a Healthy Family

Unity

Commitment	**Time Together**
Has a sense of trust traditions.	Shares family rituals and traditions.
Teaches respect for others.	Enjoys each other's company.
Exhibits a sense of shared responsibility.	Shares leisure time together.
Affirms and supports all its members.	Shares simple and quality time.

Flexibility

Ability to Deal With Stress	**Spiritual Well-Being**
Displays adaptability.	Encourages hope.
Sees crises as a challenge and opportunity.	Shares faith and religious core.
Shows openness to change.	Teaches compassion for others.
Grows together in crisis.	Teaches ethical values.
Seeks help with problems.	Respects the privacy of others.
Opens its boundaries to admit and seek help.	

Communication

Positive Communication	**Appreciation and Affection**
Communicates well and listens to all members.	Cares for each other.
Fosters family table time and conversation.	Exhibits a sense of humor.
Shares feelings.	Maintains friendship.
Displays nonblaming attitudes.	Respects individuality.
Is able to compromise and disagree.	Has a spirit of playfulness/humor.
Agrees to disagree.	Interacts with others; has a balance in the interactions.

is more than the absence of disease in an individual family member or the absence of dysfunction in family dynamics. Rather, it is the complex process of negotiating and solving day-to-day family life events and crises, and providing for a quality life for its members (Novilla, 2011). Table 6-1 lists the characteristics of healthy families, illustrating how families can promote health.

COMMON THEORETICAL PERSPECTIVES

Many models and theories are applicable to family health and family health promotion. This section introduces a variety of models or views of family health and family health promotion followed by selected models:

- Family Health Model
- Family Resilience Framework
- McMaster Model of Family Functioning
- Family Health Promotion Model
- Developmental Model of Health and Nursing
- Model of the Health-Promoting Family

Models of Family Health

Building on Smith's (1983) models of health and illness, Loveland-Cherry and Bomar (2004) suggested that there are four views toward or philosophies of family health:

- *Family Health—Clinical Model:* The family unit is viewed from this perspective. The family is healthy if its members are free from physical, mental, and family dysfunction.
- *Family Health—Role-Performance Model:* This view of family health is based on the idea that family health is the ability of family members to perform their routine roles and achieve developmental tasks.
- *Family Health—Adaptive Model:* In this view, families are healthy if they have the ability to change and grow and possess the capacity to rebound quickly after a crisis.
- *Family Health—Eudaimonistic Model:* Health care providers who use this view as their philosophy of practice focus on a holistic approach to family care to maximize the family's well-being and self-actualization in order to support the entire family and individual members in reaching their maximum health potential.

Table 6-2 shows how the four models of family health define "family health." Rather than being separate, Smith (1983) suggested that the four views can be viewed as a continuum with the person (or family),

Table 6-2	Models of Family Health
Model	**Definition of Family Health**
Clinical model	Lack of evidence of physical, mental, social disease or deterioration, or dysfunction of the family system.
Role-performance model	Ability of the family system to conduct family functions effectively and to achieve family developmental tasks.
Adaptive model	Family patterns of interaction with the environment characterized by flexible, effective adaptation or ability to change and grow.
Eudaimonistic model	The most comprehensive view of health, a holistic view. It includes the ongoing provision of resources, guidance, and support for realization of the family's maximum well-being, self-actualization, and potential throughout the family life span.

Source: Modified from Bomar, P. J. (2004). Introduction to family health nursing and promoting family health. In P. J. Bomar (Ed.), *Promoting health in families: Applying family research and theory to nursing practice* (3rd ed., pp. 3–37). Philadelphia, PA: W. B. Saunders.

going back and forth depending on the circumstances and life events. The family health models (views) are useful in three ways: (1) They provide frameworks for understanding the level of health that families are experiencing; (2) they help design interventions to assist families in maintaining or regaining good health, or in coping with illness; and (3) the specific model of family health can facilitate organization of the family nursing literature and be used to categorize family research (Loveland-Cherry & Bomar, 2004).

Family Health Model

Based on family health studies with Appalachian families (Denham, 1999a, 1999b, 1999c) and a broad base of literature and existing research about family health, Denham (2003a) proposed the Family Health Model (FHM). Family health is viewed as a process over time of family members' interactions and health-related behaviors. Denham (2011) defined family health as a "complex phenomenon comprised of diverse members, systems, interactions, relationships, and processes that hold the potential to maximize well-being, the household production of health, and contextual resources" (p. 900). The model emphasizes the biophysical, holistic, and environmental factors that influence health.

In her FHM, Denham (2003a, 2003b) suggested that family health routines offer the means of connecting with health promotion. Family routines are behavior patterns related to events, occasions, or situations that are repeated with regularity and consistency. Family routines have been identified as key structural aspects of family health that can be assessed by nurses, provide a focus for family interventions, and have potential for measuring health outcomes (Denham, 2003a). Routines supply information about behaviors and their predictability, member interactions, family identity, and specific ways families live. Denham (2003a) made the following propositions about family health routines:

- Families that tend toward moderation in family health routines are healthier than families that are highly ritualized and those that lack rituals.
- Families with clearer ideas about their goals are more likely to accommodate health needs effectively through their family routines than families that are less certain about their goals.
- Families and individuals are more likely to accommodate changes related to health

concerns when family routines are supported over time by embedded contextual systems than families whose routines are not supported.

■ Families with routines that support individual health care needs are more likely to achieve positive care outcomes in an individual with health concerns than families that do not have routines that support the needs of family members with health concerns.

■ Children who are taught routines in the home and are supported by the embedded context are more likely to practice health routines in the home than those not supported by the embedded context. *Embedded context* is defined as "the ecological environments and nested relationships that

affect the family health over the life course" (Denham, 2003a, p. 277).

Denham (2003a, 2011) identified diverse types of routines, including individual routine, family routine, family health routine, family ritual, family tradition, and family celebration. Health routines are described as interactions affected by biophysical, developmental, interactional, psychosocial, spiritual, and contextual realms, with implications for the health and well-being of members and family as a whole. Kushner (2007) defined health routines as the way that family members deal with everyday health needs in the household context, the way that they teach children health behaviors, and the way they support stress management. In the FHM, Denham (2003a) identified six categories of family health routines that are listed in Table 6-3.

Table 6-3	Types of Family Health Routines	
Family Health Routines	**Aspects of the Routines**	**Description of the Routines**
Self-care routines	Dietary Hygiene Sleep-rest Physical activity and exercise Gender and sexuality	These routines involve patterned behaviors related to usual activities of daily living experienced across the life course.
Safety and prevention	Health protection Disease prevention Smoking Abuse and violence Alcohol and substance abuse	These routines pertain to health protection, disease prevention, avoidance and participation in high-risk behaviors, and efforts to prevent unintended injury across the life course.
Mental health behaviors	Self-esteem Personal integrity Work and play Stress levels	These routines have to do with the ways individuals and families attend to self-efficacy, cope with daily stresses, and individuate.
Family care	Family fun (e.g., relaxation, activities, hobbies, vacations) Celebrations, traditions, special events Spiritual and religious practices Pets Sense of humor	These routines include daily activities, traditional behaviors, and special celebrations that give meaning to daily life and provide shared enjoyment, pleasure, and happiness for multiple members.
Illness care	Decision making related to medical consultation Use of health care services Follow-up with prescribed medical regimens	These routines are the various ways members make decisions related to health care needs; choose when, where, and how to seek supportive health services; and determine ways to respond to medical directives and health information.
Member caregiving	Health teaching (i.e., health, prevention, illness, disease) Member roles and responsibilities Providing illness care Support of member actions	These routines pertain to the ways family members act as interactive caregivers across the life course as they socialize children and adolescents about a wide variety of health-related ideals, participate in specific health and illness care needs, and support members' individual routine patterns.

Source: Denham, S. A. (2003a). *Family health: A framework for nursing.* Philadelphia, PA: F.A. Davis, with permission.

Family Resilience Framework

The Family Resilience Framework (FRF) integrates ecosystemic and developmental dimensions of experience (Walsh, 2016b). Family resiliency is defined as "the ability of family to rebound from crises and successfully overcome life challenges" (Alderfer, 2011, p. 84). The concept of family resilience refers to the family "as a functional system, impacted by highly stressful events and social contexts, and in turn, facilitating the positive adaptation of all members and strengthening the family unit" (Walsh, 2016a, p. 313). Although some families are more vulnerable or face more hardships than others, a family resilience perspective is grounded in a deep conviction in the potential of families to strengthen their resilience in overcoming their challenges (Walsh, 2016a). Walsh (2016a) identified the key processes in family resilience including: "making meaning of adversity; positive outlook, transcendence and spirituality, flexibility, connectedness, mobilize social and economic resources, clarity; open emotional sharing and collaborative problem solving" (p. 319). The Walsh Family Resilience Questionnaire (WFRQ) was developed to operationalize the nine key processes and their components (Walsh, 2016a).

A multilevel dynamic systems perspective recognizes the recursive nature of process in resilience and the bidirectionality of influences within and between levels over time (Walsh, 2016b). The key processes in family resilience are mutually interactive and synergistic. For example, a relational view of resilience (belief system) supports and is reinforced by connectedness (organizational process) and collaborative problem solving (communication process). A positive outlook both facilitates and is sustained by successful problem solving and proactive steps. Social and community resources are not simply external factors; family processes include active engagement in transactions with the environment (Walsh, 2016b).

Based on the extensive literature about family resilience, Sigman-Grant, Hayes, VanBrackle, and Fiese (2015) proposed a resiliency framework for explaining childhood obesity and intervention. They suggested that childhood obesity prevention and treatment may be found in the application of the proposed framework to the exploration of childhood obesity from a protective perspective that focuses on the family context. A FRF focuses on strengths under stress in response to crisis or with prolonged adversity. However, the FRF is also applicable to transactional processes in well-functioning families (Lebow & Stroud, 2012).

McMaster Model of Family Functioning

The McMaster Model of Family Functioning (MMFF) identifies the elements of the family group and the patterns of transactions among family members that have been found to distinguish between healthy and unhealthy families. The model specifies six domains of functioning proposed to have the greatest impact on the ability of the family to meet its basic needs (e.g., food, money, transportation, and shelter), the developmental needs of family members and the family unit, and any emerging needs such as "crises that arise for the family such as job loss, illness, etc." (Alderfer, 2011, p. 82):

- Problem solving
- Communication
- Roles
- Affective responsiveness
- Affective involvement
- Behavioral control

The McMaster Clinical Rating Scale (MCRS) and Family Assessment Device (FAD) were developed to assess family health across the six dimensions described by the MMFF. The MCRS is used by clinicians well-trained in the MMFF, and the FAD is a self-report measure that can be completed by families and scored on each of the MMFF dimensions (Staccini, Tomba, Grandi, & Keitner, 2015). Whereas the MCRS can be rated by observers during a semi-structured family interview, the FAD was designed to be completed by family members and their scores are then averaged. The FAD is widely used and has been translated into approximately 20 different languages (Alderfer, 2011).

Models for Family Health Promotion

A great need exists to encourage health promotion of the whole family unit because health behaviors, values, and patterns are learned within a family context. Family health promotion activities are crucial both during wellness and during illness of a family member. Family health promotion increases family unity and quality of life. Further, family health promotion involves a family's lifelong efforts to nurture its members, to maintain family cohesion, and to reach a family's greatest potential in all aspects of health (Pender, Murdaugh, & Parsons, 2015).

Family Health Promotion Model

Most models of health promotion focus on the individual. Adapting Pender's (1996) health promotion model, Loveland-Cherry and Bomar (2004) presented a Family Health Promotion Model (FHPM). In this model, the likelihood of a family engaging in health-promoting behaviors is influenced by the following general, health-related, and behavior-specific factors:

- *General influences*
  - Family systems patterns, such as values, communication, interactions, and power
  - Demographic characteristics, such as family size, structure, income, and culture
  - Biological characteristics
- *Health-related influences*
  - Family health socialization patterns
  - Family definition of "health"
  - Perceived family health status

- *Behavior-specific influences*
  - Perceived barriers to health-promoting behavior
  - Perceived benefits to health-promoting behavior
  - Prior related behavior
  - Family norms regarding health-promoting behavior
  - Intersystem support for behavior
  - Situational influences
  - Internal and environmental family cues

The way families define family health promotion will influence the likelihood of them planning family unit activities that promote family well-being and cohesion. Family behavioral influences, such as perceived barriers or benefits of health-promoting activities of the entire family, affect how committed a family will be to continuing or initiating activities that promote health. For example, to encourage a health-promoting family lifestyle, each family member must value and believe there is a benefit to eating together, sharing in activities to maintain the home, or balancing family power. Figure 6-1 depicts the FHPM.

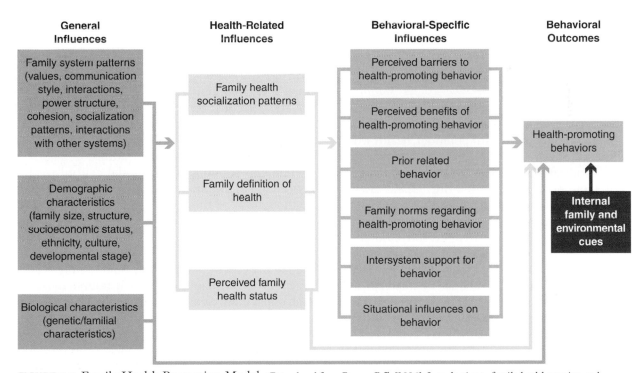

FIGURE 6-1 Family Health Promotion Model *(Reproduced from Bomar, P. J. [2004]. Introduction to family health nursing and promoting family health. In P. J. Bomar [Ed.],* Promoting health in families: Applying family research and theory to nursing practice *[3rd ed., pp. 3–37]. Philadelphia, PA: W. B. Saunders, with permission.)*

Developmental Model of Health and Nursing

The Developmental Model of Health and Nursing (DMHN) constructed by Canadian scholar F. Moyra Allen in the mid-1970s and 1980s (Allen & Warner, 2002) set the goal of increasing the capacity of families and individuals to promote their health in everyday life situations. The DMHN supports the concept of empowering partnerships with families, as the model emphasizes health as a process and the capacities that all families have, including their potential for growth and change (Black & Ford-Gilboe, 2004). In the interaction model, the nurse's role changes at each phase of the health promotion process, thereby empowering clients toward improving their health status. Examples of nursing functions include the following:

- Focuser, stimulator, and resource producer who involves clients in such tasks as clarifying concerns and goals and thinking about their learning style
- Integrator and awareness-raiser who assists clients with analyzing the situation, identifying additional resources, and seeking potential solutions
- Role model, instructor, coach, guide, and encourager as clients make decisions on alternatives and try new behaviors
- Role "reinforcer" and reviewer as clients review and evaluate outcomes (Allen & Warner, 2002, p. 122)

Ford-Gilboe (2002) summarized six studies that tested the propositions of Allen's DMHN. The studies tested four concepts: health potential, health work, competence in health behavior, and health status. Results indicated significant relationships between health potential and health work. *Health work* is defined "as a process of active involvement though which families develop or learn ways of coping with health situations and using strengths and resources to achieve goals for individual and family development" (Ford-Gilboe, 2002, pp. 145–146). *Health potential* is defined as "a reservoir of internal and external capacities (i.e. strengths, motivation, and resources) that can be drawn on to support health work" (Ford-Gilboe, 2002, p. 146). In essence, health work reflects what families do in response to health situations rather than who they are or what they have access to (i.e., aspects of health potential). The level of family health potential, health work, and health competence all were found to be significant predictors of family functioning. Ford-Gilboe also reported that health work predicted 24% of the mother's health-promoting lifestyle practices. Similarly, in another study (Black & Ford-Gilboe, 2004) moderate correlations were also shown between health work and the mother's health-promoting lifestyle practices among 41 adolescent mothers, and the mother's resilience and health work explained 30.2% of the mother's health-promoting lifestyle practices.

Model of the Health-Promoting Family

The primary focus of Christensen's (2004) Model of the Health-Promoting Family (MHPF) is the health practices of the family. The model addresses how families can play a part in promoting both the health of children and their capacities as health-promoting actors. The model draws on contemporary social science approaches to health, family, and children, suggesting a new emphasis on the family's ecocultural pathway, family practices, and the child as a health-promoting factor.

As shown in Figure 6-2, the MHPF is analytically divided into two parts to distinguish factors external to the family and factors internal to it. The external factors are further divided into societal and community-level factors. The societal factors provide the material base for the family and will to a large degree, therefore, shape the resources available to the family. These factors include, for example, income and wealth, education and knowledge, family structure and housing, ethnicity, social networks, and time. The community level is the configuration of social spheres that contribute to child health. These social spheres include the consumer society, local community, schools, health services, mass media, peer groups, and day-care institutions.

The components of the model central to the conception of the family and the processes that may be thought of as going on "inside" it are indicated with a semipermeable boundary—the circle. These are linked to and influenced by the processes and factors "outside" of the family. The internal level has the "family ecocultural pathway" and "family health practices" as the main elements. By interacting with each other, these elements lead to collective patterns of health action, practice, and forms of knowledge. An important feature of the model is that it will allow differences between families to be revealed by identifying the conditions for a family to act in an optimal way for health. It also highlights the obstacles for families in promoting the health and well-being of children, and the barriers to enabling

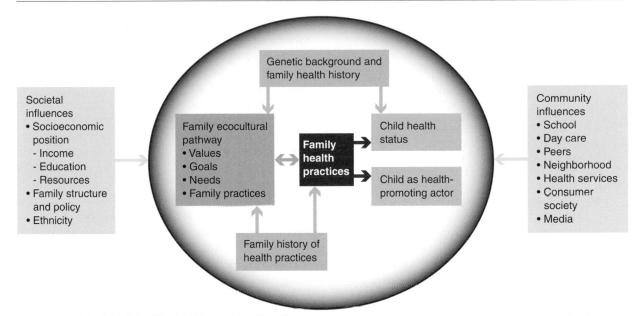

FIGURE 6-2 Model of the Health-Promoting Family *(Reproduced from Christensen, P. [2004], The health-promoting family: A conceptual framework for future research. Social Science & Medicine, 59(2), 377–387, with permission.)*

the child's development as a health-promoting actor during the child's growth.

Family health practices fall into the center of the circle (internal factors), and include all those activities of everyday life that shape and influence the health of family members. These consist of the traditional health practices around food and healthy eating, physical activity, alcohol and smoking, and care and connection, as well as other key factors that can be shown to affect young people's health and well-being.

Although family health promotion has received considerable emphasis in nursing in the past decade, reports on the effectiveness of family-focused health promotion continue to be scarce. Therefore, continued research is required using family health promotion models to evaluate the effectiveness of interventions to promote family health.

ECOSYSTEM INFLUENCES: BIOECOLOGICAL SYSTEMS THEORY

The ecological approach, first proposed by Bronfenbrenner (1977), is useful to understand the multidimensional aspect of family health promotion (see Chapter 2 for a conceptual understanding and explanation of this model). Family health promotion

is one of the byproducts of family interactions with factors and systems outside the home and internal family processes. This approach attends to the interactions among the system levels:

- Microsystem
- Mesosystem
- Exosystem
- Macrosystem

The *microsystem* pertains to individual factors, such as biology, personal experience, and general demographics (e.g., age, gender, and education). The *mesosystem* refers to the interactions between the individuals and their close relationships with partners, peers, and families. The *exosystem* refers to the community contexts for the family, such as schools, places of work, and neighborhoods. *Macrosystems* are considered the broad cultural attitudes, ideologies, and belief systems that have influence on the family health choices (Lucea, Glass, & Laughon, 2011). This section explores how the ecosystem influences the quality of family life and family health.

Exosystem and Macrosystem Influences on Family Health

Both the exosystem and the macrosystem influence family decisions, actions, and interactions that contribute to the health of family members. Some specific external influences include the national economy, family and health policy, societal and cultural norms, media, and environmental hazards such as noise, air, soil, crowding, and chemicals. We explore some specific exosystem and macrosystem influences as follows.

Economic Resources

The national economy directly affects the family's ability to promote health. As a general matter, during economic downturns, health promotion initiatives tend to take a back seat to other, more pressing needs. More pointedly, the availability of jobs and, in turn, discretionary funds, directly affects the quality of a family's lifestyle. Clear disparities exist between health promotion in middle-class families and in low-income families (Edburg, 2013). See Chapter 4 for more on family social policy and health disparities.

Socioeconomic status is a determinant of health promotion. When a family has economic health, it has the resources needed for family health promotion. Adequate family income contributes to emotional well-being and supplies resources for adequate family space, recreation, and leisure. Low-income families, by contrast, are less likely than middle- and upper-class families to engage in health-promoting and preventive activities. The cost of buying recreational and exercise equipment, for example, is often beyond the means of low-income families. The activities of low-income families (and government policy aimed at them) are often directed toward meeting basic needs—providing for food, shelter, and safety, and curing acute illness—rather than preventing illness or promoting health. Access to fresh fruits and vegetables in low-income neighborhoods is notably more difficult than in wealthier neighborhoods (Di Noia & Byrd-Bredbenner, 2014). Low-income families often have disproportionately high utilization of emergency department (ED) and hospital services, and low utilization of preventive visits (Holland et al., 2012).

Governmental Health and Family Policies

Health and family policies at all governmental levels affect the quality of individual and family health. In the United States, the Department of Health and Human Services (DHHS) is a government agency that protects and promotes the health of all Americans. *Healthy People 2020* was developed as a framework for health promotion and disease prevention with established benchmarks and goals to (1) encourage collaborations across communities and sectors, (2) empower individuals toward making informed health decisions, and (3) measure the impact of prevention activities (U.S. Department of Health and Human Services, 2017d). However, many of the objectives can be achieved only through supportive policies, access to health care, and healthy family lifestyles (Holland et al., 2012; Wang, Orleans, & Gortmaker, 2012). For example, local communities provide water and monitor its quality, maintain sanitation, develop and maintain parks for recreation, and provide health services to low-income families and families with older adults. Such local services enhance the health of individuals and, thus, enhance family health. At the state level, services include assistance with medical care through Medicaid, the maintenance of state recreational areas and parks, health promotion and prevention programs, and economic assistance for low-income families and children (Anderson & Fallin, 2014).

Government policies concerning unauthorized immigrants are among the mostly hotly debated topics in the United States (Vargas & Pirog, 2016). This intensified activity can affect various aspects of immigrant health, including family and mental health. Recently, Vargas, Sanchez, and Juárez (2017) analyzed the Robert Wood Johnson Foundation's 2015 Latino National Health and Immigration Survey ($n = 1493$) to examine the relationship between immigration and immigrant policy and Latino health and well-being. They found that those who worry about a friend or family member being deported have a higher likelihood of reporting the need to seek mental or emotional help and concluded that Latino health, regardless of immigration status, is being influenced by a concern that family members and friends may be detained or deported (Vargas et al., 2017). The findings of the previous research found that among mixed-status families the risk of being deported decreases the odds of using social services such as Medicaid and the federal Women, Infants, and Children (WIC) program (Vargas, 2015; Vargas & Pirog, 2016).

In Canada, one of the agencies charged with promoting and protecting the health of Canadians through leadership, partnership, innovation, and action in public health is the Public Health Agency of Canada (Public Health Agency of Canada, 2016). The agency is responsible for promoting health;

BOX 6-1

Historical Perspectives of Family Health Promotion: *Healthy People*

Although the majority of health care providers continue to focus their activities on prevention and treatment of illness in individuals and dysfunctional families, key social forces, including the wellness and self-care movement started in 1979, continue to stimulate the nursing profession to focus on health promotion for families. The 1980 White House Conference on Families pointed out the need to improve family functioning and encourage healthy family lifestyles. The conference brought to light the importance of disease prevention and health promotion for improving the quality of family life in the United States. Three documents from the USDHHS—*Healthy People: The Surgeon General's Report on Health Promotion and Disease Prevention* (1979); *Promoting Health/Preventing Disease: Objectives for the Nation* (1980); and *Healthy People 2000: National Health Promotion and Disease Prevention Objectives* (1990)—provided overall goals for the nation regarding health promotion for individuals and families.

Although there were many improvements in the health status of the nation as a whole, the *Healthy People 2020* framework builds on the lessons learned from the three previous initiatives (USDHHS, 2017d). The goals for 2020 are to eliminate health disparities and to increase the quality and years of life. Major objectives for the millennium include promoting healthy behaviors, promoting healthy and safe communities, improving systems for personal and public health, and preventing and reducing diseases and disorders.

Since the first report by the surgeon general in 1979 and the continued national interest in health promotion in the 1990s, health care providers, family scientists, sociologists, psychologists, religious leaders, and social workers have made considerable strides in understanding and intervening to improve the quality of family health. Another example of the continued focus on health promotion is the increasing use of parish nurses, who provide holistic care and health promotion to members of faith communities through home visiting and wellness support (Harkness & DeMarco, 2016).

preventing and controlling chronic disease, injury, and infectious disease; and applying an international research focus to the development of Canada's public health programs (Public Health Agency of Canada, 2016). Key areas of health promotion and disease prevention for the agency include infectious disease, chronic disease, travel health, food safety, immunizations and vaccines, emergency preparedness and response, laboratory biosafety and biosecurity, and public health surveillance.

An example of the work being done on a national level is the public health prevention program addressing the human immunodeficiency virus (HIV), which is a serious and preventable public health threat faced by Canadians. The government of Canada is working closely with local provinces and territories to reduce risk by (1) providing HIV screening and testing support for health providers; (2) engaging with groups and communities to provide access to screening and treatment; and (3) enhancing HIV surveillance to monitor risk and burden (Public Health Agency of Canada, 2016).

Federal-level policies and fiscal support in both the United States and Canada are needed to improve the quality of family health. Because of the number of different government agencies involved in health care and family issues, a need exists for collaboration among these policymaking bodies. Box 6-1 summarizes the brief historical perspectives of family health promotion in the United States.

Environment

Awareness of the quality of the family living environment is crucial because the family and its members are exposed to public, occupational, and residential hazards. Environmental health is one of the areas of emphasis of the *Healthy People 2020* objectives in the United States (USDHHS, 2017b). Box 6-2 lists the major environmental objectives specific to families. Many environmental hazards are not monitored consistently by families or organizations. In addition, access to green space and safe places to play is more restricted in low-income neighborhoods (Grigsby-Toussaint, Chi, & Fiese, 2011). Therefore, it is imperative to increase the capacity of families to recognize environmental hazards and to teach strategies to prevent, remove, or cope with environmental hazards such as pollution of air, water, food, and soil from numerous chemicals, occupational hazards, and violence (Nyman, Butterfield, & Lundy, 2016). For instance, to prevent exposure to lead and pesticides, families could be taught to

BOX 6-2

Healthy People 2020 Environmental Objectives Specific to Families

Objective Short Title

Water Quality

EH-4: Increase access to safe drinking water
EH-5: Reduce waterborne disease outbreaks
EH-6: Increase water conservation
EH-7: Increase safety of public swimming spaces

Toxins and Waste

EH-8: Reduce blood lead levels in children
EH-9: Reduce risks posed by hazardous sites

EH-10: Reduce pesticide exposures
EH-11: Reduce toxic pollutants in the environment

Healthy Homes and Healthy Communities

EH-13: Reduce indoor allergens
EH-14/15: Increase homes tested for radon
EH-16: Implement school policies to protect against environmental hazards
EH-17/18: Increase lead-based paint testing
EH-19: Reduce the number of occupied substandard housing

Source: U.S. Department of Health and Human Services. (2017b). *Healthy People 2020: Environmental health*. Washington, DC. Retrieved from www.healthypeople.gov/2020/topicsobjectives2020/objectiveslist.aspx?topicId=12

wash fruits and vegetables before eating. Workers should be taught to monitor chemicals and infectious materials that might be transmitted to them and their families on work clothing or skin. In addition, paint in older homes and outside play areas should be inspected for lead contamination. Families with young children and workers who work around metals and chemicals need to be especially cautious of lead poisoning, and should consult Web resources such as the Centers for Disease Control and Prevention (CDC, see www.cdc.gov) for additional information.

Media

Media influence on children has steadily increased as new and more sophisticated types of media have been developed and made available to the public. A Kaiser Family Foundation report found that children ages 8 to 10 years old spend nearly 8 hours using media each day, whereas teenagers spend more than 11 hours (Rideout, Foehr, & Roberts, 2010). Consistent evidence has been reported that violent imagery in television, film and video, and computer games has substantial short-term effects on arousal, thoughts, and emotions, increasing the likelihood of aggressive or fearful behavior in younger children (Strasburger, Jordan, & Donnerstein, 2010). Newer screen devices may have a stronger impact on sleep in particular because of the ease with which adolescents (and adults) can bring the devices into their bedrooms (Falbe et al., 2015; Thomee, Harenstam, & Hagberg, 2011).

Time spent with screen media devices, including televisions, computers, videogames, smartphones, and tablets, saturates the waking hours of most American youth. Teenagers (13 to 18 years old) spend over 6 hours daily engaged with screen devices (Common Sense Media, 2015). The types of screens that youth use have changed rapidly. Smartphone use now makes up the majority of screen engagement among teens (Common Sense Media, 2015) and most youth, even younger children, have their own device; a recent study found over one-half of 3-year-olds had been given their own tablet (Kabali et al., 2015). Falbe et al. (2014) found that, over a period of 6 years, increased total screen time, including television, digital versatile discs (DVDs), and electronic games, was associated with increased intake of sugar-sweetened beverages (SSBs), fast food, salty snacks, and total energy, as well as decreased intake of fruits and vegetables among 9- to 16-year-olds. Kenney and Gortmaker (2017) analyzed data on the use of television and other screen devices (including smartphones and tablets) and obesity risk factors for a nationally representative, cross-sectional sample of 24,800 U.S. high school students (2013–2015 Youth Risk Behavior Surveys). The authors found that approximately 20% of participants used other screen devices for ≥5 hours daily and using other screen devices ≥5 hours daily was associated with daily SSB consumption, inadequate physical activity, and inadequate sleep (Kenney & Gortmaker, 2017).

Long-term mental health risk for early childhood media exposure to violence was reported by Fitzpatrick, Barnett, and Pagani (2012). They examined whether a preschool child's exposure to what parents generally characterize as television violence predicts a range of second-grade mental health outcomes. Fitzpatrick et al. reported that child exposure to televised violence was associated with teacher-reported antisocial symptoms, emotional distress, inattention, and lower global academic achievement in second grade. Viewing televised violence also was associated with a lower child-reported academic self-concept and less intrinsic motivation in second grade (Fitzpatrick et al., 2012).

Health care providers need to grapple with how to advise families on healthy screen engagement in an age of increasing smartphone, tablet, and computer use (Kenney & Gortmaker, 2017). The American Academy of Pediatrics (AAP) (2016) offered comprehensive recommendations to address the issue of media influence on children. Included in these recommendations are suggestions for parents, health care providers, schools, the entertainment industry, the advertising industry, researchers, and the government to protect children and adolescents from harmful media effects and to maximize the powerfully prosocial aspects of modern media. In addition, the AAP urges media producers to be more responsible in their portrayal of violence. It advocates for more useful and effective media ratings. Specifically, it recommends proactive parental involvement in children's media experiences. By monitoring what children hear and see, discussing issues that emerge, and sharing media time with their children, parents can moderate the negative influences and increase the positive effects of media in the lives of their children (AAP, 2016). Recently, the AAP recommended that parents establish "screen-free" zones at home by making sure there are no televisions, computers, or video games in children's bedrooms and by turning off the television during dinner. Children and teens should engage with entertainment media for no more than 1 to 2 hours per day, and that media should have high-quality content. It is important for children to spend time playing outdoors, reading, engaging with hobbies, and using their imaginations in free play. The AAP also recommends that television and other entertainment media should be avoided for infants and children under the age of 2.

Many health promotion efforts to reduce health risks emphasize not only individual behavior change but also the importance of not ignoring the critical role of environmental and social factors. In 1969, Congress passed the Public Health Cigarette Smoking Act that prohibited cigarette advertising

in the broadcast media beginning in 1971 (CDC, 1989). Congress extended the ban on broadcast advertising to little cigars in 1973, and to smokeless tobacco products in 1986 (CDC, 1989). The federal law banning cigarette advertising on television and radio also included a clause preempting states and localities from regulating or prohibiting cigarette advertising or promotions for health reasons. In 2009, Congress enacted the Family Smoking Prevention and Tobacco Control Act, which gave the FDA authority to regulate tobacco products so as to benefit the public's health (U.S. FDA, 2009).

The federal Tobacco Act in Canada restricts anyone under 18 from buying or being supplied with tobacco products, although some provinces have increased the restrictions to anyone under the age of 19 (Canada, 2016). Canada also enforces a complete smoking ban (smoke-free environments) in all public spaces to protect the public from second-hand smoke (Canada, 2016).

Many advertisements still advocate drinking alcohol, using tobacco products, and consuming foods that are high in sugar, salt, and fat. Electronic cigarettes (e-cigarettes) have gained popularity in America, and marketers are using advertising to recruit new users to their products. Despite outright bans on traditional cigarette advertisements, e-cigarettes have no specific regulations (Willis, Haught, & Morris II, 2017). Although the use of tobacco and alcohol is legal for adults, the aggressive marketing and promotion tactics of both the alcohol and tobacco industries heavily target the youth market. The alcohol and tobacco industries create an environment in which the consumption of these dangerous products is acceptable and, within some teenage peer groups, even expected. Both alcohol and tobacco industries use similar strategies to appeal to youth and increase market share (American Public Health Association [APHA], 2016). Cigarette manufacturers altered their packs using different color schemes to convey the same misleading perceptions about the strength of their cigarettes (light colors for previously labeled light cigarettes, blue and green for mint and menthol flavorings), which means that many consumers continue to be misled about the fact that there is really no benefit to be gained by smoking a filtered or so-called low yield product as currently marketed (Paoletti, Jardin, Carpenter, Cummings, &, Silvestri, 2012).

Many health promotion efforts to reduce health risks emphasize not only individual behavior change but also the importance of not ignoring the critical role of environmental and social factors. Relatively recent tobacco advertising regulations, for instance, take a small step in the right direction toward promoting healthier families. The regulations prohibit tobacco advertisements near schools, on T-shirts, and in magazines for teens. Many states require that cigarettes not be in the reach of minors in retail stores (CDC, 2012). In fact, one of the *Healthy People 2020* objectives is to reduce the proportion of adolescents and young adults in grades 6 through 12 who are exposed to tobacco advertising and promotion (USDHH, 2017c).

Science and Technology

Advances in science and technology have increased the life span of Americans, decreased the length of hospital stays, and contributed to our understanding of how to prevent, reduce, and treat disease. The development of more effective medications and advanced medical equipment technology has greatly increased the feasibility of home health care for chronically ill family members of all ages. Families are often the caregivers for ill members and they provide the majority of care to older adults. Many valuable sources of information on health promotion for families and individuals are now available. Evidence-based family prevention programs have been reported as highly effective in preventing even inherited diseases in adolescents (Kumpfer, 2014). However, attendance barriers such as transportation and trouble with accessibility, busy family schedules and time constraints, inability to commit to multiple sessions, stigma associated with family therapy, or even variations in parental education can reduce the program retention and engagement (Kumpfer et al., 2016).

Other technological advances are changing how we provide health care. The use of remote patient monitoring, often referred to as *telehealth*, has been widely adopted by health care providers, particularly home care agencies (Suter, Suter, & Johnston, 2011). Telehealth, involving phone, e-mail, photos, and videoconferencing, is becoming a more common way of sharing health care information. It provides a forum for consultation with patients/families and health care providers when face-to-face involvement is not possible owing to barriers such as time and/or distance (Jacobson & Hooke, 2016). Most agencies have invested in telehealth to facilitate the early identification of disease exacerbation, particularly

for patients with chronic diseases such as heart failure and diabetes. For example, telehealth permits families to transmit heart rates via telemedicine to health care providers and specialists to consult with family physicians, making it easier for individuals to access health care and for practitioners to provide it (Gregoski et al., 2012). Telehealth has the potential to improve health care access, quality, and efficiency. Suter et al. (2011) proposed that the use of telehealth by home care agencies and other health care providers be expanded to empower patients and promote disease self-management with resultant improved health care outcomes. Jacobson and Hooke (2016) evaluated the use of telehealth videoconferencing in children with severe hemophilia in the home setting and concluded that telehealth videoconferencing is a feasible tool for managing bleeding disorders in the home setting. Looman and colleagues (2015) evaluated the effect of advanced practice registered nurse (APRN) telehealth care coordination for children with medical complexity (CMC) on family caregiver perceptions of health care and found that APRN telehealth care coordination for CMC was effective in improving ratings of caregiver experiences with health care and providers.

Microsystem and Mesosystem Influences on Family Health

Internal ecosystem influences on family health include family type and developmental stage, family processes, personalities of family members, power structure, family role models, coping strategies and processes, resilience, culture, spirituality, family lifestyle patterns, and nutrition. All these factors are interrelated. For example, a family's lifestyle cycle stage influences a family's structural pattern, and family structures affect the family interaction process and relationships (McGoldrick et al., 2016). Therefore, nurses working with families in the area of health promotion must be sensitive to these various factors to recommend successful family health promotion interventions.

Family Structure

Families in the 21st century are quite different structurally from the families of the 1970s. Family structures are more diverse; there are more dual-career/dual-earner families, blended families, same-sex couples, transgender family members, and single-parent families (Kaakinen & Webb, 2016).

Recently, increasing numbers of grandparents raising grandchildren have been reported (Choi, Sprang, & Eslinger, 2016). Families in both the middle and lower classes are in such economic strain that they struggle with health promotion. The number of vulnerable families has also increased, including low-income traditional families, low-income migrant families, homeless families, and low-income older adults. Included in the vulnerable population are low-income, single-parent families and single-parent teen families. Vulnerable families are coping with a pileup of stressors and may be unable to focus on activities to enhance health (Walsh, 2011). As stated earlier, low-income families may focus less on health promotion and more on basic needs of obtaining shelter, adequate food, and health care.

Health promotion for disadvantaged families presents various challenges. For example, single mothers are generally poorer, more highly stressed, and less educated compared with married mothers (McLanahan & Jacobsen, 2015). In addition, children in father-absent homes are almost four times more likely to be poor (Kumpfer et al., 2016). Unless child support is paid, children in single-parent families with little extended family support typically are negatively affected. Kumpfer et al. reported that children residing in cohabiting stepfather families experience higher rates of school suspension or expulsion, delinquency, lower grades, lack of college expectations, and increased emotional and behavioral problems than teenagers living with two married biological parents.

Data from the 2002, 2006, and 2010 Scottish Health Behavior in School-aged Children (HBSC) surveys indicate that in single-mother homes, having a working mother was also positively associated with irregular breakfast consumption (Levin, Kirby, & Currie, 2012). Similarly, the findings of the Canadian Community Health Survey indicated that there is an association between household structure and smoking among adolescents in Canada. The odds of young smokers in the single-parent household were 1.78 times greater than the odds of young smokers in two-parent households (Razaz-Rahmati, Nourian, & Okoli, 2011). Family structure is associated with a range of adolescent risk behaviors, including smoking, drinking, marijuana use, having sex, and fighting (Levin et al., 2012). Those adolescents living in a family with both parents present fared better than those who lived with single parents (Kumpfer et al., 2016).

Family Processes

Family processes are continual actions, or a series of changes, that take place in the family experience. Essential processes of a healthy family include functional communication and family interaction (Smith, Freeman, & Zabriskie, 2009). Through both verbal and nonverbal communication, parents teach behavior, share feelings and values, and make decisions about family health practices (Wallace & Spear, 2016). Positive, reinforcing interaction between family members leads to a healthier family lifestyle. For example, when family members encourage, express affection, and show appreciation to each other, the family tends to be more functional (healthier).

Family Culture

The majority of the health promotion and universal prevention programs in the United States are developed for the general American culture and focus mostly on white, middle-class values, which might not be culturally appropriate or tailored to the specific needs of ethnically diverse families (Kumpfer et al., 2016). Cultures define and value health, health promotion, and disease prevention differently (Spector, 2017). One of the most evident features of families today is the growing cultural diversity (Walsh, 2012). A mounting trend is toward a global society with ever-increasing diversity among the populations; therefore, an expanded worldview is necessary for health care students and providers (Andrews & Boyle, 2016). Clients may not understand or respond to a family nurse's suggestions for health promotion because the suggestions conflict with their own health beliefs and values. Hence, it is crucial to assess and understand the family culture and health beliefs before suggesting changes in health behavior (Spector, 2017). An important component of family assessment is the consideration of cultural health practices. These practices influence all aspects of the nursing process, and understanding them helps the nurse evaluate client behavior and plan more effective interventions that are consistent with client health beliefs.

Keep in mind with regard to the cultural background of the family members that cultural tension or an acculturation gap may emerge between immigrant children and their parents relative to beliefs about healthful behavior (Birman & Poff, 2011). Role reversal can also happen in immigrant and refugee families when children learn the new language much faster and take on the parent role, creating a familial schism (Kumpfer et al., 2016). Children become involved in the new culture relatively quickly, particularly if they attend school, but their parents may never acquire sufficient comfort with the new language and culture to become socially integrated into their new country (Andrews & Boyle, 2016). In addition, immigrant children may have few opportunities to participate in and learn about their heritage culture (Birman & Poff, 2011). There are also racial/ethnic disparities in family resources. For example, Hispanic and African American families, in general, have been found to be socioeconomically marginalized (Jiang & Peguero, 2017). Children of first-generation families are generally much more likely to live in households characterized by poverty and economic hardship (Jiang & Peguero, 2017). Children often assimilate more quickly to a new culture, creating increased family conflict because of differential generational acculturation leading to children's developmental problems such as delinquency, substance abuse, anxiety, depression, and so on (Kumpfer et al., 2016). At the same time, children may embrace the opportunity to engage in unsupervised activities and behaviors that may be normative in the host society (such as sexual activity, drinking alcohol, eating fast foods, or recreational drug use) but unacceptable in their heritage culture and to their parents (Birman & Poff, 2011). The process of children taking on unhealthful behaviors of the new culture interferes with the health promotion function of the parents, so there is a tension between society and the family socialization function. Therefore, nurses need to be aware that parents and children may misunderstand one another because of cultural differences in expectations for parent and child behaviors and family relationships.

Spirituality and Health Promotion

Illness is not generalizable, nor does it occur in a vacuum. Individuals and families experience illness in multiple ways and nurses have a role in supporting patients and families in the ways that bring meaning to their life and in witnessing their lived experience. Spirituality is one way in which nurses can facilitate health promotion because spirituality has been found to have a positive effect on the health of patients and their family members. Although there is no consensus on the definition of spirituality, for this chapter the following definition is used:

[Spirituality is] An experience that incorporates a relationship with the transcendent or sacred that

provides a strong sense of identity or direction that not only has a strong influence on a person's beliefs, attitudes, emotions and behaviors but is integral to a sense of meaning and purpose in life. (Siddall, Lovell, & MacLeod, 2015, p. 53)

Patients who have a strong sense of spirituality report that they are less likely to participate in risky health behaviors. A more religiously oriented faith identity has been identified as predictive of fewer sexual partners and less binge drinking, whereas a more commitment-oriented faith identity is predictive of less marijuana use (Walker, 2013). Connection to a religious community and strong spiritual beliefs have been associated with fewer health-risking behaviors and mental health concerns (O'Brien et al., 2013), and there tends to be a negative correlation between underage drinking and both religiousness and spirituality: the higher the spirituality, the less likely someone is to engage in underage alcohol use (Sauer-Zavala, Burris, & Carlson, 2014). College students who develop and use positive religious coping and several dimensions of spirituality engage less in hazardous drinking and marijuana use (Giordano et al., 2015).

Patients report positive outcomes when their health care providers use a holistic approach by inquiring about their spirituality in relation to the health event: Trust is built and results in stronger relationships between health care providers and patients, management plans incorporate patients' spiritual beliefs and practices, and providers see the individual as a person, as more than the disease (Best, Butow, & Olver, 2014, 2016).

Spirituality is helpful to people in many ways. In general, findings demonstrate a direct relationship between spiritual health and improved health outcomes, including disease prevention (Foley, Anderson, Mallea, Morrison, & Downey, 2016; Pilger, Molzahn, de Oliverira, & Kusumota, 2016). Higher levels of spirituality are related to better mental and physical health (MacKinlay & Burns, 2017) for both patients and their families. For example, patients report that spirituality significantly helps them cope with pain (Clayton-Jones & Haglund, 2015; Siddall et al., 2015) and family caregivers report feeling less burdened (Schillings, 2010). Their ability to find meaning in their caregiving is also enhanced when their spiritual practice is supported (Marques-Gonzalez, Lopez, Romero-Moreno, & Losada, 2012). Specifically, many Korean American older adult couples have reported that family spirituality strengthens family health by fostering family commitment, improving emotional well-being, developing new healthy behaviors, and providing healing experiences (Kim, Kim-Godwin, & Koenig, 2016).

Patients expect nurses to explore the meaning of their health event and to arrange for privacy when patients are participating in spiritual or religious practices (Drury & Hunter, 2016). Walsh (2016b) identified several specific actions nurses can use to promote spirituality and increase family resiliency:

- Help make meaning of adverse experiences
- Provide compassionate witnessing by being fully present
- Create and hold a sacred space
- Clarify ambiguity
- Rekindle realistic hope while recognizing the complexities of the situation

All nursing diagnoses relative to coping and spirituality are limited in their usefulness because they suggest that nurses need only think about this aspect of client care when distress is prevalent. Yet, spirituality is the essence of being human and should be supported in health and illness. Therefore, spirituality warrants consideration at all times.

Family Lifestyle Patterns

The importance of parents and families as an influence of healthy behaviors is well addressed in the literature. Lifestyle patterns affect family health. In North America, hundreds of thousands of unnecessary deaths occur each year that can be directly attributed to unhealthy lifestyles. These deaths can be traced back to heart disease, hypertension, cancer, cirrhosis of the liver, diabetes, suicide, mental health, and homicide. For example, parental smoking is associated with a significantly higher risk of their adolescent children smoking (Gilman et al., 2009). Alves et al. (2016) analyzed a survey administered in 2013 to students aged 14 to 17 years old in six European cities ($n = 10,526$) and found that boys and girls were more likely to smoke if they had a father who smoked. Likewise, positive lifestyle patterns affect families in positive ways. For instance, when family members engage often in leisure activities, recreation, and exercise, they are able to better cope with day-to-day problems (Smith et al., 2009). Using a multinational approach with family samples from Australia, Canada, New Zealand, the United Kingdom, and the United States, Hodge, Zabriskie,

Townsend, Eggett, and Poff (2016) found that positive relationships between family leisure (family involvement and satisfaction) and family outcomes (family cohesion, adaptability, family functioning, and satisfaction with family life) were consistent across all five countries. Time together promotes family closeness. Healthy lifestyle practices such as good eating habits, good sleep patterns, proper hygiene, and positive approaches to stress management are passed from one generation to another (McGoldrick et al., 2016). In addition, when one family member initiates a health behavior change, other family members often make a change, too. When an individual family member changes eating patterns, perhaps by going on a diet, other family members often change their eating patterns as well. For example, parents who eat more fruits and vegetables encourage their children to do the same (Wallace & Spear, 2016).

Family Nutrition

Family nutrition is a crucial aspect of 21st century family health promotion and health protection. A major issue today for North American families is the tendency toward being overweight, a lack of exercise among family members of all ages, and an increase in obesity. Major factors that influence nutritional health are societal trends (technology, media, fast food, status), the family system (rituals, mealtime, environment, culture, values, communication, finances, marital status), and individual characteristics (self-concept, age, activity levels) (Kong et al., 2013; Levin et al., 2012; Musick & Meier, 2012; Spector, 2017). "Overnutrition" in American families is often the issue rather than malnutrition (Levin et al., 2012). Parents and adult caregivers are key in the dietary choices children make and have a strong influence on their physical activity practices (Wallace & Spear, 2016). Effective parenting, health teaching about nutrition, physical activity, and consideration of the family context are reported to be essential to reducing childhood obesity. For example, setting limits with sedentary activities such as television watching encourages children to increase their level of activity, whereas having a television in the child's bedroom promotes fewer calories to be expended by children throughout the day (Wallace & Spear, 2016).

Carroll and Vickers (2014) surveyed culturally diverse families in six states in the United States through focus and discussion groups from 2011 to 2014 and found that obesity, poor nutrition, lack of physical activity, too much screen time and electronics, and stress were the top health problems faced by children today. The nurse's role in family nutrition is to assess the quality of nutrition for individuals and the family system, provide anticipatory guidance, teach about nutrition, and support changes in the individual and family nutritional lifestyle. For example, one of the primary issues for people is large portion size. To promote weight loss and control, the family cook and members could be taught the appropriate portion size according to age and nutritional guidelines. The nurse should become familiar with the most current guidelines in the *Dietary Guidelines for Americans 2015–2020* (USDHHS, 2017a) and the *Eating Well With Canada's Food Guide* (2011).

FAMILY NURSING INTERVENTIONS FOR FAMILY HEALTH PROMOTION

Family health promotion is defined as achieving maximum family well-being throughout the family life course and includes the biological, emotional, physical, and spiritual realms for family members and the family unit (Fiese & Everhart, 2011). Family nurses have a crucial role in facilitating health promotion and wellness within the family context across the life span. Enhancing the well-being of the family unit is essential during periods of wellness, as well as during illness, recovery, and stress. A primary goal of nursing care for families is empowering family members to work together to attain and maintain family health; therefore, family health promotion should focus on strengths, competencies, and resources (Gottlieb, 2013; Wright & Leahey, 2013). Family nursing that focuses on health promotion should be logical, systematic, and include the client(s). The outcomes of health promotion of the family include family unity, flexibility, communication, and quality of care (Loveland-Cherry, 2011).

A myriad of strategies and interventions facilitate family health promotion, such as empowerment, promotion of family integrity, maintenance of family process, exercise promotion, environmental management, mutual goal setting, parent education, offering information, drawing forth family support, and anticipatory guidance (Loveland-Cherry, 2011; Wright & Leahey, 2013). The interventions focus on building resources in families and promoting changes in families. Several of the interventions center on

fostering the development of parents' self-efficacy in effective parenting and accessing resources to meet family health needs (Loveland-Cherry, 2011). Findings from the focus and discussion groups and the survey conducted by *Family Voices* between 2011 and 2014 (Carroll & Vickers, 2014) provide valuable insights for nurses caring for families. Major findings from the participating families include:

- Families desire a holistic approach to health.
- Families benefit from a strengths-based approach to health care, health promotion, and health education.
- Families know a great deal about what healthy behaviors and activities look like. Participants said they try to incorporate healthy habits into their everyday life.
- Families report an interest in having additional information and support for dealing with emotional and social wellness/mental health rather than simply using medications to control the behavior of family members.
- The themes of food and nutrition were passionately discussed in virtually all the focus groups, even when the main topic of the focus group was another health promotion theme; food and nutrition is a hot topic, and a source of connection and community building.
- Obstacles to health promotion and wellness were clearly identified by participants. These obstacles are out of families' immediate control. They include lack of infrastructure in their communities for physical activity (no safe streets for walking, no parks, crime and violence in the neighborhood); lack of affordable, healthy food; low-income jobs; high stress and fatigue from untreated behavioral and mental health needs of family members; having to work so many hours outside the home in order to make ends meet; cultural and linguistic barriers; and many other issues that create social and health inequities. In short, the social determinants of health were identified by families over and over again as primary barriers.
- Obesity, mental health/anxiety, poor nutrition, lack of physical activity, too much screen time and electronics, and stress were identified as top health problems faced by children today.

- Families willingly shared many tips and strategies, and most of them were in line with evidence-based recommendations.
- Families want more health education, as well as social and recreational opportunities that are health promoting and that they can afford.

The following strategies will be discussed for promoting family health: family self-care contract (family involvement), family empowerment and family strengths-based nursing care, anticipatory guidance and offering information, use of rituals/routines and family time, and family meal and healthy eating.

Family Self-Care Contract: Involvement of All Family Members

The family and nurse must collaborate and set mutual goals by establishing a nursing contract. The nursing contract is a working agreement that is continuously renegotiable and may or may not be written depending on the situation (Anderson & Fallin, 2014). The premise of contracting is that it is under the family's control, it increases the family's ability to make healthy choices, and this process facilitates family empowerment by collaborating with a health care provider (Anderson & Fallin, 2014).

Once the nurse and family have identified family strengths and areas for growth and change, the family should prioritize its goals. The commitment of all family members directed toward achieving a goal is crucial to the family's success. Nurses can assist a family to develop a self-care contract to improve health behaviors, independently or with a nurse. Table 6-4 provides components and sample items of a family self-care contract. The contracts are more effective when the components are negotiated and signed by all family members (Kim-Godwin & Bomar, 2015).

Family provides resources for health behaviors and health care. These resources include monetary support, information, emotional support, skills to navigate systems, and direction on desirable or healthy behaviors (Loveland-Cherry, 2011). Families are responsible for the health care of their members. These responsibilities include receiving required immunizations and health checks; providing adequate shelter, clothing, and food; and seeking health care when warranted (Loveland-Cherry, 2011). Socialization of family members is another major function in families and is accomplished in a

Table 6-4 Components of a Family Self-Care Contract	
Component of the Contracting Process (Mutually Agreed on by Family Members and Health Professional or by Family Alone)	**Example of Item in a Family Contract**
Family assessment of wellness and identification of area for improvement	Our family feels a sense of always being hurried with no time to relax, and we are irritable with each other.
Set the goal, environmental planning, and reinforcement	We want to have more relaxing time together as a family and to enjoy our time together.
Develop a plan	Have a family meeting to evaluate barriers and create a plan. The outcome might be to reduce sports activities for children. Specify a family fun night/afternoon.
Assign responsibilities	Plan an evening game night with no television or phone calls allowed. All members agree on the game or recreation activity. No one else but the family should participate. Evaluate the budget for games. The family nurse will assist the family to create the plan. Family members will agree to take part in the family fun time.
Determination of time frame	We plan to do this for 2 months, one night a week on Sunday evening from 4:00 p.m. to 7:00 p.m.
Evaluate the outcomes	After each week, we will spend 5 minutes talking about what was good and what could be improved. How are we relating to each other the remainder of the week?
Modify, renegotiate, or terminate	We will evaluate the family fun time after 2 months and mutually agree on changes.

variety of ways. Parents are important role models for children.

Family members provide both negative and positive role models. For example, smoking, substance and alcohol use and abuse, poor nutrition, and inactivity are often intergenerational patterns. Stress management, exercise, and communication are also learned from parents, siblings, and extended family members such as grandparents (McGoldrick et al., 2016). One interesting finding of note to nurses is that fathers' involvement is especially important for vulnerable families. Marsiglio (2009) reported that fathers' lack of exercise, poor eating, excessive drinking, and smoking predict the same behaviors among adolescents. Shapiro, Krysik, and Pennar (2011) analyzed mother-reported data in families eligible for the Healthy Families Arizona prevention program ($n = 197$) and found that families with greater father involvement had better prenatal care, higher incomes, less maternal involvement in Child Protective Services, less physical domestic violence, and greater maternal mental health reflected through less loneliness. Therefore, nurses need to make an effort to include fathers when developing plans for family health promotion and to assist fathers to develop positive role models for their children. By teaching healthy lifestyle in the community, faith-based centers, homes, and the workplace, nurses promote positive role modeling.

Family Empowerment and Family Strengths-Based Nursing Care

A primary goal of nursing care for families is empowering family members to work together to attain and maintain family health; therefore, family health promotion should focus on strengths, competencies, and resources (Gottlieb, 2013; Wright & Leahey, 2013). The nurse collaborates with the family and provides information, encouragement, and strategies to help the family make lifestyle changes. This process is termed *empowerment*. The underlying assumption of empowerment is one of partnership between the professional and the client as opposed to one in which the professional is dominant. Families are assumed to be either competent or capable of becoming competent (Anderson & Fallin, 2014).

The primary emphasis in family empowerment is involvement of the family in goal setting, planning, and acting, not on having the nurse do this for the family. A key role of family nurses in family health promotion is to empower family members to value their "oneness," to appreciate family togetherness, and to plan activities to foster their unity (Gottlieb, 2013).

One way of empowering a family is the use of commendation because it enables families to view the family problems differently and move toward solutions that are more effective. Wright and Leahey (2013) recommend that nurses routinely commend family and individual strengths, competencies, and resources observed during the family interview. Commendations to families regarding their strengths are "powerful, effective and enduring therapeutic interventions" (Wright & Leahey, 2013, p. 150). Although this intervention is important for all families, it is especially important for vulnerable families. Often, a family has unique strengths that are temporarily overshadowed by the health needs, so these strengths lie outside of the family's awareness (Walsh, 2016b). By commending a family's competence and strengths, and offering it a new opinion of itself, a context for change is created that allows families to discover their own solutions to problems (Gottlieb, 2013; Wright & Leahey, 2013).

The strengths-based approach has been used in health promotion to enhance wellness and well-being. Working with strengths enables a person to get the most out of living in order to cope, recover, heal, and discover a new purpose and meaning in living. Strengths-based nursing care does not ignore or negate problems; neither does it turn a blind eye to weaknesses or deficits. Instead, it uses strengths to balance or overcome them (Gottlieb, 2013). Working with the person's and family's strengths allows patients to maximize and support their responses in order to deal with everyday events and difficult life challenges (including illness, injury, disability, and trauma) and to meet their goals (Gottlieb, 2013). Strengths can be biological, intrapersonal and interpersonal, and social. Biological strengths are related to the biochemical, genetic, hormonal, and physical qualities within each individual or family. Intrapersonal and interpersonal strengths reside in the person, define one's personhood, and are considered a part of a person's or a family's inner resources. Social strengths, commonly known as resources or assets, reside in the person's environment and are available to individuals or the family (Gottlieb, 2013).

Anticipatory Guidance and Offering Information

During their life course, families inevitably experience crises and normative, even non-normative, stress. The family's resilience, unity, and resources influence how it copes with crisis and stress. The goal of the family nurse is to facilitate family adaptation by empowering the family to promote resilience, reduce the pileup of stressors, make use of resources, and negotiate necessary changes to enhance the family's ability to rebound from stressful events or crises. The nurse can teach families to anticipate life changes, make the necessary adjustments in family routines, evaluate roles and relationships, and cognitively reframe events.

Nurses should offer information based on family abilities and should encourage family members to seek resources independently (Wright & Leahey, 2013). Families usually desire information about developmental issues and health promotion (Carroll & Vickers, 2014). For example, helping parents to understand and help their children is an important intervention for families (Wright & Leahey, 2013). Nurses can teach families about physiological, emotional, and cognitive characteristics, as well as identify developmental tasks or goals of children and adolescents that can be affected or altered during times of illness (Wright & Leahey, 2013).

Nurses working with well families can teach family awareness, encourage family enrichment, and provide information on community agencies and Web sites that are resources for strengthening and enriching families. The family could be encouraged to agree on a goal to attend or find out more about resources or programs. By offering opportunities for family members to express feelings about family experiences, the nurse enables the family to draw forth its own strengths and resources to support one another (Wright & Leahey, 2013). Drawing forth family support is especially important in primary health care settings (Wright & Leahey, 2013).

Use of Rituals/Routines and Family Time

Denham (2011) emphasized the use of family rituals and routines for health promotion. The findings of previous research have indicated that predictable routines and meaningful rituals are related to healthier outcomes and that establishing routines is vital to managing demands in households with many extended family members.

Family nurses know that routines are observable and repeated behavior patterns that have great consistency and regularity. Family routines are collective events that occur on a daily, weekly, or annual basis. They typically include a set time and place, assignment of roles, and an element of planning ahead. Nurses can work with families to establish or help them maintain daily routines that are created around mealtimes, taking medications, and sleep (Fiese & Everhart, 2011). Families are able to plan ahead and provide a sense of stability to daily routines, yielding lower levels of stress and better family life. Family routines can be disrupted for expected developmental transitions (such as having a new baby in the house or moving to a new geographical location) and unexpected family situations (such as a diagnosis of a chronic health condition or strained economic resources). Therefore, family nurses can help prospective parents discuss family routines so they can be established when the new family member arrives. The key preservative function of routines appears to be not only maintaining a sense of order in daily life, but also staying connected as a group (Fiese & Everhart, 2011). Routines provide family members with the opportunity to communicate about events important to them. For example, at family holiday gatherings memories about past gatherings are shared, communicating a shared heritage and sense of belonging to a larger group. Over time, these communication patterns expressed during family gatherings come to cement relationships shown to be associated with healthy family functioning (Fiese & Everhart, 2011).

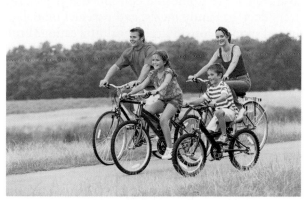

© *Digital Vision/Photodisc/Thinkstock*

Family ritual is a repetitive pattern of prescribed formal behavior pertaining to some specific event, occasion, or situation that tends to be repeated over and over again (Imber-Black, 2011). Family rituals often surround secular (such as birthday) and ceremonial occasions linked to religion (such as baby baptism), faith, or some form of canonical principles that distinguish ordinary from extraordinary and celebrate value ideals (Denham, 2011). Rituals are best introduced when there is an excessive level of confusion, as they provide clarity in a family system (Imber-Black, 2011).

Family routines/rituals may be perceived as being a fairly reliable index of family collaboration, accommodation, and synergy (Denham, 2011). To use rituals and routines as therapeutic interventions, nurses must identify ways to use intentionality to assist family members as they create, amend, and adjust routines so that they are relevant to families' unique health and illness needs. Nurses need to be educated to observe or consider the impact of family rituals and routines on the management of chronic illness. For example, diabetes is a disease greatly influenced by adherence to a prescribed medical regimen that usually includes a dietary plan, exercise, adherence to medicine usage, blood glucose monitoring, physician visits, and other care modalities. When adherence to a medical regimen is a concern, family members must identify the critical care aspects, key member duties for essential activities, and necessary actions to be included in family routines (Denham, 2011).

Family Mealtime and Healthy Eating

Factors in the family environment that promote healthful eating include the healthfulness of foods available in the home and consumed at meals, the frequency of family meals, and parental modeling of and support for children's healthful eating (Fruh et al., 2012; Haerens et al., 2008; Hammons & Fiese, 2011). Employed mothers are noted to purchase prepared foods more frequently, including fast-food and carry-out meals, consume more food away from home, and commonly report missing out on family meals (Devine et al., 2009).

Bauer, Hearst, Escoto, Berge, and Neumark-Sztainer (2012) analyzed the data from Project F-EAT, a population-based study of a sociodemographically diverse sample of 3709 parents of adolescents living in a metropolitan area in the Midwestern United States. They reported that full-time employed mothers reported fewer family meals, less frequent encouragement of their adolescents' healthful eating, lower fruit and vegetable intake, and less time spent on food preparation when compared with part-time and non-employed mothers. Full-time employed fathers reported significantly fewer hours of food preparation. In addition, higher work-life stress between both parents was associated with less healthful family food environment characteristics, including less frequent family meals and more frequent SSB and fast-food consumption by parents.

Research on family mealtime reveals that frequency of family meals is a protective factor that may curtail high-risk behaviors among youth (Fruh et al., 2012). For example, frequency of eating a family meal was associated with a reduced likelihood of all risk behaviors (e.g., smoking, drinking, marijuana use, bullying) among girls and all but fighting and having sex among boys (Levin et al., 2012). Kong and colleagues (2013) reported that although low-income families value the importance of sharing meals together, these units are often marked by more chaotic and tense social interactions.

Fruh et al. (2012) listed the following outcomes from families eating together:

- Teenagers who eat meals with their families frequently are less likely to be depressed or use drugs than those who do not eat with their families as often. They are also less likely to be violent, to have sex, and to experience emotional stress. Adolescents who eat meals with their families are likely to be more highly motivated in school and have better peer relationships.
- Regular shared mealtimes can increase children's sense of belonging and stability, and the entire family's feeling of group connection. Many adolescents in the Fruh et al. (2012) study reported that they wanted to be with their parents for most evening meals.
- Teenagers who share meals with their families on a regular basis tend to eat healthier foods than those who do not. They consume fewer high-fat, high-sugar prepared and packaged foods, and more fruits and vegetables and other foods high in important nutrients and fiber.

In addition, family mealtimes facilitate improving family communication, fostering family tradition, and teaching life skills to children. Encouraging shared meals when possible is a way nurses can enhance family bonding as this gives families an opportunity to be together and communicate with each other.

FAMILY CASE STUDIES

The following family case studies are used in the next sections of the chapter to demonstrate how different theoretical approaches can be used for assessing and intervening in the family for health promotion.

Case Study: Budd Family

Setting: Prenatal clinic (regular prenatal checkup).

Family Nursing Goals: Work with the family members to assist them in successful family transition and balance.

Family Members:
- *James: father*; 32 years old; full-time but temporarily employed without benefits, expects to be promoted to a permanent position soon with benefits (married Eleanor 3 years ago).
- *Eleanor: mother*; 33 years old; full-time employed, a school teacher at an elementary school with benefits, considering being a "stay-at-home" mother after giving birth (6 months pregnant); first marriage, married James after giving birth to Dustin.
- *Hanna: oldest child*; 8 years old; daughter (from James's first marriage), third grade, usually a good student.
- *Dustin: son*; 3.5 years old; all-day preschool (private day-care facility), developmentally on target.
- The couple is expecting a baby girl in 3 months.

Family Story:
James (32 years old) and Eleanor (33 years old) have one daughter, Hanna (8 years old), and one son, Dustin (3.5 years old). James is a full-time worker in a sales business (see the Budd family genogram in Figure 6-3). Currently, he is a full-time employee but under temporary status; he is expected to have a permanent position soon (date uncertain) that provides benefits and covers health insurance. Eleanor has a full-time position as an elementary school teacher. She wants to be a stay-at-home mother but is afraid of losing health insurance and family income if she quits now, so she wants to wait until James gets a permanent full-time position with benefits.

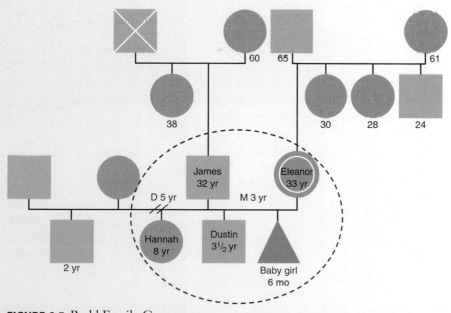

FIGURE 6-3 Budd Family Genogram

(continued)

Case Study: Budd Family *(cont.)*

The couple married 3 years ago; they recently moved from an apartment to a house because the family needs additional space for the new baby. Although the house is spacious, it is old and needs some renovation.

This is the first marriage for Eleanor and second marriage for James (James divorced 5 years ago). Eleanor states that the family has been successfully going through the remarriage cycle, and Hanna and Eleanor have a pretty good relationship. Hanna is usually withdrawn after visiting her biological mother (summer and winter school vacations, and several holidays—generally five times a year), who is also remarried and gave Hanna a new stepbrother (age 2) from her current marriage. Hanna is attending an after-school program at the same school where Eleanor works and returns home with Eleanor. On the way home, Eleanor picks up Dustin from the day care, which he attends from 7:30 a.m. to 4:30 p.m. during the weekdays. Hanna attends a piano lesson on Tuesdays and ballet class on Thursdays.

Because of the family's busy schedule, they often eat at fast-food restaurants during the evenings (at least twice a week), and meals at home are usually rushed and often eaten in front of the television. Although the family tries to eat meals together, it cannot do so because James's job requires frequent traveling, so the family often ends up eating meals without James.

When James is at home, he does outdoor chores, whereas Eleanor usually does indoor chores. The children usually watch television and play video games when the couple is working at home. The couple tries to do family activities each Sunday, and all family members attend a local Presbyterian church. But James is generally not home one Sunday each month because of the travel requirements for his job. With the exception of family vacations, holidays, and Sundays, the Budds rarely spend time together enjoying each other's company.

James and Eleanor seldom agree on parenting practices; whereas Eleanor is firm and detailed, James is laid-back. James has some guilty feelings toward Hanna, thus making him very lenient toward her. Hanna usually goes to her dad to escape her regular duties and whenever Eleanor asks her to complete assigned tasks. James usually accepts Hanna's request because of his guilty feelings, and this makes Eleanor uncomfortable and frustrated.

Eleanor was seen by a nurse in the OB/GYN clinic for her regular prenatal checkups. She is going through a normal pregnancy, but she recently has experienced serious fatigue. Her additional concern is that she has a difficult time putting Dustin to bed each night. Dustin used to go to bed easily when they lived in the apartment, where he shared a room with Hanna. After moving to the new house 3 months ago, where he has his own room, he has not been the same. Eleanor notices that he is more energetic at night and wants to stay with her before going to bed. In addition, Dustin has started visiting the parents at night and staying with them during the night, when he should be sleeping in his own bed. He has recently complained about his tummy being upset, and Eleanor is not sure whether he is sick or is just faking to get attention. Dustin is excited to have a baby sister, but he also shows some jealousy. For example, Dustin acted similar to an infant baby when his parents decorated the baby's room and bed with pink colors.

Although James helps Hanna at night, putting Dustin to bed is Eleanor's job, and she is overwhelmed with his behavior. Eleanor says that James is a good husband, but she feels that he considers parenting to be a mother's role, which sometimes leaves her feeling overwhelmed and angry. Eleanor perceives that all family members are healthy and states that they are just a busy family. Her additional concern is the family finances after she quits her job. The nurse sees only Eleanor during this time, and requests that James and the children come for the next visit. (See the Budd family ecomap in Figure 6-4.)

Assessment:

As explained in Chapter 5, models that nurses use to assess family health differ. The following illustrates how different assessments and options for interventions vary based on the theoretical perspectives of the family.

Family Systems Theory:

The focus of the nurse's practice from this perspective is family as client; therefore, assessments of family members are focused on the family as a whole. In the case study, all members of the Budd family are affected when the mother gives birth. Eleanor currently feels that her husband considers parenting as a mother's role. If James continues to be passive in his parenting role, it would cause a difficult family transition when the baby is born. In addition, the arrival of the new baby could make going to bed even more difficult for Dustin at night, if not resolved.

Developmental and Family Life Cycle Theory:

The family is a blended family and is in the stage of the "families with young children" (infancy to school age) because their oldest daughter, Hanna, is an elementary school child. The family is experiencing an additional normative developmental

Case Study: Budd Family *(cont.)*

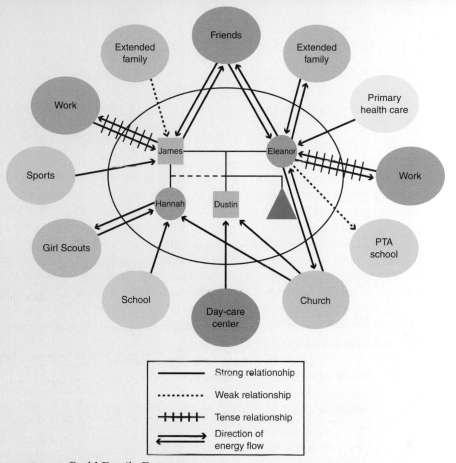

FIGURE 6-4 Budd Family Ecomap

stressor of adding a new family member. The tasks required for this family include adjusting to the addition of a new family member; defining and sharing childrearing, financial and household tasks; and realigning relationships with extended family, parents, and grandparents. In addition, although Dustin is developmentally on target, the family is experiencing a challenge to make Dustin go to bed each night and may face a challenge with potential sibling rivalry.

Bioecological Theory:

In the bioecological model, nurses need to assess the microsystem (i.e., family composition and home environment), mesosystem (i.e., external environment), exosystem (i.e., job and income), and macrosystem (i.e., community). The Budd family consists of two parents, two children, and a baby on the way. The couple has a white European heritage. The family lives in an old one-story house with four bedrooms in an older suburban section of town. During further interviews, the nurse found that the Budds' house was built before 1950 and is still under renovation.

The extended family (grandparents and siblings of Eleanor's side) live nearby, and Eleanor has a close relationship with them. The extended family gets together for most holidays; James and Hanna seem to have a tenuous relationship with Eleanor's family. The town is largely composed of white ethnicity with 30% African American. None of the parents or siblings of James lives nearby. James's dad passed away 10 years ago in a car accident; his mother remarried 7 years ago and lives 500 miles away. The Budds and James's mother usually meet once a year and talk once or twice a month via telephone. James has an older sister who lives out of the country because of her husband's military service.

(continued)

Case Study: Budd Family *(cont.)*

Family Assessment and Intervention Model:

Using the Family Systems Stressor-Strength Inventory (FS³I) of the Family Assessment and Intervention Model, the major family stressors include (1) Dustin's bedtime problem, (2) Eleanor's upcoming birth, (3) insufficient couple time and family playtime, (4) insufficient "me time" (specifically Eleanor), (5) inadequate time with the children and watching television too much (children), (6) overscheduled family calendar, and (7) parenting conflict and lack of shared responsibility. Some job stress exists because James is still in a temporary position and his work requires traveling.

Family strengths include (1) shared religious core, (2) family values and encouragement of individual values, (3) affirmation and support of one another, (4) successful family transition into a new blended family, (5) trust between members, (6) support from extended family (specifically Eleanor), (7) adequate income (current dual-career family), and (8) ability to seek help.

Interventions:

Through assessment, nurses identify family strengths that foster health promotion and stressors that impede health promotion (Pender et al., 2015). Integration of the family perspective into assessment and planning facilitates more effective plans for health promotion (Wright & Leahey, 2013). Although the family has developmentally been successfully going through the remarriage cycle, it is expecting an additional life transition of adding a new family member. For this successful transition, the couple needs to define and share childrearing and household tasks. In order to resolve the current parenting and role conflicts, the couple needs to evaluate the current roles and could experiment with being responsible for the children alternately. After the birth of the baby, the couple may face a challenge with potential sibling rivalry. Spending time together as a family would promote family closeness for this blended family. When family members engage often in leisure activities, recreation, and exercise, they are able to better cope with day-to-day problems (Smith et al., 2009). The nurse should address the hurried family lifestyle and frequent unhealthful fast-food eating habit.

Family Self-Care Contract:
- Involve all family members (including children) in establishing a family self-care contract.
- Assist the family members to share their perceived family health issues.
- Assist the family to prioritize the goals.
- Discuss the health promotion strategies.

Family Empowerment and Family Strengths-Based Nursing Care:
- Commend the family strengths and base interventions on the family strengths.
- Enhance and mobilize the family strengths for problem solving.
- Offer information/resources to help resolve parenting conflicts.
- Offer opportunities for the family members to express feelings about their family experiences.

Anticipatory Guidance and Offering Information:
- Help the family to anticipate/prepare for life changes after the birth of the baby girl.
- Encourage the family to make the necessary adjustments (e.g., role sharing).
- Offer information about resources for health promotion (e.g., smoking cessation, regular exercise).

Use of Rituals/Routines and Family Time:
- Assist the family to plan for family time, couple time, and individual family member alone time.
- Explore common family leisure activities, recreation, or exercise.
- Discuss ways to reduce the hurried family lifestyle by utilizing resources from extended family, church, or community.
- Assist the parents to establish bedtime routine.
- Discuss family mealtime and ways to improve healthy eating (e.g., reduction of fast-food consumption, avoiding meals in front of TV).

Case Study: Matthews Family

Setting: School health nurse's office (high school).

Family Nursing Goals: Work with the family to assist it for successful family transition and balance.

Family Members:
- *Andrew: father*; 52 years old; part-time lecturer at a local university (married Susan 18 years ago), first marriage.
- *Susan: mother*; 50 years old; full-time employed at a government office, second marriage with no children from the previous marriage.
- *Sophie: oldest child*; 17 years old; daughter, 11th grade.
- *Angela: middle child*; 14 years old; daughter, 9th grade.
- *Joseph: youngest child*; 11 years old; son, 6th grade.

Family Story:

Andrew (52 years old) and Susan (50 years old) have two teenage daughters, Sophie (17 years old) and Angela (14 years old), and one son, Joseph (11 years old). They have been married for 18 years. This is the first marriage for Andrew and second marriage for Susan. Susan was a survivor of domestic violence from the first marriage (which lasted less than 1 year).

Andrew is a part-time college professor. Susan has a full-time position as a director at a government office. When Andrew lost his full-time job 17 years ago, the couple moved in with Andrew's mother (Lucy, age 86) and lived with her for more than 5 years until Susan's income was sufficient to cover a mortgage and family expenses. Since moving out of Lucy's house, the couple and children visit and have dinner with her every weekend, which has become the family routine. Children are expected to spend the night with their grandmother after the dinner; however, recently Sophie has refused to spend the night at grandmother's house. Andrew's sisters and their families live in the same state and visit Lucy at least once a month. Lucy has chronic health conditions, which cause unexpected ED visits (several times a year). After divorcing her ex-husband, Susan started to study in a graduate school in a different state, where she met Andrew. Because Susan's family lives far away, she barely sees them and sometimes feels isolated and lonely.

Andrew has been a part-time employee at local colleges most of his life. Although Andrew has spent most of his time working on computers at home (online teaching), Susan has worked at a local government agency. Because Andrew has produced minimum income, Susan provides for most of the family's expenses.

The house has five rooms: master bedroom, Andrew's office (he stays at home most of the time), and three rooms for the children. The girls used to share the same room until the family added an additional room last year so the children could each have their own room. Since moving to a new room upstairs, Sophie brings her friends home frequently and a couple of close friends spend the night with her on weekends and during the summer break. The parents caught Sophie and her friend leaving the house secretly to meet a group of boys after midnight; Sophie was grounded for a month because of her actions. Last month, while she was driving to work, Susan found Sophie and her friend on the street (instead of going to school). Sophie's boyfriend lives nearby, and they meet frequently at the park or each other's home. Susan suspects that Sophie might have a sexual relationship with her boyfriend.

Because Andrew has strong family-centered values, the family eats dinner together as a family and once or twice a week with Andrew's mother (Lucy). Sophie has started skipping the family dinners frequently, stating that she is not hungry. She also has been experiencing several fainting episodes because of irregular eating habits. She frequently skips breakfast and lunch. The couple noticed that Sophie is eating fast food in her room or eating food after midnight by herself. Sophie's eating pattern is getting irregular, and Angela has begun to imitate her older sister's pattern and is refusing to participate in family dinners. Both girls are generally skipping breakfast, although Susan has made various attempts to get them to eat breakfast.

All three children are in good health. The children are generally happy, but loud at home and frequently fight and yell at each other. The girls argue about clothes and cleaning and are frequently cranky and difficult for the couple to deal with. Andrew and Susan sometimes argue because of different parenting styles: whereas Susan wants to raise the children in a Christian way, Andrew opposes Susan's parenting belief. Sophie is becoming rebellious and fights with Andrew frequently. She is losing interest in her schoolwork.

Earlier in their married life, mainly Susan was responsible for household chores. Sophie expressed resentment against her father regarding his minimal house chore contribution. Throughout the years, because of numerous heated arguments, Andrew

(continued)

Case Study: Matthews Family *(cont.)*

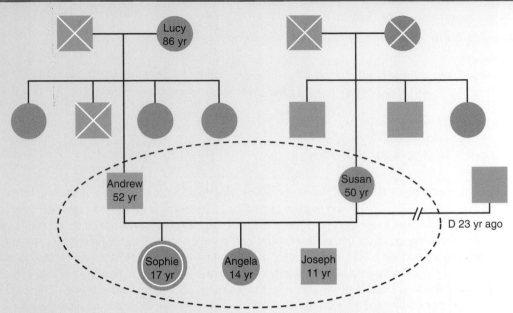

FIGURE 6-5 Matthews Family Genogram

agreed to share a significant portion of the household responsibilities, including outdoor chores. Still, Susan spends weekends doing grocery shopping, laundry, housecleaning, and attending to the children. During the weekdays, the couple takes the children to various lessons (piano, violin, cello, art, karate, and soccer), which sometimes causes schedule conflicts and builds marital tension.

Andrew and Susan have mutual friends, but seldom participate in social gatherings as a couple. Susan usually takes the children to church events, and Andrew takes Joseph to soccer practices or sports events. Susan feels social support and comfort by attending church and church-related activities, but Andrew considers it as his wife's overcommitment to religion. The family is affiliated with a Methodist church, which they used to attend every Sunday; Andrew stopped going to church 6 months ago. Sophie sometimes refuses to go to church as a family. Because of Susan's full-time job and frequent family gatherings with in-laws, as well as Lucy's frequent ED or hospital admissions, Susan has limited time to socialize with her own friends. Throughout the years, Susan has experienced chronic fatigue and stress from caring for the children and handling family responsibilities. She also experiences insomnia and hot flashes caused by menopause. Throughout the last 3 years, she has gained 30 pounds and is trying to lose weight without success. (See the Matthews family genogram in Figure 6-5 and family ecomap in Figure 6-6.)

Assessment:
Assessments of family members should be focused on the family as a whole. If Susan and/or Sophie's health status is declining and/or if Lucy's health deteriorates, the remaining members of the family will experience difficulty adjusting to the changes. Andrew and Susan experience difficult family transitions raising two teenagers who show rebellious attitudes and an unhealthy lifestyle.

Developmental and Family Life Cycle Theory:
The family is a nuclear family and is in the stage of the "families with adolescents" because their oldest daughter, Sophie, is in high school. The tasks required for this family include allowing adolescents to establish their own identities but still be part of the family; thinking about the future, education, jobs, and working; and increasing roles of adolescents in family, cooking, repairs, and power bases.

Case Study: Matthews Family *(cont.)*

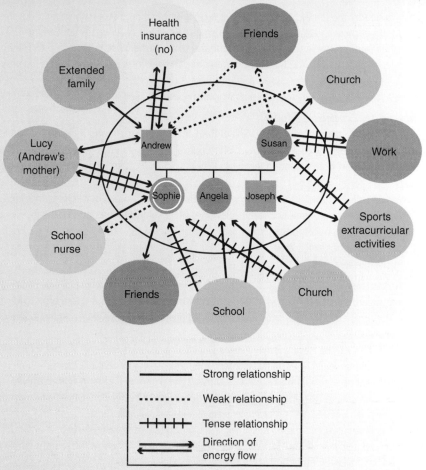

FIGURE 6-6 Matthews Family Ecomap

Family Systems Theory:

Although the Matthews family looks healthy, there is an indication of moving to family vulnerability. When family members exhibit symptoms of an illness, other family members become aware that an individual has become ill. The Matthews family does not engage in activities to improve and maintain the health of individual members and promote family functioning. Andrew and Susan exercise infrequently. Although Susan takes the children to pediatric and dental (including orthodontic) clinics for regular checkups and maintenance, Susan skips her annual checkup. Andrew is a heavy drinker and smoker. Because Andrew does not have health insurance, he only visits a clinic when he feels sick. He does not have a plan to purchase private health insurance because of financial reasons. Sophie has recently experienced fainting episodes. Susan suspects that Sophie is becoming sexually active, but Sophie denies it and refuses to receive the human papillomavirus (HPV) vaccine. Angela and Joseph usually stay home watching TV or using the computer instead of engaging in physical activities. Because of the overscheduled family calendar and work demands, they eat fast food frequently or use frozen meals. In addition, the family does not have regularly scheduled family meetings to problem solve for family risk reduction. Susan's increasing fatigue, Lucy's frequent ED visits, and Sophie's unhealthy lifestyle could lead to increased vulnerability.

Bioecological Theory:

The Matthews family consists of two parents and three children. Although the family does not live with Lucy, Lucy's influence is significant. Andrew has African American heritage with some European and Native American ancestors. Susan is biracial

(continued)

Case Study: Matthews Family *(cont.)*

(50% Asian and 50% African American). The family lives in a one-story house with five bedrooms in a middle-class neighborhood. A community park is nearby the family residence, and the children hang out there with other children occasionally. The town is largely composed of people with white ethnicity with a small proportion of African Americans and Asian Americans.

Andrew's sisters and their families live in the same state, and the family has a close relationship with them. The extended family gets together at least once a month. The Matthews family visits Lucy every week. Susan's parents passed away and she has an older sister who lives out of the country. Susan and her sister communicate with each other via e-mail or phone, talking as needed once or twice a month. Susan has two brothers whom she usually sees once every other year.

Family Assessment and Intervention Model:

Using the Family Systems Stressor-Strength Inventory (FS³I) of the Family Assessment and Intervention Model, the family strengths include (1) family values and encouragement of individual values, (2) parents' value of children's education, (3) trust among family members, (4) support from extended family and church, (5) adequate income, (6) shared religious core, and (7) ability to seek help.

The major family stressors include (1) children's poor/irregular eating habits (including skipping meals), (2) dissolved dinnertime routine, (3) insufficient couple time and family playtime, (4) insufficient "me time" (specifically Susan), (5) inadequate time with the children and spending too much time on television and the computer, (6) overscheduled family calendar, (7) Lucy's frequent ED or hospital admissions, and (8) lack of parenting skills and parental conflict. Some job stress exists because Andrew is still in a temporary part-time position.

Family Nursing Interventions:

Healthy families have both together family time and individual family member alone time (Denham, 2011; Imber-Black, 2011; Loveland-Cherry, 2011). The family experiences difficult family transitions in raising two teenagers who show rebellious attitudes and an unhealthy lifestyle.

The family needs to plan family time. Having family activities or leisure time would bring a sense of togetherness. Considering the benefits of family mealtimes for families with teenagers, the family needs to make a concerted effort to establish family mealtime routines, and each member should make that family mealtime a priority and let no other activity interfere with it.

Families with teenagers may require help in meeting both the needs of the family as a whole and members' individual needs. To find a balance, each family member should have time alone to develop a sense of self and to focus on growth. Andrew and Susan need improved couple time by modifying the overscheduled family calendar. In addition, the family needs increased sharing of household responsibilities. There is a need to redefine and negotiate the current family roles. Many of Susan's current roles could be shared by other family members.

The parents do not seem to be good role models for the children relative to physical exercise and healthy eating style. Nurses need to address healthy lifestyle practices such as good eating habits, good sleep patterns, proper hygiene, and other positive health practices, as these are passed from one generation to another. If the couple initiates a health behavior change, the children would likely make a change, too. For example, if Susan changes her eating patterns, perhaps by eating healthy meals, the children would change their eating patterns. The father's involvement is especially important for this family as a role model for the son who will be a teenager soon.

Family Self-Care Contract:
- Involve all family members (including children) in establishing a family self-care contract.
- Assist the family members to share their perceived family health issues.
- Encourage the family to discuss health promotion strategies.

Family Empowerment and Family Strengths-Based Nursing Care:
- List the family strengths and relate them to the characteristics of a healthy family.
- Use family strengths to balance and overcome existing problems.
- Offer opportunities for the family members to express feelings about their family experiences.
- Evaluate the current family roles and assist the family in establishing family role sharing.

Case Study: Matthews Family (cont.)

Anticipatory Guidance and Offering Information:
- Offer resources to resolve the current health issues (i.e., management of menopause symptoms and eating disorders).
- Offer information for health promotion (e.g., exercise and healthy eating for the whole family; healthy eating and safer-sex education for the girls).
- Offer resources for successful parenting for teenagers and conflict resolution.
- Assist individual members in health promotion.
- *Susan:* stress management skills (e.g., exercise, yoga, time for self).
- *Andrew:* weight loss strategies (i.e., exercise, healthy eating, and alcohol and smoking cessation).
- *Children:* time management (related to watching television and using the computer) and physical activities.

Use of Rituals/Routines and Family Time:
- Encourage the family to schedule weekly family time and/or family meeting.
- Help the family to explore family activities by consulting local newspapers, family magazines, and community agencies for activities that might interest the entire family, and afterward encourage them to continue these activities.
- Assist the parents in the family to arrange for couple time and individual time.
- Discuss ways to decrease the children's after-school activities.

Family Meals and Healthy Eating:
- Assist the family to establish family meal routines.
- Discuss ways to improve healthy eating (e.g., reduction of fast-food consumption).
- Experiment with premade breakfast meals (e.g., protein bars, fruit).

SUMMARY

This chapter provides an overview of family health promotion by defining family health and health promotion, introducing family health promotion models, and describing internal and external systems that influence family health promotion. The two case studies presented in this chapter illustrate family health promotion assessment and family nursing intervention strategies. The following outlines the major learning points emphasized in this chapter on family health promotion:

- Fostering the health of the family as a unit and encouraging families to value and incorporate health promotion into their lifestyle are essential components of family nursing practice.
- Health promotion is learned within families, and patterns of health behaviors are formed and passed on to the next generation.
- A major task of the family is to teach health maintenance and health promotion.

- The role of the family nurse is to help families attain, maintain, and regain the highest level of family health possible.
- Family health is a holistic, dynamic, and complex state. It is more than the absence of disease in an individual family member or the absence of dysfunction in family dynamics. Instead, it is the complex process of negotiating day-to-day family life events and crises, and providing for quality of life for its members.
- Family health promotion refers to activities that families engage in to strengthen the family unit and increase family unity and quality of family life.
- External ecosystem influences on family health include such things as the national economy, family and health policy, societal and cultural norms, media, and environmental hazards, such as noise, air, soil, crowding, and chemicals.
- Internal ecosystem influences include family type and developmental stage, family lifestyle

patterns, family processes, personalities of family members, power structure, family role models, coping strategies and processes, resilience, and culture.

- Health and family policies at all governmental levels affect the quality of individual and family health.
- Health promotion advertisements have generally targeted the more health-conscious middle class, rather than the vulnerable and underserved who are often the targets for alcohol and tobacco advertising campaigns.
- Families who are flexible and able to adjust to change are more likely to be involved in health-promoting activities.
- Vulnerable families are coping with a pileup of stressors and may be unable to focus on activities to enhance family health.
- Low-income families may focus less on health promotion and more on basic needs, such as obtaining shelter, adequate food, and health care.
- Middle-class families are skimping on health promotion, such as dental care, as they face current economic struggles.
- Through verbal and nonverbal communication, parents teach behavior, share feelings and values, and make decisions about family health practices.
- Different cultures define and value health, health promotion, and disease prevention differently. Clients may not understand or respond to the family nurses' suggestions for health promotion because the suggestions conflict with their traditional health beliefs and values.
- A primary goal of nursing care for families is empowering family members to work together to attain and maintain family health by focusing on family strengths, competencies, and resources.
- Health behaviors must be relevant and compatible with the family structure and lifestyle to be effective and useful to the family.
- The goal of the family nurse is to facilitate family adaptation by empowering the family to promote resilience, reduce the pileup of stressors, make use of resources, and negotiate necessary change to enhance the family's ability to rebound from stressful events or crises.
- Family health promotion should become a regular part of taking a family history and a routine aspect of nursing care.

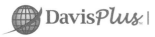 | For additional resources and information, visit **http://davisplus.fadavis.com**. References and Suggested Web sites can be found on Davis*Plus*.

Nursing Care of LGBTQ Families

Judith A. MacDonnell, BScN, RN, MEd, PhD

Mary E. Bartlett, DNP, APRN, FNP-BC, AAHIVs

Aaron Tabacco, PhD, RN

Critical Concepts

- Nurses care for families with members who have unique gender identities, sexual orientations, and family structures in a variety of settings and circumstances with increasing visibility and frequency.

- Historical, political, sociocultural, religious, and economic contexts influence the meaning of gender, gender identities, and gender expressions.

- Gender and sexuality are socially constructed concepts that vary across place and time.

- Gender, gender identity, and sexual orientation diversity are evident across ethnicities, cultures, age groups, and socioeconomic classes.

- Lesbian, gay, bisexual, transgender, and queer (LGBTQ) persons experience family through a variety of biological and social structures that include kinship ties and chosen family.

- As minorities with a historically marginalized and stigmatized population, LGBTQ individuals and families experience significant life-span barriers to health and well-being, as well as barriers to legal and social protections under the law that lead to health disparities.

- Heteronormativity, racism, sexism, ageism, and other powerful social ideals often intersect with gender diversity and result in increased barriers to care and thus increased health risks among the population. Oftentimes, nurses care for families experiencing challenges at these intersections of diversity.

- Language and social ideas about gender are ever evolving. Many cultures do not share the same language or social constructs related to gender identity, sexuality, and gender expression. Effective family nurses embrace this developing language and seek to create safe and respectful dialogue from the position of the learner when caring for LGBTQ individuals and their families.

- Families with LGBTQ members are working to achieve the same socially prescribed functions of all families to rear responsible and independent children, provide emotional and instrumental support to one another, and provide family member health care across the life span.

(continued)

■ Effective family nurses examine their own understandings and biases of gender, sexuality, and families and reflectively seek to serve LGBTQ families with efficacy and compassion.

■ Nursing care of LGBTQ families is an act of social justice, especially when focused upon health promotion and removing barriers to health care that result in health disparities in the population.

LGBTQ: AN INTRODUCTION TO DIVERSITY

Gender diversity is an umbrella term used to refer to a set of human variations that relate to biological sex, gender, gender identity, gender expression, and sexual orientation. Similar to all persons, those who identify as LGBTQ experience health and illness as members of families across the life span. Historically, this population has been underrepresented or underidentified in health and population research. During the last decade, however, new methodologies that allow better sampling and technologies that protect privacy enabled a more inclusive and focused empirical investigation (Institute of Medicine, 2011; Lambda Legal, 2010). According to the Gay and Lesbian Alliance Against Defamation (GLAAD), the preferred acronym for this immensely diverse cohort is LGBTQ for lesbian, gay, bisexual, transgender, and queer (Q may also stand for questioning) (Swartz, 2016). Most research is more narrowly directed and often refers to specific sexual minorities. In the more general discussions in this chapter, the acronym LGBTQ is used. However, much of the primary research referenced is specific to populations; therefore, in those cases the acronym is used that reflects the population of that specific study. In other words, the text will not incorrectly attribute "Q" where the researchers did not address this group.

In recent years, North American cultural and political climates gradually acknowledged and affirmed sexual minorities and LGBTQ families. Although greater acceptance promotes patients' willingness to seek care and expands access to patient-centered health services, inadequate knowledge of the unique health needs of this population may contribute to unintended outcomes including stigmatization and overall disparities in health (IOM, 2011).

Nurses have a key role in providing care to LGBTQ persons and families; however, gaps in understanding may impede the most optimal

outcomes. For example, nurses may be unfamiliar with terminology, including differences between sex, gender, sexual orientation, and sexual identity. They may be unaware of family structure and role variability. Without an adequate understanding of the population, compassionate caring is not possible. The purpose of this chapter is to provide nurses with an evidence-based foundation and to facilitate the delivery of culturally competent care, thus decreasing health risks and disparities among this most vulnerable population.

The first step in developing practice competence with LGBTQ families is to reflectively evaluate one's own background, beliefs, and biases. Reflective practice allows nurses the opportunity to open themselves to others, receive their stories and journeys, set aside biases, and ultimately be more fully and authentically present in caregiving tasks (Tanner, Benner, Chesla, & Gordon, 1993). The second step is to build cultural and personal knowledge through sensitizing oneself to relevant language, to the history of the population, and to their unique and common health needs. The third step is to understand the unique disparities of the population and, in accordance with the ethics and values of nursing, seek to develop a practice focused upon mitigating these health disparities at various socioecological levels. For most nurses, this is accomplished by offering compassionate, affirming care and advocacy at the bedside or in the community. For other nurses, this may mean finding a specific passion for LGBTQ family health and making service to this population a focus of primary care or special social justice interest.

Essential Vocabulary

Building a competent, working vocabulary related to the LGBTQ population is a complex task. At present, there are few universally accepted terms and phrases, and oftentimes the application of words can be culturally challenging. This is due, in part, to the rapidly expanding awareness of LGBTQ persons and families within the cultural, social, and political contexts. Another aspect of this challenge comes from the LGBTQ community itself as they continue to develop a shared identity and participate in social discourse. Because the unique language related to the LGBTQ population is evolving, it is essential that nurses approach the care of these families from the perspective of openness and humility. At the same time, mistakes and missteps may occur, just as they might when working with anyone whose family, culture, history, or background is unfamiliar. Effective nurses create relationships of trust and respect by offering a nonjudgmental, self-aware, and genuinely receptive attitude. In order to promote the most optimal health outcomes, it is crucial that nurses use current, relevant, respectful, and appropriate vocabulary, which are located in Box 7-1. **Sex** refers to the genetic, presenting biology of a human being in terms of anatomy and genotype (American Psychological Association, 2012; World Health Organization, 2017). Sex is typically assigned to a person at or before birth based on external genitalia (or genetic testing when external genitalia is **ambiguous**) and is most often identified as **female, male,** or **intersex**. Intersex is a biological variation of sex, which presents differently in each person along a spectrum that can include having the reproductive organs common to both female and male persons, having varying appearances of external genitalia, and/or possessing a genotype of sex chromosomes that may include an XXY variation rather than the more common XX (female) or XY (male) pattern (Intersex Society of North America, 2017). There are a large number of anatomical, genetic, and physiological variations that may be covered by the term *intersex*. It is estimated that one in 1000 to one in 2000 children are born each year with clear indications of intersex status, and although more subtle presentations are also known to exist, it is very difficult to estimate the frequency of these diversities as there is no formalized reporting process for data collection (ISNA, 2017). In the context of vocabulary, nurses may hear members of the LGBTQ community use the term **non-binary** as a way to communicate their identity as being different from the majority.

Gender is defined as the culturally held and transmitted beliefs, attitudes, and feelings that are associated with biological sex (APA, 2012; American Psychological Association & National Association of School Psychologists, 2015). Gender is largely focused on persons' behaviors in relation to their

biological sex and as such it is common to see or hear the phrases gender **conforming** or gender **nonconforming** used in relation to the LGBTQ population. Because cultural beliefs about gender are generally held to be important across cultures, social stigma is often associated with persons who challenge these social beliefs or norms. For example, in early 1990 the term *Two-Spirit* was used by First Nations and Native Americans to describe an individual with both masculine and feminine energies; these individuals were seen as sacred people (Jacobs, Thomas, & Lang, 1997) (Box 7-2). Such persons may have a different inherent gender identity or means of gender expression than what is expected of them. **Gender identity** refers to individuals' internal sense of self in respect to their sex. Persons whose gender identity and biological sex are not congruent may identify as **transgender** (APA, 2015; APA & AASP/NASP, 2015). The complementary term **cisgender** is used to denote those whose gender identity is consistent with their biological sex and personal identity (Schilt & Westbrook, 2009). **Gender expression** refers to the outward behaviors and appearance choices people make which may or may not conform to either their biological sex or gender. Some people, including a larger body of youth, may choose to identify as **queer, genderqueer**, or **gender fluid** as ways to remain open and thus not limited to the expected social beliefs about themselves (APA, 2012; 2015; APA & AASP/NASP, 2015). In modern Western cultures and histories, the root term *queer* was and may still be used as a derogatory label. However, many LGBTQ persons use the term themselves as a matter of pride; thus, terms may or may not carry the weight of stigma based on who is using them and how they are applying them in conversation. The APA (2015) and APA and AASP/NASP (2015) define *queer* and *genderqueer* as umbrella terms used by the LGBTQ community to communicate broadly that they do not identify or conform in some way to the dominant cultural definitions related to sex, gender, or sexuality.

Sexual orientation is defined as the romantic and sexual attractions people experience toward others' biological sex or gender identity (APA, 2012, 2015; APA & AASP/NASP, 2015). A person may be attracted predominantly to persons of one gender, both binary genders, to transgender or genderqueer persons, or to those who may identify as androgynous (nongendered). Most commonly, humans are **heterosexual** and are attracted to people of the

BOX 7-1

Glossary of Terms

The use of appropriate terminology is crucial when working with all patients and families as it begins to establish a respectful trusting relationship. Terms and definitions about LGBTQ have not been standardized. This box lists terms and definitions to assist nurses in capturing and documenting accurate information. The terms in this list are from the National LGBT Health Education Center.

Biphobia: the fear of, discrimination against, or hatred of bisexual people or those who are perceived as such.

Bisexual: a sexual orientation that describes a person who is emotionally and sexually attracted to people of their own gender and people of other genders.

Cisgender: a person whose gender identity and assigned sex at birth correspond (i.e., a person who is not transgender).

Gay: a sexual orientation that describes a person who is emotionally and sexually attracted to people of their own gender. It can be used regardless of gender identity, but is more commonly used to describe men.

Gender identity: a person's inner sense of being a boy/man/male, girl/woman/female, another gender, or no gender.

Genderqueer: describes a person whose gender identity falls outside of the traditional gender binary structure. Other terms for people whose gender identity falls outside the traditional gender binary structure include *gender variant, gender expansive,* and so on. Sometimes written as two words (gender queer).

Heterosexual (straight): a sexual orientation that describes women who are emotionally and sexually attracted to men, and men who are emotionally and sexually attracted to women.

Homophobia: the fear of, discrimination against, or hatred of lesbian or gay people or those who are perceived as such.

Intersectionality: the idea that identities are influenced and shaped by race, class, ethnicity, sexuality/sexual orientation, gender/gender identity, physical disability, national origin, and so on, as well as by the interconnection of all those characteristics.

Intersex: group of rare conditions where the reproductive organs and genitals do not develop as expected. Some prefer to use the term *disorders* (or differences) of sex development. Intersex is also used as an identity term by some community members and advocacy groups.

Lesbian: a sexual orientation that describes a woman who is emotionally and sexually attracted to other women.

Queer: an umbrella term used by some to describe people who think of their sexual orientation or gender identity as outside of societal norms. Some people view the term *queer* as more fluid and inclusive than traditional categories for sexual orientation and gender identity. Because of its history as a derogatory term, the term *queer* is not embraced or used by all members of the LGBT community.

Questioning: describes an individual who is unsure about or is exploring their own sexual orientation and/or gender identity.

Sexual orientation: how a person characterizes their emotional and sexual attraction to others.

Transgender: describes a person whose gender identity and assigned sex at birth do not correspond. Also used as an umbrella term to include gender identities outside of male and female. Sometimes abbreviated as trans.

Transphobia: the fear of, discrimination against, or hatred of transgender or gender non-conforming people or those who are perceived as such.

Transsexual: sometimes used in medical literature or by some transgender people to describe those who have transitioned through medical interventions.

Two-Spirit: describes a person who embodies both a masculine and a feminine spirit. This is a culture-specific term used among some Native American, American Indian, and First Nations people.

Sources: Glossary of LGBT Terms for Health Care Teams. Definitions for this glossary were developed and reviewed by the National LGBT Health Education Center and other experts in the field of LGBT health, as well as adapted from glossaries published by the Safe Zone Project and the UCLA LGBT Resource Center. June 2017.

opposite gender in a binary male/female model. **Homosexual** persons, preferring often to be called gay (males or females) or lesbian (female), are attracted to those of the same sex. Persons with a **bisexual** orientation are attracted to others of either binary sex. Some persons find their sexual orientation is somewhat fluid across the life span or is more person-dependent than it is concrete or static.

Nurses serving the LGBTQ community should be aware that sexual orientation is biologically

Two-Spirit is a group of 20+ LGBTQ groups that advocate for members of the First Nation and Native American community who identify as LGBTQ within their communities and outside their communities. An example of advocacy by the NativeOUT organization was to begin to change the negative shaming-type language within the indigenous community used to identify a person who identifies as gay. The term used in many tribal languages was *berdache*, which means, "passive partner in sodomy, boy prostitute" (dictionary.com).

The suggested new term is Two-Spirit, which means a person who has both feminine and masculine energies embodied in one person. Individuals who are Two-Spirit often hold sacred roles in their tribe, such as healer, holy person, or peacekeeper. Within most tribes there is a term, in their language, to describe a Two-Spirit person. A sample of terms in various tribes for a person who is Two-Spirit can be found on the NativeOUT Web site: https://indiancountrymedianetwork.com/news/opinions/two-spirits-one-heart-five-genders.

determined. It is a normal expression of human sexuality and not a preference over which one may exercise self-agency. Therapeutic efforts to change sexual orientation (i.e., conversion therapy, reparative therapy) have been denounced in policy statements by a majority of mainstream medical and mental health organizations (e.g., American Counseling Association, American Academy of Pediatrics, American Psychiatric Association) (Just the Facts Coalition, 2008). Indeed, it is widely held that such practices may result in reinforcement of social stigma as well as psychological, social, and family relationship damage (Just the Facts Coalition, 2008).

A working knowledge of this vocabulary will help nurses to better understand and serve LGBTQ families. This chapter is only a beginning. Nurses who are involved in serving the LGBTQ community and their families will continue to seek out learning over time; they will keep themselves informed and create the best practices possible as evidence, knowledge, and vocabulary continue to evolve.

Pronouns

Some individuals feel that gender is nonbinary, that is, not limited to male or female. For nurses who are seeking to establish a trusting relationship, it is important to ask how one prefers to be called and to note that the preferred pronoun may not necessarily match the individual's name or physical appearance. Persons who do not identify as either male or female may prefer *they/them* as their pronoun. In fact, the American Dialect Society (2016) voted the singular *they* as word of the year in recognition of several major newspapers' modifying their style guides to allow its use in reference to individuals who have

a nonbinary gender identity. Refusing to use the preferred pronouns for a transgender client is a form of microaggression that hinders empathic and therapeutic communication. As caring professionals, nurses have the unparalleled opportunity to welcome individual differences and to support the expressed or implicit needs of vulnerable patient groups.

DEMOGRAPHICS

According to one longitudinal, representative sampling survey (Gallup, Inc., 2017), at present approximately 10 million adults now identify as LGBT in the United States, a significant jump from approximately 3.5% of the overall population to 4.1% as of the year 2016. In considering further those other characteristics of significance, the prevalence of persons identifying as LGBT grew most among those who also identify as Asian and Hispanic, jumping from 3.5% to 4.9% and 4.3% to 5.4%, respectively. Of particular interest is the effect of age on the numbers of those stating LGBT identity, as the greatest increase by age group was among so-called millennials, people born between 1980 and 1998, of whom 5.8% identified as LGBT in 2012 and increased to 7.3% as of 2016 (Gallup, Inc., 2017). Although the U.S. Affordable Care Act made it possible to collect a broader base of information and the National Health Interview Survey included four questions relevant to sexual orientation (Ward, Dahlhamer, Galinsky, & Joestl, 2013), these data are very new and have yet to become useful for the development of public policy.

In Canada, the Canadian Community Health Survey (CCHS), starting in 2003, was the first to include questions about sexual orientation, and the

2001 Canadian census included questions on sexual orientation. No national survey has yet collected data on gender identity. There are challenges to defining the concepts and language used for identity categories and questions, and the CCHS was limited to asking about sexual identity. In the 2010 Ontario Health Study, similar to the U.S.-based population-based surveys, questions about sexual identity as well as sexual behavior have been included (Bauer, 2012; Travers, 2015).

It is difficult to capture a demographic picture of LGBTQ persons and families in North America, as many national level data collection efforts, such as census data, have not historically measured such diversity or have not measured it during a substantial amount of time. For example, most survey instruments use a binary male/female identifier only, limiting the knowledge about intersex persons. Additionally, very few surveys use gender or gender identity as categories for additional data. This is further complicated by the historical denial of marriage to same-sex couples and the ambiguity of data about sex, gender, and orientation in reports about domestic partnerships in lieu of marriage where such legal commitments were allowed.

In 2010 there were approximately 594,000 same-sex households (Lofquist, 2011). Among the LGB and transgender populations, 37% and 38%, respectively, reported having had a child (Gates, 2013). An estimated 5% to 15% of the Canadian population identifies as LGBTQ (Best Start Resource Centre, 2012). Data on married and common-law parents in same-sex relationships has been available in Canada since the legalization of same-sex marriage in 2005, although since 2001 the census could distinguish between children living with two parents who were either opposite-sex or same-sex parents (Bohnert & Lathe, 2014). The census reported that there were 37,885 same-sex common-law couples in 2006. Data on those who were married were not captured (Bauer, 2012). An Ontario-based study (Pyne, Bauer, & Bradley, 2015) reported that 24% of trans people are parents. Despite the belief that families are integral to overall well-being (Carr & Springer, 2010), research exploring the health of sexual and gender minorities has looked largely at individuals and has overlooked the role of family relationships and community support (Umberson & Montez, 2010).

The relationship quality reported by same-sex couples is similar to that of heterosexual married couples. Even so, unmarried same-sex couples and unmarried heterosexual couples both report a lower overall health status than married heterosexual couples (Denney, Gorman, & Barrera, 2013). The precise mechanism for this is unclear. Denney and colleagues have theorized that there may be distinct factors contributing to the reports of poorer health for LGB individuals as opposed to their heterosexual counterparts. They emphasize the need for population-based research in this area.

BIAS AND SOCIAL STIGMA

Nearly a quarter century ago, Meyer (2003) coined the term *minority stress* to describe the adverse effects of social stigma and prejudice on mental health. In the years since, minority stress is known to contribute to disparity in several health domains (Kates, Ranji, Beamesderfer, Salganicoff, & Dawson, 2016; Lick, Durso, & Johnson, 2013). In spite of broadening views and changing legislation during the last few years, institutional bias and social stigma continue to affect LGBT individuals and families (Box 7-3).

Significantly, in a review of 17 published reports of nurses' attitudes toward LGBT patients, Dorsen (2012) found that all studies revealed evidence of negative attitudes. Lambda Legal (2010) characterized the problem as follows:

> *The essential bond of trust between clinician and patient that many in the United States take for granted is not a given for LGBT people or people living with HIV. Whether because of prejudices, ignorance, outdated systems or shortsighted policies, many people across our communities are not receiving the health care they need. (p. 9)*

Patients who perceive health care providers as being uncomfortable with them may be reluctant to reveal their sexual orientation or gender identity or seek health care at all (Eliason & Schope, 2001; Espinoza, 2014). This, in turn, may result in a cycle of insufficient information leading to inadequate care, resulting in the perception of discrimination leading to fear of providing complete information (Lambda Legal, 2010). It is important for nurses to understand the patient, the family dynamic, and, most importantly, their own internalized bias (implicit bias), which is rooted in life experience and may be expressed without conscious awareness.

BOX 7-3

It's Like Coming Out All Over Again

All members of the LGBTQ community have a coming out story. Depending upon the circumstances, which are every bit as diverse as the faces, hearts, and minds of these individuals, coming out is a more or less painful experience. Fear is ever present. Telling one's friends and loved ones who you are (for real) risks rejection, isolation, discrimination, and in some cases violence. The body language of disapproval and the sympathies of ignorance are overwhelming. Familiar embraces may be suddenly withheld, long-term friendships wither, and those that remain changed. Almost everyone who knew you before coming out sees the person differently. Health care providers are no exception.

Seeking health care can be a formidable task for anyone, but for LGBTQ people there is an extra layer of vulnerability as they anticipate how they will be regarded and whether they will receive equitable care. Virtually every encounter with a new provider means that the LBGTQ person faces a kind of coming out which, depending upon circumstances, can once again be more or less painful.

- *When I go with my children to a medical appointment, I have to cross out the designation "Father" and "Mother" and insert "Parent" instead.* [A lesbian mother with five children]
- *I went to an OB/GYN and even after I told the nurse that I had a female partner, and that I do not have sex with men, she insisted on doing a pregnancy test because that was their policy.* [A lesbian nurse practitioner seeking routine gynecological care]
- *I went to a GI specialist and while I was describing my symptoms I disclosed that I was a lesbian. He appeared surprised and then muttered under his breath that he "would not have guessed."* [A lesbian seeking evaluation for acute abdominal pain]

- *I had an abnormal pap smear in my early 20s. As a trans-male I went to medical appointments for nearly 10 years before anyone ever asked me about my gynecological history.* [A transgender man seeking routine primary care]
- *When I introduced my boyfriend to the nurse who had been caring for me after my surgery, he avoided physical contact. He even passed ice chips to me on a tray so his hand would not touch mine.* [A gay man following a routine surgical procedure]
- *In the emergency room after a skiing accident, the staff continued to use male pronouns even after I had told them that I was a transgender woman.* [A transgender woman with an orthopedic injury]
- *After an emergency C-section, our baby was in critical condition and so was my wife. They had rushed her to the operating room. An aide, addressing me as "sir," swiftly escorted me to a drab waiting room. After a while the nurse came and brought me a cup of tea. She sat with me and held my hand. She stroked my head as I wept. She did not speak when they told me that my baby would probably not live. She did not have to. She was there. I think she saved my life.* [A human being, who happened to be a lesbian, on one of the worst days of her life]

When health care providers consider a person's humanness secondary to one's sexual orientation or gender identity, the person may feel classified as *other*. If they cannot relate to you as fellow humans, they cannot adequately address medical concerns or empathize with symptoms or show compassion for one's pain. All of us—us being we who are a part of the human race—are unique. Our differences are what we have in common; they make us the same. Our uniqueness should not separate us or marginalize our needs. It should not; and yet—all too often—that is what happens.

LGBTQ FAMILY STRUCTURES

The idea of what constitutes a family has changed dramatically in recent years. Today, only 22% of U.S. families fit within the *traditional* classification of two heterosexual parents with children (Movement Advancement Project, 2011). Family structures for LGBTQ people are increasingly diverse, reflecting family members across a continuum of sexual and gender identities.

The definition of *family* adopted by this textbook is as follows: *Family refers to two or more individuals who depend on one another for emotional, physical, and economic support. The members of the family are self-defined* (Kaakinen & Hanson, 2015, p. 5). A self-defined family or ***family of choice*** reflects the identification of significant persons who are not linked by blood, kinship, or legal ties, but who function as family members (Rickards, 2013). The relatively high occurrence of families of choice in the LGBTQ population may be related to the frequency with which they are alienated from families of origin who do not accept them or who refuse to acknowledge their same-sex or transidentified partners (Nelson, 2015).

Although descriptions exist of lesbian families that date historically to the era of Sappho, BCE, LGBTQ individuals and families have remained hidden from mainstream society (Zeck, 1999). It is only in the last couple of decades that LGBTQ families have been able to be more open and to thrive freely in Western cultures. In the not too distant past, same-sex families were denied access to health care options that could support reproduction and were not permitted to be named as parents of children in families they created. In emergencies or in the case of palliative and end-of-life care, gay and lesbian couples were not permitted access to their partner's health care information and were not allowed to take part in critical decisions (Best Start Resource Centre, 2012). Although current legal and societal trends have been more inclusive and LGBTQ-family-affirming, sexual minorities are still subject to social stigma and marginalization (Espinoza, 2014). In the United States, same-sex couples did not have the right to marry until the 2015 Supreme Court Ruling in the case of *Obergefell v. Hodges.* In Canada, same-sex marriage became legal in 2005 (Nicol & Smith, 2010).

It is owing to social initiatives such as the women's movement, civil rights movement, and LGBT and HIV-rights movements that gays and lesbians have gradually become more visible and have gained standing as equal members of society. It is likely that all variations of the expression of human sexuality have existed throughout time; however, those who identify as bisexual, queer, transgender, Two-Spirit (Two Spirit, 2017), and genderqueer have only recently found their way to the fore in LGBTQ family discourse (Best Start Resource Centre, 2012).

There are some 600,000 same-sex households in the United States and 220,000 children being raised by same-sex parents (Gates, 2013). According to the 2011 census report, in Canada, there are 7700 children under the age of 24 living with female same-sex parents and another 1900 living with male same-sex parents (Bohnert & Lathe, 2014). Although it is estimated that there are 600,000 transgender individuals in the United States, family-level data are not available. Similar to any other, same-sex

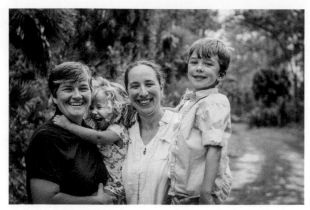
© iStock. com/Lisa5201

families depend upon one another for emotional, physical, and economic support.

In order to be effective advocates and care providers, it is important for nurses to get to know individual family dynamics, family processes, family culture, and the roles that parents play in the lives of their children (World Family Map, 2015). Nurses who understand the nature of LGBTQ family structures will be better prepared to provide holistic and culturally competent care to the diverse families they meet. They will be equipped to support changes in policy and professional practice and to participate in the evolution of health services that enhance everyday well-being for LGBTQ people (Registered Nurses Association of Ontario, 2007).

In LGBTQ families there may be some fluidity in relationships or roles (Kia, 2015; Levitt, Horne, Puckett, Sweeney, & Hampton, 2015; Stern, 2015). Kia (2015), for example, describes gay families in which a same-sex friend has the primary role of caregiver or caretaker, but is not a romantic partner. It is important for nurses, who are establishing relationships with patients, to ask about friends and family members and their respective roles.

Because of the long history of stigma and lack of social acceptance of LGBTQ individuals, one family structure specific to LGBTQ families in North America is that of a family founded through a *mixed-orientation marriage.* A mixed-orientation marriage (MOM) is typically one in which one partner identifies as heterosexual of one sex (i.e., straight female) and the other partner is a homosexual or bisexual of the opposite sex (i.e., gay male). Early scientific study of MOMs estimated that 20% of gay men married women in their lifetimes (Janus & Janus, 1993). Such marriages often occur among social groups with more generally conservative social and/or religious viewpoints that forbid same-sex relationships (Hernandez, Schwenke, & Wilson, 2010; Legerski, Biggs, Greenhoot, & Sampilo, 2015). LGBTQ individuals desiring to remain part of the community and experience "family" may enter into heterosexual marriages in order to fully participate in this experience. It is unknown how many MOMs begin with disclosure of this identity on the part of the LGBTQ spouse; however, it should not be assumed that all persons in these families concealed their orientation identities from their spouses. With the advent of more socially affirming viewpoints about LGBTQ identities, the awareness of mixed-orientation marriages has increased and many families are living through significant and difficult transitions as the LGBTQ spouse and parent "comes out" and family structure, roles, and relationships begin to be renegotiated. It is estimated that 85% of MOMs end by the third year of the marriage and the larger portion of the remaining 15% end by the seventh year (Hernandez, Schwenke, & Wilson, 2010). Spouses and children in MOM families experience grief when this occurs.

Another type of family structure sometimes seen in the LGBTQ community would be considered "living apart together" (see Chapter 1). An example of this would be when a gay man is the sperm donor for a queer couple. The gay man does not live in the household but is clearly "family" as he is involved to various degrees in parenting and different roles in that family. Health care providers cannot make assumptions about who might comprise one's family of choice. Families are self-defined and experience loss, anxiety, and depression (Hernandez et al., 2010), for which nurses should assess and offer appropriate intervention or resources for each family member with a focus on nonjudgmental compassion.

Nurses can help families evaluate their strengths and develop resilience to cope with their challenges and transitions. One of the oldest organizations that provides support to the LGBTQ community is Parents and Friends of Lesbians and Gays (PFLAG), whose mission since 1973 has been support, education, and advocacy (PFLAG, 2017). Support groups for a straight spouse or partner whose partner is LGBTQ can also be found through the Straight Spouse Network (www.straightspouse.org/).

In the United States, in response to racial minority stress, family-of-choice structures that are a variation on the mixed-orientation family structure have emerged among the African American LGBTQ, urban communities. Known as "house" families or "gay" families, these family networks developed as a form of social support in response to the homophobia, transphobia, and racialized minority stress that youth and adults can often face across their communities. They are headed by gay men or transwomen (gay, bisexual, or trans [GBT]) who parent with or without a co-parent. Adolescent children, typically not biologically related, are often "somewhat younger gay men or transwomen, or at times sexual minority women and trans men" (Levitt et al., 2015, p. 175), who the parent invites to join the family. The family relationship may be formalized or remain informal. Family life often centers around artistic performance such as dance or beauty competitions where family members' performance can represent the spectrum of constructions of gender and sexuality including hypermasculinity or femininity. In these families, parents can help children meet developmental tasks; provide shelter for those who have been ostracized by their families of origin, religious, and residential communities; and facilitate the important social support that minoritized LGBTQ youth and adults need in order to develop the resilience to achieve good health and well-being (Levitt et al., 2015). Such family structures are one response to the racialized minority stress that LGBTQ families face. However, Beal, Villarosa, and Abner (1999), writing in the *Black Parenting Book*, note that gay African American parents in general have often negotiated stereotypes about their ability to parent. They suggest that gay parenting groups can support families to deal with "societal discrimination, family rejection, finding a place of religious worship, living in a safe and accepting community, and finding supportive child care" (p. 305).

For LGBTQ family members, being able to comfortably identify and share information with nurses and other health care providers, extended family, friends, and authority figures who are a part of their lives, such as teachers and coaches, is a step forward in feeling affirmed. Nurses can advocate for assessment forms and organizational policies that support processes that affirm as relevant key members of individuals' families and open space for dialogue about the meaning of such relationships.

Becoming familiar with parenting resources to support the diversity of family structures that are found across cultural communities and understanding the complex social dynamics that influence meaningful resources for LGBTQ families can be crucial tools for supporting LGBTQ family members across ages.

LGBTQ FAMILY HEALTH ACROSS THE LIFE SPAN

Nurses often are the first to encounter LGBTQ families as they seek health care. In this section the strengths, stressors, challenges, and health concerns are discussed across the life span specific to needs for LGBTQ families. Families are presented according to a developmental aspect from a couple coming together as a family, deciding to have children and parent, families with children and teens, mid-life adults, and older adult families. In each area health disparities are described so that nurses are aware of possible issues for LGBTQ families. Although there has been a rising call to "improve the health, safety and well-being of lesbian, gay, bisexual and transgender individuals" (*Healthy People 2020*, n.d., para. 1), research in this area is lagging. Health disparities in sexual and gender minorities occur across the life span; however, the cloud of shame and secrecy has receded in the current generation. Health disparities within the LGBTQ community have as much to do with societal bias and systemic factors as they do with health outcomes. Lack of access to care, lack of insurance coverage, delaying health care, a lack of health literary, negative experiences within the health care system, overt discrimination, and inadequate cultural competence among health care providers are just a few of the challenges routinely faced by sexual and gender minorities (IOM, 2011; Kates et al., 2016; Krehely, 2009a; Krehely, 2009b). Health disparities are often amplified at the intersection of multiple minority characteristics such as when people identify as LGBTQ and are also people of color, people living with disabilities, and those who are marginalized in other ways (e.g., immigrants or refugees) (Fredriksen-Goldsen, Kim, & Barkan, 2012; Krehely, 2009b; Lambda Legal, 2010). Social acceptance and changes in law and policy have begun to ease the way for compassionate and equitable care for all. Family nurses can assist in minimizing disparities among LGBTQ families by coordinating and delivering care in a way that will minimize feelings of prejudice and stigmatization that have been internalized and may, indeed, be expected by patients who have experienced marginalization by the health care system.

Behavioral and Mental Health

In general, members of the LGBTQ community are well adjusted and they do not report mental health problems (IOM, 2011). Nevertheless, research indicates that sexual and gender minorities carry a two and a half times greater risk of depression, anxiety, and substance abuse (Lick et al., 2013). Suicide rates have been noted to be higher within the LGBTQ community and suicide has been reported as a leading cause of death among LGBTQ youth. A majority of transgender individuals have experienced suicidal ideation (Herek & Garnets, 2007).

Social stigma and discrimination give rise to chronic stress that lends to the higher rates of mental illness in sexual and gender minorities (Herek & Garnets, 2007). Although the health care community and social institutions-at-large have come a long way, 25 years ago homosexuality was listed as a disorder in the *Diagnostic and Statistical Manual of Mental Disorders* (Spitzer, 1981), and transgender identity (i.e., gender dysphoria) still is listed as a disorder (5th ed.; *DSM-5*; American Psychiatric Association [APA], 2013). Although it should be noted that use of the term *gender dysphoria* is intended to characterize a set of symptoms and is not meant to pathologize the individual (Ford, 2012), the long-standing stigma associated with these diagnoses may become internalized as a type of self-stigma with deleterious consequences to mental health (IOM, 2011).

In 2010 the first national survey was conducted addressing barriers to health care and refusal of care among LGBTQ persons and those living with human immunodeficiency virus (HIV) (Lambda Legal, 2010). Results were tabulated based on a convenience sample of nearly 5000 respondents; more than half indicated that they had experienced at least one of several discriminatory practices (e.g., refusal of care, health care providers refusing to touch them, health care providers using harsh or abusive language, and health care providers blaming them for their health status or using physical roughness). The percentage increased to 63% for patients living with HIV and to 70% for transgender individuals.

Across all categories, rates of discrimination were higher for racial minorities and those who reported low income. These findings are among the most significant causes of health disparities among LGBTQ persons and families.

Childbearing and Childrearing Families

Social acceptance of LGBTQ families has increased enormously in the United States and Canada in the years surrounding the change of the millennium. Of the parents in same-sex relationships surveyed in 1995 across regions of Ontario for a groundbreaking report (1997) by the Coalition for Lesbian and Gay Rights in Ontario, 70% were "generally open about their sexual orientation [yet] . . . almost all had to hide the fact they were parenting with a same-sex partner" (p. 85). Contrast this with the current visibility of and positive stories profiled about LGBTQ families in entertainment and news media, school curricula, and health care settings. However, these more tolerant social dynamics vary with time and place, and social acceptance is uneven. For instance, Crouch et al. (2014), who studied gay- and lesbian-headed families in Australia, report that many families and children continue to face significant stigma, which is different from similar studies from the United States and the Netherlands. Research (Rickards, 2013) on experiences of lesbian-headed stepfamilies in the three eastern Canadian provinces of New Brunswick, Nova Scotia, and Prince Edward Island suggested that lesbian families made significant strides in becoming visible in these provinces, which are largely rural with some large cities. Yet, similar dynamics of stigma and parents' need to manage disclosure of their same-sex orientation in various settings were noted.

Heterosexism, homophobia, biphobia, and transphobia pervade all social institutions, including the family, with implications for LGBTQ families across the life span (IOM, 2011). For childbearing families, a critical gender and intersectional lens can help nurses understand the deeply rooted gender norms that have contributed to the domination of the nuclear family with implications, the dynamics of stigma, invisibility, and marginalization that have marked LGBTQ families and also to consider ways of conceptualizing modern families that are more inclusive.

Research on the Well-Being of Children in LGBTQ Families

Speculation regarding the well-being of children raised by same-sex parents has been surrounded by overwhelming fear and bias. The body of available literature indicates that health and developmental outcomes of children raised by same-sex parents are at least equivalent to those who grow up with heterosexual heads of household. This holds across numerous domains including cognitive development, social development, psychological health, substance abuse, early sexual activity, and academic performance (Manning, Fettro, & Lamidi, 2014). The only published longitudinal study to date found that the 17-year-old children of lesbian mothers ranked higher on academic performance and significantly lower on social problems and externalizing behavior such as rule-breaking and aggression (Gartrell & Bos, 2010).

In the mid-1980s sociological and psychological research with a focus on gender challenged the notion that the nuclear family was uniquely ideal for social functioning and explored what was behind the often accepted negative stereotypes and myths about same-sex families. This research focused mainly on lesbians as mothers. Stereotypes that portray lesbian mothers as deviant, potential child abusers, mentally unstable, and less maternal than heterosexual women have been disproven (Patterson, 1997), but such beliefs persist in social discourse. In addition, the myths that focus on the instability of lesbian relationships, an absent father figure, and inadequate time to parent as working mothers are considered standards that may be overlooked in males (Best Start Resource Centre, 2012; DiLapi, 1989).

In 1989, Elena DiLapi created a model, the *Lesbian Motherhood Hierarchy*, to illustrate and explain how society privileged certain types of mothering that aligned with a nuclear family model and marginalized other mothering, with lesbian motherhood deemed the most marginal of all. Using concepts identified by Adrienne Rich in 1980, DiLapi showed how assumptions of compulsory heterosexuality and compulsory motherhood shaped society's attitudes toward lesbian motherhood. Society exerts enormous social pressures for women to be both heterosexual and mothers in ways that maintain patriarchal dominant values, where the male reaps social privilege as the visible head of the household and father of the children. In DiLapi's (1989) model, mothers are categorized according to their family structures and sexual orientation and are legitimized by social institutions according to their fit with the heterosexual norms. Expectant lesbians who bear and raise children may be considered more valued—and perceive or receive more support—if they hide their lesbian identity because it stigmatizes them. Single mothers, by virtue of their assumed heterosexuality, are considered marginal mothers, but more valued than openly lesbian mothers (DiLapi, 1989). This has implications for both disclosure issues and lesbian co-parents in such relationships, since they are even less visible than the biological mother. Passing as a single heterosexual mother, while reaping limited societal acceptance, contributes to "inauthentic mothering" (Abbey & O'Reilly, 1998, p. 329).

As DiLapi (1989) explained, societal approval of motherhood status is reflected in how resources are allocated to different types of mothers, especially lesbian mothers. Resources can include information, informal and institutional support systems, policies and laws that legitimize partnership status, and visibility in mainstream media. She noted that approval is highest for those mothers who fit the traditional heterosexual nuclear family structure, despite the statistics that she cited at that time, which indicated that only 36% of families met the parameters of the nuclear family (DiLapi, 1989). She noted that lesbian mothers are denied these resources and this, along with formal and informal social policies that support negative or homophobic stereotypes, contributes to their invisibility and low social status.

Dunne (2000) noted that lesbians that became mothers through donor insemination were radically challenging the heterosexual norms. By assimilating a core reproductive function of the heterosexual family, lesbians through donor insemination challenged the monopoly on parenthood held by heterosexuals. For the participants in Dunne's study, parenting was a process that was researched, negotiated, and planned to meet the needs of the lesbian couple as well as the children conceived. The pregnancies were planned around available resources including income, maternity leave, and day care. Motherhood, completely separated from the biological function of fatherhood, allowed an egalitarian division of labor based on personal strengths and not gender-defined roles (Dunne, 2000).

Most research on same-sex families is about lesbian mothers (Crouch et al., 2014). In the 1990s gay fathers became more visible and research reflected the diversity of ways that they became parents, which includes surrogacy, heterosexual parenting, adoption, and sperm donors (Best Start Resource Centre, 2012; Golombok et al., 2014; Riggs & Due, 2014). Gay fathers are becoming more openly accepted in North American society and affirmed by such key professional bodies as the American Academy of Pediatrics, based on the most current high-quality research documenting that gay fathers raise children with positive outcomes. At times, gay fathers continue to face stigma and discrimination that is related to their sexual identity. Both fathers and their children can benefit from gay-positive environments and contact with other gay fathers and children raised in similar same-sex families (Golombok et al., 2014; Patterson, 2005). Nevertheless, gay fathers are challenging stereotypes of who can parent and raise children, including the "stereotype which posits that men do not desire to become parents with the same fervor as do women . . . more likely proportionately than heterosexual men to regard full-time, at-home parenting as their calling" (Meyer, 2012, p. 479). Some research suggests that gay fathers are more likely than heterosexual fathers to exhibit a more "feminine" parenting style with a strong emotional and relationship focus (Meyer, 2012). Golombok et al. (2014) cites Gates's estimate based on the 2010 American Community Survey that "7,100 adopted children are living with male couples" (p. 457). Golombok et al. note that, whereas in the United States intercountry and interracial adoption by same-sex parents are common, this is less common in the United Kingdom. American research suggests that "adoption agencies tend to place children from the most difficult backgrounds and with the most challenging behaviors with same sex parents" (Golombok et al., p. 457), which has implications for the challenges that gay families can face in raising children and research on outcomes for children in gay families. Although some new studies on gay fathering are building on some earlier studies during the last two decades, LGBTQ family research that accounts for the diversity of gay fathering is needed.

To further redefine the appropriate mother, as well as the gender roles of parenthood, Biblarz and Stacey (2010) examined heterosexual parents, lesbian parents, and gay parents and the effect of one parent versus two parents in the family. In this review, Biblarz and Stacey demonstrated that there was little effect by gender on the psychological adjustment or social status of the children, but there may have been some impact on the parent-child relationship. On outcomes from parental displays of affection to time spent playing with the children and many others, families with two mothers were more successful than heterosexual families, and single mothers outperformed single fathers. Children were more secure about attachments to parents in two-mother and single-mother households than in heterosexual households (Biblarz & Stacey, 2010).

Alternatives to the patriarchal family model have been proposed by Margrit Eichler (1997) with her description of three versions of the family as a reflection of societal values. Of the three—the patriarchal, individual, and social justice models—only the last validates same-sex couples in a way that approaches her vision of a minimally stratified society based on gender equality. She emphasizes that families defined by function, rather than structure, will be more inclusive of same-sex couples. Lesbian families in which spousal roles are blurred and economic and affective relationships are often nonhierarchical carry out tasks common to all families (Perlesz et al., 2010). These include providing "genuine love and caring, [offering] emotional support from each family member to each member, and meeting the diverse needs of family members (residential, social, economic, sexual, procreational, etc.)" (Eichler, 1997, p. 8). As she notes, social policies based on such notions will affirm these family partnerships through more equitable sharing of public resources.

Certainly, LGBTQ research confirms that social policies such as human rights legislation, same-sex marriage, and hate crimes research, as well as health care and professional practices that promote LGBTQ cultural competency, are integral to enhancing social awareness and acceptance of LGBTQ families and their well-being. Research with LGBTQ families about their effectiveness as families enhances the effectiveness of nontraditional families when people do what they do best and are not limited by gender normative roles. This research has mainly focused on lesbian parenting and to some extent gay parents. Much more research into diverse family structures is needed to continue informing nurses and other clinicians about how to best support these unique families.

As Ross and Dobinson (2013) indicate, the "B" for "bisexual" is almost invisible in LGBTQ family research, which has implications for health providers' knowledge and strategies to support them. Care

providers and sexual minority communities alike may assume that bisexuals do not encounter the same barriers as LGTQ because they reap heterosexual privilege. Although bisexual and queer parents may find LGBTQ data informational and social support useful, research about them suggests that bisexual parents may find that neither resources geared to opposite-sex parents nor those for same-sex families necessarily meet their particular needs. This may affect decisions to disclose to providers. If bisexual parents are in an opposite-sex relationship, their experiences of the school system or becoming pregnant may be quite different from in/visibly queer parents, for instance. However, further family research with diverse groups of bisexual parents is needed that specifically differentiates B from LGBQ (IOM, 2011; Ross & Dobinson, 2013). With an understanding that parents who self-identify as bisexual have unique concerns, nurses can create welcoming spaces that can foster disclosure and discussion, and learn about existing bisexual-specific parenting resources and advocate for resources and policies that support them.

Transgender (trans) parents, although sharing commonalities with sexual minority parents, face unique issues as they further challenge heteronormative parenting and assumptions about categories of gender and the role of biology in process (Downing, 2013). Although discrimination and a lack of understanding mark family experiences for many, there are also beneficial outcomes to trans families. They are summarized by Best Start Resource Centre (2012): "An increase in their parent's happiness and well-being, leading to better parenting and improved parent-child relationships. . . . Increased open-mindedness; an understanding of oppression; pride; stronger relationships with parents; knowing a whole and healthy parent" (p. 19). Nurses can advocate for trans-positive legislation and health care policies to more inclusive environments for all family members and thus enhance their well-being.

LGBTQ parents who are raising children are not necessarily recognized as equal parents. Prospective biological and adoptive parents and those who are already raising children may find that resources for families often assume that family members reflect a traditional nuclear family arrangement (i.e., are heterosexual) and are cisgendered. These assumptions often result in the invisibility of LGBTQ families in health services and care provision and marginalization or erasure of their needs. Although they have much in common with all families across the life span, there are also unique issues related to their LGBTQ identities.

Lack of social recognition and social legitimacy for LGBTQ family members in government and agency documents, for instance, has different implications for same-sex couples (lesbian, bisexual, gay) and families with transgender members. Birth certificates have a key role in one's sense of identity, yet given the diversity of contemporary family structures with co-parents, surrogate parents, and sperm donors, birth certificates often omit key information that reflects the diversity of current families. In their study of birth registration, Gerber and Lindner (2015) concluded that:

> a birth certificate is more than a reflection of biology; it is a document that establishes a relationship of rights and obligations between a parent (or parents) and a child, and plays a vital role in a person's sense of identity . . . other family structures that should be equally recognized and respected. (pp. 228–229)

There are certainly implications for LGBTQ families, given the fact that only 15 states and the District of Columbia currently recognize same-sex second-parent adoption in the United States. For same-sex couples, there may be no place for a co-parent to be named as the adoptive parent, for instance, where two lesbian mothers are co-parenting and one is the biological mother and the other is the co-mother. Sensitivity to the language used to describe the co-parent, co-mother, co-father, "other mother," and "other father" for gay couples is important. Biological mothers and co-parents may face challenges in being recognized by health care providers as well as by institutions such as health care insurance providers and other social agencies where identification forms do not necessarily allow for the co-parent to be named as a parent. Similarly, intake and assessment forms may offer options that reflect a traditional family configuration such as mother or father. Using language of "partner" or "spouse" can create openings in conversation for individuals to identify the importance of biological or co-parent, adoptive parent, and other significant parents such as gay men who, through their involvement as sperm donors or close friends, are part of the chosen family.

For instance, at times there may be dynamics in a lesbian couple in which the biological mother is recognized by family members or health providers as the primary parent and thus the "legitimate" mother. The co-parent may be left with the sense that she is not entitled to claim motherhood status (MacDonnell & Fern, 2014). Despite society's limited recognition of the lesbian biological mother, the power perceived to be inherent in the actual experiences of childbearing and breastfeeding may confer a higher status on the biological mother. The co-parent's freedom to claim a motherhood authority may be limited by these dynamics (MacDonnell, 2001a, p. 49). Such power dynamics can contribute to relationship tensions at a time when family dynamics are already in flux with the arrival of a child. However, this information is not widely discussed in family nursing texts or curriculum, yet it is relevant to nurses in any setting where they offer health teaching, counseling, or anticipatory guidance to LGBTQ women, partners, and their families-of-choice partners from the antenatal through the postnatal periods, as well as up to the preschool years when those women may be breastfeeding. Nurses can discuss and promote prenatal education that is inclusive of LGBTQ family issues, refer to LGBTQ-specific courses where they are available, and encourage peer-to-peer LGBTQ family group support (Best Start Resource Centre, 2012; MacDonnell, 2001a, 2001b).

In 2013 British Columbia, Canada, changed the law so that up to three parents—including a sperm donor—could be named on a birth certificate (Gerber & Lindner, 2015, pp. 271–272). Although birth certificates are one way that diverse family members are recognized and socially legitimized, identification and inclusion of the relevant family members on health care assessments and interactions in planning for the provision of care, including anticipatory guidance in parenting and treatment, are crucial to inclusive family nursing care.

Both birth certificates and other important government documentation used to legitimize one's identity often reflect binary options for gender, offer two options for declaring one's gender/identity (male, female), and are the sole options for declaring the current gender identity of the parents or children or to change this at a later date. In Canada, birth certificates fall under provincial jurisdiction and changes are underway in Ontario, Canada, to expand key identity documentation in a way that affirms multiple ways of expressing gender. Throughout the United States, legal recognition of gender and parenthood continues to lag behind the constructions and reconstructions of family that are expressed by the LGBTQ community. With the landmark decision of *Obergefell v. Hodges* in 2015, same-sex couples were granted marriage equality in the United States, yet laws that affect the dissolution of these marriages and custody of children, either biological or adopted, continue to appear on the court dockets (U.S. Supreme Court, 2015). As nurses, the impact of legal actions to create or dissolve the LGBTQ family is integral to the holistic nursing assessment of that family and its members.

Twenty-five years after DiLapi (1989), LGBTQ people can still encounter barriers to creating families. Facilities to support insemination/reproductive care have been traditionally geared to infertile (and assumed to be) heterosexual couples. This was reflected in the language of material including Internet resources describing their services. Providers lacked knowledge about what aspects of their environments were perceived as creating barriers to care but there is now greater awareness for many providers in the United States and Canada in this context and increasing understanding and willingness to learn about the spectrum of LGBTQ people who are creating families, including transgender fathers. There has been a proliferation of LGBTQ online and health resources in a range of cities in the United States and Canada to support LGBTQ people who are creating families in multiple configurations (Best Start Resource Centre, 2012; MacDonnell & Fern, 2014).

LGBTQ Families From a Developmental Perspective: Birth Through Adolescence

The increasing number of lesbian- and gay-parent families directly challenges the necessity of conventional (hetero) sexual relations for reproduction (Agigian, 2004). It is a vivid example of the socially constructed nature of families as there are multiple parenthood options (Goldberg, 2010).

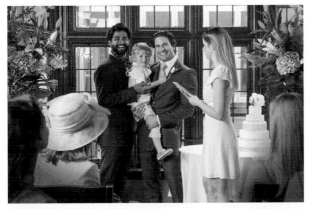

© iStock.com/SolStock

Once lesbian and gay men have made the decision to pursue parenthood, the decision then becomes how to become parents (Goldberg, 2010). These options may include sexual relations of a lesbian female with a male, surrogacy, alternative insemination, adoption, or foster care. Each one of these choices has a cascade of decisions that accompany the choice, similar to decisions heterosexual parents must determine in the path to parenthood. For example, for lesbians that elect alternative insemination, the question is which parent should carry the child (Goldberg, 2010). Another decision then is the donor type, such as acquaintance, friends, or anonymous. Then they have to decide the extent of involvement of the donor. These families must decide what to name and call each parent that communicates parental roles.

These children experience a life cycle stressor; their parents experience victimization and stigma, and must teach their children to handle homophobic encounters (Chabot & Ames, 2004; Lassiter, Dew, Newton, Hays, & Yarbrough, 2006). Lesbian and gay men families must negotiate parental roles that are usually dichotomized as mother and father (Dunne, 2000). In some cases, lesbian and gay men parents reported that they blend traditional mother and father roles to create new, hybrid degendered parenting roles (Gianino, 2008; Goldberg, 2010). An example of the struggle of understanding parenting roles in same-sex family is depicted in Box 7-4.

The preschool years are a time when rigid binary heterosexual and gender norms and related family structures and roles are explicitly and often implicitly reinforced through language, play, media, toys, and books that "invisibilize" the normativity of the nuclear family structure and relationships (Robinson, 2005). Even in the 21st century, despite the broader acceptance of gender diversity, a walk through many toy stores quickly illustrates how toys, books, videos, and video games continue to normalize stereotypical gender roles, with a preponderance of toys geared to active "boys," reflecting the dominant North American masculinity dominated by trucks and blocks. Books, games, and toys developed to encourage girls to pursue science and technology interests continue to be packaged and marketed using "feminine colors" and they are still often aligned with a white middle-class femininity that reflects a demure, more passive focus on crafts and dolls.

Nurses have roles in enhancing gender-positive and inclusive environments for children in the preschool years, whether they are informal play dates,

BOX 7-4

The Story of Mom and Mima

The following vignette illustrates some of the questions and experiences of the lived experience of LGBTQ parents. Based on true events, the names have been changed for confidentiality purposes.

It was January and pitch dark when 5:30 rolled around. The social worker had just called to say that they would be a little late. That gave us time to fidget, to plump pillows, and rearrange cookies on the plate on the kitchen counter. *Maybe we should have put out fruit instead.* We walked from room to room. The light in the family room was warm and the fire made it seem homey. There were fresh flowers on the kitchen table, clean towels in the powder room. Dining room, living room, hallway, staircase—arranged, put together, set. Upstairs, the bedrooms were magazine-ready; they were happy places, newly remodeled with 13-, 6-, and 4-year-old girls in mind.

Maya and I were confident that our house was ready, but even as we anticipated spending an evening with the three girls who would become our daughters, the hugeness of parenthood was unknowable. We had met the girls once and spent a few hours with them in the foster home where they had been living for a year. Now they were coming to our house to get the lay of the land and to see their new rooms; a sleep-over was scheduled for the weekend, and in 2 weeks they would move in.

Both in our mid-40s, we had waited a long time to become parents. We had thought a lot about the life we could give our children. We made plans that would turn out to be aspirational and fantasized futures that were not ours to design. Determined, idealistic, and hopeful, our optimism shielded us from the mountainous learning curve that stood before us. We had immersed ourselves in preparation, and during the next several weeks we negotiated a common last name, but we had not talked much about what the girls would call us. I guess I had assumed that it would be mom or mommy. I had never considered a nickname and I definitely did not want my children to call me Nichole. Maya had mentioned that she might like to be called "Mima." So there it was: we would be Mom and Mima.

For all our preparation, the knock on the door still startled us. They revealed their personalities as they inspected the house. The 4-year-old was entirely uninhibited. She ran from room to room, laying claim to a bed and to the teddy bear atop it. She approved. The 6-year-old was pensive. "Are you movie stars or something?" she asked as she silently measured our house against her experience. The 13-year-old was more reserved. She withheld emotion in the way that is implicitly prescribed by the adolescent code of cool. They ate cookies, asked a few questions, chatted, and laughed, vigilantly concealing any hint of trepidation.

When the social worker announced that it was time for them to go, the pensive 6-year-old slipped into her coat slowly. She looked around the family room, taking it all in. "I know!" she announced. *"I know!!"* She jumped up and down, obviously pleased with the fruit of her Eureka moment. She looked toward me, "I'll call *you* Mommy" and then, shifting her gaze toward Maya, "I'll call *you* Daddy!" The cool 13-year-old was the first to let go a swell of laughter and we all followed her lead.

At 6, our daughter's mind had not made space for a family with two moms. The imagery of childhood is full of possibilities, but *ideal* families are conceived as having a mommy and a daddy. Our daughter was trying to make all the puzzle pieces fit. Two weeks after that, we became Mom and Mima; 10 years later, we are still laughing at what became our first family joke. There are no rules for what children of sexual minorities call their parents. Today we appreciate it when people ask our children what they call us. It is uncomfortable when they are placed in the position of having to make corrections and, more uncomfortable still, if they feel they must acquiesce to someone's idea of what we ought to be called.

---

community activities, or day-care or co-op nursery school programs (Best Start Resource Centre, 2012). As in other environments, it is relevant to ensure the availability of posters, photos, and other online and print resources as well as teaching materials and activities that are inclusive of the diverse makeup of families that illustrate differences related to gender, race, ability, and structure, as well as language used in online and printed material. Enhancing preschool teachers' and caregivers' understanding and skills in fostering inclusive environments is important and can reduce stigma at times faced by LGBTQ families (Best Start Resource Centre, 2012). Recent research from Australia (Crouch et al., 2014) shows that the nontraditional gender roles demonstrated by same-sex families can have positive effects on the psychosocial health of children raised in these families. Reducing children's perceived stigma (i.e., providing welcoming and accepting environments) can enhance such healthy outcomes.

All publicly funded schools in Ontario use the newly revised *Health and Physical Education Curriculum* (Ontario Ministry of Education, 2015) for children in the early grades through middle school (grades 1 to 8), which introduces children to the diversity of LGBTQ families and incrementally addresses topics relevant to understanding sexual diversity and gender diversity in a context of promoting respectful, healthy relationships; health equity; and human rights. Teachers are made aware of how the social determinants of health, including oppression or discrimination, can affect health and well-being and create strategies to develop safe spaces for learning. Curriculum goals incorporate age-appropriate activities that offer opportunities to learn about gender-neutral language, teaching resources such as templates for developing family trees, videos that are LGBTQ-inclusive, and discussions of depictions of LGBTQ in the media. These are values and skills that help develop their knowledge, confidence, and sense of competence in educational success as well as develop healthy peer relationships and allow them to learn to negotiate interpersonal conflicts.

As Rickards (2013) indicates, in LGBTQ families, everyday interactions always have the potential for being judgmental, discriminatory, marginalizing, or unwelcoming. The ongoing negotiation of interactions and scanning of environments for positive acceptance, along with internalized homophobia from prevailing heteronormative institutions, can have impacts on parents, children, and extended family members (Rickards, 2013). All activities for school-aged children that are LGBTQ-affirming, from school to sports to religious and family activities, have the potential to reduce stigma and marginalization associated with homophobia, biphobia, and transphobia, and can enhance the well-being of family members including children (Best Start Resource Centre, 2012).

LGBTQ family support is not without protest from communities and organizations who decry this departure from more traditional family values. Being able to connect with allies and LGBTQ social and community supports can be integral at such times and also offer opportunities for respectful dialogue and advocacy. A recent example (Dougas, 2016) was a parent protest of a gender-nonconforming child who attended the Boy Scouts. There are implications for nurses who have examined their attitudes and values with respect to how incidents such as this influence their knowledge and practice and how they can use their privilege as nurses to take leadership and participate in creating safe and supportive health care environments and communities that are affirming of diverse LGBTQ families.

For several decades, research on and with sexual minority adolescents has been high on the radar in relation to LGBTQ family health with the development of youth-related programs and services; more recently, transgender youth have had role models and access to health-related programs and services, including online information and support (IOM, 2011; Peterkin & Risdon, 2003; Schneider, 1997). Adolescence, a time when youth are establishing their identities and negotiating peer and family relationships along the road to adulthood, can bring many challenges for parents and teens themselves. In the United States and Canada, given the high profile of LGBTQ issues in the media and greater social acceptance, LGBTQ people often come out earlier than they did in the past. For LGBTQ youth, this often happens during adolescence; many youth are now self-identifying as genderqueer or along a gender spectrum (Travers, 2015). According to a recent Canadian study by Bauer and Scheim (2015), "80% [of trans people] knew that their gender identity did not match their body . . . by the age of 14. Gender identity is often clear years before people socially transition to live in their core gender" (p. 2). It is clear that teens need safe spaces to support their coming out processes wherever they live, work, or play.

Family, peer, and community acceptance and support have been shown to be key to LGBTQ adolescents' experience of disclosure and negotiation of their LGBTQ identities across ethnicity, geographic location, and other social locations (IOM, 2011). Heterosexism may have more negative impacts for adolescents than younger children with implications for peer and community acceptance (Rickards, 2013). Family and school environments that convey nonjudgmental support for LGBTQ teens along with anti-bullying initiatives can be crucial to their mental health, as can finding LGBTQ-identified role models such as teachers and counselors who can provide needed support (Travers, 2015). Family conflict for LGBTQ youth can be a factor in their alienation from their families of origin, with significant numbers of LGBTQ youth involved in foster care, being homeless, couch-surfing, or living on the street (Nelson, 2015; Schneider, 1997).

Since 1999, the United States has taken leadership through the Gay, Lesbian, & Straight Education Network (GLSEN) to collect data on high school climates and publish biannual reports on the way that LGBTQ youth experience their schools. In Canada, a report on the first such study through an advocacy organization, Equality for Gays and Lesbians Everywhere (EGALE), was released in 2016. EGALE is comparable to GLSEN as a national advocacy organization that focuses on schools. Although it is clear that much progress has been made to alleviate overt homophobia and create more inclusive environments in schools and beyond, these surveys clearly show that high schools continue to be sites of homophobia, biphobia, and transphobia, along with racism and other oppressive dynamics that contribute to hostile environments for LGBTQ youth (IOM, 2011; Kosciw, Greytak, Giga, Villenas, & Danischewski, 2016; Taylor & Peter, 2011).

However, there is also some evidence that Gay Straight Alliances (GSA) and school supports make a difference in terms of mental health and educational outcomes. GSA (GSANetwork, 2017), which first developed in 1998 in San Francisco to provide peer support for LGBTQ-identified youth and allies in the school setting, is now found worldwide in high schools as well as some middle schools. Initiatives such as creating gender-neutral bathrooms and awareness that respecting genderqueer youth's preferred pronouns are strategies that are part of creating safe spaces in schools and are important for nurses to understand in the context of providing LGBTQ-affirming care for youth. Awareness of LGBTQ-youth-focused support organizations such as Supporting Our Youth (SOY), along with knowledge about the range of ways that youth may express their gender and sexuality (and whether or not they claim a same-sex or transgender identity), are also important in terms of creating spaces for youth and their peers. These supportive organizations help the families of origin/chosen families to find affirming health care organizations and communities that can support a sense of belonging for diverse groups of LGBTQ families with adolescents.

Health Challenges and Disparities in LGBTQ Children and Adolescents

Childhood and adolescence is a time of complex physical, mental, and emotional change. All children face a range of challenges that occur within the context of growing up. Although developmental milestones in LGBTQ youth follow the same trajectory as that of their heterosexual peers, higher rates of social stigma, homelessness, abuse, and discrimination pose threats to wellness and add to the risk of certain health problems including depression and suicidal ideation (Mustanski, Garofalo, & Emerson, 2010). Given the relative health of children and adolescents, and the rigor imposed by institutional review boards when considering studies of minors, the lack of research in this area is not surprising (IOM, 2011). Empirical investigation has also been affected by the scientific community's evolving understanding on the emergence of sexual identity and on the finding that sexual orientation and gender identity may be somewhat fluid during childhood (Kates et al., 2016). Recent research suggests that the highest rate of identification as LGBTQ among any age group occurs in high school students (Kahn et al., 2015).

In general, LGBTQ youth report being well-adjusted, but it is notable that they present a higher risk for depression, suicidal ideation, and suicide (Mustanski, Garofalo, & Emerson, 2010). LGBTQ youth have higher rates of smoking and substance abuse than heterosexual youth (Kates et al., 2016). Limited research indicates that lesbian and bisexual girls become sexually active at about the same rate as their heterosexual peers, but suggests that pregnancy rates may be somewhat higher among lesbian and bisexual girls (IOM, 2011). Gay and bisexual boys are more likely to report being sexually active than their heterosexual counterparts. In addition, they are more likely to report having been responsible for a pregnancy (Saewyc, Bearinger, Blum, & Resnick, 1999). All youth, regardless of sex, gender, or orientation, stand in need of access to high-quality, accurate information about sexually transmitted infections (STIs). Although some nurses may find it more professional to ask questions about sexual history using scientifically correct terms for anatomy and sexual practices, this may not be appropriate when interviewing an adolescent. Use of the guidelines published by the Centers for Disease Control and Prevention, the 5 **P**s for taking a sexual history will ensure an accurate and nonjudgmental approach. These include questions about **P**artners, **P**ractices, **P**ast history of STI, **P**rotection, and **P**regnancy Prevention/Reproductive Life Plan (National Coalition for Sexual Health, 2016).

In terms of families, LGBTQ youth experience significantly higher rates of being runaways, homelessness, substance use and abuse, high-risk sexual behavior, vulnerability to sex trafficking, school bullying and violence, depression, and suicide risk, especially in cases where they are rejected by their families (Russell, Ryan, Toomey, Diaz, & Sanchez, 2011; Ryan, Huebner, Diaz, & Sanchez, 2009; Wilber, Ryan, & Marksemer, 2006). A program of research led by Dr. Caitlin Ryan and her San Francisco State University-based Family Acceptance Project has produced important empirical evidence to help clinicians like nurses engage and support families with LGBTQ youth to prevent family rejection and thus improve the child and family outcomes. The program focuses on the impact of early intervention to maximize the positivity related to family acceptance (Box 7-5).

BOX 7-5

Evidence-Based Practice: The Family Acceptance Project™

Dr. Caitlin Ryan, PhD, ACSW, and colleagues at San Francisco State University (2010 to the present) used primary research strategies to engage LGBT youth and families as a means to better understand the risk factors related to mental and behavioral health risks. Through in-depth engagement with their diverse participants in a wide variety of urban and rural settings across the state of California, Dr. Ryan's team was able to better understand that LGBT youth are particularly vulnerable to family abandonment or expulsion from their homes and, as such, had much higher risks for depression, suicide, homelessness, overall deficits in well-being, substance use and abuse, poor sexual health, and HIV infection. Using their research findings, they developed several resources and initiatives to promote better outcomes for LGBT youth and their families. According to their Web site:

The project was designed to:

1. Study parents', families' and caregivers' reactions and adjustment to an adolescent's coming out and LGBT identity.
2. Develop training and assessment materials for health, mental health, and school-based providers, child welfare, juvenile justice, family service workers, clergy and religious leaders on working with LGBT children, youth and families.
3. Develop resources to strengthen families to support LGBT children and adolescents.

4. Develop a new model of family-related care to prevent health and mental health risks, keep families together and promote well-being for LGBT children and adolescents.

Findings are being used to inform policy and practice and to change the way that systems of care address the needs of LGBT children and adolescents.

From their robust program of research and clinical practice applications, the team produced an international, multiple-award-winning film detailing one typical Christian religious family's journey to accept their gay son, "Families Are Forever." In addition to their educational and advocacy work, the team created a host of tools for screening at-risk families, developed and provided educational and clinical intervention materials and practices to help families understand the critical importance of accepting their LGBT children, and consulted with other institutions including those who create public policies. Nurses who serve youth and families in schools, parishes, primary pediatric settings, and public health and community health settings should become familiar with the work of Dr. Ryan and the Family Acceptance Project™ and use the family tools and research knowledge generated to ensure reductions in risk to this vulnerable population.

Sources and Further Learning:

Always My Son. (video). http://www.familyacceptanceproject.org

Families Are Forever. (video). http://www.familyacceptanceproject.org

Family Acceptance Project. (2017). *Family acceptance project website.* San Francisco State University, CA. Retrieved from https://familyproject.sfsu.edu/overview

Ryan, C., Huebner, D., Diaz, R., & Sanchez, J. (2009). Family rejection as a predictor of negative outcomes in white and Latino lesbian, gay and bisexual young adults. *Pediatrics, 123*(1), 47–52. doi:10.1542/peds.2007-3524

Ryan, C., Russell, S. T., Huebner, D., Diaz, R., & Sanchez, J. (2010). Family acceptance in adolescence and the health of LGBT young adults. *Journal of Child and Adolescent Psychiatric Nursing, 23*(4), 205–213. doi:10.1111/j.1744-6171.2010.00246.x

Substance Abuse and Mental Health Services Administration. (2014). *A practitioner's resource guide: Helping families to support their LGBT children.* HHS Publication No. PEP14-LGBTKIDS. Rockville, MD. Retrieved from https://store.samhsa.gov/shin/content/PEP14 -LGBTKIDS/PEP14-LGBTKIDS.pdf

Positive family processes are influenced, in part, by the quantity and quality of communication between parents and children (World Family Map, 2015). For example, it has been well documented that academic achievement and certain markers of psychological well-being (e.g., substance abuse, depression, and suicide) are positively correlated with the frequency of family meals (Eisenberg, Olson, Neumark-Sztainer, Story, & Bearinger, 2004). Depending upon family culture, resilience, and the ability of the family to cope with real or perceived change, there may be more or less stress on the group as a unit when a LGBTQ youth comes out. This is an opportunity for nurses to provide reassurance, support, guidance, and direction and to inform family members of the challenges to health such stressors may evoke.

Health Challenges and Disparities in Early and Middle Adulthood

On balance, sexual and gender minorities face the same health concerns found in the population at large. There are, however, notable disparities in several specific domains (IOM, 2011) for members of the LGBTQ community, who report poorer overall well-being than those in the mainstream population. They report a higher number of acute physical symptoms and chronic conditions and indicate, at a higher rate than their heterosexual peers, that their health precludes them from participating in everyday physical activities (IOM, 2011).

In a comprehensive review of physical health disparities, Lick et al. (2013) found that compared with heterosexuals, individuals who identify as lesbian, gay, or bisexual exhibit a higher prevalence and earlier onset of disabilities (e.g., use of a cane), a greater risk of cardiovascular disease, and higher rates of asthma, allergies, osteoarthritis, migraines, and chronic gastrointestinal problems. Members of the LGBTQ community have a higher risk for and diagnosis of some cancers, with lower rates of survival reported for gay men. Lesbian, gay, and bisexual persons are 2.5 times more likely to have a mental health disorder than those in the heterosexual population (Cochran, Sullivan, & Mays, 2003) and have higher rates of tobacco, alcohol, and drug use (IOM, 2011). Higher rates of disease, especially with later-stage diagnoses, has been hypothesized to be linked to a lack of access to preventative care (Krehely, 2009a).

Patterns of risk and relative wellness differ by sex. Fewer lesbians and bisexual women report excellent or very good health when compared with heterosexual women, whereas there is no difference in health status reporting by sexual orientation among men (IOM, 2011). Lesbians are more likely to be overweight or obese (Boehmer, Bowen, & Bauer, 2007). They are less likely to have regular mammograms or Papanicolaou tests (Pap smear) screening for cancer (Lick et al., 2013). Gay men are more fit and maintain healthier weights than their heterosexual counterparts (Brennan, Ross, Dobinson, Veldhuizen, & Steele, 2010). Gay and bisexual men account for more than half of those living with HIV or AIDS; they are at an increased risk for anal cancer and some STIs (e.g., syphilis) (IOM, 2011) (Box 7-6). Similarly, a small body of research suggests that transgender women may be at a greater risk for STIs. This is perhaps owing to the increased likelihood of multiple sex partners (mainly men), casual sexual encounters, and sex while intoxicated (Herbst et al., 2008). HIV occurs in about 28% of transgender women and it is reported that most are unaware they are infected (Kates et al., 2016).

It is important to note that very little methodologically sound research has been conducted on physical health status and health disparities among transgender individuals. To date, the primary focus of research has been on the effects and side effects of hormone therapy. This research provides some evidence that transgender women are at a greater risk of venous thromboembolic disease and elevated levels of prolactin associated with feminizing hormone therapy (Weinand & Safer, 2015).

Transgender men may experience elevations in liver enzymes, loss of bone mineral density, and increased risk for ovarian cancer associated with masculinizing hormone therapy (IOM, 2011). Additionally, the Committee on Health Care for Underserved Women (2011) reported that more than half of those who identify as transgender have obtained injected hormones outside of a traditional medical setting. Overwhelmingly, the lack of access to health care insurance for transgender care and associated health issues stands as the largest barrier (Krehely, 2009a). In relation to sexual health, LGBTQ persons face similar health care and education as the rest of the population. STI prevention is a high priority, as well as pregnancy risks for those who

BOX 7-6

Pap Smears for Men?

Human papillomavirus (HPV) has been associated with the development of cancer in several common sites in the human body, most frequently in the cervix in females and oropharynx in men. HPV is the most common STI; the vast majority of adults will, at some point, contract HPV, although in most cases the body's own immune system will clear the virus within 2 years.

According to the Centers for Disease Control and Prevention, HPV is thought to be responsible for approximately 39,000 new cases of cancer among women and men in the United States per year. It is routine preventative practice for women to undergo cervical screening for abnormal cell growth that may indicate cancer, although these methods do not detect cancerous growth in the vagina, vulva, or in other reproductive organs. What is not as commonly known is that men are also at risk for HPV-associated cancers, regardless of their sexual orientation. Risk factors for HPV infection include sexual activity with a person actively infected, lack of condom use, anal sex, and oral sex. HPV is thought to be responsible for 90% of anal cancers, 70% of oropharyngeal cancers, and 60% of penile cancers. Those most at risk are HIV-positive gay or bisexual men or HIV-positive men who have sex with men (MSM), who may not identify as gay or bisexual. Since HPV-associated cellular changes can be detected with the Papanicolau (Pap) smear, men with these risk factors should be screened using this technique. HIV-positive MSM should be screened every 2 years using an anal Pap smear and those who are HIV-positive should be screened every 3 years.

Nurses caring for a MSM should ask the patient the following question: "Have you had an anal Pap smear in the last 2 to 3 years?" Although many men may sound surprised, this approach opens an important conversation about HPV-associated cancers. Nurses may provide the necessary education with these men and their partners including the risk factors, detection strategies (such as HPV blood testing and the use of the anal Pap screenings), risk reduction strategies such as the use of condoms, HPV vaccines, and also what signs and symptoms related to anal cancers they should be aware of, such as the appearance of lesions in or around the anus. Assessment and patient education could result in a reduction of risk related to HPV-associated cancers.

Early detection of cancer is paramount to preventing cancer-related deaths. As more gay and bisexual men are creating families that include children, the impact of lower cancer-related deaths in the population will have the direct effect of keeping these families from the loss of a parent and spouse or partner.

Sources and Further Learning:

Centers for Disease Control and Prevention. (2015). *HPV and men: CDC fact sheet.* Washington, DC. Retrieved from https://www.cdc.gov/std/hpv/stdfact-hpv-and-men.htm

Centers for Disease Control and Prevention. (2016). HPV-associated cancer statistics. Washington, DC. Retrieved from https://www.cdc.gov/cancer/hpv/statistics/index.htm

Lindsey, K., DeCristofaro, C., & James, J. (2009). Anal Pap smears: Should we be doing them? *Journal of the American Academy of Nurse Practitioners, 21*(8), 437–443.

possess female reproductive organs (regardless of their gender identity and sexual orientation) and typical screenings for reproductive cancers regardless of sex or gender identity.

Health Challenges and Disparities in Late Adulthood

There are at least 3 million persons aged 55 and older who identify as LGBTQ. That number is expected to double within the next 20 years (Espinoza, 2014). As is the case for earlier phases of development, the health concerns of LGBTQ adults are not distinct from those of heterosexuals and available research is minimal. It appears that lesbians and bisexual women in this age cohort have slightly higher rates of breast cancer than heterosexual women.

HIV remains a significant risk factor, particularly for men and transgender women. In 2015 17% of new HIV diagnoses were in individuals older than age 50 (AIDS.gov, 2016). This is a particularly salient finding for family nurses as most HIV prevention campaigns are not directed toward older adults (IOM, 2011). Older LGBTQ people living with HIV are another such group, which is especially relevant to aging men and transgender women, who have unique needs (IOM, 2011). With antiretroviral therapy, HIV-positive individuals are living longer. Seventy percent of those living with HIV are 40 or older, and since this is anticipated to increase significantly in the coming decade this issue will continue to be relevant to aging populations (IOM, 2011). Worldwide, about 20% of trans people are living with HIV; this number increases to 27% for transgender women who are sex workers (Poteat et al., 2015). Although LGBTQ people comprise a subgroup of older HIV-positive individuals, a small Canadian qualitative study of persons living with HIV who are age 50 and living in Quebec (Wallach & Brotman, 2012) identified concerns that include employment and living conditions, premature aging, shrinking social networks, and challenges to maintaining intergenerational relationships or finding acceptance in older peer networks. Disclosure to family, peers, and providers that results in nonaffirming responses can exacerbate experiences of stigma, social isolation, and mental health issues (Daley, MacDonnell, & St. Pierre, 2016a; Daley et al., 2017).

Many LGBTQ adults believe that their status as sexual and gender minorities helped them to prepare for older age. Although they are twice as likely as their heterosexual peers to be single and living alone, they report having developed greater resilience and better support networks. More than 75% report that they rely on close friends for social and emotional support (MetLife Mature Market Institute, 2010).

Access to, and utilization of, health care for older LGBTQ adults is particularly troubling. A large percentage (40%) report that they have not disclosed their sexual orientation to their primary care provider (Espinoza, 2014). They fear that they will not be treated fairly or will be denied care. In fact, 65% of transgender adults fear that they will have limited access to adequate health care as they get older (Espinoza, 2014). Additionally, prior or present discrimination among chronically ill LGBTQ older adults is positively correlated with an increase in physical and emotional symptoms for them and for their caregivers (IOM, 2011). This highlights the need for nurses to consider even unrelated caregivers within the context of LGBTQ family care.

A groundbreaking and award-winning American documentary released in 2011, *Gen Silent* (Maddox, 2011), pointed to the importance of understanding the particular concerns, including isolation, stigma, and discrimination, that are part of the lives of six older single and partnered LGBTQ people and caregivers. In that film, the lives of an older gay couple, a single trans woman, and an older lesbian couple are profiled in light of their health and social care needs, including their chosen families and the need for LGBTQ-affirmative community. A key focus of that movie highlighted the resilience and resistance in LGBTQ communities. As Espinoza (2011) indicates, although LGBTQ older adults have often experienced years of invisibility and discrimination, they have also been witnesses to LGBTQ activism during their lifetime and have seen incredible movement in social acceptance and policy development for LGBTQ people in the United States, Canada, and many countries. Individual LGBTQ people and allies across diverse communities and geographic areas are spearheading health policy change at the federal level for LGBTQ people through collectives such as the Diverse Elders Coalition (Espinoza, 2011) in the United States, which includes communities of Southeast Asians, Hispanics, Native Americans, and Asian Pacific people. Similarly, in Canada, Rainbow Health Ontario (Travers, 2015) and seniors-specific networks such as the Senior Pride Network (n.d.) in Toronto, along with nursing and other health provider networks, have been active in advocating for program and policy change to support LGBTQ older people locally and provincially.

Although LGBTQ-specific supports, including social groups for older people or welcoming LGBTQ seniors groups, are now becoming available to some extent in large cities in North America, the vast majority of social or health supports for older people assume that older people are heterosexual and cisgendered. Even though LGBTQ people are diverse with respect to age, culture, ethnicity, and language, organizations and providers who create seniors-focused programs and services geared to specific language or cultural groups are unlikely to have considered the relevance of LGBTQ diversity in the communities they serve. Seniors-focused services, whether they are faith-based or provided through other social agencies, must consider that their diverse communities across ethnicity and language include lesbians, gay men, bisexuals, and trans people (Brotman et al., 2007; Daley et al., 2017). Increasingly, LGBTQ seniors-focused social and recreational networks are emerging in the United States and Canada, and such resources for older people are becoming aware of the value of undertaking needs assessments and policy change to create welcoming environments and relevant programs to meet the needs of the often hidden LGBTQ groups they serve (National Hispanic Council of Aging, 2013; Services and Advocacy for GLBT Elders and National Center for Transgender Equality, 2012; Teng, 2015).

As health issues surface for older people that require them to engage with health and social services, seniors-focused programs, or condition-specific programming, they may be more likely to use home care services and may be anticipating the need for some sort of congregate care such as assisted living or long-term care for themselves or their partners. Most older LGBTQ people have established care providers and, to varying extents, support networks and prefer to age in place, even if safety is relative. To move to another place entails coming out again and learning the perils of that new environment. However, with few exceptions, LGBTQ people are invisible in long-term care, residential, and congregate facilities, and it is with trepidation that most LGBTQ people plan for the possibility of institutional care (Daley et al., 2017). Fear and anxiety mark thoughts of planning for long-term care for many older LGBTQ people, a life transition that is often difficult for many individuals and families in any context (Stein, Beckerman, & Sherman, 2010). Health care providers, families, and others providing support in planning for long-term care may not be aware of the individuals' LGBTQ identities. LGBTQ people worry that because care providers may lack knowledge or understanding about older LGBTQ people they will neglect them, express overt disapproval or more subtle hostility, and that this may result in being neglected, excluded, or ridiculed (Teng, 2015). Since few long-term care or residential facilities are openly LGBTQ-positive in terms of the material provided to prospective patients and families, and assessment forms are unlikely to have categories to ask about sexual orientation or gender identity, older LGBTQ folks—even those who have been open in many aspects of their lives—may go back into the closet (Daley et al., 2017). McIntyre and McDonald (2012) described environments that LGBTQ people face in residential and long-term care institutional facilities where "the place of home as the private domain is replaced with an 'intimate public space' rife with heteronormative assumptions" (p. 132). In addition, sexuality is often assumed to be irrelevant to older people, and sexual orientation and gender identity may be assumed to be narrowly associated with one's sexuality, rather than relevant to the holistic health and well-being of LGBTQ people. Health care providers; staff, including volunteers; families; and other residents often lack knowledge and understanding about LGBTQ people and are unaware of the needs of LGBTQ-identified older people and the importance of being able to create an environment that reflects their personal priorities, as well as one that can include partners and visible markers of LGBTQ community. Given such dynamics in residential care facilities where individuals may be increasingly dependent on care providers for physical, social, and spiritual support in relation to complex personal care needs, palliative care, and dementia care, the importance of LGBTQ-affirming providers and organizations cannot be underestimated (Finkenauer et al., 2012; IOM, 2011; McGovern, 2014; Teng, 2015). Although currently no LGBTQ-specific long-term care facilities are available in Canada, advocacy initiatives are underway to develop these in the future (Teng, 2015).

Recent Canadian research on LGBTQ home care in Ontario, Canada, showed that home care providers were unlikely to have received training in the home care environment explicitly on LGBTQ-focused health issues and that the curriculum in their professional programs lacked LGBTQ-focused content, with the result that providers and patients identified concerning gaps in LGBTQ-affirming home care. However, when care providers and home care agencies were made aware of the specific health issues that are important to LGBTQ people, they were often receptive to making policy changes and promoting service provider education to enhance the LGBTQ-affirmative environments (Daley et al., 2016a). LGBTQ communities stress that building health care provider and organizational LGBTQ cultural competence is essential. LGBTQ-identified individuals are otherwise bearing the burden of constantly teaching providers about LGBTQ health issues and affirming environments, adding to the everyday minority stress that affects their lives (IOM, 2011).

Aging, Older Adults, and LGBTQ Families

LGBTQ seniors comprise anywhere from 2 to 7 million of the U.S. population and more than 335,000 Canadians (Fredriksen-Goldsen, 2011;

Lim & Bernstein, 2012). However, older LGBTQ families have often been invisible in communities of older people as well as to the health and social service providers, the policy and decision makers whose focus is to enhance the health and well-being of older populations. It is estimated that the older LGBTQ population, age 50+, will double between 2000 and 2030 in the United States as the population as a whole ages (Fredriksen-Goldsen, 2011). Similar to other subgroups of LGBTQ populations, there is very limited health and health service research on older LGBTQ people and their families, but it is needed to inform responsive and relevant health and social care. Nurses and interdisciplinary health care providers will interact with older LGBTQ people and their families in all health care settings, from primary care to long-term care.

Most older LGBTQ people dwell in the community and, similar to other older people, many hope to age in place, often having established a level of comfort and familiarity in what they call "home." Several factors shape the aging experience for LGBTQ people. First, the historical context of LGBTQ people in society is relevant. Because they have grown up in eras where sexual orientation was considered a pathology and same-sex sexual activities were criminalized, older LGBTQ people, especially older than 75 years old, are unlikely to be "out," whereas those who are somewhat younger may be more likely to disclose their sexual orientation, although many still remain in the closet in some aspect of their lives. For many, there is an ongoing need to manage disclosure because they fear discrimination or victimization (Fredriksen-Goldsen, 2011). Secondly, since they grew up at a time when traditional family structures prevailed and same-sex marriage was not an option, they are less likely to have a spouse or children and thus face isolation. Older trans people are particularly invisible (Daley et al., 2017; Fredriksen-Goldsen, 2011).

Older LGBTQ people are diverse in many ways, including ethnicity, language, and socioeconomic status, although as the IOM (2011) has indicated, research is very limited in this regard. Ageism is a reality in our social worlds, and for LGBTQ people, sexuality and gender interact with other social dynamics such as racism to affect the availability of social support, housing, and experiences of stigma that diverse groups of older LGBTQ people may face (IOM, 2011). Thus, although older LGBTQ people are often seeking care for chronic diseases such as cancer, diabetes, and heart disease, they may also be dealing with social determinants such as discrimination, housing, and social support, which influence the possibility of achieving good mental well-being (IOM, 2011; Kertzner, Barber, & Schwartz, 2011). In contrast with the general population in which older women are more likely to live alone, older gay and bisexual men, more than older lesbian or bisexual women, are more likely to live alone with implications for their mental and emotional well-being (Fredriksen-Goldsen, 2011). Older women in general often face financial vulnerability and older lesbian women, who worked at a time when employment for women was less likely to provide them with pensions and benefits, may face particular financial challenges (Daley et al., 2017). Similarly, older adults of color, many of whom have often faced poverty or who have been and continue to have precarious work in low-income sectors, live with economic insecurity, which can affect their access to health care as well as their health outcomes (Espinoza, 2011). The experiences of aging for ethnic and racial LGBTQ minorities, such as African Americans, Two-Spirit First Nation and Native Americans, or Aboriginal trans people seeking housing or health care, can reflect multiple dynamics of discrimination based on race, sexuality, and gender (Brotman & Ryan, 2004; IOM, 2011). A recent needs assessment (National Hispanic Council on Aging, 2013) completed with older LGBTQ Hispanic individuals across the United States identified employment dynamics, housing discrimination, and social isolation as relevant to their income security and their mental health and ability to thrive independently and in community.

Older transgender people, either those who transitioned years before or the increasing number who are transitioning in their older years, often face health care systems and networks for older people that are not prepared to meet their needs. Concerns about being able to access meaningful care from a health care provider who is nonjudgmental and knowledgeable about trans-specific clinical care, networks, and resources for social support and other strategies that can enhance their mental health and well-being is crucial for trans people to thrive as they age. This can be particularly important since trans people can be disenfranchised on many levels, such as being alienated from families of origin including their children and grandchildren (Finkenauer, Sherratt, Marlow, & Brodey, 2012).

Family Caregiving for Older Adults

There are virtually no empirical reports on disability within the LGBTQ community, although loss of independence with aging or illness is a concern for sexual and gender minorities just as it is for members of the heterosexual community (IOM, 2011). Many older LGBTQ people are themselves caregivers for partners, friends, and family of all ages (Brotman et al., 2007).

Twenty percent of LGBTQ persons between 40 and 61 report that they do not know who would take care of them if they became ill or disabled; this number increases to more than one-third for those who do not have a partner or a spouse (MetLife Mature Market Institute, 2010). LGBTQ individuals are three to four times less likely to have children than heterosexuals (Espinoza, 2014). Indeed, among those who serve as caregivers, more heterosexual individuals report caring for family members (65%) when compared with their LGBTQ counterparts (53%). This underscores the importance of close relationships with friends and families of choice and should be noted by nurses who are involved in planning or coordinating in-home care or who are communicating with care providers. The use of genograms and ecomaps are useful to home care nurses to develop the client story and visualize the resources and challenges of LGBTQ families (see case study in this chapter and Chapter 5 for further explanation).

It is important for nurses and other health care providers to understand that the structure of caregiving appears to be different within sexual and gender minority populations. For example, half of LGBTQ caregivers are men, whereas 75% of heterosexual caregivers are women (Institute on Aging, n.d.). Gay men also report spending more time in caregiving tasks. They spend an average of 41 hours per week; their lesbian counterparts spend 26 (MetLife Mature Market Institute, 2010). The sensitivity of nurses to what may seem to be small or insubstantial differences in caregiving goes a long way in reducing perceived bias for patients, thereby making experiences of care more satisfying. An effective means of empowering LGBTQ caregivers is the completion of advance directives, including medical proxy or power of attorney forms to clearly delineate each family member's role, especially in states where there are no other forms of legal protection or acknowledgment of family relations and responsibilities.

Certainly, beginning with the need to support HIV-positive members of the LGBTQ community when no services existed, LGBTQ communities often developed circles of care to offer the health care and personal support that individuals required (Brotman et al., 2007; Maddox, 2011; Sinding, 1999). LGBTQ older adults have distinct networks of support from peers, who are often older themselves. Yet, as Fredriksen-Goldsen (2011) has noted, "Despite the fact that their support systems differ and they often lack legal protection for their loved ones, an alarming 30 percent do not have a will and 36 percent do not have a durable power of attorney for healthcare" (p. 6). As indicated in a recent Canadian study, given barriers to home care services, families, friends, and communities are often relegated to provide postsurgical support for trans people, for instance (Daley, MacDonnell, & St. Pierre, 2016a).

In Canada, health care providers and LGBTQ communities have collaborated to create tools for interdisciplinary service providers. In 2008, the City of Toronto collaborated with LGBTQ seniors and care facilities to develop the LGBT Long Term Tool Kit (City of Toronto, 2008), which offers health care providers and organizations a systematic approach to creating positive space in long-term care facilities. In a home care context, researchers created two tools for provider organizations based on Ontario-wide research (Daley et al., 2017) with home care providers and LGBTQ home care users. The LGBTQ Access and Equity Framework (Daley, MacDonnell, & St. Pierre, 2016a) is a user-friendly tool that offers home care organizations a way to systematically and comprehensively assess their organizations and strategies to work toward providing LGBTQ-affirmative care. These tools both emphasize the need for engaging leadership across the organization and for developing partnerships with LGBTQ communities in meaningful ways in order to develop and evaluate programs that serve sexual and gender minorities by building LGBTQ community capacity.

A second resource, *Queering Home Care* (Daley, MacDonnell, & St. Pierre, 2016b), is a one-page tool created when home care findings were mapped onto an existing home care patient values statement. To support the development of welcoming health care environments for LGBTQ people, each section of the original patient values statement was revised to illustrate the unique concerns of LGBTQ people in order to align with high-quality care. Sections included a focus on high-quality care, partnering in decision making, being respected in the health care encounter, and having the necessary information. For instance, in the following section on Being Respected, the italicized phrases were added in the *Queering Home Care* version:

To receive care that respects cultural, ethnic, spiritual, linguistic and regional preferences . . . having your home including chosen art work and photos and partner(s) and friends respected and having your chosen language including pronouns for yourself and your chosen supports respected. (p. 1)

Strategies to move LGBTQ family care forward in a context of aging include:

- Building nurses' knowledge and understanding of LGBTQ health issues for diverse groups of older people and LGBTQ histories of oppression and resilience
- Building LGBTQ-affirming cultural competency that includes the use of affirmative language; opportunities to examine attitudes and values including how ageism and racism intersect with heterosexism, biphobia, and transphobia; and holistic clinical assessments that take a strengths-based approach to high-quality care
- Engaging with LGBTQ communities in needs assessments to support responsive LGBTQ-focused programs and services, as well as LGBTQ-affirmative programs and services to serve broader populations
- Developing LGBTQ-aging-focused curriculum in nursing education and training opportunities such as professional orientations and in-services in long-term care facilities
- Advocating for LGBTQ-affirmative policies and programs in health and social care and broader communities

To assist the reader with the process of integrating and applying nursing knowledge to the care of LGBTQ families, the following case study about the Boyle family is presented.

Case Study: Boyle Family

An Older Woman in Transition:

Robin Boyle was raised as a biological female who, at the age of 48, began exploring gender identity and the process of transitioning to a transgender man. During this time, Robin challenged many traditional notions of family to support *their* (Robin's chosen pronoun) care during the transition process. Nurses providing care to families with transgender members must first identify the pronouns preferred by the transgender members by simply asking. Often, transgender people will identify and introduce themselves as John (he, him, his) or Chris (they, them, their) when in social situations.

Today, Robin Boyle (they, them, their) is a 53-year-old Asian transgender man. Robin was raised in a closely knit family in a rural area of Texas. Robin's parents came to the United States as refugees at the end of the Vietnam War and came to live in Texas through a sponsorship by the Southern Baptist Church. Robin was the younger of the family's two daughters. At age 22, Robin married a heterosexual African American man, David, and had two children through this marriage; a son named Jonathan and a daughter, Alexandra. Robin and David were high school sweethearts while growing up in Texas and moved to Southern California after they married to escape the conservative beliefs back home. They believed that Southern California would allow their children to live a life filled with diversity and support for their mixed race family. For the first 10 years of this marriage, Robin was a stay-at-home mother and was very active in their children's lives. Robin and David were active members of the United Church of Christ in their hometown because of its open and affirming doctrine. They participated in numerous rallies throughout California to show their support for same-sex marriage for their fellow church members. As Robin became more active in the LGBT community, they became close friends with Tony, a transgender man who was very open with Robin about his struggles in transition. During the next few years, Robin began counseling with a social worker that had several clients in the LGBTQ community and had been recommended by Tony as someone that Robin could trust. Robin began to reflect on the many different experiences of childhood and youth, and began envisioning life without the fear and repression that had been routine in Texas. At the age of 48, Robin began exploring their gender identity and sought support from their primary health care providers for hormones in the process of transitioning.

At the time of the transition, Robin's daughter Alexandra, now 24, was pregnant with her first child. She was overwhelmed by her mother's announcement of her transition and struggled to know how to explain things to her in-laws. Alexandra, during

Case Study: Boyle Family *(cont.)*

an argument with Robin, told them that this was an attempt to refocus attention away from what should be Robin's support for Alexandra's pregnancy. Alexandra was angry and stated: "I wanted my mother to be with me during my delivery, not some man I don't know!" Robin is a trained *doula* and had planned to provide direct support during Alexandra's delivery but now feels unwelcome. Alexandra's husband, Chris, has been very supportive of Robin's transition as many of his classmates from Stanford self-identified as members of the LGBTQ community, including his best friend. Chris believes Robin should be Alexandra's doula, leading to friction and conflict in their relationship.

Robin's son Jonathan, now 26, is pursuing his Master's in Nursing to become a family nurse practitioner and has been very supportive of his parent's transition but continues to use "Mom" when talking about Robin. He was fortunate enough to have several classes in his primary care course that focused on issues of LGBTQ health but never expected to have to apply this information to his own family. Jonathan has been living at home with his 2-year-old son Iggy since the death of his partner during childbirth. Robin has been helping Jonathan to raise their grandchild, providing day care while Jonathan is at school. Robin, Jonathan, and Iggy have been living with David in a three-bedroom home. When gender transition began, Robin moved into Alexandra's empty bedroom as David did not identify as being gay and felt this is what he would have to be to remain intimate with Robin. Robin and David had individual and joint sessions with Robin's counselor for the past year. Although these sessions helped them to live together amicably, David felt strongly that their relationship cannot continue through Robin's transition and filed for a divorce. Robin had insurance through David's company but will not be covered once the divorce is finalized. Currently, testosterone injections are covered by David's insurance; after the divorce, however, Robin will need to apply for Medicaid because of their limited income (see the Boyle family genogram and ecomap in Figures 7-1 and 7-2, respectively).

Robin's friend Tony has helped with resources about Medi-Cal and the process that must be completed to receive coverage for testosterone injections and gender-affirming surgery. Medi-Cal will cover the hormones and surgery but coverage is decided on a case-by-case basis, and there is no guarantee that Robin's medical needs will be covered. Robin needs to file a Treatment Authorization Request (TAR), explaining why their hormones and surgery are medically necessary. It can take several months for this application to be considered; if denied, the appeal will entail legal expenses and further time. When Medi-Cal expanded its Medicaid coverage with the Patient Protection and Affordable Care Act, many more services for the transgender population became available. Robin is concerned that with the new political environment this access will be lost. Like many of their friends in the LGBTQ community, Robin considered moving to Ontario, Canada, where there is access to universal health care that covers all physician and hospital services except elective surgery. If Robin moves to Canada, the concern becomes that they

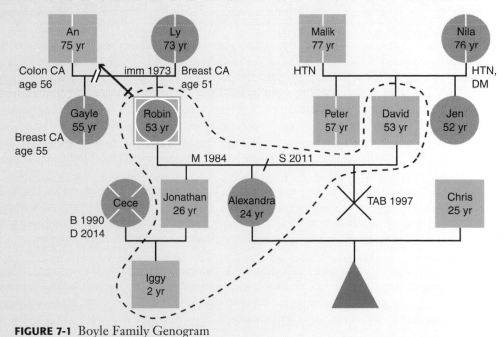

FIGURE 7-1 Boyle Family Genogram

(continued)

Case Study: Boyle Family *(cont.)*

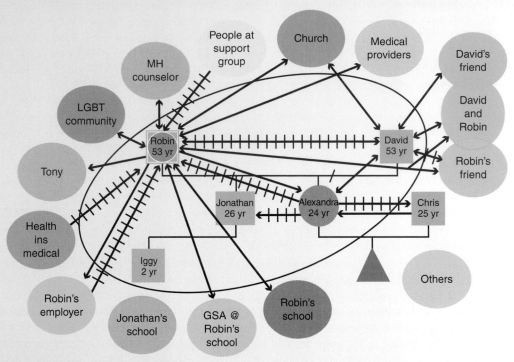

FIGURE 7-2 Boyle Family Ecomap

will no longer be able to have a nurse practitioner as their primary care provider as testosterone is considered a controlled substance that must be prescribed by a physician. In addition, Robin will need to get support from their providers to show that this surgery is medically necessary.

Robin has decided to have top surgery only—that is, a double mastectomy—and has begun the process of applying for Medi-Cal. Unfortunately, as long as Robin is living with David, David's income is considered a part of the household income and they are over the limit by $1000 monthly for Robin to qualify for assistance. David's insurance company stated they will terminate Robin's coverage as soon as the divorce is final no matter the living arrangements. Robin estimates they will be uninsured for at least 6 months before qualifying for state assistance. Robin wanted to arrange for as much of the transition as possible to happen during summer vacation from school as they had arranged a transfer to a new school where fewer explanations would need to be made about Ms. Boyle becoming Mr. Boyle. Robin knows faculty are not exempt from bullying, teasing, and transphobic remarks from students and others at high school. Fortunately, there is a gender-neutral bathroom available at the new high school and the administration has encouraged its use. At the current place of employment, all the bathrooms are labeled for faculty/staff or students with male or female. Robin has continued to use the women's restroom but feels increasingly out of place.

Robin's church and its members remain very supportive during the transition but there are a few friends who have begun to take sides as they learned of the impending divorce between Robin and David. Some of these friends expressed concern for the confusion that Iggy may feel, which Robin sees as a projection of how these friends are feeling. Iggy used to call Robin "Nana," but recently has switched to "Bobin"; overall, Iggy just seems content to have his favorite playmate around the house baking cookies.

Robin has begun taking testosterone during the last 2 years. Since undergoing the transition and beginning testosterone, Robin has been growing more body hair, their voice deepened, and their relationship with their female body parts has become strained. Robin has been using binders since beginning the transition to minimize their large breasts but developed an ongoing problem with candidiasis, often with chafed, raw, intertriginous areas that sometimes have a foul odor. The daily routine

Case Study: Boyle Family *(cont.)*

of binding their breasts, the fear of an embarrassing odor, and the pain lead to Robin's decision for a double mastectomy. Robin's primary care provider scheduled a mammogram, but Robin has been cancelling and rescheduling these appointments. Robin hoped the mastectomy would eliminate the need for mammograms but recently learned this will not be the case. Although the procedure will reduce the risk by 90% to 95%, Robin carries the *BRCA1* gene and will need ongoing surveillance (Domchek et al., 2010). Robin is beginning to understand the psychological term *gender dysphoria* in a very personal sense. Although Robin has been using this diagnosis as they were preparing the TAR, it was not until these body changes that Robin felt any unease with transitioning. Robin knows this transition is essential to their psychological well-being to become the man they have known to be inside but deciding how much surgery to have or not based on financial concerns has worn Robin down. Robin had no Pap smear in more than 10 years, with the last one being slightly abnormal. Even with a strong family history of colon cancer, Robin was trying to avoid a colonoscopy. The thought of going to an outpatient procedure center, filling out the registration forms with male identification, and then having to answer questions from the nurses and doctors before and after the procedure explaining the transition was overwhelming for Robin. With Robin's insurance situation in limbo, limited income, and family demands, these routine health maintenance procedures seemed low priority.

Robin began mourning the loss of the relationship with David and feels isolated. While at the transgender support group, a woman began to show an interest in Robin but the advances were deftly deflected. Robin has been reading a lot online, chatting with others, and is considering living an asexual lifestyle. Robin learned over time that intimacy does not need to include sex and does not feel safe to explore their sexuality until the transition is complete.

Questions to consider as the nurse provides care to this family:

- What are your own biases that may affect the way you provide care for Robin?
- What are the stressors and barriers for this family?
- What are the strengths and facilitators for this family?
- What practices and nursing interventions would you prioritize in caring for this family were you to be caring for Robin as a nurse on an inpatient surgical unit at the time of double mastectomy?
- What practices and nursing interventions would you prioritize for this family if you were caring for Robin in a primary care setting when doing an intake and history to establish care?
- How would you find resources for LGBTQ families in your community?
- How would you, as Robin's nurse, either in the United States or Canada, be able to act as an advocate for transgender health rights affecting the experience of this family?

SUMMARY

Nurses provide direct care to LGBTQ families in a variety of health care and community settings. In order to be most effective providing care that meets the specific needs and concerns of LGBTQ families across the life span, nurses must:

- Begin with the close examination of their own belief systems and biases.
- Apply an attitude of openness and develop an appropriate vocabulary, consulting with the families they care for from the position of learner.
- Recognize that LGBTQ families are at increased risk for several health and health-related problems that range from physical and psychological illnesses to social, political, and health care access barriers.
- Provide direct, compassionate, and competent care to the LGBTQ family population by engaging in and developing practice to meet the specific needs of the community.

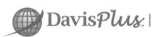 **DavisPlus** | For additional resources and information, visit **http://davisplus.fadavis.com**. References can be found on Davis*Plus*.

Chapter 8

Genomics and Family Nursing Across the Life Span

Marcia Van Riper, PhD, RN, FAAN

Louise Fleming, PhD, RN

Critical Concepts

- Advances in genomics and technology have dramatically altered the landscape of health care by providing the tools needed to determine the hereditary component of many diseases and conditions, as well as to improve our ability to predict susceptibility to genetic conditions, onset and progression of genetic conditions, and responses to medications.

- Genomics refers to the study of all genes in the entire genome, whereas genetics refers to the study of a particular gene.

- Genomic medicine (also called genomic health care) is an emerging discipline that involves using genomic information about an individual as part of that person's clinical care and the health outcomes and political implications of that clinical use.

- Biological members of a family may share the risk for disease because of genetic factors.

- Families respond to genetic discoveries in their own unique way; even within the same family, members react differently.

- When a genetic risk is identified in a family, the two major nursing responsibilities are to help family members understand that the genetic risk is present and to make sure decisions about testing, management, and surveillance are well-informed decisions that fit with individual and family beliefs, desires, values, and circumstances.

- Results of genetic tests are considered to be private and thus should not be disclosed to other family members without the tested individual's consent.

- Nurses play a critical role in helping individuals and families with concerns about genetic and genomic health risks find accurate information and access resources.

- All nurses, regardless of their areas of practice, need to be able to apply an understanding of the effects of genetic risk factors when conducting assessments, planning, and evaluating nursing interventions; ideally, a family perspective should be used.

Some illnesses "run in families" and people commonly wonder if they, or their children, will develop a disease or condition that is present in their parents or grandparents. This is especially true now that stories about advances in genomics and the experience of living with genetic conditions appear in the popular media on a regular basis (Angier, 2017; Lappe, 2016). Nurses are likely to be among the first health care providers that individuals and families go to with questions about genomics and health because nurses are typically viewed as trusted health care providers with a long history of providing holistic family-focused care (Daack-Hirsch et al., 2013; Van Riper, 2016). Moreover, they have traditionally shown expertise in bridging gaps among health care providers, individuals, families, and communities (Lee, Gill, Barr, Yun, & Kim, 2017). Therefore, the ability to apply an understanding of genetics and genomics in the clinical setting needs to be a priority for all nurses. This helps to ensure that individuals and families that might benefit from genetic services receive appropriate education and referral (Boyd, Alt-White, Anderson, Schaa, & Kasper, 2017).

During the past two decades, there has been growing recognition throughout the world that genomic knowledge and skills need to be incorporated into nursing education and training. Because of this, there have been ongoing efforts to provide genomic education and resources to nursing faculty (Calzone et al., 2011; Jenkins et al., 2015; Kirk, Tonkin, & Skirton, 2014; Lee et al., 2017; Tonkin, Calzone, Jenkins, Lea, & Prows, 2011; Van Riper, 2011). In addition, in some countries, there have been national efforts to require basic competencies in genetics and genomics for all nurses (Boyd et al., 2017; Kirk, Calzone, Arimori, & Tonkin, 2011; Kirk et al., 2014). For example, in the United States, an independent panel of nurse leaders from clinical, research, and academic settings developed a set of guidelines called the *Essential Nursing Competencies and Curricula Guidelines for Genetics and Genomics.* These guidelines were originally endorsed in 2009 and updated in 2011 by nearly 50 organizations in the United States (Greco, Tinley, & Seibert, 2011). All nurses need to have minimal competencies in genetics and genomics regardless of their academic preparation, practice setting, or specialty (Van Riper, 2016). Nurses in all areas of practice are expected to participate in genetic risk assessment, play a pivotal role in explaining genetic risk and genetic testing to patients and families, and support informed health decisions and opportunities for early intervention (Lee et al., 2017). Essential genetic and genomic competencies for nurses with graduate degrees were developed by a consensus panel in 2011 and published shortly thereafter (Greco, Tinley, & Siebert, 2011). These advanced competencies are based on the assumption that nurses with graduate degrees will have already achieved the core essential competencies.

Genetic conditions are often described as "family diseases or conditions" and genetic testing is often considered to be a family experience (Van Riper, 2006). However, much of what is known about the experience of being tested for or living with genetic conditions has focused on the individual. Relatively few researchers have used a family perspective to illuminate the meaning of living as a family in the midst of a chronic condition (Arestedt, Benzein, & Persson, 2015).

It is important for nurses to be aware of the effect of genetics and genomics on families because biological family members share genetic risk factors. In addition, families function as systems with shared health risks that affect the whole family, and family processes mediate how individual family members and the family as a whole respond to these health risks. Family members inevitably have an effect on each other's lives, and in many cases they support each other in seeking and maintaining healthy growth and development, regardless of their biological kinship. All nurses, regardless of their areas of practice, must be able to apply an understanding of the effects of genetic risk factors when conducting assessments, planning, and evaluating nursing interventions; ideally, a family perspective should be used (Van Riper, 2011).

This chapter describes nursing responsibilities for families of persons who have, or are at risk for having, genetic conditions. These responsibilities are described for nurses working with individuals and families across the life span. Genetic conditions are lifelong, so families living with genetic conditions need ongoing care and support (Kirk & Marshallsay, 2013). The goal of the chapter is to describe the relevance of genetic information within families when there is a question about genetic aspects of health or disease for members of the family. Family nursing knowledge is incomplete without an understanding of how families influence and are influenced by the way in which individual family members adapt to the experience of being tested for or living with a genetic condition.

GENETICS AND GENOMICS

Advances in genomics and technology have dramatically altered the landscape of health care and nursing practice by providing the tools needed to determine the hereditary component of many diseases and conditions, as well as to improve our ability to predict susceptibility to genetic conditions, onset and progression of genetic conditions, and responses to medications (Calzone et al., 2013; Green & Guyer, 2011; McCarthy, McLeod, & Ginsburg, 2013). *Genomics* refers to the study of all the genes in the entire genome, whereas *genetics* refers to the study of a particular gene (National Human Genome Institute, 2016). Genomic medicine (also known as genomic health care) "is an emerging discipline that involves using genomic information about an individual as part of their clinical care and the health outcomes and political implications of that clinical use" (National Human Genome Institute, 2016, p. 1).

The human genome consists of approximately 3 billion bases of DNA sequence and more than 99% of these bases are the same in all individuals (National Institutes of Health, 2017), making individuals more genetically similar than different. Individuals inherit genetic material from their parents and pass it on to their children. Some conditions result from a change or mutation in a DNA sequence of a gene. A *gene* is defined as the basic physical and functional unit of heredity (National Institutes of Health, 2017). For example, Huntington's disease results from a specific change within the DNA sequence in a particular gene. This is an example of a condition traditionally referred to as a Mendelian or single-gene disorder and is one that follows an identified pattern of traditional inheritance in families, in this case, autosomal dominant inheritance. Persons who are biologically related may have inherited many of the same DNA sequences in addition to having shared common environments with other family members; this combination ultimately increases risks for having similar specific illnesses.

Researchers also identify common genetic variations known as single-nucleotide polymorphisms. These variations may not cause an actual disruption in the DNA coding but can often be used as tools that help scientists and clinicians recognize DNA variations that may be associated with disease. These conditions include common disorders, such as diabetes, that are observed to occur more frequently in families but do not follow a traditional pattern of inheritance.

A core competency for nurses is to maintain knowledge of the relationships of genetic and genomic factors to the health of individuals and their families. Cancer provides an example of the relationships between genes, environment, and health. The development of a malignant tumor is the result of a complex series of changes at the cellular level. Several genes protect against cancer by regulating cell division (during mitosis); mutations in those genes can occur during the course of a person's lifetime, affecting one's predisposition to cancer. A person may be at increased risk of developing cancer if an inherited mutation occurs in one of those genes or if he or she is exposed to environmental factors that influence genetic mutations. For example, tumor suppressor genes help protect against the development of breast cancer. If a woman inherits a mutation in a tumor suppressor gene (such as the *BRCA1* gene), she has lost some of her protection against breast cancer from birth, but she will not necessarily develop cancer unless other cellular changes (some of which are influenced by factors such as her reproductive history) occur during her lifetime (Bougie & Weberpals, 2011). Others in her family also may have inherited the same mutation and are similarly at risk. If she subsequently becomes a smoker, she has an additional increased risk for lung cancer because of the environmental influence of smoking on cell division in her lungs. In families where smoking is the norm, there may be a perceived "familial" condition because of the shared environmental and genetic influences on several members of the family. Box 8-1 lists inherited and multifactor inherited genetic conditions.

GENETIC TESTING

Types of Genetic Testing

Genetic testing can be performed for several purposes, including prenatal diagnosis, diagnosis of a genetic condition in a newborn, detection of carrier status,

BOX 8-1

BOX 8-1
Examples of Inherited and Multifactor Inherited Genetic Conditions

Inherited Genetic Conditions	Multifactor Conditions—Combination of Genetics and Environment
■ Huntington's disease ■ Cystic fibrosis ■ Sickle cell anemia ■ Familial hypercholesterolemia ■ Congenital adrenal hyperplasia	■ Heart disease ■ Diabetes ■ Most cancers ■ Alzheimer's disease ■ Neural tube defects

confirmation of a genetic diagnosis, predictive testing for familial disorders, and presymptomatic testing. See Table 8-1 for types of genetic tests. In addition, the National Human Genome Research Institute (2015) has a Web page (http://www .genome.gov/19516567) with answers to frequently asked questions about genetic testing plus links to a list of other sites offering information about genetic testing. Prenatal testing is offered during pregnancy to help identify fetuses that have certain genetic conditions. The most common conditions tested for prenatally are neural tube defects (NTDs), Down syndrome, trisomy 13, and trisomy 18. Carrier testing can tell people if they have (carry) a gene alteration for a particular kind of inherited disorder called an autosomal recessive genetic disorder, such as cystic fibrosis, sickle cell anemia, or congenital adrenal hyperplasia (CAH). Predictive testing can identify individuals who have a higher chance of getting a disease before the symptoms appear. Predictive testing is available for inherited genetic risk factors that make it more likely for someone to develop certain cancers, such as colon or breast cancer. Presymptomatic genetic testing can indicate which family members are at risk for a certain genetic condition that is already known to be present in their family. This type of testing is performed for people who have not yet shown symptoms of a disease, such as Huntington's disease (National Human Genome Research Institute, 2015).

In an effort to bridge the transition from the development of a genetic test to diagnostics and treatment, the National Institutes of Health launched the Genetic Testing Registry (GTR), a free online tool that can be used to obtain a comprehensive list of available genetic tests (www.ncbi.nlm.nih.gov/ gtr/). The GTR Web site includes links to a variety of clinical resources such as *GeneReviews*, MedGen,

Online Mendelian Inheritance in Man (OMIM), and Orphanet, as well as links to consumer resources including Genetics Home Reference (National Institutes of Health, 2012). *GeneReviews* is a collection of peer-reviewed, expert-authored descriptions of genetic conditions presented in a standardized format. The reviews provide clinically relevant and medically actionable information regarding diagnosis, management, and genetic counseling (Van Riper, 2016). MedGen is a Web site where you can search for specific genetic conditions, related genes, and clinical features. It also includes practice guidelines. OMIM is an online catalog of human genes and genetic disorders. Orphanet is a portal for rare diseases and orphan drugs. As far as the consumer resources, they provide consumer-friendly information about genetic conditions and links to support organizations.

The National Comprehensive Cancer Network (2017) continually updates guidelines that specify what kind of screening is indicated for a person who has a gene mutation that increases the chances of

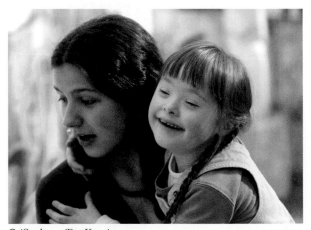

© *iStock.com/DenKuvaiev*

Table 8-1	Types of Genetic Tests
Diagnostic	Performed when signs and/or symptoms of a genetic condition are present. Confirms whether or not an individual has the suspected condition.
Carrier	Detects whether a person is a carrier of either an autosomal recessive or an X-linked disorder.
	A carrier of an autosomal recessive condition usually has no signs of the condition and will be at risk for having an affected child if the other parent is also a carrier. He has one normal copy of the gene in question and one mutated copy.
	A female carrier of an X-linked condition has one normal copy of the gene on the X chromosome and one mutated copy of the gene on the other X chromosome, and generally has no signs or very mild signs of the condition. Her sons have a 50% chance of having the condition, and her daughters have a 50% chance of being carriers.
Predictive or presymptomatic	Performed on healthy individuals; detects whether they inherited a mutation in a gene and, therefore, whether they will or may develop a condition in the future.
Prenatal diagnosis	Genetic test performed on the fetus. Indicates whether the fetus has inherited the gene mutation that causes a specific condition and, therefore, whether the child will develop that condition.
Pharmacogenetic (PGx) testing	Analyzes a person's genes to understand how drugs may move through the body and be broken down. The purpose of PGx testing is to help select drug treatments that are best suited for each person.
Direct-to-consumer (DTC) genetic testing	DTC genetic tests are marketed directly to the general public, usually via the Internet. DTC genetic testing provides access to an individual's genetic information, usually without involving a health care provider.

cancer developing. For example, family members may seek testing if they are at greater risk for familial colon cancer. In some cases, clinical practice guideline criteria recommend that genetic testing be done to determine whether a person is at risk.

Another type of genetic testing that is rapidly being integrated into clinical practice is pharmacogenetic (PGx) testing (Haga & Mills, 2015). PGx testing is performed to examine an individual's genes to determine how medications are absorbed, move through the body, and are metabolized by the body. The purpose of PGx testing is to allow health care providers to create tailored individualized drug treatments that are specific to each person. For example, before starting a patient on warfarin (one of the most commonly prescribed drugs in the United States and many other countries), PGx testing can be done to figure out what starting dose would work best for the patient. Adjusting the dose based on the patient's genotype can help avoid toxicity and improve efficiency (McCarthy et al., 2013).

Certain gene mutations can affect how an individual's body metabolizes some medications. For instance, patients can be tested to see if they are ultrarapid metabolizers (1% to 10% of population),

extensive metabolizers (majority of the population), intermediate metabolizers, or poor metabolizers. Ultrarapid metabolizers may need a higher dose of a medication because they metabolize drugs so quickly that they may never reach a therapeutic concentration. Intermediate and poor metabolizers may require a lower-than-normal dose.

As of 2015, the Food and Drug Administration (FDA) included pharmacogenomics information on the labels of more than 150 medications (National Institute of General Medical Sciences, 2015). Herceptin (trastuzumab) is an example of a drug for which obligatory genetic testing has been developed (McCarthy et al., 2013). The purpose of this obligatory testing is to identify a subset of women with breast cancer who overexpress HER2/neu, because these women are likely to be the only patients with breast cancer who will benefit from taking Herceptin (http://www .herceptin.com/). Nurses need to understand PGx testing so they can provide comprehensive care, especially at the time of discharge (Haga & Mills, 2015). Nurses who have a good understanding of PGx testing can play a critical role in making sure that drug doses are optimized and drug reactions are avoided (Cheek, Bashore, & Brazeau, 2015).

Direct-to-Consumer Genetic Testing

Traditionally, the only way a person could undergo genetic testing was to go through health care providers such as physicians, nurse practitioners, and genetic specialists. However, it is now possible to undergo genetic testing in one's home. Direct-to-consumer (DTC) genetic testing is a type of genetic testing that is marketed directly to consumers via television, the Internet, or print media (National Institutes of Health, 2017). Once the genetic test is ordered by the consumer, a test kit is mailed directly to the person's home. The test kit typically includes instructions for how the DNA sample is to be collected (often by swabbing the inside of the cheek) and a return envelope. Consumers are notified of their results either by mail or by phone, or the results are posted online. With some DTC companies, a genetic specialist or other health care provider is available to discuss the results by phone.

There are several companies offering DTC testing, with one of the most well-known being 23andMe. In 2013, the FDA sent the CEO of 23andMe a cease and desist order because they had determined that 23andMe was marketing a 23andMe Saliva Collection Kit and personal genome service without marketing clearance or approval; because of this, they were in violation of the Federal Food, Drug and Cosmetic Act. The company, 23andMe, responded by shifting their focus more toward ancestry testing. Currently, 23andMe offers consumers two options: (1) ancestry testing or (2) health + ancestry service. According to their Web site (https://www.23andme.com/), if a person orders the health + ancestry service he or she receives 65+ online reports on his or her ancestry, traits, and health.

It is important for nurses to be aware of DTC genetic testing so that they can advise their patients who are interested in DTC to meet with a health care provider or a genetic specialist to learn more about this type of testing and its accuracy and applicability to health care. Furthermore, nurses and other health care providers should be aware of the reliability (or unreliability) of DTC genetic testing. The main concern with DTC genetic testing is that without guidance from a health care provider or genetic specialist, the individual may make significant decisions about prevention or a particular treatment that is based on incomplete or inaccurate information (National Human Genome Research Institute, 2016; National Institutes of Health,

2012). There have been studies that demonstrated that DTC testing is not always done in a uniform manner, which leads to results that are unreliable and inaccurate (Kutz, 2010; Webborn et al., 2015). There have also been reports indicating that if an individual submits his or her DNA sample to multiple companies, the results may be contradictory. For example, one DTC company might say the person is at increased risk for developing prostate cancer, whereas another DTC company says the person is at moderate risk and a third DTC company says the person is at low risk. Obviously these results would be difficult for even a genetic specialist to interpret.

Potential Advantages and Disadvantages of Genetic Testing

Nurses should understand the differences in the types of genetic tests that families may consider and the potential advantages and disadvantages of genetic testing summarized in Box 8-2. Nurses who participate in discussions about genetic testing must maintain current knowledge on these tests, as well as on new technology for testing and interpretations of results.

Genetic tests have limitations that vary according to the specific test. For some tests, not all persons who want the test may qualify, which occurs when their family history does not suggest that the disease has a major genetic component, or where the genetic mutation that causes the disease has not been identified. For some tests, it is possible that a result may be difficult to interpret. For some conditions, genetic mutations have been discovered that are associated with the disease in that family. Because many genes may be associated with one condition, or several different mutations may be possible in a gene, it is often necessary to test an affected family member first to try to identify which gene is involved and which type of mutation is causing the condition in that family. A sample is taken from the affected person to determine whether a genetic mutation can be identified that is associated with that condition. This may not be possible if the affected person in the family has passed away or if the affected person refuses to undergo the genetic testing to help other family members.

Another limitation of genetic testing is that the results may not be definitive. This is especially true

BOX 8-2

Potential Advantages and Disadvantages of Genetic Testing

Potential advantages of testing include:

- Opportunity to learn whether one has an increased likelihood of developing an inherited disease; in those who prefer certainty, this can help resolve feelings of discomfort, even if the result shows the person has inherited the condition
- Relief from worry about future health risks for a specific disease if the test is negative
- Information that can be used for making reproductive decisions
- Information to inform lifestyle choices (e.g., food choices, smoking, alcohol use, contraceptive choice)
- Information to guide clinical surveillance or management of the condition
- Information for other family members about their own status

- Confirmation of a diagnosis that has been suspected (i.e., that early or nonspecific signs and symptoms are caused by a specific condition)

Potential disadvantages are that the test results may provide:

- A source of increased anxiety about the future
- Guilt at having survived when others in the family are affected, if the result is negative ("survivor's guilt")
- Concern about potential discrimination based on genetic test results
- Regret about past life decisions (such as not having children)
- Changes in family attitudes toward the person who has been tested (such as less reliance on them for support)

---

with any type of genetic screening such as prenatal and newborn screening. For example, a mother who undergoes prenatal screening may be told that she is at increased risk for having a child with Down syndrome. Or, new parents may be informed that their infant's test results from newborn screening for cystic fibrosis are in the positive range for that screening test. A positive result to a screening test simply means, however, that a diagnostic test is required to determine if the results of the screening are correct (e.g., the fetus has Down syndrome or the newborn baby has cystic fibrosis). It is important for parents to understand that, in some infants who test positive, a diagnostic test result can indicate that the infant has a genetic condition and will need further evaluation and treatment; in other cases, however, subsequent tests will be normal. When an infant has further evaluation and is found not to have the condition, the first test result is sometimes referred to as a false positive, or an out-of-range result that requires further testing.

In many cases, families first learn of an abnormal screening result either by phone or during a follow-up visit. Families often respond with fear and distress to the news and many turn to the Internet for information about the genetic test or condition (DeLuca, Kearney, Norton, & Arnold, 2012; DeLuca, Zanni, Bonhomme, & Kemper, 2013). Nurses can help guide parents to credible Web sites concerning condition management and help them disseminate information obtained online (DeLuca et al., 2013).

DISCLOSURE OF GENETIC INFORMATION TO FAMILIES

Down Syndrome

Much has been written about parental satisfaction with family-provider interactions surrounding the diagnosis of Down syndrome, and there have been ongoing efforts to help health care providers become more prepared to share positive results from prenatal screening and diagnostic testing (Van Riper & Choi, 2011). However, reports of parental dissatisfaction with the informing process continue to appear in the popular literature. There continue to be reports of health care providers giving families inaccurate, out-of-date information about what life is like for individuals with Down syndrome and their families. Nurses need to be well informed about types of prenatal testing being offered and they need to know the difference between prenatal screening and diagnostic testing (Prows, Hopkin, Barnoy, & Van Riper, 2013). Additionally, they need to be prepared to give expectant parents more than just technical information about the genetic test. Nurses need to provide information about choices that will need to be made by expectant parents following a positive test result, resources for families who receive a positive result, and up-to-date information about life with Down syndrome in the 21st century (Van Riper, Knafl, Duarte, & Choi, 2016). Findings from an ongoing cross-cultural study about adaptation and resilience and adaptation in families of individuals with Down syndrome (Van Riper, Knafl, Duarte, & Choi, 2016) revealed that parental preference concerning the informing process match fairly well with the guidelines proposed by Skotko, Kishnani, and Capone (2009) and recommended by the National Society of Genetic Counselors (Sheets et al., 2011). Therefore, nurses are encouraged to become familiar with these guidelines.

Results of Genetic Testing and Communication Between Nurses and Caregivers

A 2012 study by Salm and colleagues examined parents' reactions to newborn screening and their recommendations for improving communication (Salm, Yetter, & Tluczek, 2012). Interviews were conducted with 203 parents of 106 infants with positive newborn screening results. Diagnostic testing confirmed that 37 of the infants had congenital hypothyroidism, 26 had cystic fibrosis, and 43 were cystic fibrosis carriers. Reactions from the parents ranged from "very scary" to "not concerned." Common emotions reported by parents include shock, panic, and worry. In addition, some parents reported feeling guilty. Concerning recommendations for improving communication, seven main themes were identified:

- *Provider characteristics:* The provider should be knowledgeable, known to the family, and an effective communicator.
- *Provider approach:* The provider should be calm and reassuring, answer questions, be honest, not downplay results, be sensitive, use simple language, speak to both parents, take their time, and address the parents' questions.
- *Timing of the notification:* Inform the parents as soon as possible, but not on a Friday afternoon. Some parents specified that they would have preferred to not be notified until the diagnosis was confirmed, not suspected.
- *Communication channel:* Parents desired to be told in person, rather than on the telephone and that providers not leave a message on the answering machine.
- *Care coordination:* Parents preferred being referred to an appropriate specialist as soon as possible and that there was direct communication between the primary care provider and specialist.

- *Information:* Parents wanted written materials and a follow-up process in place if additional questions arose in the first few weeks following being told.
- *Family support:* Parents wanted access to other families having a child with the condition, adults with the condition, and support groups to hear life experiences.

Certain genetic conditions, such as salt-wasting CAH, are life threatening without proper treatment. Families learning of their child's CAH diagnosis in the first few weeks following birth may become overwhelmed because not only are they learning their child has an inherited, genetic condition, but also that their failure to treat the CAH adequately can result in the death of their child (Boyse, Gardner, Marvicsin, & Sandberg, 2014; Fleming, 2016; Fleming, Rapp, & Sloane, 2011; Speiser et al., 2010). CAH requires parents to administer oral steroids, typically hydrocortisone, up to three times daily to affected children. Additionally, parents must supplement maintenance steroid doses with oral "stress dosing" during times of illness and an emergency intramuscular (IM) injection of hydrocortisone when a child is unable to tolerate oral medications and/or if signs of adrenal crisis are present. This need for stress dosing, either orally or by injection, related to simple viral and bacterial childhood illnesses is frequent and unpredictable, often requiring parents to make complex treatment decisions (Speiser et al., 2010). Moreover, girls born with CAH often experience virilization, which results in atypical genitalia at birth, caused by elevated testosterone related to adrenal dysfunction (boys born with CAH have typically appearing male genitalia) (Witchel & Azziz, 2011). Nurses and other health care providers must be sensitive to families during this challenging time and be willing to provide needed support. This support may include repeating management instructions, putting families in touch with local and national support groups, and referring families to pediatric endocrinologists and pediatric urologists in a timely and clear manner.

FAMILY DISCLOSURE OF GENETIC INFORMATION

Access to genetic information gained from genetic testing, as well as from family history, raises a host of questions for the family regarding confidentiality that includes the following: who to tell, what and when to tell them, and how much to share. Nurses must maintain the confidentiality of each family member's genetic testing information. It is completely up to the individual to determine whether or not to reveal information about genetic risks, testing, disease, or management. Results of genetic tests are private, so they should not be disclosed to other family members without the tested person's consent. In the United States, the Health Insurance Portability and Accountability Act (HIPAA) permits disclosures of health information if there is an immediate and serious threat to the person and if the disclosure could reasonably lessen or prevent the threat (U.S. Department of Health and Human Services, 2017). In most cases, however, the choice of disclosure of genetic information is an individual decision that is made in the context of the family.

Family members may prefer to maintain privacy regarding their decision to undergo testing, even within the family. This decision may reflect an attempt to avoid disagreements within the family, an attempt to protect others in the family from sadness or worry, or an attempt to prevent discrimination or bias. For example, people who have predictive Huntington's disease testing may be reluctant to share this information with their primary care provider. This reluctance may be because they fear that any notation in their medical record may be accessed by an employer or insurance provider, which may lead to loss of employment or insurance. Although there are laws that prohibit insurance or employment discrimination based on a person's genotype, some individuals may remain concerned that revealing their genetic information may place them at risk for future discrimination (Klitzman et al., 2013).

When one person in a family has a condition that is caused by an alteration in a single gene, such as a gene associated with hereditary breast or ovarian cancer, the person with the mutation is asked to notify others in the family that they too may have this same DNA mutation. In general, the family members themselves pass on this information, but occasionally, with the consent of all concerned, direct conversations can occur between the nurse and other family members. It is up to the individual family members and the family as a whole as to how, when, and to whom to share their genetic information. Concerning

hereditary breast cancer, mothers report anxiety about upsetting their children and causing unnecessary worry with disclosure; however, avoiding disclosure has profound effects on their children including children developing blasé and conflicting attitudes toward breast reconstruction surgery as well as misunderstandings of the full implications of risk management decision making (Rowland, Plumridge, Considine, & Metcalfe, 2016).

Both individual and family relationship factors can influence communication among family members. Therefore, nurses should have a good understanding of their patient's personal beliefs about sharing genetic risk information with family members. Typically, close relatives are told of the new diagnosis shortly after it has been made; however, there are times when a longer period of time is needed so that the affected person can make sense of the genetic test result for himself or herself (Gaff & Hodgson, 2014). Nurses should be patient, empathetic, and caring during conversations with the family as disclosure decisions are made. Box 8-3 depicts an example of family communication of genetic information.

Parents: To Tell or Not to Tell

Parents form views about how and when to tell their children early on after a diagnosis and typically feel responsible to communicate this information to their children themselves (Ulph, Cullinan, Qureshi, & Kai, 2014). Parents of a child with a genetic disorder take into consideration what to tell their children about the condition based on the developmental level of the child and the child's extent of interest in knowing about the genetic condition. Parents who are unsure about informing their children may feel that it would be better coming directly from a health professional (Ulph et al., 2014). Parents of children with genetic conditions may choose not to share information because they have concerns about school issues, obtaining health care for their children, and insurability or employability of their children. Nurses have a significant role in helping parents decide what information to share with their children about their genetic condition based on their developmental level. Another role of family nurses is helping parents determine how much information to share with outside sources, such as schools, day care, or employers, about their child's genetic condition.

BOX 8-3

Family Communication of Genetic Information

Brian, a 46-year-old man, is the oldest of three siblings. He is married but has no biological children. Brian was aware that his mother died of bowel cancer at the age of 38 years, and although this worried him, he hid his anxiety from both friends and relatives. He never discussed his mother's death with his wife or siblings. Brian had been experiencing abdominal pain for some months when he collapsed at work one day and was taken to his local hospital emergency department. He was found to be anemic and suffering a bowel obstruction. A tumor located near the hepatic flexure of the large colon was removed successfully. Brian was informed that his family and medical history indicated that it was likely he had inherited a mutation in an oncogene that predisposed him to bowel cancer. He was advised to share this finding with his siblings, and recommend that they seek advice and screening for themselves. Brian was reluctant to discuss the issue with his siblings but did tell his wife. Brian chose not to disclose this information to his siblings. Several months later, at the encouragement of his wife, they met with the cancer nurse to discuss the situation. The cancer nurse helped Brian decide what information to share with his siblings. They created a plan for how and when to share the information. Subsequently, both Brian's sister and brother had genetic testing. Brian's sister was found to carry the mutation. She was screened, and she worked with the nurse to devise a plan to tell her children about their possible risk when they reached 18 years of age.

Concealing Information: Family Secrets

Families choose to keep genetic information quiet for a variety of reasons. Sometimes information is kept a secret out of a desire to protect other family members. Some keep a secret because they feel shame. Still other families may choose to keep information confidential because the exploration of genetic inheritance may reveal other personal information. For example, consider a family with four sisters who want health advice because their father has a form of familial colon cancer. In the course of obtaining the family history, the mother confides to the nurse that her husband is not the biological parent of the oldest daughter, and that others in the family do not know this history. In this situation, the nurse recognizes that the oldest daughter does not share the same risk for this disease as her sisters, but the nurse would not be permitted to reveal that information to any family member without the mother's permission. This family secret can create conflict for the nurse, because the lack of disclosure might mean the eldest daughter is exposed to unnecessary procedures, such as a colonoscopy (which carries a risk for morbidity). The nurse would discuss the issue of risks for procedures with the mother so that she can consider all the information in deciding to tell her daughter the family secret. The mother would have to decide if the benefits of disclosure outweigh the distress the daughter may experience by learning about her parentage.

Family Reactions to Disclosure of Genetic Information

Families are unique and respond to genetic discoveries differently. Even within the same family, the responses of family members may vary. Some members may seek predictive testing to determine whether they have inherited the genetic condition. Others choose not to seek testing. Some members react to genetic discoveries with grief, loss, and denial. The nurse's role is to support all family members in their reactions and ultimate choices.

Children, regardless of age, may wonder if they will have the same condition as their parent. For example, this may be the case for teens who have a parent or grandparent with Huntington's disease, an autosomal dominant condition. Guidelines do not recommend predictive testing until a teen is old enough to provide informed consent. However, delayed disclosure to children can lead to increased family tension which results in misunderstanding, blame, and secrecy (Rowland & Metcalfe, 2013). Teenagers should be given the opportunity to discuss concerns about genetic testing, but parents should be involved in and support the adolescent's final decision (Botkin et. al., 2015). Nurses should offer the opportunity for them to ask questions and discuss their concerns, including offering to facilitate a family discussion. Box 8-4 depicts a family working with an adolescent about genetic testing.

Older adults may have varied experiences with genetic conditions that they have seen in their

BOX 8-4

Working With an Adolescent About Genetic Testing

Susan is a 17-year-old young woman whose mother developed breast cancer at age 42 and had to have a double mastectomy. Susan's mother is now recovering from her surgery and doing well. Susan's maternal grandmother and one of her maternal aunts died from breast cancer in their forties. Susan's mother chose to have genetic testing to learn about the possible genetic cause of her breast cancer. The test results revealed that she has a *BRCA1* gene mutation, which significantly increases a woman's lifetime risk of developing breast cancer. At her annual health care appointment, Susan tells the nurse about her family history of breast cancer and that her mother has a *BRCA1* gene mutation. Susan says that she would like to know what her risk is for inheriting this gene and that she would like to have the genetic testing to find out if she carries the same *BRCA1* gene as her mother. She says that she is worried about her younger sister, too. Susan tells the nurse that she does not want to worry her mother or family by talking with them about her concerns. The nurse informs Susan that she is free to express her concerns with her and her physician and that they can talk with her about how best to discuss the issue with her mother and express her concerns. The nurse also lets Susan know that when she is 18 she will be old enough to provide informed consent to have genetic testing for the *BRCA1* mutation that her mother has. The nurse recommends that when Susan is 18, she consider genetic counseling with a genetic specialist to learn more about her risk and the *BRCA1* genetic testing.

BOX 8-5

Preselection Beliefs

John is a 21-year-old young man who has recently graduated from college and is trying to decide what career he wants to pursue. John has a family history of Huntington's disease (HD) on his mother's side. His mother's brother and her father have both passed away from HD. His mother, age 45, is currently in good health. John is very worried that he will develop HD because it is in his mother's family. John makes an appointment with his health care provider so that he can talk with him about his concerns. As the nurse is taking his vital signs, John tells her about his concerns that he will develop HD. He says that he doesn't know if his mother has it and he is worried because it seems to be in the males of the family, and he resembles his uncle who died from HD. John says that he would like to go to medical school but he is scared that he will develop HD when he is young and it will greatly affect his career. He also tells the nurse that he has a girlfriend to whom he is very attached, but he is afraid to consider getting married because he does not want to put her through the experience of losing him to HD. He says that he has not even told her about his family history. The nurse tells John that she understands his concerns and encourages John to talk with his doctor about how he can learn more about his risk for HD. She tells him that he could consider having genetic counseling to talk further about his risks and available genetic testing for HD to learn more. John thanks her for her support and suggestions and says that he will surely talk with his doctor further about his concerns and options.

families over the years and serve as a valuable source of information regarding family history of genetic conditions. Advances in genomics will make susceptibility testing for common diseases of middle and old age (such as coronary artery disease or cancer) more common.

Family members possess beliefs about their own risks and who in the family will develop a genetic condition. These beliefs are termed *preselection* (Tercyak, 2010). Preselection beliefs are often based on the family's previous experience. For example, if only male relatives have been affected by an autosomal dominant condition that could affect either

sex, female members in the family may believe they are not at risk. Sometimes preselection beliefs are based on the fact that the person thought to have inherited the condition physically resembles the affected parent or shares a physical characteristic (such as hair color) with other affected relatives. A preselection belief may influence the person's self-image and overall functioning. For example, those who believe they will develop a condition may make different career choices, avoid long-term relationships, or decide not to have children. Box 8-5 depicts a case study that demonstrates preselection beliefs.

DECISION TO HAVE GENETIC TESTING

In some circumstances, family members may want to know the likelihood that they will develop a condition in the future, which is referred to as either *predictive* or *presymptomatic* testing. Typically the physical risk for undergoing genetic testing is minimal, but not so for the emotional risk. The test results may have a significant effect on a person emotionally, influence medical decisions, and result in discrimination. Undergoing genetic predictive testing requires nurses to work with clients so that they make this decision in a way that meets their specific needs, alert to the nonphysical risks. Nurses involved with these families should be able to identify the sources of emotional distress and offer effective strategies to help mediate distress, make informed decisions about medical interventions, and handle possible discrimination (Williams et al., 2009).

Emotional Health

Family members seek or avoid genetic testing for a variety of reasons. Some elect to know whether or not they carry a mutation so they can reduce their fear of the unknown, or make life choices, such as having children. Some people decide not to have predictive testing because they believe this knowledge would increase their level of anxiety and would prompt a constant watch for developing symptoms (Soltysiak, Gardiner, & Skirton, 2008). Test results mean different things in different situations, which makes these decisions to undergo testing even more complex and multifaceted. For example, a positive test for a *BRCA1* or *BRCA2* breast cancer mutation does not mean the individual has a 100% chance of developing breast cancer, so taking precautionary measures requires weighing costs and benefits. In other situations, such as in the case of Huntington's disease, if an individual carries the autosomal dominant condition, he will develop the disease. Some choose not to be tested for fear that they would lose hope.

Even adjustment to a negative result—meaning that a person does not have the genetic pattern of the disease—can be difficult. Some people who find that they are not at risk of developing a genetic condition experience "survivor guilt," which can be described as a sense of self-blame or remorse felt by a person who, in this case, will not develop a condition that others in the family will develop.

Evidence exists that when individuals have a genetic test that indicates that they will develop a condition, other family members may rely on them less than previously, in an emotional sense. These individuals experience feelings of loss of place in the family well before developing disease symptoms (Williams & Sobel, 2006). Some experience a deep sense of grief and loss of a potential future.

Medical Decisions

Physicians and nurse practitioners are in an excellent position to work closely with individuals and families in making well-informed decisions about their health based on genetic and genomic information. These health care providers have the ability to refine and personalize medical care that is based on the client's genetic makeup. For example, there is an increased probability that treatment outcomes will result in fewer adverse effects from medications, such as pain management being determined on the basis of whether a client is a known fast metabolizer or slow to metabolize certain kinds of drugs. But just because there are many tests available does not mean that the best option is for the individual to have genetic testing done. Advanced practice nurses need to work closely with the individual and family in deciding to have genetic testing that would include what the test would show, how specific the results might or might not be, and explore what options are possible based on the outcome of the testing.

After conferring with the health care provider, some individuals may not choose to have genetic testing at that time. Instead, these individuals may elect to undergo regular checkups and screenings, such as more frequent mammograms. In contrast, when a person has genetic testing and tests positive for a specific disease, a cascade of decisions then befalls that person, including and involving preventive or prophylactic treatments, degrees of treatment, risks of treatment, and benefits of treatment. For example, a woman may decide to undergo surgery, such as sterilization, so as to not pass on to offspring a condition such as cystic fibrosis or sickle cell anemia; or someone with positive results for *BRCA1* breast cancer mutation may elect to have a bilateral mastectomy.

Discrimination

Even though there is little evidence that genetic discrimination is a current problem (Feldman, 2012), many individuals choose not to undergo genetic testing because they fear discrimination. For example, a person may have concerns that she may be bypassed for promotion if it was known she tested positive for a medical condition. In the United States, the Genetic Information Nondiscrimination Act (GINA) of 2008 protects individuals from discrimination initiated by an employer or health insurance company.

Under GINA, insurers may not use genetic information to set or adjust premiums, deny coverage, or impose pre-existing conditions, and they may not require any genetic testing. Unfortunately, the GINA law does not apply to employers with fewer than 15 employees and it does not include protection against discrimination when an individual seeks to obtain life insurance, short-term disability insurance, or long-term care insurance. GINA does not protect members of the military, veterans, federal employees, or the Indian Health Service. Each of these sectors of society is protected against discrimination by other laws and statutes.

Under GINA, an employer may not make any decisions about hiring, firing, promoting, or pay or assignment based on any genetic information. The Patient Protection and Affordable Care Act of 2010 also prohibits denial of insurance coverage based on genetic information. The GINA law is significantly more stringent and specific in preventing discrimination by employers and health care insurance agencies (Feldman, 2012), however, because it defines genetic information as including medical history.

ROLES OF THE NURSE

When a genetic risk is identified in a family, nurses, together with others on the health care team, have two major responsibilities: (1) help family members understand that the genetic risk is present and (2) make sure decisions about testing, management, and surveillance are well-informed decisions that fit with individual and family beliefs, desires, values, and circumstances.

This section suggests ways that nurses should review their own beliefs and values when working with families. It covers how to conduct a risk assessment and genetic family history, the importance of working with a couple in preconception education, and the role of nurses as genetic information managers.

Personal Values: A Potential Conflict

Nurses must become aware of cultural values that differ from their own family cultural values. Cultural awareness allows nurses to tailor their practices to meet the needs of the family. Box 8-6 demonstrates how a nurse who does not understand a family's cultural values could contribute to a poor outcome.

It is a difficult emotional situation when nurses' personal values conflict with those of families. One example of this type of conflict occurs when the nurse personally does not agree with the family decisions relative to the potential risks of having a child who is genetically predisposed to having a terminal disease. It is unethical, however, for nurses to try to influence the decisions of the family or family members because of their own personal views.

BOX 8-6
Cultural Awareness for Working With Families

Kate is a genetic nurse working in a pediatric clinic for children with inherited metabolic conditions. She was scheduled to see a family whose son had a rare inherited metabolic disorder to discuss the parents' future reproductive options, including prenatal diagnosis. When the family entered the room, she noted with surprise that the parents and the child were accompanied by both sets of grandparents. She quickly arranged for more chairs to be brought into the room. Kate was quite disconcerted to find that the paternal grandfather repeatedly answered questions that were directed to the parents, and she continued to address the parents. Eventually, the child's father explained that, according to his culture, the oldest male relative on the father's side was responsible for making the decision that would affect the family; therefore, it was critical that the grandfather be fully involved in all discussions. While reflecting with her mentor, Kate realized that, in the future, she would ask the family at the beginning of the family conference to share any specific cultural needs she should know about in order to help meet their family needs.

Another type of conflict occurs when opinions within the family vary. In this type of situation, the role of the nurse is to facilitate family members expressing their views. In clinical genetics, more than one family member may be involved in decision making, and nurses should respect each person's autonomy.

Conducting a Genetic Family History

As described in Chapter 5, a genogram collects useful information about family structure and relationships. Nurses can use a three-generation family pedigree to provide information about a potential genetic inheritance pattern and recurrence risks. The genetic risk assessment enables nurses to identify those family members who may be at risk for disorders with a genetic component so that they can be provided appropriate lifestyle advice, screening recommendations, and possibly reproductive options. Information on standardized pedigree symbols and the construction of a genetic family pedigree is available to the public through the U.S. Surgeon General's Family History Initiative with resources available through the National Genetics Education and Development Centre (U.S. Department of Health and Human Services, 2016).

The purpose of drawing the family tree using a genetic family pedigree is to enable medical information to be presented in the context of the family structure. Obtaining a genetic family history in this systematic manner helps ensure inclusion of all critical information in the analysis (Skirton, Patch, & Williams, 2005). The process of obtaining a detailed health history and causes of family deaths is as follows:

- Start with the client
- Client's immediate family members
- Client's mother's side of the family
- Client's father's side of the family
- Relatives who have died, including their cause of death

Relatives who are not biologically related, such as those joining the family through adoption or marriage, should also be noted with the appropriate pedigree symbol. The reason that relatives who are not biologically related are noted in a pedigree with a special symbol is to identify them as family members who are not at risk for passing on or inheriting harmful genes from the family they have joined.

Obtaining a family genetic history is a nursing skill that requires technical expertise and knowledge of what needs to be asked, as well as sensitivity to personal or distressing topics and an awareness of the ethical issues involved. Box 8-7 outlines the components of a genetic nursing assessment. Information given by patients is considered part of their personal health record and should be treated as personal and private information.

Drawing the genetic family pedigree or family tree for at least three generations often provides important data about the potential inheritance pattern. When a condition affects both male and female members, and is present in more than one generation, a *dominant condition* is suspected (Figure 8-1). Conditions that affect mainly male relatives, with no evidence of male-to-male transmission, increase suspicion of an *X-linked recessive condition* (Figure 8-2). When more than one child is affected of only one set of parents, it may be evidence of an *autosomal recessive condition* (Figure 8-3).

BOX 8-7

Components of a Genetic/Genomic Nursing Assessment

A genetic nursing assessment includes the following information:

- Three-generation pedigree using standardized symbols
- Health history of each family member
- Reproductive history
- Ethnic background of family members (as described by the family)
- Documentation of variations in growth and development of family members

- Individual member and family understanding of causes of health problems that occur in more than one family member
- Identification of questions family members have about potential genetic risk factors in the family
- Identification of communication of genetic health information within the family

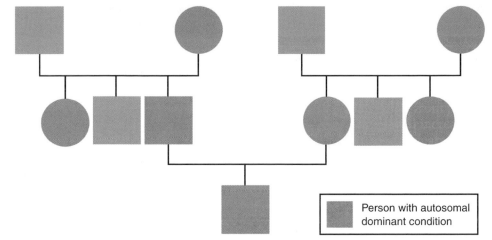

FIGURE 8-1 Pedigree of Autosomal Dominant Genetic Condition

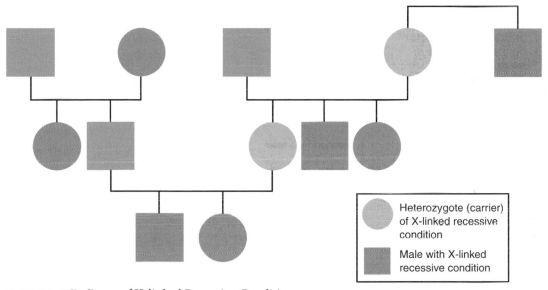

FIGURE 8-2 Pedigree of X-linked Recessive Condition

Nurses should not assume that a condition is genetic merely because more than one family member has it. Family members who are subject to similar environmental influences may have similar conditions without a genetic basis. One such example is a family with a strong history of lung cancer. Bob, a 62-year-old man, was affected by lung cancer. His two brothers and father all died of lung cancer. Bob expressed deep concern about having a genetic predisposition that he could pass on to his grandsons. The family history revealed that Bob's father and every male member of his family worked underground as coal miners from the age

of 14 years. In addition, they all smoked at least 20 cigarettes a day from when they were teenagers. None of the women smoked, nor did they work in the mines, and none developed lung cancer. In this family, the cancer could likely be attributed to environmental rather than inherited causes.

Preconception Assessment and Education

Preconception counseling is an intervention that includes providing information and support to individuals before a pregnancy to promote health

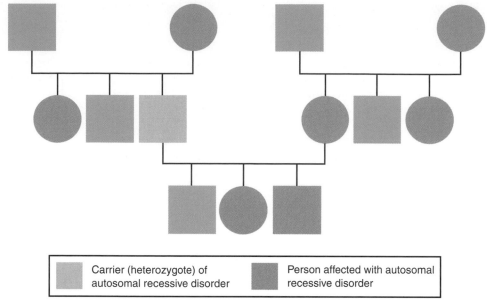

FIGURE 8-3 Pedigree of Autosomal Recessive Genetic Condition

and reduce risks (Walfisch & Koren, 2011). It is ideal when a family has the opportunity to discuss difficult genetic decisions before a pregnancy. During a pregnancy, the emotional ties to the existing fetus may complicate the decision-making process for the parents. Preconception counseling enables a couple to explore options without time pressures.

One aspect of preconception education is conducting a health risk profile that includes family history, prescription drug use, ethnic background, occupational and household exposures, diet, specific genetic disorders, and habits such as smoking, alcohol, or street drug use. When nurses identify information that may

present a health risk in future offspring, they should explore whether the woman or family wants a more extensive evaluation from a genetic specialist. Box 8-8 provides an example of preconception education for a couple concerned about genetic risks for offspring.

In addition to identifying inherited conditions, preconception counseling includes education regarding other risk factors that could change the outcome of a pregnancy. During preconception counseling, family nurses explain the importance, for instance, of taking an adequate amount of folic acid, one of the B vitamins, which is known to decrease the number of babies born with NTDs (Centers for Disease

---

BOX 8-8

Preconception Education

Jay and Sara are college students who are planning to be married. Both are of Ashkenazi Jewish ancestry. Although both have heard about Tay-Sachs disease, and the availability of carrier testing, neither has had the carrier test. When Sara visited the student health office, she talked with the nurse about her fears that she may not be able to have healthy babies. She knew that Tay-Sachs disease, a degenerative neurological condition, is more common in Ashkenazi Jewish families, and that no treatment will alter the course of the disease. Sara was interested in learning more about the carrier test.

The nurse offered to refer Sara to a genetics specialist, who would help the couple explore the following childbearing options:

- Decide to have or not have biological children
- Have a pregnancy with no form of genetic testing
- Have a preimplantation genetic diagnosis
- Have a pregnancy and have a prenatal genetic diagnosis with an option to terminate an affected fetus
- Have a pregnancy using a donor gamete from a noncarrier donor
- Adopt a child

BOX 8-9

Folic Acid Recommendations to Prevent Neural Tube Defects

In 1992, the U.S. Public Health Service recommended that all women capable of becoming pregnant take 0.4 mg/400 g folic acid daily, which is the amount of folic acid in most multivitamins. Although a daily intake of folic acid does not completely rule out the possibility that an infant will have NTDs, studies have reported an 11% to 20% reduction in cases of anencephaly and a 21% to 34% reduction in cases of spina bifida since this recommendation was issued (Mosley et al., 2009).

Control and Prevention, 2017). Box 8-9 provides more information about NTDs.

Risk Assessment in Adult-Onset Diseases

Genetic history taking is important in the adult population to assess for risk factors that are pertinent to common diseases, such as cancer and coronary heart disease. The risk assessment is based on the genetic family pedigree, but additional genetic or biochemical testing may be used to clarify the potential risk to each individual. To ensure privacy, health care providers must obtain consent from all living relatives before accessing their medical records and confirming relevant medical history. Family members who are seeking information are advised of their risks and options for clinical screening and follow-up. One example is the assessment of risk for cancer when there is a strong history of cancer in the family. Nurses must explore feelings of grief and anxiety about the future, as well as beliefs about the inheritance pattern. Providing explanations enables families to understand the information and helps them learn possible options to reduce the risk for cancer in their family members.

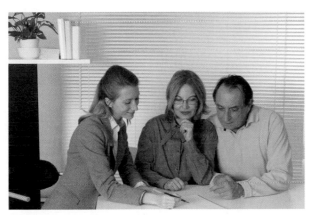

© iStock.com/Lisa-Blue

Increasingly, women with a family history of breast or ovarian cancer, or both, are seeking to reduce their risks for these conditions. All women have a risk for breast cancer (13% of women in the general population) and may be offered mammography screening according to the standards of care or regional health policy (Leonarczyk & Mawn, 2015). For women with a genetic family history that is consistent with familial breast and ovarian cancer, genetic and familial cancer specialists should discuss earlier and more frequent screening. The challenge of decision making with hereditary breast cancer is heavily found in the complicated process of weighing risks and benefits (Leonarczyk & Mawn, 2015).

With appropriate treatment, some health problems with a major genetic component may improve or at least remain stable. But many genetic conditions lead to increasing loss of health and function throughout the person's life span. These genetic conditions require more and more complex care from both health care providers and the family. In the chronic phase of a genetic condition, individuals and the family not only come to terms with the permanent changes that come with the onset of illness symptoms (Biesecker & Erby, 2008; Truitt, Biesecker, Capone, Bailey, & Erby, 2012), but also must adapt their family routines and roles, and locate needed resources to meet changing health care needs.

Providing Information and Resources

An essential nursing competency includes the need for nurses to be able to identify resources that are useful, informative, and reliable for patients and families. It is the role of nurses to ensure that recommended Web sites include relevant and evidence-based information. Patients and families have a need for psychosocial and medical information about genetics; therefore, any information that is prepared for distribution should include material on both types of needs (Salm et al., 2012).

BOX 8-10
Evaluation of Nursing Intervention

Fiona is a 5-year-old child who is attending kindergarten. Her teacher is concerned that she does not appear to be progressing as well as expected, and asks the school nurse, Cindy, to check her hearing. Cindy arranges for Fiona's parents to bring her for a hearing test. She asks Fiona's mother about her medical history; the mother says she has always been a well child and has not had any ear infections but has developed some "funny patches" on her skin. They have not caused a problem, but the mother has wondered what they are and if they could turn cancerous. Cindy checks these and notes that they seem to be café-au-lait patches—small, pale brown pigmented areas of the skin. She reassures the parents that the café-au-lait patches are not harmful but could indicate an underlying cause for Fiona's slight learning problems. She draws a genetic family pedigree or family tree (Figure 8-4) and notes that Fiona's father and his mother (Fiona's paternal grandmother) had unusual skin lumps, but no other medical problems.

When the pediatrician sees the family, she measures Fiona's head circumference and examines her skin. She confirms that the skin marks are café-au-lait patches and that Fiona has eight of them. Fiona's head circumference is larger than average, on the 97th percentile for her age. A diagnosis of neurofibromatosis type 1 is made. The pediatrician explains that this is a genetic condition, but that it could have arisen for the first time in Fiona or may have been inherited from one of her parents. Neither parent is aware of the condition in the family. The pediatrician examines both parents and finds that Fiona's father has a large head circumference and has several raised lumps on the skin, called *neurofibromas*. He tells the pediatrician he needed extra help with math at school, but he finished college and works teaching French. He has never been concerned about the lumps because his own mother had dozens of them, and apart from having one removed because her shoe was rubbing against it, they did not cause her a problem.

The pediatrician is aware that children with this condition may have learning problems. She recommends that Fiona be evaluated to identify whether Fiona would benefit from extra help at school. As high blood pressure and malignancies can occur because of the condition, she also makes arrangements for Fiona and her father to have an annual checkup. Fiona's brother, James (9 years old), is also examined but has no signs of the condition and does not require any further assessment.

When Cindy is informed of the diagnosis, she helps the family to identify reliable sources of information on the Web and provides Fiona's parents with information about neurofibromatosis organizations.

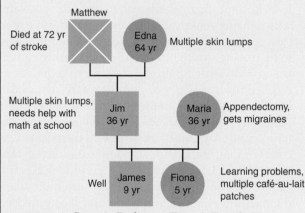

FIGURE 8-4 Genetic Pedigree: Fiona's Family Tree

Evaluation of Genomic and Genetic Nursing Interventions

Genomics and genetics are relatively new fields in nursing, but some work has assessed the value of genetic services, including nursing input, for patients and their families. Nurses must expand their assessment skills to include detailed family histories, understand the elements of genetic testing, and facilitate care coordination for genetic and genomic conditions and therapies (Boyd et al., 2017). Nurses should aim not only to be knowledgeable about genomics but also provide individualized care, and address the needs and specific agendas of each family. Box 8-10 provides an example of a nurse's evaluation of interventions with a family whose child has a genetic condition.

Although it is not possible for health care providers to have current knowledge about every condition, nurses exhibit competence in this area by having an awareness of their limitations, being open to discussion, finding appropriate resources, and referring to specialists when required. It is essential that nurses working in all types of settings be prepared with an adequate knowledge base to explain the basis and implications of genetics and genomics.

SUMMARY

The following major concepts were discussed in this chapter:

- Families share both social and biological ties. Identifying biological risk factors is an essential component of professional nursing practice, and a nursing assessment is incomplete without identifying biological factors

that may place individuals or their offspring at risk for genetic conditions.

- Nurses providing care to families across all health care settings and throughout the life span must maintain current knowledge of genomic aspects of health and risks for illness to assist families in obtaining information and further evaluation if needed.

- Nurses work with families on assessment, identification of issues influencing family members' health, facilitating appropriate referrals, and evaluating the effect of these activities on the family's health and well-being.

- Family values, beliefs, and patterns of communication are integral components of how families cope with and respond to family members with medical conditions that have a genetic component.

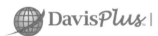 | For additional resources and information, visit **http://davisplus.fadavis.com**. References can be found on Davis*Plus*.

Chapter 9

Families Living With Chronic Illness

Jacqueline F. Webb, DNP, FNP-BC, RN

Maria Elena Ruiz, PhD, RN, FNP-BC

Kimberly E. Kintz, DNP, ANP-BC, RN

Critical Concepts

- Chronic illness is a global phenomenon with the potential to worsen the overall health of the nation's people and limit the individual's capacity to live well.

- Healthy lifestyle behaviors and early detection or screening may prevent some forms of chronic disease.

- Chronic illnesses that occur at birth or early childhood are most likely to be genetic and require special attention during developmental changes and across the life span.

- Nurses must use evidence-based knowledge to empower families with the information, skills, and abilities to manage chronic diseases over the life course and prevent complications and comorbidities.

- Family-focused care is important for prevention and management of chronic illness when it occurs; this involves intentional nursing action that meets both the individual and family needs.

- Knowledge about disease self-management and adherence to a therapeutic medical regimen is essential for individuals and their family members if they are going to prevent additional complications.

- Nurses use various actions (e.g., teach, coach, demonstrate, counsel) to assist individuals and their family members to cope with the stress of uncertainty, powerlessness, and anticipatory and ambiguous losses that accompany chronic illnesses.

All members of the family are affected when one member of the family has a chronic illness. When an individual is diagnosed with a chronic illness, it becomes necessary for the individual and the family to learn to manage the disease or disorder while living a quality life. Individuals with a chronic condition often battle to stay healthy, live active lives, retain a high quality of life, and prevent complications.

This battle primarily is waged within the confines of the family. When an individual is diagnosed with a chronic illness, whatever it might be, family members must incorporate unexpected changes into their roles and daily processes, manage disabilities imposed, and identify ways to do it with the resources they have available and within a context of uncertainty. Managing uncertainty is a significant concern for individuals and families living with chronic illness (Hummel, 2013b). Family members are challenged to balance the needs of the ill family member with their own needs and the needs of the family as a whole.

Chronic illnesses often require complex care, and many people have more than a single condition. People with chronic illnesses can experience complications or comorbidities that make situations even more difficult. For example, a person diagnosed with type 2 diabetes may also have hypertension, hyperlipidemia, and neuropathy. A person with Parkinson's disease may also have a serious sleep disorder, constipation, chronic pain, and Lewy body dementia. Often, with a chronic illness, individuals require care from multiple health care providers. Nurses are crucial in helping families coordinate care provided by multiple providers and among potential resources. The complex needs can create havoc for families, especially those with limited access to care and resources as they attempt to manage many thorny situations faced daily. The holistic approach of nurses is crucial to the individual and family adaptation and management of living with chronic illnesses across the life span. Chronic illnesses have an impact on the lives of infants, children, adolescents, young adults, older adults, and the old-old. Chronic illnesses affect the physical, emotional, intellectual, social, vocational, and spiritual functioning of the person with the condition as well as the family members. Wide variations exist in the ways different chronic illness conditions affect individuals, and the family's physical, mental and spiritual health, employment, social life, and longevity.

Differences in the ways families accommodate a chronic illness exist and are influenced not only by the level of disability and associated symptoms, but also by individual, family, and systemic factors. Families differ in their perceptions about disability, in their backgrounds, cultural and spiritual beliefs, and in their access to needed resources. Care responses differ depending on whether the symptoms are constant (cerebral palsy), episodic (migraine headaches), relapsing (sickle cell anemia), worsening or progressive (diabetes, Parkinson's disease, or certain types of cancer), or degenerative (Alzheimer's disease or Rhett syndrome). Details of the unique individual situation vary with the age of the individual, previous family experiences, level of disease complexity, individual's motivation or ease in managing the illness, unique family member relationships, and distinct personalities and values. Response to an illness may also be associated with the individual and family's explanatory models for understanding and coping

with an illness (Kleinman, 1980). Regardless of the type of chronic illness experienced, one thing remains the same: Various family members are likely to be involved at several levels.

Because family members are the most enduring care providers, they might be viewed as the biggest resource for individual care over time. Family members generally offer the constancy and continuity of care needed for the most optimal health outcome. Most health care providers come and go in the lives of persons with chronic conditions, offering medical management, education, and counseling for brief times. But it is generally family members that provide the needed ongoing and persistent care across time.

The purpose and focus of this chapter is to describe ways for nurses to think about the impact of chronic illness on families and to consider strategies for helping families manage chronic illness. The first part of this chapter briefly outlines the global statistics of chronic illness, the economic burden of chronic diseases, and three theoretical perspectives for working with families living with chronic illness. The chapter begins with the importance of integrating ethnoculture in family health care and the impact of chronic illness on family life. Four theoretical approaches are introduced for assisting nurses to think about the best way to assist the family living with chronic illness. The rest of the chapter captures a variety of nursing actions possible to assist these families. Two case studies are presented in this chapter: one family who has a family member living with type 1 diabetes and another family helping an older parent and grandparent manage Parkinson's disease. Although every family and illness experience is completely individual, many of the trials that these two families demonstrate are universal to other families supporting members living with different chronic illnesses.

WHAT IS CHRONIC ILLNESS?

Definitions for what constitutes chronic diseases vary widely although most definitions seem to address duration and limitations in function (Goodman, Posner, Huang, Parekh, & Koh, 2013). Different approaches used to measure the prevalence and consequences of chronic diseases and health conditions in children contribute to the lack of uniformity and acceptance of a definition (van der Lee, Mokkink, Grootenhuis, Heymans, & Offringa, 2007). The terms *chronic disease* and *chronic illness* are often used interchangeably by health care providers and researchers. Larsen (2012) differentiates between condition and illness, as *"condition* refers to the pathophysiology of a disease" whereas *illness* is referred to as "the human experience of a disease and refers to how the disease is perceived, lived with, and responded to by individuals, their families and health care professionals" (p. 4). This chapter will utilize the term *chronic illness* as much as possible.

The term *chronos* is the root word for "chronic" and refers to time; however, *chronicity* has various definitions. Chronic illnesses have been defined as conditions that last or are expected to last more than 3 to 12 months and result in functional limitations and/or need ongoing medical care (Freid, Bernstein, & Bush, 2012; Friedman, Jiang, & Elixhauser, 2008; Hwang, Weller, Ireys, & Anderson, 2001). Another definition describes a chronic illness as a health condition that lasts longer than 6 months, is not easily resolved, and is rarely cured by a surgical procedure or short-term medical therapy (Miller, 2000). The World Health Organization (WHO) uses the term *noncommunicable diseases* (NCDs) interchangeably with chronic diseases that are not passed from person to person, generally have a slow progression, but have a long duration. The WHO (2014) primarily describes four main types of NCDs; cardiovascular diseases (such as heart attacks and stroke), cancers, chronic respiratory diseases (such as chronic obstructive pulmonary disease and asthma), and diabetes.

INTEGRATING ETHNOCULTURE IN FAMILY NURSING

With the rapidly changing world today, nursing care must be understood not only in the local context, but also with a global (international) vision as nurses strive to meet the needs and demands of individuals and families experiencing chronic illnesses. Both Canada and the United States are experiencing demographic shifts because of growing multicultural and multilingual communities. The rapidly changing population patterns require nurses who can assess and effectively meet the needs of diverse family groups that are living longer with complex chronic health conditions.

Population Shifts: Growing Diversity

According to the U.S. Census Bureau, approximately 314 million people live in the United States, and this figure is projected to grow to over 400 million by midcentury (Colby & Ortman, 2015). An increase in racial/ethnic diversity is also projected, as the minority population is expected to rise from today's figure of 36%, to 56%, with more than half of the children classified as children of minority parents. At the same time, all baby boomers (the cohort born after World War II, between 1946 and 1964), will be 65 years or older by 2029. This means that one out of every five individuals in the United States will be a senior citizen, an increase from today's figure of one out of seven. By midcentury, it is anticipated that the foreign-born population will rise from today's 13% to almost 19%.

Similarly, Canada's population is projected to continue to increase during the next 50 years, growing from 35.2 million in 2013 to a high of 63.5 million by 2063, with migration being the main driver of population growth (Bohnert, Chagnon, & Dion, 2015). By 2031, the proportion of foreign-born people will grow from 20% to almost 28%. What this means is that within 15 years, population diversity will increase and visible minority groups could comprise as much as 63% of the population of Toronto, 59% of Vancouver, and 31% of Montreal. As the largest recognized minority group, South Asians could represent 28% of the minority population (Bohnert et al., 2015). Allophones (people whose mother tongue is neither English nor French) accounted for less than 10% of Canada's population in 1981. It is projected that by 2031 they could represent as much as 32% of the minority population in Canada (Bohnert et al., 2015).

Demographic shifts are not isolated trends, and the changes have not occurred slowly. For example, in the last 30 years, more than 90% of major cities and small towns experienced a rise in migration and increasing diversity in their communities. With the increasing diversity in metropolitan and rural communities, there has also been a declining trend for white-dominant communities. Thirty years ago, the U.S. Census Bureau estimated that almost 80% of the population was white, 11.5% African American, 6.2% Hispanic, and 1.5% Asian. In contrast, recent census projections show increasing racial/ethnic diversity, with 62% identified as white, 13% African American, 17% Hispanic, and 6% Asian (Colby & Ortman, 2015). These population changes point out an increase in communities where a specific group is no longer the majority (Lee, Iceland, & Sharp, 2012). However, diversity has not filtered through all cities in the United States, Canada, and other nations, as there are regions where families from diverse backgrounds tend to concentrate. For example, in the United States more than half of all African Americans live in the southern states, whereas Hispanics/Latinos and Asians are more concentrated in New York, Florida, and various southwestern states (Lee et al., 2012). What this means is that residents are living and interacting in communities with a greater number of foreign-born residents and multiracial/ethnic, multicultural, and multilingual families (Passel & Cohn, 2008). For nurses, these demographic shifts are important, as nurses are the first responders and the glue that bridges individuals and families with the complex health care system today.

Nursing: Addressing Health Needs of a Multicultural Society

The increasing migration between and within nations suggests that health care providers may experience both benefits and challenges in today's health care arena. For many, life in the United States is an international experience. For nursing, what this means is that in order to meet the health needs of diverse communities, nurses must not only be qualified, but also must be culturally knowledgeable and ready to adapt to the changing needs of a rapidly diversifying population with multiple cultural, language, and varying health beliefs and health needs. Beliefs and self-management are a combination of cultural beliefs and traditions. Patients and their families are best served when nurses focus not only on the differences but also on the similarities within and among various cultural groups. Family nursing focuses on the strengths of individuals, families, and their communities. Global population shifts require that nursing meet the needs of diverse communities. Ethnocultural frameworks assist nurses to make client-centered assessments and inclusive management plans:

- Nurses achieve cultural knowledge by first desiring the knowledge and by actively engaging in cultural encounters with patients from diverse backgrounds.
- Nurses must self-reflect and acknowledge biases and discriminatory practices that prevent meaningful communication and interactions with unfamiliar community members.

- When working with individuals and their families, nurses must consider the client's worldview, environmental context, values, beliefs, religious patterns, and health practices.
- When developing plans of care, nurses assess and include longstanding culture-bound traditional beliefs and practices.
- Nurses must be knowledgeable of biocultural variations, disease incidences, and health inequities in the populations they are serving.
- Nurses must become familiar with the historical, political, economic, and public policies that affect chronic illness management.

Addressing the needs of diverse communities is not a new phenomenon, but it has become a focal point for nurses and other health care providers. Examining the integration of diversity in health care is timely and warranted, especially as the nursing profession in the United States, as in other nations, is limited in the number of nurses from racial/ethnic backgrounds with the skills to navigate health matters in diverse environments. In the United States today, 83% of nurses self-identify as white (American Association of Colleges of Nursing, 2015). What this means is that the percentage of U.S. nurses of racial/ethnic minority backgrounds is at odds with the increasing national and global demographic shifts.

Canada lacks studies that evaluate nursing workforce racial/ethnic backgrounds in health care settings (Premji & Etowa, 2014). The Canadian Nurses Association (2009) expressed the need to describe the diversity profile of nurses in order to help human resource planning. In 2011 Canadian men represented 6.6% (17,961) of the total employed registered nurses (252,763) (Canadian Nurses Association, 2013). The National League of Nursing (NLN) suggests that a lack of racial, ethnic, and gender diversity in the health professions limits our ability to provide appropriate care for families in a changing environment, and further limits nursing's ability to assist families to navigate a complex and fragmented health care system (NLN, 2016).

CHRONIC ILLNESS: A GLOBAL CONCERN

Chronic illness is a global issue and is the leading cause of mortality and disability in the world, representing 38 million or 68% of all deaths and projected to increase to 52 million by 2030 (WHO, 2014). From 1999 to 2014, four of the five leading causes of death in the United States were from chronic diseases, two of which (heart disease and cancer) accounted for approximately 46% of all deaths (Moy et al., 2017). Canada has very similar statistics, with cancer accounting for 30% and heart disease for about 20% of all deaths (Ellison, 2016). Worldwide chronic conditions such as cardiovascular diseases, cancer, chronic respiratory disease, and diabetes are responsible for 82% of these deaths (WHO, 2014). These four prominent chronic diseases are linked by common and preventable biological risk factors, notably high blood pressure, high blood cholesterol, and overweight, and by related major behavioral risk factors: unhealthy diet, physical inactivity, and tobacco use (WHO, 2014).

Various factors such as a growing older population, an increasing life expectancy related to advances in public health and clinical medicine, along with lifestyle-associated modifiable behaviors such as tobacco use, excessive alcohol use, insufficient physical activity, and poor nutritional habits, have all contributed to the increase in chronic illnesses (Goodman et al., 2013; Johnson, Hayes, Brown, Hoo, & Ethier, 2014; WHO, 2016c).

WHO (2015a) estimates that out of the 38 million people who died from chronic disease in 2012, 17.5 million were under the age of 70 years and 82% of those premature deaths occurred in low- and middle-income countries. Projections are that the number of people worldwide older than the age of 60 years and living with chronic illness will increase between 2015 and 2050 from 12% to 22%. By the year 2020, the number of people older than the age of 60 years will outnumber children under the age of 5 years. As people age, the risk for developing a chronic illness increases.

Common chronic conditions associated with aging include diabetes, hypertension, chronic obstructive pulmonary disease, hyperlipidemia, depression, cancer, and osteoarthritis. Many older individuals live with multiple chronic illnesses and complex conditions. As individuals get older and experience more chronic illnesses, they are at risk for geriatric syndrome. Geriatric syndrome is not a chronic illness or specific disease diagnosis but a cluster of five clinical symptoms: incontinence, pain, malnutrition, cognitive impairment, and frailty. The presence of geriatric syndrome is associated with a higher mortality rate when present in older adults

(Chang & Lin, 2015; WHO, 2015a). Cardiovascular disease is the number one cause of death globally, with 46.2% of all global deaths attributed to it (WHO, 2016a). Cardiovascular disease morbidity and mortality could be reduced by addressing risk factors such as tobacco use, unhealthy diet, obesity, physical inactivity, high blood pressure, diabetes, and elevated lipids (WHO, 2016a). Worldwide, obesity has more than doubled since 1980. In 2014 approximately 11% of men and 15% of women 18 years or older were obese. It is estimated that in children 5 years and younger obesity rates will rise to 11% worldwide by 2025 (WHO, 2016d).

Globally, cancer is the second leading cause of death and accounts for approximately 8.8 millions deaths a year (WHO, 2017). The most common cancer deaths are cancers of the lung, liver, colorectal region, stomach, and breast (WHO, 2017). According to the WHO, tobacco use is the most important risk factor for cancer as it is estimated to cause 22% of global cancer deaths and 70% of the global lung cancer deaths (WHO, 2017). In addition, tobacco use is the primary cause of chronic obstructive disease, such as emphysema and asthma, worldwide.

In 2014, about 422 million adults worldwide were living with diabetes, with the majority affected by type 2 diabetes (WHO, 2016b). When diabetes is not well managed it leads to complications that include heart attack, stroke, kidney failure, limb amputation, vision loss, and nerve damage. In 2012, diabetes caused approximately 1.5 million deaths, with many of these deaths (43%) occurring in those under the age of 70 (WHO, 2016b).

When pain becomes comorbidity, the challenges to individuals and their family increase tremendously. Many chronic conditions involve chronic nonmalignant pain (Chou et al., 2015; Chou et al., 2009). Chronic nonmalignant pain is one of the most prevalent and costly health care problems addressed in primary health care settings (Anderson, Wang, & Zlateva, 2012; Bair, 2008; Robinson & Rickard, 2013). Chronic pain affects about 100 million American adults, which is more than the total number affected by heart disease, cancer, and diabetes combined (Institute of Medicine [IOM], 2011b).

The United States has very high rates of chronic health conditions. When compared with 10 other industrialized countries, the United States has the highest rates of chronic health conditions such as heart disease and diabetes (Osborn, Moulds, Squires, Doty, & Anderson, 2014). About 87% of older adults report at least one chronic illness and 68% report two or more. U.S. older adults are more likely to face financial barriers to care than their counterparts in 10 other industrialized countries (Osborn et al., 2014).

The United States and Canada are nations experiencing increased racial/ethnic, language, cultural, and family system changes. Coupled with the increase in life expectancy, rising health care costs, a greater number of individuals living longer with chronic diseases, and the increasing need for family health support, nurses experience unprecedented challenges in providing care to families.

Family Health: Why Diversity Matters

It is well recognized that racial/ethnic minority populations suffer disproportionally from not only chronic debilitating conditions, but also preventable acute ailments and social conditions associated with poor health outcomes. According to the Office of Minority Health (2016), Hispanics/Latinos suffer disproportionately from obesity, asthma, liver disease, diabetes, and related complications. Diabetes is a major concern among subgroups of Hispanics, because of visual and renal impairment, higher rates of amputations, and premature death. Among African American populations, heart disease, strokes, cancer, asthma, diabetes, lung diseases, human immunodeficiency virus/acquired immune deficiency syndrome (HIV/AIDS), and homicide are of greater concern at younger ages. Among American Indians/Alaska Natives, the leading causes of death are diabetes, heart disease, cancer accidents, strokes, and infant death. Asian Americans share some of the health risks as for other minority groups, including cancer, heart disease, strokes, and accidents. A special concern among this population is smoking, as they have a higher rate of tuberculosis compared with the overall U.S. population. Although the risk factors, morbidity, and mortality rates vary among and within these underserved populations, a concern is the paucity of health data available on minority health. For nurses, it is imperative that evidence-based measures be increasingly available to assist individuals, their families, and communities managing disabling chronic conditions. Without adequate data and tools for improving health care, nurses may not be able to assist the growing number of individuals and families from diverse backgrounds, and all citizens living with and managing chronic debilitating conditions.

Surveillance of Chronic Illness

How do we know how many people have chronic illness and whether the problem is getting better or worse? In public health, one approach is the availability of surveillance data that are systematically collected over time. This information is used to analyze a problem and help identify trends of change over time. The following are examples of some of the surveys and surveillance systems that are used in the United States:

- Behavior Risk Factor Surveillance System (BRFSS)
- National Ambulatory Medical Care Survey (NAMCS)
- National Health Interview Survey (NHIS)
- National Healthcare Safety Network (NHSN)
- National HIV Surveillance System
- National Hospital Discharge Survey (NHDS)
- National Notifiable Disease Surveillance System (NNDSS)
- National Vital Statistics System (NVSS)
- Youth Risk Behavior Surveillance System (YRBSS)

In the United States and Canada, the BRFSS is a survey used to collect national information regularly. This is a state-based or province-based system of health surveys conducted through phone surveys. The survey tracks health risk factors and uses the findings to improve the health of the nation's people who are 18 years of age and older. For example, in 2015 when asked, "Have you ever been told by a doctor that you have diabetes?" participants from southern states such as Oklahoma, Arkansas, Louisiana, Mississippi, Alabama, South Carolina, Tennessee, Kentucky, and West Virginia had the highest prevalence of "Yes" responses with an average of 11.6% to 16.5%, compared with 10% as the national average (BRFSS, 2016). These types of statistics assist health care providers in developing target population-specific programming. In 2013 more than half of the U.S. adult's population drank alcohol in the past 30 days, with approximately 17% reporting binge drinking and 6% reporting heavy drinking (BRFSS, 2016). The Centers for Disease Control and Prevention (CDC, 2011) defines *binge drinking* as a pattern of drinking that brings a person's blood alcohol concentration (BAC) to 0.08 grams percent or above.

This typically happens when men consume five or more drinks, or when women consume four or more drinks, in about 2 hours. During the next few years, surveys will collect additional data about alcohol use and the problem of binge drinking. Therefore, it will be possible to compare and analyze alcohol abuse and binge drinking as a risk factor on chronic illness trends and concerns.

Another survey instrument used to collect information about chronic illness risks is the National Health and Nutrition Examination Survey (NHANES, 2016) in the United States and the Food and Nutrition Surveillance in Canada. The National Cardiovascular Data Registry is a database used to capture information about particular individuals. The National Program of Cancer Registries in the United States and the Canadian Cancer Registry are both surveillance organizations that focus on collecting, monitoring, and interpreting trends in cancer risks among a variety of populations. Large cohort studies, such as the Framingham Heart Study (2017), provide retrospective information about groups of people that share similar experiences. The Canadian Tobacco Use Monitoring Survey (CTUMS) (2015) describes the smoking trends in Canada from 1999 to 2013. Other data regarding chronic diseases are identified through individual records, from insurance companies, and with reviews of death certificates.

Internationally, surveys have revealed that the burden of chronic disease in adults and children is increasing in low- and middle-income countries, and despite increasing awareness and commitment to address chronic illness, global actions to implement cost-effective interventions are inadequate (Alwan et al., 2010; WHO, 2016c). The cause of the increase of chronic diseases in these countries is not easy to pinpoint. Most of the research on chronic illness factors has been conducted in developed countries.

Economic Burden of Chronic Illness

Chronic diseases are not only common; they are costly for families and society. During the next 20 years it is estimated that chronic illnesses globally will cost more than $30 trillion; thus, millions of people will be below the poverty line (Bloom et al., 2011). In 2010, cancer medical costs were estimated to cost $154 billion, with nonmedical costs at $67 billion and income losses at $69 billion. The global cost of cardiovascular diseases is at $863 billion and it is estimated to rise to $1.044 trillion by 2030 (Bloom et al., 2011). Diabetes costs the global economy about $500 billion, and this figure is also projected to rise to $745 billion by 2030.

The national economic burden of Parkinson's disease exceeded $14.4 billion in 2010 (approximately $22,800 per patient) (Kowal, Dall, Chakrabarti, Storm, & Jain, 2013). Indirect costs of Parkinson's disease (e.g., reduced employment) were conservatively estimated at $6.3 billion (or close to $10,000 per person with Parkinson's disease) (Kowal et al., 2013). When chronic illness is considered, it is useful to recognize that besides the associated dollar costs of various chronic diseases, there is also a loss in productivity and wages because of absenteeism.

Cardiovascular diseases are the most costly for Canada, costing roughly $21.2 billion in direct and indirect costs (Tarride et al., 2009). In 2012, the economic burden of diabetes in Canada was about $12.2 billion and expected to rise by another $4.7 billion by 2020. In Canada, the economic burden of the three major lung diseases—cancer, asthma, and chronic obstructive pulmonary disease—was $12 billion in 2010 (Theriault, Hermus, Goldfarb, Stonebridge, & Bounajm, 2012). Given the growing number of older adults in Canada, this economic cost for chronic lung disease is expected to double by 2030.

In 2014, 18.1% of Canadians aged 12 and older (roughly 5.4 million people) smoked. However, this is a decrease from 2013 when roughly 19.3% of Canadians aged 12 and older smoked (Statistics Canada, 2015). Each year more than 230,000 Canadians continue to die from smoking-related illness (Health Canada, 2011). Worldwide, tobacco use causes nearly 6 million deaths per year, and current trends show that tobacco use will cause more than 8 million deaths annually by 2030 (WHO, 2015b). In the United States more than 480,000 deaths occur annually from cigarette smoking and from secondhand smoke (CDC, 2016). Indirect costs, including loss of productivity when an ill person cannot work and the loss of productivity in the workplace when family leave is taken, was estimated to be $8.6 billion. There are approximately 2 million informal family caregivers with an economic burden contribution estimated at $25 billion (Hollander, Lui, & Chappell, 2009; Keefe, 2011).

Economic costs for chronic illnesses such as diabetes are continuing to increase. The WHO estimates that the direct global annual cost of diabetes is more than $827 billion (WHO, 2016b). In Canada, the economic cost of diabetes was approximately $12.2 billion in 2010, which accounts for about 3.5% of public health care spending in Canada (Canadian Diabetes Association, 2009). In 2012 diabetes was reported to cost Americans $245 billion. Direct medical costs were $176 billion and indirect costs, such as disability, work loss, and premature death, were $69 billion (CDC, 2017). A disproportionate percentage of these costs result from treatment and hospitalization of persons with diabetes-related complications. One of every five health care dollars is spent caring for someone diagnosed with diabetes (Dall et al., 2010). Financial costs for this disease are even greater when the family pays for additional health care needs, such as over-the-counter medication and medical supplies, additional visits to optometrists or dentists, health complications that occur before the diabetes is diagnosed, lost productivity at work for the individual and family members, and costs for informal caregiving. Because of continued emphasis on treatment of disease and related complications, rather than prevention, the cost of diabetes continues to climb. In fact, only a small amount of the money spent on diabetes is on research, education, or prevention (Dall et al., 2010).

DeVol (2008) found that the seven most common chronic diseases—cancer (broken into several types), diabetes, hypertension, stroke, heart disease, pulmonary conditions, and mental disorders—affect 133 million Americans. These diseases have large-ticket economic costs of $1.3 trillion annually, along with potential for lost work and productivity. Findings from the DeVol (2008) study also have the following indications:

- At the current rate, a 42% increase in cases of the seven chronic diseases is predicted by 2023, with $4.2 trillion in treatment costs and lost economic output.
- Modest improvements in preventing and treating diseases could avoid 40 million cases of chronic disease by 2023, with the economic effect of chronic illness decreased by 27% or $1.1 trillion annually from the current cost.
- Decreased obesity rates, a large risk factor linked with chronic illness, could result in productivity gains of $254 billion and avoid $60 billion in annual treatment expenditures.

Many with chronic illnesses fear they will be unable to afford needed medical care, a fear not unfounded as medical costs for those with chronic illness tend to be higher. Families with a child or an adult member with a chronic condition often face economic challenges. For example, in diabetes management, although medical insurance may cover the costs of medications and supplies such as syringes and glucose testing strips, other health-promoting activities might require out-of-pocket expenses. A person with diabetes needs to eat a balanced diet, which requires the purchase of foods high in nutritional value, food that might be more expensive than less healthy foods.

Lay caregivers, although posing far less of an economic burden on the health care system, come with their own set of costs. Still, the cost of funding caregiver services and support is small compared with the value of their contributions (Feinberg, Reinhard, Houser, & Choula, 2011). Policy recommendations that can make these economically friendlier unpaid caregivers' services (Family Caregiver Alliance, 2012; Feinberg, 2014) less burdensome to families include the following:

- Implement "family-friendly" workplace policies (e.g., flextime, telecommuting).
- Expand the Family and Medical Leave Act (FMLA) and include the definition of eligible employees under FMLA beyond the care of immediate family members to include care for siblings, in-laws, and grandparents.
- Expand funding for the National Family Caregiver Program, which was established in 2000 to provide funding to states and territories based on the number of people older than 70 years of age. It supports families and informal caregivers to keep loved ones at home as long as possible (U.S. Department of Health and Human Services [USDHHS], 2012).
- Provide adequate funding for the Lifespan Respite Care Act (2006). This program coordinated systems of accessible, community-based respite care services for family caregivers of children and adults of all ages with special needs (Administration for Community Living, 2013).
- Provide a tax credit for caregiving.
- Permit payment of family caregivers through consumer-directed models in publicly funded

programs (e.g., Medicaid home, community-based services waivers).

■ Assess family caregivers' own needs through publicly funded home and community-based service programs and referral to supportive services.

Costs Associated With Children With Special Health Care Needs

In addition to the health care provided in clinical settings, children with chronic special health care needs (SHCN) often require illness management and health maintenance in the home. The increased time and care demands of SHCN can make it difficult for family caregivers to be employed fully; emotional stress and financial burdens can result. A child might need special therapy such as physical, speech, or occupational assistance. Certain illnesses require constant out-of-pocket health care (such as autism, cystic fibrosis, or mental health needs) that can range from $2669 to $69,906 per year, compared with $676 to $3181 for families with non-SHCN children (Lindley & Mark, 2010). In addition, these families may have to pay more for everyday living expenses, such as water, heating, or special clothes or equipment, that are not included in their health plan. Parents of SHCN may lose pay as they need to take days off from work to care for their child (Lindley & Mark, 2010).

Parents working in low-income jobs often do not receive adequate health insurance benefits. Some families earn too much money to qualify for public subsidies but not enough money to cover the health care expenses of raising a child with SHCN. Compared with children in higher-income (and also lowest-income) households, children living in such "near-poor" families are more likely to have gaps in insurance coverage and more likely to be uninsured (Looman, O'Conner-Von, Ferski, & Hildenbrand, 2009). Eleven percent of uninsured children did not receive needed family support services related to chronic illness care, compared with 7.7% of children with public insurance and 2.7% of privately insured children (USDHHS, HRSA, Maternal and Child Health Bureau, 2008). Families who lack health insurance are more likely to report that although health and family support services are needed, they were not received. In addition, families can be greatly challenged as they try to balance chronic illness costs against other member and household needs.

Keep in mind that costs for the individual and his or her family can also be measured in loss of quality of life.

THEORETICAL PERSPECTIVES: WAYS TO UNDERSTAND CHRONIC ILLNESS

Family health care works best when it moves beyond an individual or cultural focus (Arestedt, Benzein, & Persson, 2015). Understanding illness beliefs on a family level enhances the nurses' ability to work with family members to develop a plan of care that works for the entire family. Few ethnocultural models address the application of transcultural assessment when working with families dealing with a chronic illness. Nursing is well positioned to use transcultural models that integrate multiple worldviews, with a greater emphasis on the strengths of individuals managing chronic conditions and the nurses who assist in their care.

By using an ethnocultural model as an overarching perspective of working with families, nurses strengthen their ability to establish relationships with families in context as they apply chronic illness models in their practice. The Ethno-Cultural Gerontological Nursing Model, or ECGNM (Phillips et al., 2015), is one of the few transcultural models that include family care. By using multiple theoretical perspectives, nurses have more flexibility to offer options to families in the management of their chronic illness. Three additional models specific to living with chronic illness are briefly explained: Rolland's Chronic Illness Framework (1987), the Family Management Style Framework (FMSF; Knafl & Deatrick, 1990, 2003), and the Family Health Model (FHM; Denham, 2003). These models provide unique perspectives on assessment, goal planning, nursing actions, and outcome evaluation using a family-focused point of view in chronic illness.

Ethnocultural Model

The ECGNM lays the groundwork for focusing on diversity with an aging population (Phillips et al., 2015); however, it is also applicable to other populations. A central principle of this model is that patients are best served when nurses focus not only on the differences but also on the similarities within and among cultural groups, with particular focus on

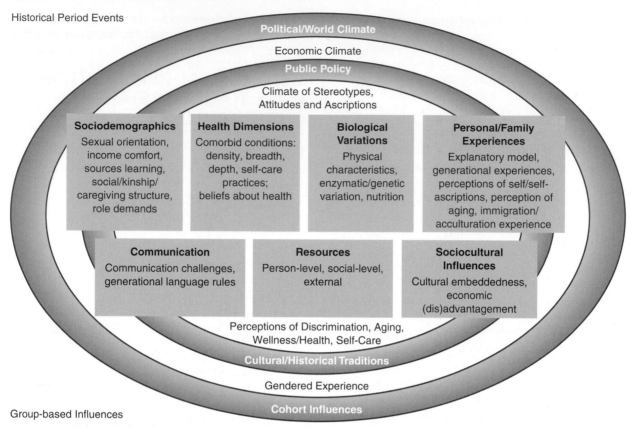

Historical Period Events

Group-based Influences

FIGURE 9-1 Ethno-Cultural Gerontological Nursing Model (ECGNM) *(Reprinted with permission from Phillips, L., et al. [2015].* Developing and proposing the Ethno-cultural Gerontological Nursing Model. *Journal of Transcultural Nursing, 26*(2), 121).

the strengths of individuals, families, and generational cohorts in the communities in which they live. By assessing various macrosocial and microsocial forces, family nurses working with individuals and families dealing with a chronic illness are better able to assess the needs and resources available to families.

A review of the ECGNM model demonstrates the interrelationship between macro- and microsocial influences, thus assisting nurses to assess how various forces intersect and influence individual, family, and ethnocultural groups' interpretation of health, illness, and life events in various phases of their lives (Figure 9-1). The top and lower frames of the model list various macrosocial factors, including historical, political, economic, and public policy factors, as well as the environmental climate and stereotypes. On the lower frame, group influences are outlined including discrimination, health and self-care, traditions, and how gender and cohort influences interact with historical events and the meaning ascribed to these

elements by individuals and family. Running across the center of the model are microsocial (personal) dimensions such as health, biological and generic variations, individual and family experiences, modes of communication, resources, and sociocultural factors that in turn influence the interpretation, responses, and ultimately health experiences and health outcomes. In an analysis of the utility of the ECGNM for working with diverse Latino populations, Ruiz, Phillips, Kim, and Woods (2016) demonstrated how health, culture, language, and aging intersect and contribute to health outcomes for this population.

As proposed, this ECGNM offers nurses an expanded framework for conducting a more comprehensive assessment of individuals and families. For nurses, the model provides an expanded framework for gaining insight on the strengths of a family, as well as exploring a wider net of creative resources that may be utilized by families living with a chronic illness or other challenging life event.

Rolland's Chronic Illness Framework

Chronic illnesses can be categorized by their traits, as outlined in Rolland's (1987) Chronic Illness Framework. This framework outlines how the following aspects come together in families and explains how families with similar illness stories adapt differently:

- Onset of the illness (acute or gradual)
- Level of disability resulting from the conditions (capacitating or incapacitating)
- Outcome of the illness (fatal, unpredictable, nonfatal)
- Stability of the disease (progressive, constant vs. relapsing symptoms)
- Time phase of the chronic illness (diagnosis, mid-illness, or terminal phase)

In Rolland's framework, the preceding elements of chronic illness affect family functioning, strengths, and vulnerabilities. For example, although some chronic conditions involve primary disabilities, such as those occurring from birth anomalies, other conditions, such as strokes, myocardial infarctions, secondary blindness, or kidney failure, are acquired disabilities resulting from lifestyle patterns or delayed or ineffective treatment of other conditions. The reaction and adaptation of the individual and family to a chronic condition differs according to whether the disability is considered on-time and expected versus off-time and unexpected. Likewise, although some people with chronic conditions have lives fraught with pain, depression, and mental or physical difficulties, others experience satisfying lives with only minimal difficulties.

Family Management Style Framework

The FMSF was designed to help nurses understand how families who have a child with a chronic condition integrate management of the chronic illness for the child into the everyday living needs and routines of the family as a whole. The original work on the development of the FMSF was conducted by Knafl and Deatrick in 1990. This original work has been refined over time to be one of the most significant longitudinal studies of a family assessment instrument. The assessment instrument helps nurses understand the needs of families who have children with specific chronic conditions, such as brain tumors (Deatrick et al., 2006), children undergoing palliative care at home (Bousso, Misko, Mendes-Castillo, & Rossato, 2012), and adolescents who have spina bifida (Wollenhaupt, Rodgers, & Swain, 2011). In addition to investigating families with children, Beeber and Zimmerman (2012) used the FMSF to increase understanding of challenges for families who have an older adult with dementia.

Understanding the family's responses to a chronic condition provides ways for family nurses to offer effective interventions to meet both the needs of the individual and family. In this framework, there are five family management styles: thriving, accommodating, enduring, struggling, and floundering. The management style a family adopts is based on how the family members define the situation, manage the situation, and perceive the consequences of the situation. In the FMSF, the parents each define what the child's chronic condition means for them individually and their family. Included in this definition is how the parents view the child. Does the parent view the child as a child who has a health issue that can be managed, or does the parent focus on the condition before the child and see the management of the health condition as tragic and difficult to manage? Influencing the definition are the parents' personal beliefs about the cause, the seriousness, the predictability, and the course of the condition. Another component in defining the illness is how disparate or similar the two parents' perceptions are on how they view their child, the condition, parenting philosophy, and overall approach to management. Table 9-1 briefly outlines the five family management styles.

Managing the child's condition is another piece to establishing a family's management style. To manage illness, parents combine their philosophy of parenting with their beliefs about their ability to parent a child with a chronic condition. One management approach may be that of being confident in their ability to parent and manage a chronic health condition. A second management approach may be when the parent views the child and situation as burdensome. A third approach is when parents feel they are inadequate in their abilities to parent a child with a chronic condition.

Another element of management concentrates on how the parent balances the ability to manage the chronic health condition with other aspects of

Table 9-1	Family Management Style Framework			

View of the Child

Thriving	Accommodating	Enduring	Struggling	Floundering
Parents view child from the lens of normalcy. They see the child as just as capable as other children. Their child has a chronic health condition that is incorporated into everyday life of the child and the family as a whole.	Parents usually see their child from the lens of normalcy and being capable of living everyday life.	Parents fluctuate in their view of the child between that of normalcy and tragic. Sometimes see them as capable and other times focus on vulnerabilities.	Parents are inconsistent in how they view the child relative to normalcy capabilities and vulnerabilities.	Parents have primarily a negative view of their child and see the situation as tragic. They see the child as not capable and as vulnerable.
Parents view life as normal and incorporate the management of the health condition into everyday life of the child and family.	Parents tend to view life as normal and caring for the child with a chronic condition as part of life.	Parents vary on how they view life between normal or focused on the management of the health condition.	Parents are variable in how they view everyday life, but primarily see it from a negative lens and the management overtakes their everyday life as a family.	Parents view the situation as a burden and have a sense of hatefulness about having to manage their child's chronic health condition.
Parents mutually agree in their viewpoints and definition of the child and their management approach.	Parents usually share the same viewpoints, definition, and management choices.	Parents usually share the same viewpoints, definition, and management choices.	Parents do not share the same viewpoints and definition and do not agree on management approaches, which creates much conflict between the parents.	Parents differ significantly on how they view the child, how they define the situation, and the management plan.

Management Behaviors

Thriving	Accommodating	Enduring	Struggling	Floundering
Parents are confident in their management abilities and incorporate management regimen into the life of the family. They are proactive in their problem-solving approach.	Mothers are confident in their abilities to manage the chronic condition. Fathers are not as confident as the mothers in their abilities to manage the illness. They are usually proactive in problem solving, but sometimes are reactive.	Parents are confident in their abilities but have the viewpoint of the management regimen as burdensome. They are usually proactive in problem solving, but sometimes are reactive.	Parental conflict is the overriding theme. Mothers see the management as burdensome. Fathers express more confidence in their ability to manage the chronic condition. Neither parent anticipates problems that are routine; therefore, they are reactive to problems.	Parents view the management regimen as burdensome. They feel inadequate and overwhelmed. They are reactive to problems and often are overwhelmed or put into crisis mode when a problem occurs.

Perceived Consequences

Thriving	Accommodating	Enduring	Struggling	Floundering
Parents view the child in the foreground and see the stress and hassles of the chronic health condition in the background. Parents have a positive outlook and create a new sense of "normal" for the family as a whole.	Parents usually place the child in the foreground and the stress and strains of the chronic condition in the background. In general, the parents have a positive outlook for the family as a whole.	Parents fluctuate in how they perceive the outcome and stress/strains of the chronic condition on the child and the family.	Mothers typically have a negative view of the situation and future outlook for the child. Fathers tend to be more positive in their view of the future for the child.	Parents have a negative outlook and view of the future. They worry that their future as parents will be less happy and limited.

family life. Parental management behaviors linked with chronic illness are often aligned with their ability to establish consistent and effective treatment routines. Parents may not be well prepared to handle the caregiving responsibilities shortly after receiving a chronic illness diagnosis; they might require some coaching (Sullivan-Bolyai, Knafl, Sadler, & Gilliss, 2004). Stable routines that allow for balance or equilibrium in daily life are essential for optimal disease management over time and through life course changes. For example, if the chronic illness requires dietary changes, family members must learn ways to balance personal food preferences and prior eating patterns with the medical needs of the ill member. Although specific management or routine activities may vary, a predictable and consistent routine is beneficial.

Finally, the ways parents focus attention on and perceive consequences of a chronic illness is an important consideration in determining the family's management style. Chronic illness can be viewed as a central feature of the family, an organizing focus, or a life aspect balanced with other responsibilities.

The FMSF not only identifies cognitive and behavioral family aspects, but also points to factors that may be predictive of family strengths or problems (Knafl & Deatrick, 1990, 2003; Knafl, Deatrick, & Havill, 2012). Nurses using this model are urged to consider the unique needs of individuals within the family, those of family members or member dyads, and the family as a whole. Family nurses should use this model as a guideline that outlines ways to think about how a family is responding to having a child with a chronic illness. Nurses can use this model to help think of interventions that may help a family in the management of the situation and adaptation to living with a chronic condition. Nurses need to understand member dynamics and family processes as they assess care needs, provide education, and offer counseling.

Family Health Model

Connections between chronic illness and families are tied to ideas suggested within the FHM (Denham, 2003). This ecological model provides a lens to consider the multiple traits, interactive processes, and life experiences that influence the health and illness of interacting and developing persons. Families and individual members have infinite ways to define themselves as they interact and exchange information with larger societal systems and institutions. The family household is the hub of action where members depart and return as individual members are nurtured and socialized. The FHM identifies member connections to each other and those beyond the household boundaries that have relevance to chronic illness. The FHM uses three domains—contextual, functional, and structural—in which nurses perform assessments, plan care, provide nursing actions, and evaluate outcomes. This model encourages nurses to consider ecological factors relevant to the family members and their household. Things such as the neighborhood, community resources, community demographics, political milieu, and social environment are factors that also influence families' responses to chronic illness and disease management, and affect outcomes.

Operational definitions suggest ways to describe the complex relationships among the biophysical and holistic aspects of a chronic illness and how these aspects affect family, health, and family health. In the FHM, health is defined as an adaptive state experienced by family members as they seek to optimize their well-being and wrestle with liabilities found within self, family, households, and the various environments where they interact throughout the life course (Denham, 2003). This definition guides nursing practice roles useful for family care when a member has a chronic illness. Even when one has a chronic illness, health can still be possible and well-being can be maximized. Family health suggests that member transactions occur through system and subsystem interactions, relationships, and processes that have the potential to maximize processes of becoming, enhance well-being, and capitalize on the household production of health. Families strive to achieve a state where members are content with themselves and one another. That is, family health includes the complex interactions of individuals, family subsystems, family, and the various contexts experienced over the life course. The household becomes the pivotal point for coping with health and family health needs.

Context

Family health is depicted with contextual, functional, and structural dimensions (Figure 9-2). The *contextual domain* includes all the environments where family members interact or have potential to be acted on, but also includes the characteristics or traits of the family (e.g., socioeconomic, educational attainment,

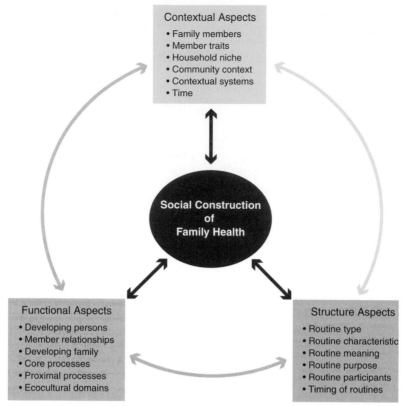

FIGURE 9-2 Contextual, Functional, and Structural Aspects of Family Care

extended kin relationships). The contextual domain is affected by the internal household environment (e.g., membership traits and qualities, culture, traditions, values) and external household environment (e.g., neighborhood, community, safety, larger society, historical period, political context). An ecological model helps nurses understand that nested life aspects can challenge or strengthen one's abilities to discern causes and outcomes. Over time, it is difficult to decipher the many powerful influencers; things overlap, intersect, and potentiate or negate important health factors.

The *family household* is a key family environment or context. The household refers to the physical structure(s), immediate neighborhood surroundings, material and nonmaterial goods, and tangible and intangible family resources of the members that live together. As people age, they often reflect back on many households where they lived and the various influences impressed upon self from those settings. The family context pervades all life aspects and affects personal interactions, values, attitudes, access to medical resources, and availability of support

systems, and has influence on individual and family health routines. For example, a family living in poverty or lacking adequate health care insurance is unlikely to have the same access to medical care as a more affluent family. A rural family with a long tradition of cultural values about health or illness might minimize physical symptoms and be slower to seek medical care than an urban family with great confidence in science and the abilities of health care providers.

Function

The *functional domain* refers to the individual and cooperative processes family members use as they interact with and engage one another during the life course. This domain includes individual factors (e.g., values, perceptions, personality, coping, spirituality, motivation, roles), family process factors (e.g., cohesiveness, resilience, individuation, boundaries), and member or family processes (e.g., communication, coordination, caregiving, control). These dynamic factors mediate the actions of individuals, family subsystems, and families as a whole as they seek to attain, sustain, maintain, and regain health. The core family functions of caregiving, celebration, change, communication, connectedness, and coordination alter as health and illness are faced; these are areas nurses can assess, plan nursing actions, and collaborate with family members to improve chronic illness outcomes (Denham, 2003).

The experiences linked with chronic illness can test and burden the functional capacities of the family and its members. In some families, individual and group strengths can be rallied to address pressing concerns, whereas other families might have member conflicts that threaten the capacities of effective disease management.

Structure

The contextual and functional domains are the situational and behavioral antecedents that family members use to construct family habits or patterns linked with health and illness outcomes. The third aspect of the FHM is referred to as the *structural domain*; it is composed of six categories of family health routines: self-care, safety and precautions, mental health behaviors, family care, illness care, and member caretaking. Each routine category is comprised of complex multimember habitual actions that form interactive patterns that describe the lived health and illness experiences of family households (Denham, 2003). *Family health routines* are relatively stable but still dynamic actions or habitual patterns that can be recalled, described, and discussed from individual and family perspectives. What might initially appear as random or chaotic patterns to an outsider may represent to family members regularity, purpose, and value of individual routines.

Although routines have unique qualities and involve all household members, some aspects of them change and evolve over time. This evolution can be a voluntary and intentional act or it can be a consequence of other things occurring in the family's life. Family members tend to maintain the integrity of routines as long as they are viewed as meaningful. New life situations can cause some adaptations to occur, however. Health routines tend toward steadfastness, but the diagnosis of a chronic condition that demands medical management and the availability of new or different support or resources (i.e., contextual factors) can challenge prior valued routines. During a chronic condition, if the family uses effective modes of communication, has abilities to share roles, and

is comprised of resilient personalities, it might be more capable of handling the changes than those lacking these qualities. Family members might be able to cooperate and deconstruct ineffective routines and reconstruct new ones better than a disorganized family or one where member conflict rules. Health and illness routines are ways family members can support or thwart the management of a chronic illness. Family-focused nurses who partner with individuals and families can collaborate with them to plan care, strategize ways to implement changes, and evaluate outcomes. The creation and stability of healthy family routines and lifestyles can be strengthened through cooperative efforts. Family health routines are dependent on the human and material resources needed for the individual and family to make needed changes. Functional perspectives give insight into ways families optimize health potentials and use resources to balance diverse and conflicting needs.

Well-Being

Family-focused nurses strive to assist individuals and families make the most of available resources to achieve health and well-being. *Well-being*, in the Family Health Care Model (Denham, 2003), is defined as a health state with actualized opportunities, minimized liabilities, and maximized resources. Well-being includes many dimensions, including biophysical, psychological, emotional, social, spiritual, and vocational. Well-being is achieved through accomplishment of family goals such as risk reduction, prevention, health maintenance, and self-actualization. Nurses aim to provide holistic care that enhances well-being and to partner with families to empower them when chronic illness is the concern. Nurses who provide family-focused care aid individuals and families to achieve their health goals. They also empower members to devise plans and identify ways to implement strategies, and evaluate whether goals are met. Nursing encounters become a means to target the household production of health, or holistically address related or potentially related health attributes or threats.

In chronic illness, family-focused care assists multiple family members to adapt, accommodate, and use household resources to achieve well-being for the entire family. Based on the FHM, family-focused nurses can use what are identified as core processes to consider family aspects relevant to chronic disease management and identify ways to empower individuals

Table 9-2	Core Family Processes and Chronic Illness		
Core Processes	**Definition**	**Areas of Concern**	
Caregiving	Concern generated from close intimate family relationships and member affections that result in watchful attention, thoughtfulness, and actions linked to members' developmental, health, and illness needs	Health maintenance Disease prevention Risk reduction Health promotion	Illness care Rehabilitation Acute episodic needs Chronic concerns
Cathexis	Emotional bonds between individuals and family that result in members' emotional and psychic energy investments into needs of the loved one	Attachment Commitment Affiliation Loss	Grief and mourning Normative processes Complicated processes
Celebration	Tangible forms of shared meanings that occur through family celebrations, family traditions, and leisure time that might be used to commemorate special times, days, and events; these times are often used to distinguish usual daily routines from special ones; they often occur across the life course and have special roles, responsibilities, and expectations	Culture Family fun Traditions Rituals	Religion Hobbies Shared activities
Change	A dynamic nonlinear process that demands an altered form, direction, and/or outcome of an expected identity, role, activity, or desired future	Control Meet expressed needs Meanings of change Contextual influences	Compare and contrast Similarities/differences Diversity
Communication	The primary ways children are socialized and family members interact over the life course about health beliefs, values, attitudes, and behaviors, and incorporate or apply health information and knowledge to illness and health concerns	Language Symbolic interactions Information access Coaching Cheerleading	Knowledge and skills Emotional needs Affective care Spiritual needs
Connectedness	The ways systems beyond the family household are linked with multiple family members through family, educational, cultural, spiritual, political, social, professional, legal, economic, or commercial interests	Partner relationships Kin networks Household labor Cooperation Member roles	Family rules Boundaries Tolerance for ambiguity Marginalization
Coordination	Cooperative sharing of resources, skills, abilities, and information within the family household, among members of extended kin networks, and larger contextual environments to optimize individual's health potentials, enhance the household production of health, maintain family integrity or wellness, and achieve family goals	Family tasks Problem solving Decision making Valuing Coping Resilience	Respect Reconciliation Forgiveness Cohesiveness System integrity Stress management

Source: Modified from Denham, S. A. (2003). *Family health: A framework for nursing.* Philadelphia, PA: F. A. Davis, with permission.

and families to meet care goals (Table 9-2). The FHM suggests a variety of ways to understand what happens when a member has a chronic illness from contextual, functional, and structural perspectives (Denham, 2003). Table 9-3 identifies several areas a family nurse might assess using this conceptual model.

PREVENTION OF CHRONIC ILLNESS THROUGH HEALTH PROMOTION

Many chronic conditions are preventable. Others, though not preventable, may be able to be delayed, thus ensuring more quality years of life. Prevention is an important factor to consider when understanding chronic illnesses. There are various prevention programs at the local, national, and federal levels. For example, the Robert Wood Johnson Foundation (2008) estimated that every $10 invested per person per year in community-based programs to increase physical activity, improve nutrition, and prevent smoking and other tobacco use could save the United States more than $16 billion annually within 5 years. For each dollar spent on the Safer Choice Program (a school-based HIV, other sexually transmitted infections, and pregnancy-prevention program), about $2.65 is saved on medical

Table 9-3	Assessment Using the Family Health Model
Categories to Assess	**Specific Areas Within Each Category**
Contextual	• Developmental stage
	• Family traits
	• Availability of health insurance
	• Access to care
	• Demographics (age, education, sex, employment)
	• Social support
	• Culture and ethnicity
	• Political, historical, and environmental factors
Functional	• Stressors
	• Coping skills
	• Family roles
	• Member responsibilities
	• Communication patterns
Structural	• Illness characteristics
	• Family organization or chaos
	• Routines established
	• Ability and willingness to alter routines

and social costs (Wang, Davis, Robin, Collins, & Coyle, 2000).

A 2010 CDC Communities Putting Prevention to Work (CPPW) program allocated $403 million to communities to reduce obesity, tobacco use, and exposure to secondhand smoke and saved $2.4 billion in direct medical costs (Soler et al., 2016). For example, a 35% tax on sugar-sweetened drinks ($0.45 per drink) led to a 26% decline in sales, with the conclusion that a 20% tax on these drinks would reduce obesity levels by 3.5% in U.S. adults (Mytton, Clarke, & Rayner, 2012).

In looking at gaps of current data collection systems, the IOM (2011a) suggests that individual and collective data are needed that help understand the continuum of prevention, disease progression, treatment options, and their outcomes. A troubling aspect of all surveillance efforts is that we have little to no information about family roles, inputs, or outcomes in the prevention or management of chronic illness.

Nonetheless, chronic illness is often linked to behavioral and environmental risk factors that could be effectively addressed through prevention programs.

For example, the increasing rates of obesity, leading to several chronic complications, could be prevented with changes in dietary and exercise behaviors and changes in our environment that encourage exercise. A 2017 Prevention and Wellness Trust Fund (PWTF) report highlights what has been accomplished when Massachusetts lawmakers created PWTF by directing health care funding into disease prevention programs. Hypertension screening increased from 58% to 62% with a projected 5-year, $2 to $3 million health care cost averted. In the 0- to 9-year-old population, asthma rates decreased from 13% to 10% in communities that instituted PWTF school-based education programs (Zotter, 2017). These changes could reduce the climbing chronic illness rates and reduce related complications through preventive care.

The IOM (2012) suggests taking a "health in all policies" approach to federal regulations, legislation, and policies that improve opportunity for health and physical function for those living with chronic illness. This report also recommends that community-based services available for persons with chronic disease align with health care services and insurance reform legislation. If such an approach were to be taken, legislators and those involved in policy writing would be more conscious about health risks and the ultimate costs resulting from legislative decisions. To curb the chronic illness epidemic, it is critical to initiate innovative approaches in the ways these diseases are prevented and managed now.

HELPING FAMILIES LIVE WITH CHRONIC ILLNESS

Family-focused nurses understand that when individuals have a chronic illness, whether they are young or old, family is always involved in the care. Family members influence decision making, engage in family planning, and play roles that positively and negatively influence disease management.

Some people manage their chronic illness without much difficulty or help from others, whereas others require a great amount of assistance and significant family involvement. Many need little medical care, but others require extensive medical services that may include care from special health care providers, regular treatments or testing, multiple medicines, or intense therapies. Life can be completely disrupted when confronting long-term or chronic illnesses that affect physical abilities, appearance, and independence.

Diminished endurance capacities; continual discomfort in physical, emotional, and social realms; and financial problems are just a few of the challenges that families face. New medical procedures, diagnostic tests, screening, and pharmacologic therapies have improved health and the ability to live with chronic conditions and an extended life span so families are living longer with chronic illness.

The IOM (2012) considered what it takes to live well with chronic illness and determined that it requires more than medical care and pharmacologic therapies. The IOM suggests that there are a variety of health determinants that affect the life course (i.e., biology, genes, behavior, coping responses, physical environment, sociocultural context, peers, and family). Some of these aspects are linked with learned behaviors, family households, and the communities where families live. One might classify persons as healthy, at risk, chronically ill, functionally limited, disabled, or nearing the end of life. These health outcomes are influenced by several factors; some are intrinsic or controlled by the individual, and some are beyond the individual and live in the larger society (e.g., environmental risks, public policy, population surveillance, media, public health, community organizations, health care, social values). This section focuses on how to work with families to support the person with the chronic illness to participate in his or her own self-management, and ways to help families adapt to living with a chronic illness and working with the family care provider.

Helping to Support Self-Management

Self-management is a crucial aspect to quality living and successful management of a chronic illness. Self-management includes self-efficacy, self-monitoring of illness, and symptom management that is conducted by self or as the person directs others to do for him or her (Richard & Shea, 2011). Self-management is both a process and an outcome of family nursing care. The "Self-Management Support for Canadians With Chronic Health Conditions" report (Health Council of Canada, 2012) outlines the following four recommendations to help the Canadian health care system support people living with chronic illness in a more systematic way (p. 7). These recommendations should be applied to those living with chronic illness regardless of country:

■ Create an integrated, system-wide approach to self-management support.

■ Enable primary health care providers to deliver self-management support as a routine part of care.
■ Broaden and deepen efforts to reach more Canadians who need self-management supports.
■ Engage patients and informal caregivers as a key part of any systematic approach.

Family nurses work with the individual and family to support self-management of the illness. For example, adolescents/young adults who engage in self-management at the time they transition from pediatrics to adult medical care are known to have improved health outcomes (Henry & Schor, 2015; van Staa, van der Stege, Jedeloo, Moll, & Hilberink, 2011).

Diabetes is a clear illustration. Diabetes self-management, similar to self-management for any chronic illness, entails adhering to a prescribed medical regimen and making lifestyle behavior changes. Most of these actions largely occur outside nurses' and other health care providers' observation. Self-management calls for integration of prescribed treatments into the daily experience. Self-management requires highly motivated individuals to follow medically prescribed treatments and protocols that may not be understood fully. This means that the individuals must have some confidence that their health care providers know what they are doing and trust that following these directions will improve one's quality of life.

The last several decades have produced a large body of research findings that suggest that self-efficacy is an important factor linked with a willingness to participate in specific behavior (Richard & Shea, 2011). Persons with higher self-efficacy are more likely to engage in more challenging tasks, set higher goals, and achieve them (Bandura, 1977). Individuals with the chronic illness and their family members will have different levels of self-efficacy and may differ in their level of readiness for change. Nurses who understand self-efficacy and readiness to change can use these concepts as they collaborate with families to set goals and plan strategies for meeting them. Nurses assess families on their perceptions and abilities to make the changes and then assist them as they agree on what changes they can make together. Nurses can explore family members' desires and confidence in their ability to alter lifestyle habits that might support their family member with a chronic illness to adhere to lifestyle changes, such as diet.

A nurse-led family conference might be a way for the nurse to share more information about why changes are needed, benefits that might be realized, and risks if no changes are made. Some agreement might arise on trying a few things differently each week and moving toward the goals by using small steps each week. Nurses should not be simply telling the family what needs to be done, but asking them what they need, identifying their concerns, and helping them identify what they believe will be a plan they are willing to achieve together.

Self-Management in the Older Adult Population

Although many older adults are able to manage their chronic illnesses without additional family or external support, some older adults have difficulty with self-management of their care independently and require additional support. One of the major aspects of nursing is to assist patients in self-management ability. Self-management of care is not disease management, but rather the ability of an individual to direct and maintain control over his or her chronic illness (Richard & Shea, 2011). A metasynthesis of the literature identified five factors affecting self-management of care: (1) personal/lifestyle characteristics, (2) health status, (3) resources, (4) environmental characteristics, and (5) health care system (Schulman-Green, Jaser, Park, & Whittemore, 2016). See Table 9-4 for a list of barriers and facilitators that affect self-management.

Personal/Lifestyle Characteristics

Personal/lifestyle choices are influenced by knowledge, beliefs, motivation, and life patterns. Individuals who successfully self-manage their care are knowledgeable about their medications and treatment plan, and are able to successfully apply that knowledge to their daily lives (Richard & Shea, 2011; Schulman-Green et al., 2016). Nurses who use motivational interviewing assist patients in their self-care.

In order for individuals to successfully self-manage their care, they need knowledge about their disease, medication/treatment, and how to apply that knowledge to their own care. When there is a lack of understanding about their chronic illness, medication, or treatment, self-management is impeded and individuals are less likely to be successful with self-management (Griva, Ng, Loei, Mooppil, McBain, & Newman, 2013; Henriques, Costa, & Cabrita, 2012; Ploughman et al., 2012).

Motivation and self-efficacy are intertwined and influenced by an individual's self-discipline or control over his or her personal choices. Stigma was identified as a motivating factor for individuals to take care of themselves to avoid additional health care services and accommodations (Audulv, Norbergh, Asplund, & Horsten, 2009; Ploughman et al., 2012).

Life patterns and the ability to establish a routine influence an individual's ability to successfully self-manage (Savoca & Miler, 2001). The ability to establish positive self-management routines is correlated with prior positive self-management experiences and subsequent positive health outcomes (Griva et al., 2013). Establishing daily routines is associated with improved self-management behaviors such as eating healthy and exercising. Conversely, unstructured or disrupted routines negatively affect self-management and the ability of individuals to establish routines (Griva et al., 2013). Additionally, aging is associated with impaired self-management primarily because of cognitive impairment and forgetting to take medication (Song et al., 2010).

Health Status

Health status and comorbidities influence self-management. Self-management is hampered by multiple factors including: severity of symptoms, length of illness, adverse effects from treatment including medication, complex treatment/medication regimens, and cognitive function (Schulman-Green et al., 2016). When combined with physical comorbidities, effective self-management is hampered (Griva et al., 2013; Ploughman et al., 2012). Using a family ecomap is an excellent instrument to help patients and families manage multiple illnesses.

Resources

Resources that influence self-management are financial resources, equipment, and psychosocial support (Lundberg & Thrakul, 2011; Newcomb, Mcgrath, Covington, Lazarus, & Janson, 2010). Limited financial resources impair an individual's ability to self-manage. Many individuals experiencing chronic illness frequently have multiple medications they need to take daily (polypharmacy). Additionally,

Table 9-4	Barriers and Facilitators to Self-Management	
Self-Management Behavior	**Barriers**	**Facilitators**
Personal/Lifestyle Characteristics	Lack of knowledge about: medication/treatment and chronic disease	Knowledge about: medication/ treatment and chronic disease
	Unstructured routine	Stigma as a motivator to improve health
	Disrupted routine	Motivation and self-efficacy
		Self-discipline
		Personal choices (self-determination)
		Establishing a routine
Health Status	Aging and associated cognitive impairment resulting in forgetting medication	
	Symptom severity	
	Length of illness	
	Adverse effects from treatment including medication	
	Complex treatment regimens	
	Complex medication regimens (i.e., frequent dosing or medication changes or complex regimen such as with warfarin), polypharmacy	
	Multiple comorbidities	
Resources		
Financial	Lack of insurance, underinsured, or limited insurance coverage	Financial support from family and friends
	Limited financial resources	Political systems that do not discriminate
	High cost of medication	
	High cost of healthy foods	
	Cost of supplies	
	Loss of employment	
Equipment	Internet	Internet
	Inability to obtain assistive devices such as glucometers and pill boxes either because of cost or lack of awareness	
	Inability to obtain equipment	
Psychosocial	Lack of support (family, parental, peer)	Perceived positive support (family, parental, peer)
	Isolation	Access/participation in support groups
Environmental Characteristics		
Home	• Different dietary preferences among family members	
	• Conflict among family members over food served in the home	
	• Competing demands of family members experiencing chronic illness	

Table 9-4	Barriers and Facilitators to Self-Management *(cont.)*	
Self-Management Behavior	**Barriers**	**Facilitators**
Work	• Time and schedule constraints impairing ability to self-manage diet, exercise, and medication • Food environment while at work (short lunch break, limited access to healthy foods)	
Community	• Lack of transportation to medical appointments or to the gym • Unhealthy food choices when dining out at restaurants	
Health Care System Access	Lack of access to: • Specialists • Nursing care • Self-management programs • Alternative therapy	Access to: • Specialists, nursing care, self-management programs, alternative therapy • Educational resources outside health care system (information from books, radio, brochures)
Navigating system/ continuity of care	• Long wait lines for appointments • Unreturned phone messages • Confusing communication with clinic staff • Multiple health care specialists • Seeing different providers at every appointment hampered obtaining prescriptions • Inconsistent advice from providers	
Relationships with providers	• Avoiding conflict by not being honest • Limiting communication with provider • Language barriers (not speaking or reading English)	• Positive patient-provider relationship where the patient had time to share concerns with provider • Patient trusted provider • Patient felt supported by provider • Empathy from the provider • Collaborative approach where patient and provider problem solved together • Shared goals • Adequate time to discuss changes in plan of care • Adequate time for the patient to ask questions and obtain feedback • Confidence in provider's competence important when following provider recommendation • Good communication by provider and avoiding use of medical jargon or technical language • Having regularly scheduled visits • Provider recommending culturally sensitive self-management strategies

Source: Adapted from Schulman-Green, D., Jaser, S., Park, C., & Whittemore, R. (2016). A metasynthesis of factors affecting self-management of chronic illness. *Journal of Advanced Nursing, 72*(7), 1469–1489.

older adults and the chronically ill are often on a limited, fixed income and are forced to choose between refilling their medications or choosing to pay for housing, electricity, food, and transportation (Newcomb et al., 2010; Vest et al., 2013).

Equipment, specifically the Internet, is both a barrier and facilitator in self-management. The Internet provides a wealth of information to individuals and can connect them with peer support and information about health conditions (Brand, Claydon-Platt, McColl, & Bucknall, 2010; Wellard, Rennie, & King, 2008). Conversely, the Internet provides an overwhelming amount of health information that may not be from reliable and credible sources, causing the patient undue stress (Balfe, 2009). It is the role of the nurse to help patients and families use credible Web sites in their search for current information.

Psychosocial support can be perceived as a barrier and facilitator in self-management. Psychosocial support was perceived as positive and influential in self-management when received from peers or partners (Brand et al., 2010; Henriques et al., 2012). A lack of partner support was perceived as a barrier to self-management, especially with regard to new dietary changes. Social isolation (lack of support) is also a barrier to self-management (De Brito-Ashurst et al., 2011). Support groups with members experiencing the same health condition was a facilitator to self-management and provided opportunities for individuals to connect with communities and resources (Lowe & McBride-Henry, 2012; Rasmussen, Ward, Jenkins, King, & Dunning, 2011). Many families connect with support groups online, especially when the family caregiver finds it difficult to get out of the home. Nurses have an important role in connecting patients and family members with support groups to attend in person or online.

Environmental Characteristics

Environmental characteristics of home, work, and community influence self-management. Barriers affecting self-management in the home include different dietary preferences among family members, differences/personal preferences among family members over food served in the home, and competing demands of family members experiencing health problems (Orzech, Vivian, Torres, Armin, & Shaw, 2013; Wu, Juang, & Yeh, 2011). Work barriers identified include time and schedule constraints that impair the ability to self-manage diet, exercise, and medication (Lundberg & Thrakul, 2011; Oftedal, Karlsen, & Bru, 2010). Community barriers to self-management are complex and multifaceted. Lack of transportation to medical appointments or to the gym were identified as barriers as well as limited or unhealthy food choices served at restaurants and convenience stores (Lundberg & Thrakul, 2011; Pascucci, Leasure, Belknap, & Kodumthara, 2010). One technique used by family nurses is to help patients and families conduct a needs assessment.

Health Systems

Health system factors that influence self-management include access to health care, ability to navigate the health system, continuity of care, and relationship with providers. Access (or lack of access) to specialists, nursing care, self-management programs, and alternative therapies were perceived as essential elements of self-management (Brand et al., 2010; Lundberg & Thrakul, 2011; Ploughman et al., 2012). Additionally, educational resources outside the health care system (information from books, radio, brochures) was a facilitator (Brand et al., 2010; Lundberg & Thrakul, 2011). If at all possible, the nurse working with the family should connect the patient and the family with a nurse navigator (see Chapter 1), whose role is to assist families that have multiple health care providers.

Barriers for individuals experiencing chronic illness include navigating a complex health care system and continuity of care. Additionally, long wait lines/times for appointments, unreturned phone messages, and confusing communication with clinic staff were identified as barriers to effective self-management (Brand et al., 2010; Newcomb et al., 2010). Inconsistent continuity of care with multiple providers/specialists, inconsistent recommendations from providers, and difficulty obtaining prescriptions from different providers was identified as a barrier to care and self-management (Brand et al., 2010; Newcomb et al., 2010).

Relationships with health care providers and the influence on self-management are seen in Box 9-1. Too often, persons with chronic conditions see numerous clinicians who order treatments without considering how they might affect the whole family. Individuals and families benefit from coordinated care; this means providing treatments and medical visits in ways that integrate services and relevant

BOX 9-1

How Health Care Providers Influence Self-Care Management for Chronic Conditions

Positive Influences*

- Positive patient-provider relationship
- Patient trusts the provider
- Patient feels supported by the provider
- Provider expresses empathy
- Collaborative approach to care and shared goals/decision making
- Adequate time for the patient to ask questions and obtain feedback
- Confidence in a provider's competence when following provider recommendations
- Provider uses good communication skills and avoids medical jargon and technical language
- Regularly scheduled visits

- Provider recommends culturally sensitive self-management strategies

Negative Influences

- Conflict by not being honest or limiting communication with a provider [†]
- Language barriers (not speaking or reading English) [‡]
- Inadequate time to discuss changes in plan of care [‡]

*Brand et al., 2010; JoWu, Chang, & McDowell, 2008; Lundberg & Thrakul, 2011; Ploughman et al., 2012; Vest et al., 2013; Wu et al., 2011

[†] Lundberg & Thrakul, 2011; Newcomb et al., 2010

[‡] De Brito-Ashurst et al., 2011; Griva et al., 2013

communication among those providing care. Goals of coordinated care include improving health outcomes, identifying risks or problems early, avoiding crises, and ensuring cost-effectiveness of service delivery. Poorly coordinated care has risks for preventable health complications, conflicts among health care providers, increased stress for the individuals and their families, unnecessary hospitalizations, added expenses, and even death. Persons who experience even a single chronic illness can receive conflicting information, numerous diagnoses, or multiple medications by different health care providers. Nurses are in positions where they can facilitate care management and help individuals and family members sort out the conflicting information or directions in developing a family-focused management plan. By helping the family to develop a management plan, the nurse empowers the family and the person with the chronic illness to participate in and control self-care, with the goal of improving health outcomes for all members of the family.

Family Adaptation

Living with chronic illness is described by Arestedt, Persson, and Benzein (2013) as an ongoing process of adaptation, co-creating ways for the family members, both individually and as a family, to achieve a sense of well-being. By using this in-depth research methodology (i.e., phenomenological hermeneutic analysis), nurses can work with families to help them adjust to everyday living by developing a new rhythm

of adaptation. (Hermeneutic phenomenology is a qualitative research methodology whose basic tenet is that our most fundamental and basic experiences of the world have meaning. Phenomenology is a method to study the individual and how the individual ascribes meaning to an experience.)

With many chronic illnesses, the family is continually shifting between illness being the primary focus of the family and wellness being the primary view of the family. For example, when there is an exacerbation of the illness that requires the family member to be hospitalized, the family is reminded that the illness is present and needs attention. At other times, the family is focused on the wellness of everyone by, for instance, having family dinner together once a week. Co-creation of ways the family adapts and flows with this movement allows for some overlapping of these two family situations (Patterson, 2002). Nurses working with families living with chronic illness who understand this process of evolving family adaptation empower families to move from a viewpoint of "victim" of circumstances to a viewpoint of "creator" of circumstances (Arestedt et al., 2013; Patterson, 2002).

Nursing Interventions to Assist Families Living With Chronic Illness

One person's chronic condition has great potential to influence the lives of many others. Those living with a family member with a chronic disability can become fatigued by the constant vigilance required to perform normal everyday activities of daily living

(ADLs) and the stress of uncertainty (Hummel, 2013b). This fatigue is influenced by the volume of help required, the emotional strain that accompanies the daily hassles, and the relationship strain of constantly giving to another. The following nursing interventions assist the family with adaptation to living with chronic illness.

- *Co-creating a context for living with illness:* When families are confronted with the reality of living with a family member having a chronic illness, they spend time learning how to develop different ways of accomplishing the tasks of the family and meet the needs of the family members. They accomplish this through discussion of the situation. After this initial adjustment and the establishment of how to maintain daily functioning, families report that the illness and situation are not always on their minds.
- *Communicating the illness within and outside the family:* Families learn to balance discussion about the illness, the situation, and the future with chronic illness with other life events for the individual family members and the family as a whole.
- *Co-creating alternative ways for everyday life:* Families learn to operate at a slower pace than before chronic illness. Families note that they are more focused on the present as there is an ever-present awareness of an uncertain future.
- *Altering relationships:* The members of the family develop or adapt their relationships to include chronic illness as they have to get to know each other in a different way. In some situations, family members are interacting more often than before the onset of the chronic illness. In other situations, families report being stronger and pulling together more when the illness has exacerbations.
- *Changing roles and tasks:* All roles in the family require adjustment when living in the midst of chronic illness. The family struggles to reestablish a balance in getting the needs of the family accomplished.

One aspect of family nursing that is crucial to helping these families is assisting the family members to adjust to new roles, such as caregiver and care receiver. Nurses can help families explore who does what role in the family and how to use resources to help the family function well by using outside resources

to fill some of the family roles. See Chapter 5 for more detail about how to work with families about role negotiation.

Social Support

Social support can be categorized into four types of supportive behaviors: emotional, instrumental, informational, and appraisal (House, 1981). The family's capacity to mobilize social support to manage crisis periods and chronic stressors related to a family member's health condition contributes to the well-being of all family members (Bellin & Kovacs, 2006). Table 9-5 provides examples of the four types of social support for families who have a member with a chronic illness condition.

Community contexts, such as the neighborhood, school, or church, support the family's development of positive values and foster strengths (Bellin & Kovacs, 2006). Social capital is a concept that can be useful in understanding the community context of health for those with chronic illness and their families. Similar to social support, social capital is about resources that come from relationships with other people and institutions. Social capital includes features of social life, such as norms, networks, and trust, that enable people to act together toward shared objectives (Putnam, 1996). Looman (2006) defines social capital in terms of investments in relationships that facilitate the exchange of resources. For families who have a chronically ill family member, social capital is especially relevant.

Unique community building activities are now possible through the Internet through social media such as support *logging*. Huh, Liu, Neogi, Inkpen, and Pratt (2014) analyzed 72 vlogs on YouTube by users diagnosed with HIV, diabetes, or cancer and found that this unique video medium allows for intense and enriched personal disclosures to viewers, which in turn leads to strong community building activities. They found vlogs allowed small groups to form, providing implications on how future technologies can provide support for chronic illness management.

When an individual has a chronic illness, the members of the family (particularly caregivers) are required to engage with numerous professionals and institutions in the process of managing the condition and exchanging resources. The family benefits when a mutual investment exists in their relationships with nurses, physicians, teachers, other families, and neighbors. For example, a mother might invest in

Table 9-5	Helpful Support for Families With a Chronically Ill Member		
Type of Support	**Definition**	**Activities**	**Example From Case Studies**
Emotional support	Provision of love, caring, sympathy, and other positive feelings	Listening Offering commendations Being present	The nurse working with the Yates family commends them by saying, "I am impressed by the commitment that your family has made to making life as 'normal' as possible for Chloe and her siblings."
Instrumental support	Tangible items, such as financial assistance, goods, or services	Assisting with household chores (e.g., laundry) Providing respite care Providing transportation Assisting with physical care	Devon's parents offer to take Chloe's siblings for a weekend, providing respite for the family and giving the siblings an opportunity to share time with their grandparents.
Informational support	Helpful advice, information, and suggestions	Sharing resources (e.g., books, Web sites, provider names) Educating family members on the health needs of the ill family member Informational support groups	Sarah's brother David, who also has type 2 diabetes, recommends a Web site that provides healthy recipes for individuals with diabetes.
Appraisal support	Feedback given to individuals to assist them in self-evaluation or in appraising a situation	Reviewing daily logs Sharing written feedback from providers (e.g., laboratory results)	The nutritionist provides appraisal support to Sarah during her regular appointments, offering feedback on how Sarah is doing with her lifestyle and dietary changes.

her relationship with her child's teachers by providing them with information about her child's health condition, or by helping the teacher understand the child's unique learning style. The teacher, in return, might invest in a relationship with the child's family by scheduling additional parent-teacher conference sessions or by learning more about the child's specific health condition. The benefit of this investment in the family-school relationship, where the common goal is the success of the student, is an exchange of resources. The benefit of this investment may also reach other students and families if this pattern of communication becomes a norm in the school, and if the general level of trust among parents and teachers increases. In this way, social capital facilitates the family's ability to acquire emotional, instrumental, informational, and appraisal support in many contexts.

CAREGIVING IN FAMILIES

A caregiver, sometimes referred to as an informal caregiver, is an unpaid individual such as a spouse, partner, family member, friend, or neighbor who is involved in assisting with ADLs and with the management of an illness (Family Caregiver Alliance, 2016). According to the National Alliance for Caregiving (2016) approximately 43.5 million caregivers in the United States have provided unpaid care to an adult or child in the last 12 months. This unpaid labor force is estimated to be at least $306 billion annually. Evidence shows that most caregivers are not well prepared for their role and may be providing assistance with very little support. Caregivers are at risk of experiencing emotional, mental, and physical health problems themselves from the strains of caring for family members. Higher levels of stress, anxiety, and depression are common among family members who are caring for a member with chronic illnesses. Studies of caregivers show that ethnic minority caregivers provide more care to families than their white counterparts and report worse physical health than white caregivers (McCann et al., 2000). Additional findings indicate Asian American caregivers made less use of professional support services than other groups of caregivers. Nurses have an important role identifying the caregiver, and providing support and effective education when working with families who are living with a chronic illness.

Family Caregiving

Family caregiving is a crucial role that provides support for those living with chronic illness. Several chapters in this book touch on family caregivers caring for family members with chronic illness. Glasdam, Timm, and Vittrup (2012) reviewed

32 studies of professional interventions with family caregivers. Few studies targeted the caregivers of family members with cancer, cardiovascular disease, or stroke. They concluded that health care providers lack knowledge about the effects of interventions on caregivers. There is a need for accurate descriptions of the intensified interventions used with caregivers and the outcomes achieved in order to identify the benefits of nursing actions for caregivers. It is clear, however, that soon after the diagnosis of a chronic illness of a family member, caregivers must become proficient in many areas, including managing the illness, coordinating resources, maintaining the family unit, and caring for self. Nurses assisting families can incorporate the following educational and counseling needs into a treatment plan, making clear who is responsible for what in the family:

- Monitoring conditions and behaviors
- Interpreting normal and expected behaviors from different and serious ones
- Providing hands-on care
- Making decisions
- Developing care routines
- Problem solving
- Teaching self-care management
- Identifying resources to assist with respite care

Child Caregiving for an Adult

One population that is growing around the world is that of young children providing care for a chronically ill adult. In the United States, there are approximately 1.3 to 1.4 million child caregivers who are between the ages of 8 and 18 (Hunt, Levine, & Naiditch, 2005). The following list provides an estimated number of children providing care for adult family members in countries or commonwealths of the United Kingdom (Becker, 2007; Clay, Connors, Day, Gkiza, & Aldridge, 2016):

- *England:* There are nearly 5 million caregivers; of these, 166,000 are children ages 5 to 17.
- *Scotland:* There are 657,000 caregivers in Scotland; of these, 16,701 are children.
- *Wales:* There are 340,745 people who are caregivers; of these, 11,000 are children.
- *Northern Ireland:* There are 185,066 people who are caregivers; of these, 2300 are children.

In Australia, it is estimated that there are almost 2.7 million caregivers; of these, about 72,000 were younger than 15 years of age (Australian Bureau of Statistics, 2013). A 2010 Canadian high school study of 483 ethnically diverse students in grades 8 through 12 found that 12% of youth between the ages of 12 and 17, with a mean age of 14 years, self-identify as "Young Carers" (Marshall & Stainton, 2010). In response to a rising number of young caregivers, Canada created an action task force to investigate the invisible population of the young caregiver population and its needs (Bednar et al., 2013). In a similar study in the United States, Bridgeland, DiIulio, and Morison (2006) found that a third of high school dropouts (32%) said they had to get a job and make money, 26% said they dropped out because they became a parent, and 22% said they had to care for a family member. Many of these young people reported doing reasonably well in school and had a strong belief that they could have graduated if they had stayed in school. Childhood caregiver statistics in the United States identified by Hunt et al. (2005) are noted in the following list:

- Three in ten child caregivers are ages 8 to 11 (31%), and 38% are ages 12 to 15. The remaining 31% are ages 16 to 18.
- Child caregivers are almost evenly balanced by gender (male 49%, female 51%).
- Caregivers tend to live in households with lower incomes than noncaregivers, and they are less likely than noncaregivers to have two-parent households (76% vs. 85%).

There are both negatives and positives to being a young family caregiver. The positive effects are that they report feeling appreciated for their help and that they like helping their family member (Hunt et al., 2005). Negative outcomes from assuming the family caregiver role at a young age are reported in the literature, however. Young caregivers between 8 and 11 years old are more likely than noncaregivers to feel at least some of the time that no one loves them (Hunt et al., 2005). A 2012 study found significant effects on caregiving teens' mental health, specifically, significantly higher risk for anxiety and depression (Cohen, Greene, Toyinbo, & Siskowski, 2012). Nurses should be aware that there are several young caregiver support groups that are offered online and there are camps offered for these children where they can have some carefree time away from family responsibility. Family nurses should inquire about the involvement of children and teens in caring for family members with chronic illness.

The population of young caregivers remains an invisible population and the exact numbers are unknown. Some reasons this caregiver population is growing include the following:

- Decreasing family size
- Geographical dispersion of families
- High divorce rates
- Increasing number of single parents
- Multiple marriages and reconstituted families
- In African countries, it may be related to the number of adult deaths caused by AIDS

These students and young caregivers live a stressful life that has many more responsibilities when compared with peers. In addition, the young caregivers are found to have significantly more anxiety and depression and less satisfaction when compared with noncaring age-related peers (Cohen et al., 2012). Caregiving has a negative influence on the emotional well-being of youth with dual student-caregiver roles (Cohen et al., 2012).

Countries in the United Kingdom have several major national laws that provide for a wide range of services and programs that include financial allocations to assess vulnerable children; provide community- and home-based services for care recipients, families, and youths; and have several support programs and resources for youth caregivers. The United States has no national policies or programs to support this vulnerable population. The American Association of Caregiving Youth (2015) was established by Connie Siskowski, a nurse. This is the only program in the United States that addresses any concerns about this vulnerable population. She designed an after-school program to help these young caregivers meet others living in similar situations, learn how to provide care for their family member safely, and learn how to seek help or resources (American Association of Caregiving Youth, 2015). This nurse also designed a week-long onsite summer camp for these young caregivers to attend so they could experience a normal childhood event and get away from the stress of everyday caregiving.

As this population of vulnerable caregivers continues to grow, one role of the family nurse is to be alert and recognize when a young child is providing care for an adult in the family. When this situation is present, the nurse should work to find supports for this caregiver and remember that the caregiver is also a child or adolescent who has normal developmental needs in addition to this caregiving family role.

Families Caring for Children Living With a Chronic Illness

According to the *National Survey of Children With Special Health Care Needs 2009–2010* (Data Resource Center for Child and Adolescent Health, 2012), 11.2 million children from 0 to 17 years of age have SHCN, which translates to one in five American households. Children with SHCN have a wide range of conditions and risk factors that underlie many shared health conditions. Based on survey results, the six conditions that require the most average hours of caregiving at home each week are: (1) cerebral palsy, (2) muscular dystrophy, (3) cystic fibrosis, (4) traumatic brain injury or concussion, (5) intellectual disability, and (6) epilepsy or seizure (Romley, Shah, Chung, Elliott, Vestal, & Schuster, 2017). SHCN who are most likely to receive the greatest amount of family care at home are children with severe chronic conditions, age 5 or younger, Hispanic families, and families that live below the poverty level.

Children with SHCN are similar to typical children in many ways: They are actively growing and developing, enjoy playing and being with peers, and thrive in cohesive family environments. Children with chronic conditions, however, have limitations that affect daily lives and contribute to challenges uniquely different than peers without chronic conditions. More than half of the children with SHCN report that they experience four or more functional disabilities that are related to everyday living, such as respiratory problems, eating problems, vision issues, difficulty using their hands, and communication issues.

Out-of-pocket health care costs that exceed $250 are often perceived by the family as burdensome, and even lower amounts affect families with lower socioeconomic status (Lindley & Mark, 2010). Twenty percent of families of children with SHCN report that they spend 2 to 7 hours a week providing health care for the child at home and 14% spend more than 11 hours a week. Caring for the child at home is associated with a significant increase in the odds of having a family member reducing or quitting employment outside the home because of the child's health care needs (Looman et al., 2009).

Families with children with SHCN have many needs, caregiving and otherwise. Studies have shown that mothers of chronically ill children often have greater levels of distress than fathers, a concern

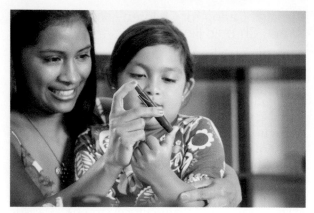

© iStock.com/Fertnig

thought to be related to the greater care demands placed on the mothers (Spilkin & Ballantyne, 2007). It is also not unusual for parents to differ in their perceptions about the impact of the chronically ill child on the family as a whole and on the marital relationship. Although mothers may find that caregiving demands influence their role performance, fathers may perceive the impact most in their expression of feelings and emotions (Rodrigues & Patterson, 2007). A study of 173 parent dyads of children with chronic conditions found that mothers' marital satisfaction was influenced more than fathers' by perceptions about the effects of their child's condition on the family (Berge, Patterson, & Rueter, 2006). Parents' perceptions of the negative effects of the child's chronic condition were measured in terms of family social strain, role strain, and emotional strain. If parents differed in perceptions about the effects of the illness on the family or marital relationship, an increase in stress and frustration resulted. Nurses can assist couples to identify differences in perception between parents, and facilitate discussions about the effects on roles and the benefits of sharing caregiving tasks (Berge et al., 2006; Spilkin & Ballantyne, 2007).

Family-focused care involves active participation between families, nurses, and other health care providers. Family-focused care supports partnering or collaborative relationships that value and recognize the importance of family traditions, family beliefs, and family management styles. When considering the general population of children with SHCN, approximately 35% of them received care that lacked one or more of the essential components of family-centered care (USDHHS, Health Resources and Services Administration, Maternal and Child Health Bureau, 2008).

In general, families raising children with chronic illnesses face the joys and challenges that most typical families face, and are as unique and varied as families of typically developing children (Drummond, Looman, & Phillips, 2012). These families want their children to be happy, have a high quality of life, grow, and develop into caring adults who can live independently and contribute to society. These families face additional stressors, and many researchers acknowledge that the children and parents in these families who care for their children at home are at increased risk for stress-related health conditions and psychosocial problems (Barlow & Ellard, 2006; Berge et al., 2006; McClellan & Cohen, 2007; Meltzer & Mindell, 2006; Mussatto, 2006). Box 9-2 provides a list of stressors likely to be experienced by families caring for a chronically ill child. Despite the risks for problems, however, most children with chronic conditions and their families, including siblings, demonstrate incredible resilience and capacity for finding positives amidst the challenges.

One approach to helping these families is to help them understand the concept of normalization. Normalization is a lens through which families of children with chronic conditions focus on normal aspects of their lives and deemphasize those parts of life made more difficult by chronic conditions (Bowden & Greenberg, 2010; Protudjer, Kozyrskyi, Becker, & Marchessault, 2009; Rehm & Bradley, 2005). The following five attributes of normalization for families of children with chronic conditions offer foundational knowledge for nurses working with such families (Deatrick, Knafl, & Murphy-Moore, 1999):

- Acknowledge the chronic condition and its potential to threaten their lifestyle.
- View all the management of the chronic illness as just normal daily activities in the family.
- Engage in parenting behaviors and routines that are consistent with a normalcy lens.
- Develop treatment regimens that are consistent with normalcy.
- Interact with others based on a view of the child and family as normal.

Although normalization is a useful conceptual and coping strategy for many families of children

BOX 9-2

Potential Stressors When Raising a Child With Chronic Health Conditions

Following are potential stressors for those raising a child with a chronic health condition:

- Care regimen in meeting daily caregiving demands
- Grief, loss of anticipated child events or activities
- Financial and employment strains
- Uncertainty about future
- Access to specialty services
- Reallocation of family assets (e.g., emotional, time, financial)
- Recurrent crises and crisis management
- Foregone leisure time and social interactions
- Social isolation because of stigmatizing policies and practices
- Challenges in transporting disabled children (e.g., when architectural and other barriers restrict their inclusion)
- Physiological stress of caregiving
- Fragmented health care systems
- Planning for additional space if health-related equipment is required (i.e., wheelchairs)
- Multiple medical, home health care appointments
- Respite care needs for caregivers

with chronic conditions, in families whose children have both complex physical and developmental disabilities, normalization as a goal may be neither possible nor helpful (Rehm & Bradley, 2005). When developmental delays compound the effects of a child's physical chronic conditions, a family's ability to organize and manage its daily life is affected significantly. In this case, parents often recognize normal and positive life aspects, acknowledge the profound challenges faced by their family, and accept a "new normal" (Rehm & Bradley, 2005). This capacity to normalize adversity and to define challenging experiences as manageable and surmountable fosters family resilience.

Families with members with chronic conditions, especially those whose conditions are complicated and require care from multiple specialists, often spend a great deal of time interfacing with multiple specialists and systems. For example, a family who has a child with Down syndrome may require regular visits for cardiac, ophthalmological, developmental, and immunological evaluations; physical and occupational therapy; and orthopedic assessments. In addition, parents typically spend a significant amount of time and energy advocating for their child within the school system, attending individualized educational program meetings, meeting with academic support professionals, and coping with worries about what

is occurring when the child is out of sight (National Association for Down Syndrome, 2012).

In addition, children with chronic conditions still need well-child care similar to those without such an illness. Further, these children are susceptible to other infectious diseases or risks for injuries. It is important for children with chronic conditions to receive regular health maintenance visits with a primary health care provider for anticipatory guidance, routine illness, and injury prevention discussions. Parents of children with chronic conditions expect to discuss illness concerns during the well-child care visit. Many primary care providers report that they are coordinating care in their practices. However, evidence indicates that approaching coordination that involves distributing tasks across personnel is not an effective approach (Looman et al. 2013). Instead, research indicates coordinating care with nurses who have content expertise, interpersonal skills, and knowledge of systems is essential to the success of care coordination as an important intervention for SHCN and their families (Looman et al., 2013). For parents of children with SHCN and other parents, as more illness topics were discussed, more prevention topics were also discussed.

Whether the chronically ill person is a child or an adult, family members require useful information that can be applied directly to real family needs. A trusting environment must exist, with easy information exchange, communication directed toward meeting individual and family needs, and respect.

Families want information that will help them provide adequate care for their member with chronic illness and that will help them to anticipate future needs. A decade ago, Ray (2003) noted that excellent informational resources are available, but are not used by families because professionals assume that someone else has provided the family with the information. Parents' and others' needs for information and support change over time as they move through phases of the illness and the family life cycle (Nuutila & Salantera, 2006). At the time of diagnosis, parents want clear and consistent information, and possibly a more directive approach from the provider. For example, when a child with Down syndrome is born, the parents may want to know the immediate implications for the child's health and how that will affect their ability to care for the child at home. As the child grows older and the family gains experience in the care of the child, parents may want a less directive approach from the provider and more of a mutual exchange of information in a collaborative partnership (Nuutila & Salantera, 2006). The nurse who encounters this family at a 3-year well-child examination, for example, should acknowledge the parents' intimate understanding of the child, her reactions to the environment, and her unique needs during the clinical encounter. At this point, the most helpful advice from the nurse is likely anticipatory guidance and planning for entry into the school system. Nurses must recognize that individual and family needs will greatly differ for this child as she becomes 16, 28, or 46 years of age.

Adolescents With Chronic Illness Transition to Adult Services

Transition of care issues have been discussed in the health care industry for decades, but little attention has been allotted to studying and resolving transition problems. Transitions occur in health care in a variety of ways; for example, when a patient moves from one health care provider to a different provider, when a person is sent home from the hospital, when a person who lives in a nursing home needs to be hospitalized, or when a person must switch

from private pay to being on Medicaid. Basically, a transition is any time there is a major change in the health care management.

Transition of care issues for adolescents, who are required to switch from pediatric health care providers to the adult providers of care, is a global health care problem (Kralik, Visentin, & van Loon, 2011; Lugasi, Achille, & Stevenson, 2011; Sonneveld, Strating, van Staa, & Neiboer, 2013; Steinbeck, Brodie, & Towns, 2007, 2008; Wong et al., 2010). Family nurses are in a prime position to address transition issues because they work closely with families and children who have chronic illness (Jalkut & Allen, 2009). As survival rates have improved with many children who live with a chronic illness, this aspect of family nursing requires even more focus. The transition is not just about the medical care from a pediatric physician to an adult specialist. The transition also needs to include psychosocial, educational, cultural beliefs, and vocational needs of the young adult. It also needs to consider the parents who, up until that point, have orchestrated the management of the illness, communicated with the health care team, made appointments, and interfaced with school. The transition period causes anxiety for the whole family and involves leaving long-term health care provider relationships, developmental psychosocial stressors of Adolescents, uncertainty about health insurance coverage and issues of the Health Insurance Portability and Accountability Act (HIPAA) relative to parental knowledge, and involvement in the care process and communication (Peter, Fork, Ginsburg, & Schwarz, 2009).

What compounds the difficulty of this transition period for the family and the individual members is the fact that the adult health providers who are assuming care of the young adults with chronic illness often lack understanding of normal adolescent growth and development (Bowen, Henske, & Potter, 2010). This lack of understanding on the part of adult health care providers was recognized as a problem by the American Academy of Pediatrics (2011).

Osterkamp, Costanzo, Ehrhardt, and Gormley (2013) developed an online educational program for nurses about the transition of care for adolescent patients with chronic illness. The modules in the program are HIPAA, family-centered care and its core concepts relative to transition of care of the adolescent patient, and healthy versus chronically ill adolescent development (including information

BOX 9-3

Principles of Successful Transition to Adult-Oriented Health Services

The following are principles of successful transition from child-to-adult-oriented health care:

1. Health care services for adolescents and young people need to be developmentally appropriate and inclusive of the young person's family where appropriate.
2. Young people with chronic illnesses and conditions share the same health issues as their healthier peers. Health services therefore need to be holistic and address a range of concerns, such as growth and development, mental health, sexuality, nutrition, exercise, and health-risking behaviors, such as drug and alcohol use.
3. Health care services require flexibility to be able to deal with young people with a range of ages, conditions, and social circumstances. The actual process of transition needs to be tailored to each individual adolescent or young person.
4. Transition is generally optimized when there is a specific health care provider who takes responsibility for helping the adolescent or young person and his or her family through the process.
5. Active case management and follow-up helps optimize a smooth transfer to adult health services, as well as promote retention within adult services.
6. Engagement with a general practitioner can address holistic health care needs and help reduce the risk of failure of transfer to adult services.
7. Close communication between pediatric and adult services will help bridge the cultural and structural difference of the two health systems, resulting in a smoother transition of young people to adult services.
8. An ultimate goal of transition to adult health care services is to facilitate the development of successful self-management in young people with chronic conditions.

Source: Adapted from: Nakano, K. T., Crawford, G. B., Zenzano, T., & Peralta, L. (2011). Transitioning adolescents into adult healthcare. *American College of Preventive Medicine*. Retrieved from http://www.medscape.com/viewarticle/755301_1; Rosen, D., Blum, R., Britto, M., Sawyer, S., & Siegel, D. (2003). Transition to adult health care for adolescents and young adults with chronic conditions. Position paper of the Society for Adolescent Medicine. *Journal of Adolescent Health, 33,* 309–311.

about decrease in adherence to medical regimens and feelings of isolation by being different than other teens). Box 9-3 lists the Principles of Successful Transition to Adult-Oriented Health Services that have been endorsed by the Society for Adolescent Medicine in 2003.

Nurses who work with families and their teenagers with chronic illness should establish a process of "getting ready" for the transfer at least a year or so in advance—long before the situation occurs (van Staa et al., 2011)—and work with the family to design a well-thought-out purposeful plan of transition. One difficult part of this care process is working with the family and the health care team to determine when is the best time for the transition to occur. To base this transition decision solely on chronological age is not sufficient (van Staa et al., 2011). Typically, the transition occurs sometime between years 18 and 21 (American Academy of Pediatrics, 2011). The abilities of the young adult to demonstrate responsibility and to participate as much as possible in self-care management (self-efficacy) are better predictors than age of readiness to transfer (American Academy of Pediatrics, 2011;

van Staa et al., 2011). Other factors nurses need to consider and address besides self-efficacy and age in this transition plan are the adolescent's attitude toward transition and the complexity of the illness and treatment plan. The transfer plan should also entail:

- Introducing the concept of transition early in the care relationship with the family. Stress that the transfer is a normative process that reflects achievement of an additional developmental task (Lugasi et al., 2011). Assure the family that transition is not a form of abandonment.
- Holding family meetings to discuss expectations regarding the move to adult care. Explore what they think will be the same or different. Discuss the timing of the transfer. Use these meetings to uncover concerns and needs of the family and each family member about the transition process (Lugasi et al., 2011).
- Assessing the adolescent's ability to provide self-care (Lugasi et al., 2011).
- Designing educational programs to meet the needs of the adolescent/young adult about

the illness, how to self-monitor, how to self-manage illness and situations, and how to ask for help when needed. This should include helping the young adult to learn how to develop communication skills.

- Holding discussions about the adult health care environment, insurance coverage, and health policy changes that will affect the care once the adolescent becomes 18 years of age and is considered a legal adult. This discussion should include differences between pediatric and adult health models of care.
- Having discussions about how the parents may need to move from acting as the primary decision makers to a more supportive and collaborative model of decision making with the young adult.
- Providing the family with a list of adult health providers they may want to consider in their selection process.
- Introducing independent visits with the pediatric health care provider without the parents present.
- Arranging for an introductory visit with the adult provider so that the first interaction is not about an exacerbation of the chronic illness, but one that is about health maintenance. If possible, plan for a joint visit of the family, the pediatric health care team, and the adult health care team.
- Identifying a transition coordinator or someone in the adult health care team who can serve in this role for the family and young adult (Lugasi et al., 2011).

Siblings of Children With Chronic Illness

Younger siblings often strive to model the behaviors of older siblings, including illness behaviors. A study focusing on participants who identified themselves as growing up with an ill sibling found they reported acting out and alienation behaviors as well as social withdrawal. However, the majority of participants also reported that the experience affects their lives positively with a greater appreciation of life and greater awareness of family bonding and support (Fleary & Heffer, 2013). Focus groups held with parents, siblings,

and health care providers resulted in a comprehensive list of psychosocial concerns specific to the experience of school-age siblings of children with chronic illness (Strohm, 2001). These conversations identified seven significant feelings of siblings of children with chronic health care conditions (Strohm, 2001, p. 49):

- Feelings of guilt about having caused the illness or being spared the condition
- Pressure to be the "good" child and protect parents from further distress
- Feelings of resentment when their sibling with special needs receives more attention
- Feelings of loss and isolation
- Shame related to embarrassment about their sibling's appearance or behavior
- Guilt about their own abilities and success
- Frustration with increased responsibilities and caregiving demands

Other studies reveal more positive sibling outcomes, pointing out that siblings develop improved empathy, flexibility, pride in learning about and caring for a chronic illness, and understanding of differential treatment from parents based on ability and health. Siblings are noted to be more caring, mature, supportive, responsible, and independent than their peer counterparts who do not have siblings with chronic conditions (Barlow & Ellard, 2006). Siblings are reported to have high levels of empathy, compassion, patience, and sensitivity (Bellin & Kovacs, 2006). Siblings demonstrate learning about the disease and being supportive of their ill brother or sister, and sometimes assume parental roles (Wennick & Hallstrom, 2007). Children who learn about their chronically ill sibling's illness and its mechanisms tend to feel more confident and competent in their ability to support their sibling (Lobato & Kao, 2005; Wennick & Hallstrom, 2007).

Families face the challenge of balancing the needs of the child with a chronic condition with those of the surrounding family, including siblings. It has long been demonstrated that parents of siblings of children with disabilities often lack the ability to give needed time and attention to siblings because of the demands of caring for the child with a disability; this sometimes results in siblings resenting the child with disabilities (Rabiee, Sloper, & Beresford, 2005). Some parents rely on siblings to entertain or assist in the care of the child with disabilities, an action that puts additional stress on the other children.

FAMILY NURSING INTERVENTION DURING CHRONIC ILLNESS

The role of the family nurse is to assist multiple family members to interact in ways that optimize abilities and strengths. Although chronic illness care requires consideration of individual outcomes, it must be addressed within the family environment, with consideration of long-term caregiver needs and family outcomes. Across the life span, families use management styles, functional processes, and family health routines to address actual problems, minimize risks, and maximize potentials. Nurses who assess for these styles, processes, and routines, and who then tailor their interventions accordingly to empower and collaborate with families, will be most effective in meeting chronic care needs.

Nurses assist families by discussing things such as family strengths, couple time, balancing illness and family needs, developmental milestones, sibling needs, economic restraints, and caregiver well-being (Kieckhefer et al., 2013). Moreover, family-focused nursing care should address prevention or reduction of additional health risks, maintenance of optimal wellness levels for all family members, development of therapeutic care management routines, goal-setting that enhances individual and family well-being and integrity, assessments of ethnocultural influences including macro- and microsocial factors, and accommodating unplanned changes. The FHM (Denham, 2003) suggests that families have *core processes* (i.e., caregiving, cathexis, celebration, change, communication, connectedness, coordination) or ways families interact with one another. Nurses can use these ideas as guides to working effectively with families who have a member with a chronic illness (see Tables 9-2 and 9-3).

In chronic disease management, family-focused care needs that equip these individuals and their families with knowledge and tools to be effective self-managers have long been lacking (Wagner et al., 2001). Use of an empowerment model and integrative processes to respond to unique needs has been most successful (Hummel, 2013a; Phillips et al., 2015; Tang, Funnell, & Anderson, 2006). An empowerment model involves the following types of care:

- Patient-centered care
- Problem-based care
- Strengths-based care
- Evidence-based care
- Culturally relevant care

Moreover, empowerment acknowledges that the person is central to chronic care self-management. As nurses seek to empower families for chronic illness management, they should encourage flexibility, coordinate actions of multiple caregivers, use evidence-based guidelines, help families identify community resources, and provide education that builds confidence and skills in multiple family members. A need exists for more evidence about empowerment interventions (Henshaw, 2006; Hummel, 2013a).

Family nurses will be well served by keeping in mind that families typically vary in four systematic ways in their abilities to incorporate medical regimens into their daily routines: remediation, redefinition, realignment, and reeducation (Fiese & Everhart, 2006). *Remediation* refers to a need to make slight alterations in daily routines to fit illness care into preexisting routines. *Redefinition* refers to a strategy whereby the emotional connections made during routine gatherings need to be redefined. *Realignment* occurs when individuals within the family disagree about the importance of different medical routines, and routines need to be realigned in the service of the child's health. The fourth form, *reeducation*, arises when the family has little history or experience with routines and family life is substantially disorganized (Fiese & Everhart, 2006).

Research about family health suggests that structural behaviors or family health routines are visible activities that family members can readily recall and discuss from multiple perspectives (Denham, 1997, 1999a, 1999b, 1999c). Although family members may report similarities in routines, unique variations are common. The nested family context is a powerful, persuasive, and motivating determinant that influences ways health information is shared within a family and then incorporated into daily routines. Routines have unique characteristics, they vary in rigidity and timing, and members have different expectations across families because of response to member beliefs, values, and perceived needs. Information that fits with perceived family needs is probably the most likely to be incorporated into daily actions. Thus, nursing assessment of chronic care management extends beyond the disease and should also include ways members interact and the life patterns already established.

Family health routines include several categorically different foci. Self-care routines involve habits linked with usual ADLs such as hygiene. Safety and prevention routines are primarily concerned with health protection, disease prevention, prevention of unintended injury, and avoidance of unsafe situations. A nurse assessing this routine area might also be interested in discerning less healthy habits and considering the impact of high-risk behaviors, such as smoking, alcohol, and misuse of other substances, on a chronic condition. Mental health routines are related to self-esteem, personal integrity, work and play, shared positive experiences, stress, self-efficacy, individuation, and family identity. Family-care routines are related to valued traditions, rituals, celebrations, vacations, and other events tied to making meaning and sharing enjoyable times. Illness-care routines are related to decisions about disease, illness, and chronic health care needs, and often determine when, where, and how members seek health care services and incorporate medical directives and health information into self-care routines. Family caregiving routines pertain to reciprocal member interactions believed to assist with health and illness care needs and support during times of crisis, loss, and death.

Families use routines to arrange ordinary life and cope with health or illness events (Fiese & Wamboldt, 2000). These routines are embedded in the cultural and ecological context of families, and highlight ways to focus on family processes and individual and family dynamics (Fiese et al., 2002). Nurses aiming to provide education and counseling to individuals with a chronic illness need to understand the unique family routines of multiple household members and the ways chronic care management is going to alter patterns that are revered, cherished, and comfortable. Nurses who collaborate with families during assessment, goal setting, and outcome evaluation increase the likelihood of providing effective nursing actions that get results that are sustainable over time.

CASE STUDIES: FAMILIES LIVING WITH CHRONIC ILLNESS

It is important to recognize that all chronic diseases are not the same. When diagnosis differs, individual and family needs can differ as well. Other factors also enter into the picture. For example, the race/ethnicity, primary language, cultural background, age, gender, educational level, socioeconomic factors, health resources, health and illness beliefs, health practices, and availability of family members can be critical factors in ways diseases are managed in family situations.

This section explores the ways the Yates and the Current families address chronic illness management. The Yates family represents a diverse family unit, with two generations living together. The father is white, the mother is Latina of Mexican origin, and the grandmother recently moved in to the household. The family is focused on the young daughter, who has been diagnosed with type 1 diabetes, and the family has been living with this situation for a while. The second family, the Currents, provides an example of a rural working family with an older member living with Parkinson's disease. Although these two chronic diseases share some similar characteristics for the families living with chronic illness, some unique qualities also emerge. The values and beliefs about illness and ways for managing illness need to be explored. The timing of diagnosis can differ, and access to health care, treatment options, and financial and other resources can also be different. Living with the disease during several decades could mean that new treatments become available. Families living with these two conditions often face different challenges because of individual motivation and knowledge, demographics, family member characteristics, family developmental stage, and family community resources. Family-focused nurses recognize that multiple factors enter into understanding why some individuals successfully manage their disease whereas others may not, and reasons why they are at risk for complications.

Case Study: Yates Family

Chloe Yates, age 13, was recently admitted to the pediatric intensive care unit with ketoacidosis, a complication of type 1 diabetes. She passed out at school after vomiting and complaining of fatigue and was transported to the hospital via ambulance. On her hospital admission, her serum glucose level was 350 mg/dL. Her glycosylated hemoglobin (Hba1c) was 11%, indicating poor metabolic control during the past 3 months. Chloe has been in the hospital for 2 days and is getting ready to be discharged home today.

Chloe's parents, Devon and Bonita Yates, were surprised when they found out how poorly Chloe's metabolic control had been before her admission. (See Figure 9-3 for a detailed Yates family genogram.) They believed that their family had open communication and that they knew what was happening with their children. Chloe told her parents that her glucose levels were "fine." Chloe is an honor-roll student at school, active in basketball and soccer, and well liked by her peers. Devon, a white male, is college educated and works for a thriving law firm. Bonita, a college-educated female, is a first-generation Mexican American and is employed as a business manager in a large firm.

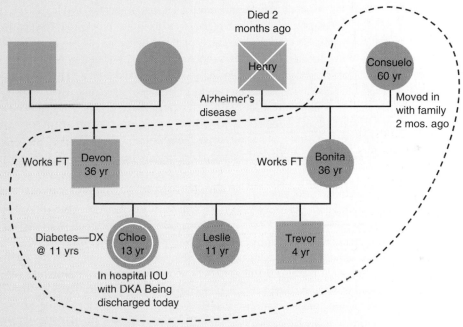

FIGURE 9-3 Yates Family Genogram

The Yates family recently experienced several stressors besides this new hospitalization. Bonita's father, Henry, passed away 2 months ago after a long bout with Alzheimer's disease. Bonita's mother, Consuelo, is now living with them. The family recently moved into a new and larger home in a racially diverse urban neighborhood. The children are enrolled in a private school, so the move did not affect their school relationships. Chloe and her younger siblings, Leslie and Trevor, appear to have adjusted to the new living location and seem content with their new neighborhood friends. Chloe has continued to receive primary care services in the clinic where the long-term pediatric nurse practitioner has come to know the family quite well.

Chloe was diagnosed with diabetes 2 years ago and was 11 years old at the time. When diagnosed, she spent several days in the hospital. Bonita accompanied her to a series of diabetes education classes, and they shared what they learned with the rest of the family. Chloe easily assumed responsibility for monitoring her glucose levels and administering her insulin when she was diagnosed. At first, the family struggled to make needed changes to their family health routines based on Chloe's medical needs—changes in Chloe's dietary needs, daily regulation of her insulin, bouts with hypoglycemia, and frequent monitoring of blood glucose levels that required significant management. The family has tried to adopt dietary patterns that support Chloe's needs. Bonita has continued her mother's Mexican cooking traditions but understands she needs to change the family's carbohydrate intake. Bonita learned some new things about counting carbohydrates, avoiding processed foods with high fructose, and preparing foods in nutritious ways. For example, Bonita avoids buying chips and now shops for more nutritious snack items that will not elevate Chloe's blood glucose level. The family incorporated the management of her diabetes into the family

(continued)

Case Study: Yates Family *(cont.)*

routines, and it seems less foreign to them now. Leslie and Trevor were unhappy with the dietary changes at first, but they have made a positive adjustment over time. The family makes a point of eating at least one meal together daily, which allows each family member to talk about his or her day. The family recently started "highlight/lowlight" time at dinner, during which each family member shares one high point and one low point about his or her day. Chloe's highlights have focused on her new friend at school, Brian. Her lowlights have focused on the "hassle" of checking her glucose and having to eat differently than her friends, something she is finding embarrassing. Having Consuelo move in with the family added some stress to the family, but the children are enjoying having their grandmother present when they come home after school.

Leslie and Trevor are staying at home with Consuelo while Bonita and Devon prepare to take Chloe home from the hospital today. Leslie and Trevor have been asking about Chloe for several days, because they are worried about her "sugar." Leslie, age 11, has been especially concerned about Chloe. She and Chloe have been arguing lately and Leslie feels it might be her fault that Chloe became ill. Trevor, age 4, has been asking if he can use Chloe's "finger pokers" and saying, "I have diabetes too!" Devon and Bonita share with the nurse their beliefs that he wants some of the special attention that his sister is getting at the hospital. These parents are worried about being "spread too thin" as they try to fulfill their employment responsibilities, attend to each child's unique needs, understand Consuelo's emotional needs after the loss of her husband, and also provide Chloe with the medical care she needs to manage the diabetes. Bonita is also concerned that her mother may not be ready to assist with Chloe's medical management so soon after caring for her husband for several years before he died from Alzheimer's disease.

Chloe's parents are meeting with the nurse today as they prepare for Chloe's discharge home. When the nurse asks whether they thought Chloe fully understood how to manage her diabetes, Devon said, "She not only understands, she could teach it! We just can't figure out why she had such a setback recently." This family is experiencing a transitional stress that is typical of adolescent behavior and also typical of adolescents living with a chronic illness.

Family Nurse's Reflection on the Yates Family Using Evidence-Based Practice:

Adaptation to type 1 diabetes is more effective when there is ongoing communication between parents and children regarding treatment management. Continued involvement of parents in treatment management is associated with better health and psychosocial outcomes in children and adolescents (Jaser, 2011). The American Diabetes Association (ADA, 2017) makes specific recommendations for the transfer of responsibility for treatment management. They recommend that school-age children (ages 8 to 11 years) can begin to assume more tasks such as insulin injections/boluses and blood glucose monitoring, but need significant assistance and supervision when making management decisions. The ADA also recommends that adolescents (ages 12 years and older) are able to perform most of the tasks of diabetes management on their own, but will still need assistance with decision making regarding insulin adjustments. Adolescents' increasing need for autonomy may conflict with ongoing parental involvement. Several studies found that when parents give up responsibility for treatment management too early, adolescents have poorer adherence to the regimen and deteriorating glycemic control (Anderson et al., 2002; Hegelson, Siminerio, Escobar, & Becker, 2009; Jaser, 2011). Parents of children diagnosed with type 1 diabetes are more likely to experience distress. Studies found as many as 23% to 29% of parents of children with type 1 diabetes have significant depressive symptomatology (Whittemore, Urban, Tamorlane, & Grey, 2003; Williams, Laffel, & Hood, 2009).

Studies that have looked at the role of race and ethnicity in diabetes management suggest that minority youth with type 1 diabetes are at greater risk for poor glycemic control than white youth; however, the mechanism of risk is not well understood (Gallegos-Macias, Macias, Kaufman, Skipper, & Kalishman, 2003; Swift, Chen, Hershberger, & Holmes, 2006). Differences in parental involvement may influence glycemic control. For example, Mexican culture is generally more likely to emphasize the needs of the family than Anglo American culture, which traditionally promotes the development of more autonomy during adolescence. Research has shown Mexican youth have better adherence when they have greater family support and when parents are involved in the responsibility for diabetes management. Conversely, parents of African American youth with type 1 diabetes had significantly lower levels of monitoring adolescents' diabetes management than parents of white youth (Gallegos-Macias et al., 2003; Hsin, La Greca, Valenzuela, Moine, & Delamater, 2010; Swift et al., 2006). What these findings help nurses understand is that race/ethnicity and the impact of culture are important to consider when assessing the effects of family adaptation to type 1 diabetes.

Bonita hesitated involving her mother in the care of Chloe's diabetes management needs, thinking that caring for her grandchild may have negative effects on her own health. However, large scale studies note that there is no evidence that caring for grandchildren has negative effects on the grandparent's health and health behavior (Hughes, Waite, LaPierre, & Luo, 2007). According to a Pew Research report, a record 60.6 million Americans lived in multigenerational households in 2014 (Cohn & Passel,

Case Study: Yates Family *(cont.)*

2016). Some of the benefits of multigenerational households include family members experiencing high levels of emotional bonding and closeness across generations. Grandparents become important role models and children learn how to care for their elders. Depending on the health care needs of the grandparents, multigenerational households can help reduce financial strains.

Although nurses should be aware of the potential for family conflict around diabetes management, they should not assume that poor medical adherence is a product of the conflict observed, because conflict and poor medical adherence are developmentally normal processes in families with adolescents (Dashiff, Bartolucci, Wallander, & Abdullatif, 2005). It is important to keep in mind that conflict occurs in all families, regardless of the age of individual family members. What is vital is the way conflict is handled and resolved. Nurses can assist families by suggesting effective communication techniques and developmentally appropriate strategies to address problems and areas of conflict linked with healthy functioning and development. Studies of psychosocial well-being in families of children with chronic conditions too often focus on psychopathology and lack of adjustment, with less attention given to well-functioning and positive growth after childhood illness (Barlow & Ellard, 2006). More recent research on sibling relationships measures the positive attributes that occur in families with a child with a disability, instead of only pathologizing this experience (Fleary & Heffer, 2013). Little is known about the best ways to educate caregivers about how to manage this disease in the family household and little to no consideration is given to individuals' social background (Glasdam et al., 2012). Findings from a 2012 study that considered family support and adherence to medical regimen identified that persons with diabetes felt sabotaged by family members when members knew what was needed to manage the disease, but were unmotivated to provide the support needed to make changes or offered temptations to indulge in contradictory activities (Mayberry & Osborn, 2012). These researchers concluded that there is a need for nursing actions that enhance family members' motivation and assist them to choose behavioral skills that empower their family member diagnosed with diabetes.

In families with adult members who have diabetes, family health routines are instrumental in self-management (Collier, 2007; Denham, Manoogian, & Schuster, 2007). A diabetes diagnosis affects previously constructed health routines; these old behaviors often need to be deconstructed and new ones formed in accord with unique family needs (Denham & Manoogian, unpublished). In diabetes self-management, differences in family members (e.g., gender, age, motivation, relationship) have implications for member support or threats to dietary and other care routines (Schuster, 2005).

As a nurse working with persons with various types of diabetes, it is important to note that a one-size-fits-all solution is not appropriate. Nursing assessments must consider the various ways conditions might affect individual members and the family as a whole. Chronic diseases may involve similar diagnostic factors and symptoms might be similar, but the human and family response of different households can be very different. Therefore, developing plans of care, nursing actions, and ideas about family empowerment must be based on the unique circumstances experienced by each family.

The Yates family case study illustrates the multiple factors that face multigenerational families who have a child with a chronic illness. The Yates family has three children, ages 13, 11, and 4. Chloe, the oldest child, has had diabetes for 2 years and has done well with parental guidance and self-management until recently. As a young teen, Chloe is moving into a new developmental stage. Chloe's disease management is threatened by things outside the family household, such as peer pressure and larger periods outside of the home environment with friends that involve food choices. However, her grandmother's involvement may provide additional support. Overall, Native-born Mexican grandparents seem to encourage greater adherence to parental rules, productive use of time, and self-reliance (Buriel, 1993; Knight et al., 2011).

In the Yates family case study, Leslie's and Trevor's reactions are typical for siblings of children with chronic conditions. Leslie, for example, feels responsible for Chloe's hospitalization, and has expressed possible guilt linked with recent arguments. Trevor's desire to have diabetes similar to his sister may represent his recognition that Chloe's diabetes is the source of much attention from their parents, attention that may be drawn away from him.

Chloe's parents have rearranged their lives to incorporate the management of her diabetes, but they also face the continued needs of their other children. Bonita and Trevor are also facing challenges of having extended family members living under one roof. The family recently became a multigenerational household and must learn to balance the joys as well as the difficulties of this living arrangement. These parents also need to recognize the ways Leslie's and Trevor's developmental needs influence their actions and consider possible ways the psychosocial development of children at different ages will be attended to in the future (Bellin & Kovacs, 2006). The experience may catalyze these siblings' abilities to tap into inner resources and develop empathy, compassion, patience, and sensitivity. Leslie and Trevor will benefit from age-appropriate, accurate information about Chloe's diabetes and from knowing that their responses are normal.

(continued)

Case Study: Yates Family *(cont.)*

The Yates family demonstrates several examples of a cohesive family unit. For example, the family members value time together at meals and encourage shared feelings. Now they must learn to incorporate an extended family perspective to their family unit. They opened their home to Bonita's mother and experienced the benefits and challenges of a multigenerational household. Several studies have shown that high family cohesion is associated with adherence in children and teens with treatments for type 1 diabetes (Cohen, Lumley, Naar-King, Partridge, & Cakan, 2004; Leonard, Jang, Savik, & Plumbo, 2005). Cohesiveness allows for shared understanding, respect for differences of opinions, and an emotional investment in keeping the family together (Fiese & Everhart, 2006).

An ethnocultural framework perspective will assist the family nurse working with the Yates family to assess and recognize the interrelationship between macro- and microsocial aspects that are influencing this family (see Table 9-6 for a comprehensive framework evaluation). For example, some of the macrosocial influences include the political/world climate that would affect research of type 1 diabetes and access to new pharmacologic approaches. The family's economic climate is such that both parents are working, which limits their ability to directly supervise their children. With both parents working, attending medical appointments may be difficult; thus, they are not routinely scheduled. Public policies affecting Chloe would pertain to school-based policies related to syringe use and disposal, providing emergency medical services, and development of safety plans during school and school-related outings. Additionally, Chloe and her friends' attitudes toward a chronic illness such as type 1 diabetes will have an impact on their ability to communicate and assist with things such as healthy food choices and adherence to management plans. Gender and cohort influences play a role as well, especially during the adolescent years.

Microsocial or more personal influences, such as Chloe's multicultural family dynamics and changes to the caregiving structure since her grandmother moved in with them, are important to assess. Comorbidities such as hyperlipidemia and

Table 9-6	**Select Features of the Ethnocultural Gerontological Nursing Model: Comparing the Yates and Current Families**	
ECGNM Elements	**Case Study 1: Chloe Yates Family (selected primary dimensions for this family)**	**Case Study 2: Ben Current Family**
Macrosocial (Outside) Influences		
Political/World climate	Uncertainty with new political administration, new type 1 research	Uncertainty with new political administration, new PD research
Economic climate	Two working parents Three children in private schools Explore implications of adding a maternal grandmother to the household	Ben is retired and his health insurance and family's financial status needs to be explored. Financial struggles prevent family from hiring a full-time caregiver.
Public policy	Safety requirements at school Policies at school with syringes Providing EMS services with hypoglycemic events	Ben agrees to stop driving and surrender his license.
Climate: Stereotypes, attitudes, ascriptions	Children/adolescent with type 2 diabetes	What are Ben's beliefs re: assisted living? How does Grace, his sister, feel with providing personal hygiene?
Perception of discrimination; illness; self-care	Assess Chloe's perception of her illness among her peers	Stigma of PD in community?
Cultural/historical traditions	Multicultural household Role of grandparents Mix of American and traditional Mexican diet	Explore Ben's belief and values systems as his elder role is compromised; close knit family. Patriarch structure now shifting with grandsons taking a caregiving role.
Gendered experience	Bonita raised in traditional Mexican household; adjusting to her mother and caregiving role; adjusting to having a parent living in the home	Ben as a patriarch Provider of family

Case Study: Yates Family *(cont.)*

ECGNM Elements	Case Study 1: Chloe Yates Family (selected primary dimensions for this family)	Case Study 2: Ben Current Family
Cohort influence (generational, etc.)	Maternal grandmother primarily Spanish speaking; children may or may not speak Spanish	Multigenerational home: grandsons and sister living in ranch
Microsocial (Personal) Influences		
	Need to assess multicultural personal influences for the father, mother, and grandmother	Need to assess shift in roles; Ben needing assistance from grandsons
Sociodemographics; income comfort, caregiving structure	How will caregiving be affected by adding a grandmother to the household?	Daughters, sister, and grandsons take on role of caregiver. Who takes leadership?
Health dimensions; comorbid conditions	Hyperlipidemia is common with diabetes Annual checkups to assess for retinopathy, nephropathy, and neuropathy	Scheduling and coordinating continued evaluations for nonmotor PD symptoms: depression, constipation, sleep changes
Biological variations	Latinos at higher risk for delayed diagnosis of diabetes and complications; will need to assess nutritional practices further	PD is a genetically heterogeneous condition and, most likely, accounts for about 30% of familial PD; complex disorder.
Personal/family experiences		
Communication	Language: Grandmother speaks Spanish; what is the language of children at home? What resources are used for communication? Who communicates with the providers? Can Chloe communicate with the providers?	What resources are used for communication? Who communicates with providers? Can Ben communicate with providers?
Resources: Additional Considerations for the Yates and Current Families		
Sociocultural; including economics	Who provides education regarding hypoglycemia to Chloe's peers? Who provides language-appropriate educational material for the grandmother?	Who manages Ben's bank account? Who has executive function?
Others-chronic illness focus	Explore cross-cultural beliefs and practices, grandmother's perspective Explore younger children's beliefs and knowledge about diabetes and family risk	Explore the family's perspective and practices with progressive chronic illnesses Discuss concerns with possible familial/genetic component to PD
Health insurance (private, state aid, etc.)	Two working parents; need to explore options	Need further exploration of insurance coverage, referral services
Employment		
Family structure; caregiving support Transportation needs	Multigenerational household, roles and responsibilities need to be assessed; explore if grandmother drives, and if she is participant in the child's care and medical appointments; parents and grandmother may need to be included in nutritional guidance appointments	Multigenerational household, roles and responsibilities need to be assessed. Explore if all members have transportation and who takes responsibility for getting Ben to his appointments.
Housing/space Equipment needed for health care	Housing: Is additional space needed for extended family members? Explore parental, mother, and grandmother roles; determine space needed to accommodate adolescents; assess knowledge of glucometers and potential insulin pump use	Home needs to be assessed for potential fall risk for Ben, with resources to keep him safe such as rails in the bathroom; assess knowledge and use of CPAP machine, battery, and maintenance.

(continued)

Case Study: Yates Family *(cont.)*

complications of hyperglycemia, such as diabetic neuropathy, nephropathy, and retinopathy, would all be variables the family nurse needs to assess. An ethnocultural framework allows the nurse to recognize the higher risk for delayed diagnosis of diabetes and its complications for Mexican American children (Ureña-Bogarín et al., 2015).

The FMSF could be useful for nurses in considering the Yates family (Knafl & Deatrick, 1990, 2003; Knafl et al., 2012). Chloe's parents attempt to focus on the normal aspects of Chloe's early adolescence, and they see her as normal in many ways. For this reason, the Yates family might be viewed as accommodating. They have, up to this point, felt confident about Chloe's ability to manage her diabetes independently, but perhaps Chloe's transition into adolescence will require the family to reassess their assumptions. The Yates family has the resources and cohesiveness to negotiate the developmental changes that occur along the way.

An early adolescent who has successfully managed diabetes may find it difficult to continue to manage the condition while simultaneously negotiating a move to social independence. Chloe's desire to fit in with her peers may be at odds with her need to check her blood glucose levels before meals, especially at school, and with her dietary limitations. Chloe's communication with her parents is particularly important at this transitional time. Parents are challenged to provide the adolescent with a level of autonomy that is developmentally appropriate while simultaneously monitoring abilities to adhere to complex medical regimens. This family will also need to explore how having the grandmother living with them may affect Chloe's behaviors. Studies have shown that the more teens (particularly girls) perceive their mothers as controlling, the greater the negative effect on adherence (Fiese & Everhart, 2006).

It is possible that health care providers and parents may overestimate adolescents' desire for autonomy and confidentiality, especially when illness-related (Britto et al., 2007). Adolescents, who tend to be more peer oriented, may wish to reduce the power differential between themselves and their health care providers. They might prefer that providers use direct communication styles. Adolescents with chronic illnesses may actually have fewer expectations for confidentiality and greater needs for parental involvement in care than healthy peers (Britto et al., 2007). Thus, nurses should not assume that all teens are seeking independence and autonomy just because they have reached the adolescent stage. In fact, nurses should consider the uniqueness of individual and family situations before giving advice and avoid passing judgment.

The family nurse should work with Chloe's parents' mobilized resources to help them meet the needs of all their family members. See the Yates family ecomap in Figure 9-4. The grandparents provided care for their two younger children while the parents prepared to take Chloe home from the hospital. In addition, the nurse could facilitate a parents-and-Chloe meeting with the school nurse and teachers. By helping families to assess their resources and determine what they still need, the whole family will enjoy improved health outcomes.

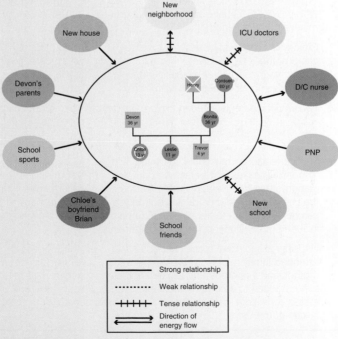

FIGURE 9-4 Yates Family Ecomap

Case Study: Current Family

Ben Current, a 68-year-old white widower, was diagnosed with Parkinson's disease at the age of 58. He owns and farms his 500-acre family ranch in eastern Oregon on which he raises cattle and hay. Several years ago, Ben managed a small group of cattle and this provided the family income. Since his wife Sarah's death 2 years ago, the number of cattle decreased, as well as the household income. This case study is presented through the lens of the Rolland's Chronic Illness Framework.

Illness Onset:

Parkinson's disease is a slowly progressive neurodegenerative brain disorder with motor symptoms of slowness, rigidity, and tremor. There are also a host of nonmotor symptoms that include autonomic, neuropsychiatric (e.g., dementia and depression), and sleep complaints. The cause of Parkinson's disease is not known and treatment is aimed at minimizing disability and maintaining optimal quality of life. At this most recent visit to the Movement Disorder Clinic, Ben presents with several motor and nonmotor concerns. In addition, he has low adherence to treatment recommendations and his family is expressing strain from the growing burden of care.

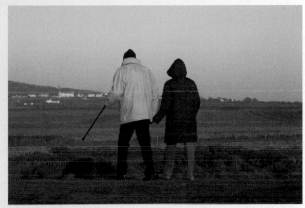

© *iStock.com/tirc83*

Course of Illness:

When individual family members have a progressive chronic illness, such as Ben with Parkinson's disease, the increasing disability requires families to make continual changes in their roles as they adapt to the losses and needs of the family member. Ben's family is at the Movement Disorder Clinic today to seek help with Ben's increasing symptoms. Several family members express feelings of stress and are exhausted with the routine and ongoing demands of his progressive symptoms.

There are two assessment tools used to evaluate the progressive aspects of Parkinson's disease. The first is the Hoehn and Yahr scale. This instrument identifies five stages based on motor symptoms: Stage 1 is unilateral motor involvement; Stage 2 is bilateral movement involvement; Stage 3 is mild-to-moderate disease with impaired balance; Stage 4 is severe disease with marked disability; and Stage 5 is confinement to bed or a wheelchair. It is important for family nurses to know that any reference to staging of Parkinson's disease is a quick look at the condition at that point in time during that visit and is not meant to suggest a time frame of progression. It is also worth noting that it only evaluates motor symptoms and it is important to realize that nonmotor symptoms, such as depression, can cause as much (or more) disability as the motor symptoms. The second instrument, the Unified Parkinson's Disease Rating Scale, is a detailed instrument that assists family nurses to assess the daily needs of the ill family member and the family caregiver in six areas of function: functional status, level of ADLs, motor function, mood, cognition, and treatment-related manifestations.

Outcome—Trajectory of Illness and Incapacitation:

Typically, people with Parkinson's disease can live 20 years or more from the time of diagnosis. Death is usually secondary to symptoms of immobility. It is the 14th leading cause of death in the United States. There is currently no cure for Parkinson's disease. The stages of the illness, as previously discussed, are progressive in nature. Ben has been in Stage 3 of the disease and symptoms suggest he is progressing to Stage 4. The focus of this visit is to minimize disability through symptom management and to help the family find resources in its local community to support Ben and minimize caregiver strain. If these interventions improve his adherence to medication, the family may maintain Ben in his current Stage 3.

(continued)

Case Study: Current Family *(cont.)*

Time Phase: Brief Review of Ben's Initial Diagnosis:

At initial diagnosis, Ben, 58 years old, was, in his words, "just not doing well." He was worried about a tremor in his left hand, but at that point it did not interfere much with his daily work or activities. Sarah, his wife, had taken over writing the paychecks for their three ranch hands and all the bills because Ben's handwriting had started to deteriorate. He noticed that he was slowing down, but attributed his increasing stiffness of legs and arms to "getting old" and his demanding physical lifestyle. What brought him in to see his health care provider was dizziness and falls. Sarah was worried that he would get dizzy while operating the farm machines. When he came home with a cut lip, swollen ankle, and scraped-up shoulder, Sarah demanded he see the family nurse practitioner (FNP), who was located 50 miles from his ranch. The FNP suspected Ben had PD, but sent him to the Movement Disorder Clinic and specialists in Portland, Oregon, which was 330 miles from where Ben lived. Since then, Ben has been managed primarily by his FNP with consultation and supportive assistance from the specialists, who see Ben every 6 months. Because of weather, declining family resources, and other family events, however, Ben and his family have not been to the clinic for a year.

Mid–Time Phase and Family Functioning:

Ben and his extended family have been living and adapting to his progressive PD for 10 years. See Figure 9-5, which shows the Current family genogram. Early on, the adaptation was relatively smooth as Ben responded well to medication intervention and his wife Sarah was the major support person. The family experienced a major change in the family involvement and management of Ben's illness when Sarah died 2 years ago from a heart attack at age 66. Since that time, 27-year-old Logan, Ben's grandson, has been living at the ranch and helping to provide support and care for Ben.

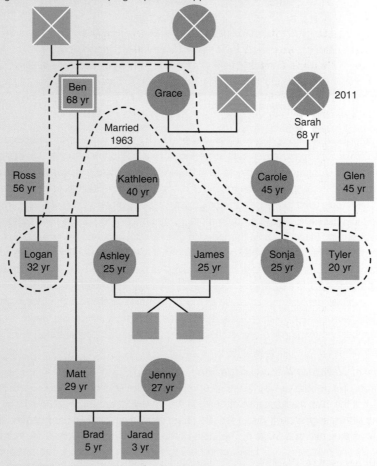

FIGURE 9-5 Current Family Genogram

Case Study: Current Family *(cont.)*

Julie, the NP specialist in the Movement Disorder Clinic, consulted the detailed family genogram in the chart. She noted that the family genogram had not been updated since Sarah's death; therefore, she updated it. At this visit, the family members who are present include Ben, his daughter Kathleen, his daughter Carole, and his grandson Logan, who is the primary caregiver. Logan expresses feeling overwhelmed with his caregiver role and work-time conflict. He feels that Ben needs more assistance. As both Kathleen and Carole are worried about Ben's safety while Logan is working on the ranch during the day, they report alternating days they come to spend with Ben. In order to facilitate uncovering the family stressors as well as the current medical condition of Ben, Julie decides to write issues in a table format that may then easily be used as a decision-making grid for the family. Julie completes her physical assessment of Ben's motor abilities, which are incorporated into the table. Ben fills out a geriatric depression assessment instrument. Logan completes a caregiver strain assessment instrument. Julie also recognizes that a change in income has occurred since Sarah's death, and this change in household income, availability of health insurance, and changes in the household will need to be explored and incorporated into the care plan for Ben.

Salient family issues in this phase for the Current family as it struggles to find a balanced family life and normalcy in functioning include the following:

1. Pacing and avoiding burnout: Logan is overwhelmed with being the primary caregiver for Ben. When Ben was more independent and the Parkinson's disease medications worked well at relieving Ben's motor problems, Logan primarily had to focus on cooking and being sure that Ben took his medications. With advancing executive function (short-term) memory issues, the increased number of falls, and concerns about his grandfather's safety, Logan feels that he cannot manage his own work on the ranch and take care of Ben. In the last month, Kathleen and Carole have been alternating days at the ranch to provide care for Ben during the day while Logan is working.

2. Reorganization of family roles: Logan, Kathleen, and Carole are all experiencing role overload as they all spend considerable time as the caregiver. Logan has expressed that he cannot continue to provide care for Ben in the home in the same way that he has in the past. The whole Current family is committed to keeping Ben at home as long as possible. Ben is clear that he does not want to leave the ranch. Tyler, 20-year-old grandson and Logan's cousin, stated that he would move into the ranch to help as he has begun working there and this would save him time commuting to and from work. Logan would like Tyler to live at the ranch, but insists that caring for Ben requires more than the two of them could provide.

3. Sustaining autonomy for all members of the family: Ben is struggling with the advances in his Parkinson's disease that he sees in himself; therefore, he continues to drive and tries to do some work on the ranch knowing that he is not safe. Logan is stressed to the maximum with role strain overload in the caregiver role.

4. Successfully grieve the loss incurred from the disability or chronic condition: All the family members present shared concerns about the "declining" status of Ben's health. The Current family is a close-knit family that is actively involved in Ben's life and care. Ben has held a strong patriarchal role for the family. Each family member is grieving the loss of Ben in this role and having to adjust to changes that are brought about by the progressive nature of Parkinson's disease.

The family discussed several options for seeking additional help and other interventions during the family meeting:

- The family discussed having Ben move to an assisted-living facility that is about 30 miles from the ranch. Ben vetoed this option of care at this time. He insists that he will stay on the ranch as long as possible. The Current family needs to explore finances and the cost of this option further.
- The second option was to hire a full-time caregiver who would either live at the ranch or in the town. This approach would mean that Logan would provide nighttime care for Ben. The cost of this avenue was considered too much at this time. All family members agreed that they would like to save financial resources for when Ben may need nursing home placement.
- The third option considered by the family was to ask Ben's sister Grace if she would like to come live on the ranch where she grew up, and to help provide care for Ben. Grace, who was recently widowed and has no children, has a solid relationship with Ben. This option would relieve Logan, Kathleen, and Carole of many of the immediate daily caregiver responsibilities. Tyler could also move to the ranch and assume some of the caregiving tasks or home maintenance in the evenings along with Logan. Carole mentioned that she had briefly brought up this idea with Grace.

The family decided to have Aunt Grace come out for a trial run and determined that they would explore having a home health aide come to the ranch a couple of days a week to help with Ben's hygiene. The family also agreed that they would

(continued)

Case Study: Current Family *(cont.)*

explore having a shower with a chair installed, along with other home adaptations that may be required. Ben may require a cane or a walker in the near future because of balance, decreased strength, and a history of falls. The family genogram was updated to include Grace and to show Grace, Ben, Logan, and Tyler all living in the same household.

After a visit to the physical therapist during their time at the Movement Disorder Clinic in Portland, Logan was excited about the possibility of all the grandsons working together to build a flat walking trail not far from the ranch house for Ben that would incorporate many of the physical therapy exercise strategies that may help strengthen his muscles, improve agility, and help decrease the freezing episodes. They would put several logs at varying heights for him to practice high stepping. They could increase his stride by placing stepping stones across the creek. They would make the trail so that it had several direction changes and have Ben walk between two trees that were shoulder width. Logan agreed that he would spearhead this venture with all the cousins.

Julie worked with Logan and Ben on medication reconciliation. Together they designed a medication administration chart to help the family caregiver and Ben improve medication adherence. See Table 9-7.

Julie made referrals to speech therapy to assist Ben with his soft voice (hypophonia). Kathleen agreed to accompany Ben to this part of the visit in an attempt to alleviate Logan of some caregiving responsibilities.

Julie sent a written summary of the visit to the FNP, who is Ben's primary care provider. The summary included a suggestion to address Ben's sleep problems and repeat the study at the sleep clinic, perhaps fitting him with a different continuous positive airway pressure (CPAP) mask, as many more are available now.

Ben agreed to stop driving and surrender his license only if he could still drive on the ranch, See the Current family ecomap in Figure 9-6.

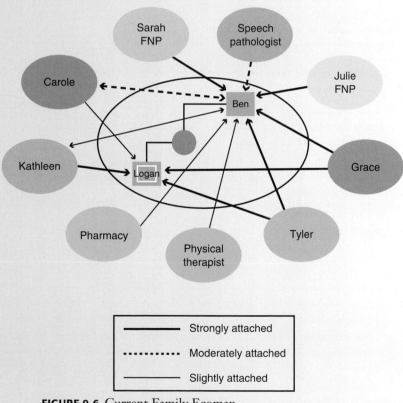

FIGURE 9-6 Current Family Ecomap

Case Study: Current Family *(cont.)*

An ethnocultural approach begins by first desiring the knowledge and actively engaging in cultural encounters with patients from diverse backgrounds. The Current family is a ranching family living in rural Oregon. Their daily lifestyle choices and approaches to problem solving chronic illness concerns may differ from a family living in an urban setting. Nurses must self-reflect and acknowledge biases and discriminatory practices that prevent meaningful communication and interactions with unfamiliar community members. Results from a recent survey on behalf of The Michael J. Fox Foundation Harris Poll (Partners in Parkinson's, 2014) found only about half of patients feel "informed or very informed" about living with Parkinson's disease (53%) and how to determine if their disease is progressing (51%). Only 48% of Parkinson's patients and 38% of caregivers reported feeling informed about where to turn for support or information, and even fewer (43% of patients and 36% of caregivers) felt informed of ways to get connected with their local Parkinson's community. Only about two-thirds of patients, who see a general neurologist (66%) or primary care physician (60%) as their primary doctor for Parkinson's, reported feeling informed about their disease, compared with a substantial 92% of Parkinson's patients who currently see a movement disorder specialist (Partners in Parkinson's, 2014).

The nurse working with Ben and his family must assess his family's longstanding culture-bound traditional beliefs and practices. The various political, economic, and public policies that have an impact on this family's chronic illness management also need to be examined. Changes to the Affordable Care Act may influence the medical benefits that affect Ben's ability to continue seeing Julie, the NP specialist in the Movement Disorder Clinic in Portland, and possibly having access to management strategies beyond the scope of practice of his primary care provider. See Table 9-6 for a comprehensive ECGNM framework evaluation sample.

Table 9-7	Presentation of Ben's Mid-Phase Parkinson's Disease Symptoms Using Unified Parkinson's Disease Rating Scale		
	Ben's Presentation and Score	**Family Concerns/Problems**	**Suggested Actions**
Mentation, Behavior, and Mood			
IQ impairment	Score of 2: moderate memory loss with disorientation and moderate difficulty handling complex problems: needs prompting for some ADLs.	Ben wants to continue to drive during the day to do some errands, especially as Logan works during the day on the ranch. Ben is not driving safely, especially with skills such as pulling out on the highway or turning left when traffic is present. In addition, Ben got lost on the ranch last week while trying to check on an area of fencing.	Discuss Ben surrendering his license. Allow him to continue to drive during daylight on the ranch as long as someone is with him.
Thought disorder	Score of 0: no problems.		
Depression	Score of 2: sustained depression (1 week or more). When asked, Ben reports feeling sad and depressed. He has made several statements of low self-esteem and how he is useless on the ranch anymore.	Family asks if Ben should be started back on an antidepressant medication. He was taking one right after Sarah, his wife, died 2 years ago, but he stopped quite a while ago.	Start on an SSRI medication. The prescription has been faxed to the local pharmacy in Joseph, Oregon, and will be there for the family to pick up when they get home. Need to build this into medication daily schedule.
Motivation-initiative	Score of 1: less assertive than usual; more passive. See the previous entry. Ben does report feelings of anxiety at times.	Logan reports that Ben repeatedly asks about the same aspect of work on the ranch, such as completing the corral repair.	Consider adding an anxiety medication, but will hold off for now. Discuss next visit or during phone call with local FNP.
Activities of Daily Living			
Speech	Score of 2: when "on" and "off" or at end of dosing period as Ben has hypophonia because of his PD.	Family reports that Ben is hard to hear and they feel as though they are always asking him to repeat what he says.	Referral to speech therapist while here during this visit to review with family some simple vocal exercises that will help Ben speak louder.

(continued)

Case Study: Current Family *(cont.)*

Table 9-7   Presentation of Ben's Mid-Phase Parkinson's Disease Symptoms Using Unified Parkinson's Disease Rating Scale *(cont.)*

	Ben's Presentation and Score	Family Concerns/Problems	Suggested Actions
Salivation	Score of 1: slight but definite excess of saliva in mouth; has nighttime drooling.	Ben says this is annoying but not a problem.	Suggest Ben chew gum or suck on hard candy if this bothers him as it will stimulate swallowing.
Handwriting	Score of 3: severely affected; not all words are legible.	Kathleen has assumed bookwork for the ranch.	No further interventions at this time.
Cutting food and handling utensils	Score of 2: can cut most food, although clumsy and slow; some help needed; this is becoming more of an issue and before Ben didn't need any assistance from Logan.	Logan and Ben eat breakfast and dinner together. Logan helps Ben when this is an issue. Logan has been doing all the cooking.	Kathleen and Carole agreed to both bring home cooked meals for Logan to heat up. Kathleen and Carole take turns food shopping.
Dressing	Score of 2: occasional assistance with buttoning, getting arms in sleeves.	Logan helps Ben in the morning and at night with changing clothes. Ben struggles some at home in getting pants zipped and buttoned after toileting.	Suggest overalls that don't require buttons or pants with Velcro closures. Use slip-on shoes. Because of balance concerns, suggest Ben sit down when dressing.
Hygiene	Score of 2: needs help to shower or is very slow in hygienic care.	This is new development. Logan is embarrassed by having to help his grandfather shower. In addition, this adds increased caretaking time to Logan's day.	Discuss safety adaptations in the shower (i.e., chair, grab bars). Discuss not bathing every day. Refer to Occupational Therapy to see if there are assistive devices for brushing teeth.
Turning in bed and adjusting bed clothes	Score of 2: can turn alone or adjust sheets, but with great difficulty.	Logan was concerned as he didn't even think about this aspect of help his grandfather might need.	He will use silk PJ bottoms to decrease the friction of turning. Explore if a bed rail can be placed on the bed. Discuss the weight of the covers or blankets used at night.
Falling	Score is between a 2 and 3: Ben falls often but not daily. Sometimes he has fallen more than once in a day. Ben reports being dizzy when he stands (orthostatic hypotension).	All family members are very concerned about Ben falling and the difficulty he has getting up from the fall. Ben walks on a regular basis. He has not kept up with his physical therapy in the last year. Ben seems to be stiffer and has more abnormal movements even on his medications.	Family will increase fluids and get some support stockings to keep blood from pooling in his extremities. Have Kathleen and Carole complete a fall safety check in the home environment to help identify hazards. Check to be sure Ben has his cell phone on him or a cordless phone is within reach so he can call if he falls when alone.
Freezing when walking	Score of 3: Ben frequently freezes and occasionally falls from freezing.	See the previous entry. Explore more to see when Ben is freezing, such as during a turn, going through doorways, at the start of walking, or when he is doing something that requires him to take a step back.	Review strategies with Ben to help him get going when he freezes while walking.

Case Study: Current Family (*cont.*)

	Ben's Presentation and Score	Family Concerns/Problems	Suggested Actions
Walking	Score of 2: moderate difficulty. Ben refused to use a cane, but his grandson Tyler made Ben a walking stick, which he now uses. Ben has bradykinesia with a weak push off, reduced leg lift, small stride length, lack of right arm swing, and a narrow stance.	See the previous entry. After much discussion, Ben admitted that he had trouble following his medication regimen during the day when Logan was at work. He also noted that he had been taking more Sinemet when he wanted to go out.	See the previous entry. Refer to PT for assistance in walking.
Pain	Score of 2: Ben complains of numbness, tingling, and frequent cramps and constant ache in his calves and lower back.		Starting Ben on SSRI for depression may help decrease pain sensations. Stretching and heat may relieve pain in calves.

Other Complications

Sleep	Ben reports that he has insomnia. He has difficulty staying asleep. Before being diagnosed with PD, Ben was assessed for sleep apnea in a sleep clinic. He reports that he dislikes the CPAP machine and the mask on his face, so he does not use it. He thinks he sleeps about 4 hours a night. He has daytime sleepiness.	Logan hears Ben up at all hours of the night, which interferes with his sleep. Ben has fallen at night too, which adds to Logan's vigilance of getting up to check on Ben.	Will discuss with FNP about having Ben reassessed for sleep at the sleep clinic in Pendleton, Oregon. Have Ben keep a simple sleep log if possible. Check on medications that Ben is taking and make sure that the timing is not affecting sleep.
Excessive sweating	Ben reports that he has been having periods of excessive sweating . . . similar to if he was caught in a rain storm.		Check the timing of medications as these may be happening as the dosing is ending or the "off" periods.
Constipation	Ben has a long history of constipation, even before diagnosis.		As Ben is sweating excessively at times, consider he may be dehydrated. Set up a plan so he drinks about 1500 mLs of fluids a day. Continue daily dose of Miralax.
Urinary problems	Ben reports nocturia, which might contribute to his insomnia.	Note that Ben was given a diuretic for hypertension. Explore the time of day he is taking this medication.	Be sure there is a nightlight in the bathroom and rugs in the bathroom.

SUMMARY

A family focus on care should not be considered optional when it comes to chronic illness. The long-term effects of chronic health conditions affect individuals and families differently than acute health events.

- Although the needs families experience may be similar initially, the duration of the illness alters the ways care is managed and perceived during a long life course.

- The severity, complexity, and longevity of care needs associated with chronic conditions can alter a desired or expected future into one that dramatically revolutionizes the lives of entire households.
- Financial costs and family resources are often highly taxed by years of debt and stress that would not be expected if a chronic condition had not occurred. Some conditions may worsen over time or require endless amounts of attention that can become especially

burdensome as the chronically ill person ages and economic or family resources are exhausted.

- Some children with SHCN and adults may require extraordinary adaptations by parents, siblings, and others that strain relationships.
- Although the chronic illnesses of children may be primarily genetic or environmental in nature, many of the adult chronic conditions are linked with lifestyle behaviors.
- Healthier lifestyles can reduce risks for some chronic conditions and can prevent or delay many complications from these diseases.

- Family-focused care aimed at meeting family needs when a member or members have a chronic illness requires nurses equipped with knowledge about families and their interactions.
- Optimal nursing care for those with chronic illness involves nurses who are knowledgeable about developmental alterations, willing to hear and listen to the voiced needs without judgment, and able to become collaborators that empower multiple household members to reorganize routines and manage existing resources.

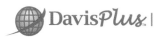 | For additional resources and information, visit **http://davisplus.fadavis.com**. References can be found on Davis*Plus*.

Chapter 10

Families in Palliative and End-of-Life Care

Carole A. Robinson, PhD, RN

Rose Steele, PhD, RN

Kimberley A. Widger, PhD, RN, CHPCN(C)

Melissa Robinson, PhD, RN

Critical Concepts

- Palliative care is both a philosophy and a type of care.
- Palliative care is "whole person" care that involves a focus on quality of life, or living well, for all family members when they are dealing with a life-limiting illness. It can start long before the end-of-life period, as early as at the time of diagnosis of a life-limiting illness, and extend beyond death to bereavement.
- The principles of palliative care are applicable in a sudden, acute event—such as an accident, suicide, or myocardial infarction—though the context is different because there is a shorter time span in which to work with a family. A palliative approach complements the disease orientation that is often the focus of acute care.
- The majority of palliative care is provided by family caregivers.
- Skilled nursing interventions and relationships between nurses and families are crucial in creating positive outcomes in palliative and end-of-life care.
- Interprofessional teamwork is essential in palliative and end-of-life care and the team is inclusive of family members.
- People who have advanced, life-limiting illnesses worry about being a burden on their families and about the consequences of their death on their families. Family members worry about burdening their ill member. Everyone involved is often afraid. This fear can lead to communication problems, isolation, and lack of support within the family.
- Barriers to nurses providing quality end-of-life care may be ameliorated when the nurse understands palliative care principles.
- Nurses need strong patient and family communication, assessment, and intervention skills to provide optimal palliative and end-of-life care.
- End-of-life decision making is a process that involves all relevant family members identified by the ill person and evolves over time. Advance care planning is an important part of this process.
- A "good" death is one that happens in alignment with patient and family preferences.

Nurses encounter families who are facing end-of-life issues in virtually all settings of practice. From newborns to seniors in their nineties and older, people die, and their families are affected by the experience. Nurses are in an ideal position to influence a family's experience, either positively or negatively. Ideally, nurses facilitate a positive experience for families, one that will bring them comfort in the future as they recall the situation when their loved one died. Unfortunately, not all families have a positive experience, and it is often because health care providers do not know how to work effectively with families at this challenging time (Andershed, 2006). Yet, palliative and end-of-life nursing can be extremely rewarding and professionally fulfilling. It offers an opportunity for personal growth in patients, families, and health care providers; interactions among all concerned are especially meaningful (Anderson, Kent, & Owens, 2015; Davies et al., 2017).

Providing and improving palliative care should be a goal for all nurses, regardless of educational level. As more people live longer with chronic, life-limiting conditions, nurses increasingly require knowledge and skills in palliative care, particularly because nurses spend the most time with patients and families compared with any other health care providers. Even at the undergraduate level, nursing students require education about palliative care so they can deliver quality care (Ferrell, Malloy, Mazanec, & Virani, 2016).

This chapter details the key components to consider in providing palliative and end-of-life care, as well as families' most important concerns and needs when a family member experiences a life-threatening illness or is dying. It also presents some concrete strategies to assist nurses in providing optimal palliative and end-of-life care to all family members. More specifically, the chapter begins with a brief definition of palliative and end-of-life care, including its focus on improving quality of life for patients and their families. The chapter then outlines principles of palliative care and ways to apply these principles across all settings, regardless of whether death results from chronic illness or a sudden or traumatic event. Three palliative care and end-of-life case studies follow.

PALLIATIVE AND END-OF-LIFE CARE DEFINED

Palliative care and *end-of-life care* are not synonymous terms. End-of-life care focuses exclusively on the immediate period surrounding death, whereas palliative care includes end-of-life care but extends for many months, even years (especially in children), and can coexist with treatments aimed at curing an illness (World Health Organization [WHO], 2006). This difference in meaning is confusing to many health care providers, patients, and families who share a common misconception that palliative care is end-of-life care, which then underpins the significant problem of late referral and acceptance of palliative care (Fox et al., 2016; McIlfatrick et al., 2014). Another misconception, identified previously, is that health care providers cannot actively treat disease while concurrently engaging in palliative care. Palliative care focuses on improving the quality of life of patients and their families facing problems associated with life-limiting illness. Palliative care helps families in these situations live well by preventing and relieving suffering through early identification and excellent assessment and treatment of pain and other physical, psychosocial, or spiritual problems (WHO, 2006). Employing a team approach, palliative care offers a support system to help patients live as actively as possible, and to help families cope during the patient's illness and their own bereavement. Life is affirmed and dying is regarded as a normal process (WHO, 2006).

Focus on the family as a unit is a key principle in palliative care. Nowhere is this more evident than when a child is the patient. Support targets both individual family members and the family as a whole. The age range of patients receiving pediatric palliative care, typically 0 to 19 years of age, requires that children's developmental, social, educational, recreational, and relational needs be considered. The developmental stage of the family must also be considered, regardless of the patient's age.

Palliative care in adults developed primarily around care for patients with cancer. The current trend in palliative care, however, is an expanded focus on life-threatening illnesses beyond cancer. Patients and their families have similar needs for information, care, and support in a wide variety of chronic illnesses, including heart disease (Barnes et al., 2006), muscular dystrophy (Abbott, Prescott, Forbes, Fraser, & Majumdar, 2016), motor neuron disease (Aoun et al., 2012), dementia (Reinhardt, Chichin, Posner, & Kassabian, 2014; van Soest-Poortvliet et al., 2015), Parkinson's disease (Fox et al., 2016; Goy, Carter, & Ganzini, 2007), and neurodegenerative diseases (Kristjanson, Aoun, & Oldham, 2006), as well as when patients are simply of an advanced age (Jackson et al., 2012; van Eechoud et al., 2014).

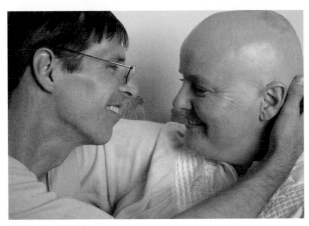

© *iStock.com/lisafx*

Palliative care is about nurturing and maintaining quality of life from diagnosis of life-limiting illness through bereavement. The approach encompassed by palliative care principles can be used in any setting with any family, regardless of how long a person has to live or how sudden the death is. Murray and Sheikh (2008) described three main trajectories of decline at the end of life. Awareness of these trajectories (Murray & Sheikh, 2008) helps nurses recognize when palliative care may best be introduced. Palliative care can be offered alongside care that is curative in intent (Murray, Kendall, Boyd, & Sheikh, 2005). At some point in the illness trajectory, the primary goal of care shifts from curative to palliative intent. This point often occurs when there are no available curative treatments, or treatments are no longer effective or are associated with a burden that is no longer tolerable to the patient. It is well recognized that communication about the transition of care from curative to palliative intent is difficult but crucial (Marsella, 2009). It requires discussion about shifting the focus to quality of life rather than quantity of life. When a sudden or traumatic event occurs, there is little time to hold such discussions. But when someone has a protracted illness, this discussion can be introduced gradually and can be repeated over time.

Unfortunately, in many clinical settings, palliative care is raised only in the last few days or weeks of life, even when death has been anticipated (Widger et al., 2016). This late introduction of palliative care may have a significant negative effect on quality of life. For example, the early introduction of palliative care, alongside disease treatment, has been shown to enhance quality of life and reduce depressive symptoms among patients with metastatic lung cancer (Temel et al., 2010). An unexpected finding of this research was that the early palliative care patient group lived longer than the standard care group despite choosing less aggressive end-of-life care. This outcome challenges the myth that palliative care shortens patients' lives.

The introduction of palliative care is particularly challenging for health care providers when patients suffer from illnesses that are difficult to prognosticate, such as advanced lung, heart, and liver disease. One way of determining if a patient and family is in need of palliative care is to use the "surprise" question: "Would you be surprised if this patient died in the next 12 months?" Research has shown that this simple question is an effective way of identifying patients who are at higher risk of dying (Moroni et al., 2014; Moss et al., 2008). When the answer is "no," these patients and families should be a high priority for initiating conversations about palliative care and offering palliative interventions. It is important to ensure that patients, family members, and health care providers are aligned in their goals for care (Kitko, Hupcey, Pinto, & Palese, 2015; Thompson, McClement, & Daeninck, 2006) and have a common understanding of what quality of life means for the patient and family. Goals of care and the meaning of quality of life will be unique in each situation and care should be tailored to the needs of each particular family (Heyland, Dodek, et al., 2006).

Death occurs in many settings, from various causes, and across the life span. Some differences can be expected in families' experiences depending on the context, for example:

- Where the death takes place (e.g., home versus intensive care unit [ICU])
- The cause of death (e.g., natural progression of a chronic illness versus an unexpected, acute event; increased progression versus suicide)
- The dying trajectory (e.g., over a period of years versus sudden)
- The age of the family member who is dying (e.g., a 3-year-old child versus an 85-year-old person)
- The cultural and spiritual backgrounds of families (e.g., white versus Chinese; religious faith versus no faith)

No matter the context, the principles of palliative care should be consistent, with implementation tailored to address the particular family and the family's context. Consistent use of these principles contributes to high-quality palliative and end-of-life care. See Box 10-1 for some of the basic principles of palliative care.

BOX 10-1
Palliative Care Principles

- Palliative care begins as soon as there is a diagnosis of life-limiting illness.
- Palliative care can occur concurrently with care that is curative in intent.
- The focus of palliative care is on supporting and enhancing quality of life.
- Patient and family are cared for as a unit.

- Attention is paid to physical, developmental, psychological, social, and spiritual needs and concerns.
- Education and support of patient and family are crucial.
- An interprofessional approach is required.
- Care extends across settings.
- Bereavement support is part of good palliative care.

Identifying Relevant Literature

The amount of research about the provision of palliative and end-of-life care to adults is growing. Research in pediatric palliative care is much more limited, but many of the reported issues for families are similar across the life span. An electronic search of the Cumulative Index to Nursing and Allied Health Literature (CINAHL) database from 2002 until June 2012 uncovered more than 2000 articles that reported on some aspect of patient or family perceptions of the palliative, end-of-life, or bereavement care provided to the family by health professionals. Despite the number of articles in existence, only about a third presented research findings or a systematic review of research findings, and most of the research had been published in the previous 4 years. An updated search in October 2016 revealed 1291 additional publications, 594 of which were research studies. Thus, though the proportion of research studies appears to be increasing, the pattern of limited research remains prevalent. Virtually all areas of palliative care continue to need more research to strengthen the evidence base.

The studies included exploration of patient and family concerns and needs in relation to different diseases (cancer being the most common); causes of death (sudden deaths, deaths after illness); care settings (long-term care, acute hospital care, critical care, home, and hospice); ages (pediatric to older adult patients); countries; and cultures.

Often, great variation existed in beliefs and needs within a given cultural or other type of group, as well as within individual families (Adames, Chavez-Duenas, Fuentes, Salas, & Perez-Chavez, 2014; Aspinal, Hughes, Dunckley, & Addington Hall, 2006; Davies, Contro, Larson, & Widger, 2010; Heyland, Dodek, et al., 2006; Nielsen, Angus, Howell, Husain, & Gastaldo, 2015; Pergert, Ekblad, Enskar, & Bjork, 2008).

Therefore, one cannot determine from the literature what the exact needs of, for example, family members of an older African American person living with Alzheimer's disease in a long-term care setting will be. But the literature does highlight the key considerations in providing palliative and end-of-life care, important areas to assess for any family facing life-limiting illness, and interventions that may be helpful for many families or that can be adjusted to fit with a particular family's assessed needs. The literature found through this search, plus seminal articles, forms the evidence base for the remainder of this chapter.

KEY CONSIDERATIONS IN PALLIATIVE AND END-OF-LIFE CARE

In order to provide optimal palliative and end-of-life care, there are key areas that must be considered, such as the following: nurses' own personal assumptions and biases about death and dying, nurses' personal assumptions about people and their backgrounds, the involvement of the family in all aspects of care, the involvement of the interprofessional team, the inclusion of bereavement care as part of palliative care, and potential barriers to optimal palliative and end-of-life nursing care.

Personal Assumptions and Biases About Death and Dying

To provide optimal palliative and end-of-life care, nurses need to be aware of their own assumptions and biases about death and dying (Sousa & Alves, 2015). As a nurse, it is important to explore personal beliefs, attitudes, and personal and professional experiences to understand how they may influence your attitudes toward death, dying, and bereavement. For example, if a nurse believes that a family member should be physically present with someone who is dying, he or she may find it difficult to work with family members who choose not to be present. It is neither possible nor wise to separate the "nurse as person" from the "nurse as professional," because if personal reactions are ignored, then being able to focus on meeting the needs of patients and their families is more difficult (Davies & Oberle, 1990).

Many nurses do not know how to deal with dying and death. They are afraid, nervous, or anxious when faced with a dying patient and grieving family. But, some nurses experience great satisfaction when working with dying patients. They have developed their palliative knowledge and skills, not simply through caring for many dying patients, but through reflecting on their experiences with those patients and in their personal lives, on the meaning of life and death, and on their own behavior (Hendricks-Ferguson et al., 2015). They are able, therefore, to provide competent physical care and be a welcomed presence to those who are dying and their family members. All nurses, from novice to expert, need to develop basic competencies in the area of death and dying, from how to provide effective symptom management, using both pharmacological and nonpharmacological therapies, to being comfortable enough with death and dying that they can be present for family members.

See Box 10-2 for some key areas of focus when seeking education about palliative and end-of-life care.

Novice nurses can develop these competencies by building on personal strengths and learning ways to become more comfortable with death and dying. It is often helpful to begin with reflection on personal experiences surrounding loss, death, and dying. Reflecting on personal beliefs about life and death will help clarify understanding of and appreciation for the human condition—the only thing certain in life is that everyone will die. This reflection will form the foundation for the inner strength that will enable optimal palliative and end-of-life care (Davies & Oberle, 1990). Furthering education on death, dying, and providing care at life's end through one of the many available resources, such as workshops, books, and conferences; best practice guidelines (Registered Nurses' Association of Ontario, 2011); or even popular movies (e.g., *Life as a House; One True Thing*) can help a nurse transition from novice to competent palliative caregiver. Gaining knowledge through formal education can also help improve comfort with providing care to patients facing a life-threatening illness and their families (Kehl, 2014; Kwak, Salmon, Acquaviva, Brandt, & Egan, 2007).

Novice nurses often remember their first experience of patient death, and that memory can have a lasting impact, both personally and professionally. Preparing for this experience in advance through education, seeking out a supportive mentor and peer

---

BOX 10-2

Key Areas of Focus for Education in Palliative and End-of-Life Care

The Registered Nurses' Association of Ontario (2011) recommends that entry to practice nursing programs and post-registration education should incorporate specialized end-of-life care content that includes the following areas:

- Dying as a normal process, including the social and cultural context of death and dying, dying trajectories, and signs of impending death
- Care of the family (including caregiver)
- Grief, bereavement, and mourning
- Principles and models of palliative care
- Assessment and management of pain and other symptoms (including pharmacological and nonpharmacological approaches)

- Suffering and spiritual/existential issues and care
- Decision making and advance care planning
- Ethical issues
- Effective and compassionate communication
- Advocacy and therapeutic relationship-building
- Interprofessional practice and competencies
- Self-care for nurses, including coping strategies and self-exploration of death and dying
- End-of-life issues in mental health, homelessness, and the incarcerated
- The roles of grief and bereavement educators, clergy, spiritual leaders, and funeral directors
- Knowledge of relevant legislation

Source: Registered Nurses' Association of Ontario. (2011). *Best practice guidelines: End-of-life care during the last days and hours.* Toronto, ON: Author. Retrieved from http://rnao.ca/sites/rnao-ca/files/End-of-Life_Care_During_the_Last_Days_and_Hours_0.pdf

support at the time of a death, taking time to participate in debriefings that may be offered following the death, and reflecting on the experience can all facilitate a more positive experience that offers the opportunity for personal and professional growth, reduced anxiety, and development of positive attitudes to care of the dying (Anderson et al., 2015; Hendricks-Ferguson et al., 2015).

Personal Assumptions and Biases About People and Their Backgrounds

An underlying principle in palliative care is respect for persons. As a nurse, it is helpful to be aware of the assumptions and stereotypes that are held about the people cared for because assumptions and stereotypes get in the way of person- and family-centered care. For example, bereaved lesbians reported that health care providers often disrespected or ignored their relationship with the patient; after death, their loss was often unacknowledged or devalued (Jenkins, Edmundson, Averett, & Yoon, 2014). Part of good palliative and end-of-life care is recognizing that every person is valuable in his or her own right; however, this is sometimes negatively influenced by judgments about a particular person's or family's worth. Valuing appreciates the possibility that every human being has the potential for actualization or optimal development (Davies & Oberle, 1990; Widger, Steele, Oberle, & Davies, 2009).

Sometimes, assumptions and biases about people relate to their cultural or spiritual background. Similar to exploring personal assumptions and biases about death and dying, it is important to recognize one's personal cultural or spiritual background or previous experiences with other cultures and how they might influence practice, as well as one's expectations of others (Huang, Yates, & Prior, 2009). For example, if the importance of an Aboriginal smudging ceremony to a family is not understood, the nurse may be unwilling to create an environment that allows for such a ceremony within a hospital setting. The cultural and spiritual implications discussed elsewhere in this text also are relevant to quality palliative care. Effectively implementing the palliative care philosophy means that the nurse must be sensitive to diversity and able to deal with issues that arise when caring for people with varied cultural and spiritual backgrounds (Davies & Oberle, 1990). Cultural beliefs, as well as spirituality, spiritual beliefs, or faith, significantly influence how patients

and families cope with advanced illness (Aspinal et al., 2006; Blank, 2011; Donovan & Williams, 2014; Donovan, Williams, Stajduhar, Brazil, & Marshall, 2011; Knapp et al., 2011; Robinson, Thiel, Backus, & Meyer, 2006; Thrane, 2010). Some may find strength and renewed connection to their cultural or spiritual background, whereas others may question previously held beliefs. It is very important that the nurse avoid imposing his or her own beliefs on the patient and family, but rather determine what is most important to the family. Although across cultures different needs may exist, there is likely more similarity than differences among cultures in terms of basic human needs for connections with others, physical care, dignity, and support (Kongsuwan, Chaipetch, & Matchim, 2012). On the other hand, it is important to remember that there may be a great deal of diversity *within* cultures or faiths. This means there will never be a single approach that is appropriate for all people from a particular culture or faith group, so one of the best strategies is to ask families about their beliefs and preferred way of doing things (Kleinman & Benson, 2006). From this place of understanding, nurses can negotiate care so that it aligns as closely as possible with the family's values and beliefs and demonstrates a fundamental respect for people.

Involvement of the Family

Life-threatening illness affects all family members, not just the patient. When the ill person is having a "good" day, so is the family caregiver (Stajduhar, Martin, Barwich, & Fyles, 2008). If the ill person is in emotional or physical pain, has a low quality of life, or has difficulty coping with the illness, the caregiver's suffering dramatically increases as well, both during the illness and into bereavement (Abbott, Prigerson, & Maciejewski, 2014; Milberg & Strang, 2011). Siblings too may suffer if parents are too focused on the ill child to meet sibling needs (de Cinque et al., 2006; Horsley & Patterson, 2006; Price, Jordan, & Prior, 2013; Rodriguez & King, 2014). Therefore, interventions directed at one family member can also be supportive to other family members, and this is the case whether the ill person is a child or an adult. Family members feel supported when they believe that professionals have the best interests of their loved one at heart. Therefore, nurses need to ensure that the patient is well cared for, but also keep in mind that interventions directed at family members as a group and individually have been found to be most effective in supporting families and achieving the best outcomes (Northouse, Katapodi, Song, Zhang, & Mood, 2010).

Among the top concerns of dying patients is the well-being of their family members in terms of caregiving burden and their ability to cope after the death (Aspinal et al., 2006; Broom & Kirby, 2013; Fitzsimons et al., 2007; Jo, Brazil, Lohfeld, & Willison, 2007; Kristjanson, Aoun, & Yates, 2006). Even ill children may make decisions based on what they believe is best for their family rather than what they particularly want (Weaver, Baker, Gattuso, Gibson, & Hinds, 2016). Patients do not want to become a burden to their families (Fitzsimons et al., 2007; Heyland, Dodek, et al., 2006). If patients know that their family is well supported, it may reduce their own suffering.

Family members provide the majority of care for persons with life-threatening illness, and a home death relies on their strong involvement (Grande et al., 2009; Morris, King, Turner, & Payne, 2015; Stajduhar, Funk, Jakobsson, & Ohlen, 2010; Stajduhar, Funk, Toye, et al., 2010). Family members carry a variety of burdens when a family member is dying (Totman, Pistrang, Smith, Hennessey, & Martin, 2015), including compromises in their own health (e.g., depression, back pain, shingles, difficulty sleeping, and pre-existing chronic illnesses), conflicting family responsibilities (e.g., caring for the ill parent or spouse plus caring for their own children), little time to meet their own needs, cumulative losses, fear, anxiety, insecurity, financial concerns, loss of physical closeness with a spouse, and lack of support from other family members and health professionals (Corà, Partinico, Munafò, & Palomba, 2012; Funk et al., 2010; Grande et al., 2009; Jo et al., 2007; Kenny, Hall, Zapart, & Davis, 2010; Osse, Vernooij Dassen, Schade, & Grol, 2006; Riley & Fenton, 2007; Robinson, Pesut, & Bottorff, 2012; Wollin, Yates, & Kristjanson, 2006).

Moreover, the work of caregiving can be both physically and mentally exhausting (Riley & Fenton, 2007; Robinson et al., 2012). There also may be an ambivalent sense of waiting for the person to die but not wanting the person to die (Riley & Fenton, 2007). Family members may experience these issues whether their relative is mostly at home (Andershed, 2006; Totman et al., 2015) or in an institutional setting (Martz, 2015). They often have increased responsibilities and may view the situation as burdensome (Andershed, 2006; Mehta, Chan, & Cohen, 2014). Yet, family caregivers often are more concerned about the care of the dying person than about their own health (Robinson et al., 2012; Ward-Griffin, McWilliam, & Oudshoorn, 2012), so as not to burden the patient or take focus off the patient (Fridriksdottir, Sigurdardottir, & Gunnarsdottir, 2006; Grande et al., 2009; Konrad, 2008; Riley & Fenton, 2007). A recent study found that one of the most effective ways of supporting family caregivers is to help them fulfill their need to be excellent caregivers (Robinson et al., 2012).

Although patients may want to remain at home, family members often have to assume extra responsibilities, such as administering medications, which can lead to a great deal of anxiety (Mehta et al., 2014; Rosenberg, Bullen, & Maher, 2015; Totman et al., 2015). Further, when patients choose to receive care or die at home—perhaps to increase their quality of life through greater normalcy; increased contact with family, friends, and pets; and the familiar, comfortable surroundings (Hansson, Kjaergaard, Schmiegelow, & Hallström, 2012)—this location may not be the caregiver's first choice. For some families, a home death brings additional burdens, worry, and responsibility, and the home becomes more similar to an institution or may even feel similar to a prison (Funk et al., 2010; Mehta et al., 2014). The caregiver may forego breaks in caregiving in order to honor the patient's desire to stay at home. Decisions related to care location must be made with family members because the course chosen has a profound impact on the well-being of both the patient and the family (Cipolletta & Oprandi, 2014; Kinoshita et al., 2015; Morris et al., 2015). Recognize too, however, that family caregivers often do not express their preferences if they differ from those of the ill person and may need assistance from a nurse to navigate the competing demands and priorities (Robinson et al., 2012).

Further, family members may not be available or able to give care at home. Patients and family members may perceive that hospitals or hospices are able to provide a higher quality of end-of-life care than can be given at home, or the patient and family may prefer hospital or hospice care because they feel a close connection to the health care providers in the institution (Cipolletta & Oprandi, 2014). Some family members may experience profound guilt if they are not able to provide end-of-life care at home. Health care providers can alleviate some of this guilt if they alert patients and families early on that plans for location of care may need to change as time goes on to ensure provision of the best possible care that meets the needs of all family members, not just the dying person (Martz, 2015).

Burnout from caregiving is a common risk if family members are not able to cope with the caregiving requirements (Totman et al., 2015). The risk may be increased by the physical and emotional demands of the patient; reduced opportunities for the caregiver to participate in usual activities; and feelings of fear, insecurity, and loneliness (Totman et al., 2015). Caregiver strain may increase when patients need more assistance with activities of daily living or have greater levels of psychological and existential distress. Differences may exist in needs based on age and sex, with younger caregivers having more concerns about finances and maintaining social activities and relationships when compared with older caregivers (Osse et al., 2006). Female caregivers may have more difficulties with their own health (lack of sleep and muscle pain), with transportation, coordinating care, and feeling underappreciated when compared with male caregivers (Osse et al., 2006). Although there is conflicting evidence in the literature about parental mortality and morbidity following the death of a child, there is agreement that bereaved parents are at higher risk for completed suicide when compared with the general population (Hendrickson, 2009).

On the other hand, many people report positive aspects of caregiving (Cadell et al., 2014), such as feelings of satisfaction, greater appreciation for life, greater purpose and meaning to life, increased closeness and intimacy, newfound personal strength and ability, and the opportunity to share special time together and show their love for their dying family member (Andershed, 2006; Grande et al., 2009; Hudson, 2006; Jo et al., 2007; Riley & Fenton, 2007; Steele & Davies, 2006). Some family members may view care provision as an opportunity and a privilege (Hudson, 2006; Jo et al., 2007; Ward-Griffin et al., 2012). Hudson suggested a link between the caregiver's ability to see the positives in the situation and both better coping and less traumatic grief. It is important, therefore, to help families uncover the positive aspects and help families recognize the value in what they are doing because it may contribute to their overall well-being and may enhance their experience. Similarly, some researchers have found links between parents' satisfaction with care, or assessment of care quality, and their coping

ability or emotional state in the years after the child's death (Aschenbrenner, Winters, & Belknap, 2012; Kreicbergs, Lannen, Onelov, & Wolfe, 2007; Rosenberg, Baker, Syrjala, & Wolfe, 2012; Surkan et al., 2006). Nurses are in an excellent position to identify and foster a family's strengths, as well as to identify, prevent, and alleviate many of the negative aspects of caregiving. Through provision of optimal palliative and end-of-life care, nurses can have a significant, lifelong effect on the well-being of family members.

Involvement of the Interprofessional Team

Although the focus of this chapter is on the role of the nurse, provision of care through an interprofessional team approach is one of the principles of palliative care (Kelley & Morrison, 2015). The composition of the team may look quite different depending on the care setting. For example, in a rural setting, the team may be comprised of a family physician and a nurse, whereas in a large urban setting there may be a team of palliative specialists including palliative physicians, advanced practice nurses, psychologists, spiritual care advisors, pharmacists, social workers, and volunteers. In all settings, nurses are core team members. The *interprofessional* team approach focuses on health care providers collaboratively working with each other and with a patient/family as members of the team to develop a plan of care to achieve common goals (Davies, Baird, & Gudmundsdottir, 2013; Kelley & Morrison, 2015). Despite sharing common goals, each team member will bring different ideas and skills to the team, which is both the strength and the challenge of the interprofessional approach. Multiple perspectives contribute to holistic care and the ability to meet the multiple complexities of the patient and family needs that arise in palliative care. The challenge is how to make best use of each health care provider's and family member's contributions while negotiating differences in perspective and respectfully managing tensions around professional and personal boundaries and expertise. Palliative care is known for blurring of team member roles in order to meet the current needs of the patient and family members.

An interprofessional model of care is different from a multiprofessional model. Interprofessional care refers to professionals working and collaborating together to achieve common goals, with expected overlap in roles, whereas multiprofessional teams work with the same family, but focus on distinctly different aspects of care with little overlap in roles. For example, an interprofessional team often meets regularly to review and revise the care plan, discuss changes in care regularly, and share ideas in a collaborative manner. In contrast, multiprofessional teams rarely meet to discuss care planning and tend to have separate roles and goals in care dependent on professional expertise. In health care settings, traditional roles and expectations among the professionals involved in providing care can raise barriers to integrated and effective teams. Traditional medical services have been based on a *multiprofessional* model that has tended to hinder the development of an effective team. See Box 10-3 for a summary of the differences between the interprofessional and multiprofessional approaches.

For nurses, being an effective member of an interprofessional team often means that they share information and consult with others on the team, mediate on behalf of patients and families when necessary, and act as a liaison between various members, institutions, and programs. Novice nurses can effectively contribute to the interprofessional team by eliciting and understanding the patient's and family members' hopes, preferences, beliefs, fears, and goals and sharing this understanding with the team. Knowledge about group dynamics is invaluable in learning how to become a successful team member. Everyone needs to know and accept that each member of the team is unique and valuable,

and good communication skills are crucial so that supportive rather than defensive communication can be fostered. A lack of communication among health care providers is common and frustrating for families because they then receive conflicting information or need to repeat information and relay decisions that have been made already (Hudson, 2006; Widger & Picot, 2008; Wiegand, 2006).

Bereavement Care

One of the principles of palliative care is that care continues after the death and into bereavement. The need for follow-up with the family after the death by involved health care providers is considered by many families to be a crucial component of end-of-life care, but unfortunately one that is often missing (Aschenbrenner et al., 2012; D'Agostino, Berlin-Romalis, Jovcevska, & Barrera, 2008; de Jong-Berg & Kane, 2006; Meyer, Ritholz, Burns, & Truog, 2006; Price et al., 2013; Widger & Picot, 2008; Wisten & Zingmark, 2007; Woodgate, 2006). Families sometimes feel abandoned after the death, which adds to the grief they experience (D'Agostino et al., 2008; de Cinque et al., 2006; Meert et al., 2007; Widger & Picot, 2008). Bereavement care is important because family caregivers may experience negative effects, such as feelings of loneliness, sadness, and physical exhaustion caused by difficulty sleeping, as well as the aftermath of the demands of caregiving (Funk et al., 2010). These feelings may be juxtaposed

---

BOX 10-3
Interprofessional Versus Multiprofessional Teams

Multiprofessional Team	Interprofessional Team
■ Medical treatment model; fragmented approach to care	■ Holistic, "patient-centered" approach to care
■ Centralized control	■ Group control
■ Autocratic team leader	■ Facilitative team leader
■ Decision making by team leader	■ Decision making by consensus
■ Vertical communication between professionals	■ Horizontal communication between professionals
■ Treatment geared toward intraprofessional goals	■ Treatment geared toward interprofessional goals
■ Separate goals among professionals	■ Common goals among professionals
■ Professional goals are basis of plan	■ Patient goals are basis of care plan
■ Families are peripheral	■ Families are integral
■ Meetings/rounds involve individual professional reporting	■ Meetings/rounds involve group problem solving and decision making

with feelings of relief that the patient's suffering has ended and that everything possible was done to keep the patient comfortable (Hudson, 2006; Wollin et al., 2006). After the death, some caregivers may be at risk for impaired quality of life and mental health issues (Song et al., 2012; Thomas, Trauer, Remedios, & Clarke, 2014). Support for families after the death may help prevent or alleviate prolonged suffering. Specific interventions for bereavement care are highlighted later in the chapter and in the second and third case studies.

Barriers to Optimal Palliative and End-of-Life Nursing Care

A major barrier to optimal palliative and end-of-life care for patients and their families arises from the limited formal education and training nurses receive (Espinosa, Young, & Walsh, 2008). Although some improvements have been made, historically little attention has been given to palliative and end-of-life care in nursing and other health care providers' curricula. Health care providers are often uncomfortable or too afraid to initiate conversations about palliative care because they feel unprepared and are concerned about diminishing the patient's or family's hope (Fox et al., 2016; Shirado et al., 2013). However, research has shown that even difficult conversations about preferences for care at the end of life do not disrupt hope (Robinson, 2012; Shirado et al., 2013). It is critical that health care providers participate in dispelling myths and raising awareness of palliative care (McIlfatrick et al., 2014), but this approach requires adequate professional education. Further, health care providers report being unprepared to treat pain and symptoms effectively, emotionally support the dying person and his or her family, or deal with the ethical issues that may be present at end of life (Davies et al., 2008; Feudtner et al., 2007).

Another barrier to optimal palliative care is the availability and usage of palliative services. Specialist palliative care services may not be available in all care settings, particularly at home or in more rural and remote areas, to provide support to practicing health care providers in addressing learning needs or providing care to patients and families. Even when appropriate hospice and palliative care services are available, a lack of understanding of palliative care on the part of health care providers can lead to delayed, or even a lack of, referral to these services.

Involvement of the patient and family members in the interprofessional team is a critical component of palliative care, yet barriers may exist that limit this involvement. In many cases, the program setup and lines of communication do not allow for families to be included to the extent they could and should be, nor do they allow for provision of bereavement care by the health care professionals who provided care before the death. Although work needs to be done to remove the identified barriers, it is possible for nurses to practice high standards within constraining contexts. It is important to seek out opportunities to improve your knowledge and skills in palliative and end-of-life care and to be an advocate for the needs and views of patients and families regardless of barriers that may present themselves.

A different type of barrier that can be even more challenging to manage is the moral distress that can arise for nurses when they provide end-of-life care to patients and their families (Espinosa et al., 2008; Pattison, Carr, Turnock, & Dolan, 2013). Moral distress occurs when a person is powerless to carry out an action that he believes to be ethically appropriate. Some situations common to the provision of palliative care that may cause moral distress include the following:

- Patients receiving medical treatments that are believed to be inappropriate and/or contributing unnecessarily to patients' suffering (e.g., a ventilator, providing artificial nutrition and hydration) (Cheon, Coyle, Wiegand, & Welsh, 2015)
- Inadequate management of pain or other symptoms (Gagnon & Duggleby, 2014)
- Lack of communication with family members about prognosis (Cheon et al., 2015)
- Provision of false hope to family members (Epstein & Degado, 2010)
- Difficulty providing palliative care in acute care because of organizational constraints (e.g., task-oriented curative culture of care that devalues the emotional dimension of care, lack of time, and poor communication within the interprofessional team (Gagnon & Duggleby, 2014)

Moral distress can affect nurses' job satisfaction, physical and psychological well-being, self-image, spirituality, and decisions about their own health. Such distress may lead to burnout and leaving the work environment (Burston & Tuckett, 2012).

FAMILY NURSING PRACTICE ASSESSMENT AND INTERVENTION

Nurses must possess strong patient and family assessment skills if they are going to provide optimal care (e.g., excellent pain and symptom management, psychosocial support), because the most appropriate interventions can be designed and implemented only once a family's needs and goals have been assessed accurately. A nurse's assessment will help determine what a specific family or family member needs, and the care can then be tailored with an individual approach in consultation with the family. Assessment and intervention are, therefore, intertwined and are discussed together in the following sections.

Keep in mind that assessment should be ongoing and sequential, building on what is known about the family and shaping interventions to meet the family's changing needs and preferences throughout the palliative and end-of-life process. This section is organized around interventions that may be helpful to families. Unfortunately, definitive research with high-quality designs to identify the best interventions for promoting optimal long-term outcomes for family members is limited (Grande et al., 2009; Harding, List, Epiphaniou, & Jones, 2012; Hudson, Remedios, & Thomas, 2010; Rosenberg et al., 2012; Stajduhar, Funk, Toye, et al., 2010). The interventions discussed are informed by existing research evidence and have been used successfully in the authors' clinical practices. The most important thing to remember is that each family is unique. Although practice should be evidence-informed, it is important to apply theory and research critically and in alignment with individual family needs. What works for one family or family member may not be right for another. The need to assess and critically analyze each situation on its own merits and actively involve the family in the process is especially important in palliative care. Because a nurse cannot know in advance if an intervention will be useful to a particular family, interventions should always be offered tentatively and then evaluated regularly from the family perspective. An intervention is only helpful if a family or family member experiences it as helpful.

It is not possible to cover every potential scenario in palliative and end-of-life care; therefore, the focus is on discussing the main assessment and intervention concepts that are needed for palliative and end-of-life care. Most deaths encountered when providing end-of-life care occur as the result of chronic disease rather than an acute event. Therefore, these situations are the focus of the remaining discussion and the case studies.

Connections Between Families and Nurses

The relationships that families develop with health care providers have a significant effect on how families manage palliative and end-of-life events (Davies et al., 2017). In nursing education, characteristics of a helping or therapeutic relationship are often discussed, but in practice, nurses often speak of their "connections" with families rather than their "relationships" with families. Making a connection with family members helps uncover what is meaningful to them and builds a bridge between the nurse and the family member as human beings (Davies et al., 2013; Davies et al., 2017).

Understanding the family's situation apart from the illness is important (Benzein & Britt-Inger, 2008; Steele & Davies, 2006; Surkan et al., 2006; Tomlinson et al., 2006). Asking about the family's previous experiences with death, any recent or concurrent life changes (e.g., new job, new house, new baby), or work and school responsibilities (e.g., self-employed, supportive work environment, nearing final examinations) may allow a more in-depth understanding and appreciation of the complex influences on the family's palliative experience.

Connecting allows a nurse to apply her general palliative knowledge in ways that are more likely to be successful for individual patients and their families. Connecting is a two-way process where both the nurse and the patient/family members get to know one another as individuals and begin to establish reciprocal trust (Robinson, 2016). With trust comes a greater sense of comfort and ease for the family, and an increased ability for nurses to offer effective interventions and to act as advocates (Davies & Oberle, 1990; Davies et al., 2017).

Communication and interpersonal skills can facilitate or hinder connecting with patients and families (Davies et al., 2017). Therefore, nurses need to be aware of how their personal styles of interaction and communication can make, sustain, and break connections. These connections need to be attended to and nourished over time. Families typically are not used to talking about death and dying (Andershed, 2006). The presence of a mutual, trusting relationship is foundational to palliative assessment and intervention (Davies & Oberle, 1990; Davies et al., 2017; Robinson, 2016; Widger et al., 2009) and is crucial in providing a safe environment for difficult and emotional conversations to occur.

Nursing interventions that promote connections and trusting relationships include the following: careful listening to the family's experience with illness and suffering, valuing their expertise as caregivers, asking good questions that encourage family members' understanding of the differences in their perspectives, demonstrating compassion by showing that you are touched by the family's suffering, remaining nonjudgmental, offering a new perspective or information through open and honest communication, working *with* the family, acknowledging family strengths, and being reliable and accessible (Aspinal et al., 2006; Cronin, Arnstein, & Flanagan, 2015; Davies et al., 2017; Dosser & Kennedy, 2012; Heyland, Dodek, et al., 2006; Kristjanson, Aoun, & Oldham, 2006; Seccareccia et al., 2015). It is important to show families through your attitude and behavior that you not only have the knowledge to assist them, but also that you are willing and able to do so. The sense of security and trust a family experiences in relationships with health care providers can add to and strengthen the family's resources (Andershed, 2006). Simple acts, such as addressing family members by name, smiling, making eye contact, showing emotion, and appropriate physical contact, such as a hand on the shoulder, can foster connections between family members and the nurse (Butler, Hall, Willetts, & Copnell, 2015; Davies et al., 2017; Seccareccia et al., 2015). Family palliative caregiving is hard emotional work and responsive empathetic communication is critical (Wittenberg-Lyles et al., 2012).

It is the nurse's responsibility to take the lead in developing a trusting relationship with families and to provide an environment of openness where all family members feel comfortable asking questions (Robinson, 2016). Completion of a brief family genogram is one effective way of learning family members' names, relationships, and level of involvement in care, including decision making. Social support, including shared caregiving, is a key aspect of managing well, yet primary family caregivers may be reluctant to ask for help (Wittenberg-Lyles, Washington, Demiris, Oliver, & Shaunfield, 2014).

A genogram, and also an ecomap, will help you see gaps in support.

Getting to know each family member demonstrates respect for the patient's and family members' individuality, dignity, needs, concerns, and fears (Aspinal et al., 2006; Dwyer, Nordenfelt, & Ternestedt, 2008; Gordon et al., 2009; Hinds et al., 2009; Kristjanson, Aoun, & Oldham, 2006; Midson & Carter, 2010; Monterosso & Kristjanson, 2008; Riley & Fenton, 2007). Further, it enables recognition of differences within the family. Box 10-4 provides some questions to help open up communication and learn about family members' perspectives to build connections with the family.

Making a connection does not necessarily happen instantly, nor does it have to take a lot of time; however, it does require attention and cannot be taken for granted (Davies et al., 2017). Sometimes a connection easily exists between a nurse and a family; other times, the nurse may need to make an extra effort to get to know the family and to establish a relationship. You might feel as if you have to "prove" your trustworthiness to the family (Robinson, 2016) or set aside your own negative reaction to a particular family or family member. Developing a reflective practice and consulting with experienced professionals may be helpful when making connections proves difficult (Hendricks-Ferguson et al., 2015).

Unfortunately, all too often, families report lack of support, not being valued and respected, and a poor sense of connection with a nurse, which can in turn contribute to negative experiences and dissatisfaction with care (Andershed, 2006; Aschenbrenner et al., 2012; Dosser & Kennedy, 2012). Even single incidents related to poor communication and interpersonal skills on the part of health care providers can contribute to intense emotional distress in family members, including anxiety, depression, and guilt, often long after the event occurred (Gordon et al., 2009; Meert et al., 2007; Rini & Loriz, 2007; Surkan et al., 2006; Widger & Picot, 2008). Understanding this pattern leads some nurses to worry about saying the wrong thing. Listening carefully may assist in knowing where to start. Sometimes there are no "right" words to say, but simply being present and staying with the family can be helpful.

Humor may be another way to facilitate a connection with families, but it is important first to assess receptivity to humor (Ridley, Dance, & Pare, 2014). Generally, when families use humor, it is fine

BOX 10-4

Key Questions to Ask Families to Open Up Communication and Obtain Family Members' Perspectives

Ideally, questions to open up communication and obtain family members' perspectives should be asked with all involved family members present, including the patient. Keep in mind, however, that family members may not want to burden their ill member with their emotions and concerns, so you may find that some of these questions need to be asked of family members when they are alone. You will need to finesse questioning depending on where the ill family member is in the palliative care experience.

Start by saying, "I'd like to understand what it has been like for your family to live with [illness]." Then, use the following key questions to invite communication and obtain family members' perspectives. It is often helpful to indicate that you expect different family members will have different views about things. So you may need to ask a question multiple times in order to have all family members' views.

- What is your understanding of what is happening with [ill family member]?
- What experience do you have as a family in dealing with serious health problems? With death and dying?
- If you were to think ahead a bit, how do you see things going in (the next few days, the next few weeks, the next few months [use the time frame that is most appropriate])?
- How are you hoping this will go?
- What is most important for me to know about your family?
- What are you most concerned or worried about?
- When you think about your loved one getting really sick, what fears or worries do you have?
- I've found that many families caring for someone with this condition think about the possibility of their loved one dying. They have questions about this. Do you have questions?
- Who is suffering most?
- How do they show their suffering?

- How are you managing?
- I understand that different family members will have different talents or strengths: How do you most want to be involved?
- How can I be most helpful to you at this time?
- How does your family like to talk about challenging things?
- How have you been talking about the situation you find yourselves in? Who has been involved?
- Is there anyone involved who is important and who I haven't met?
- How are important decisions made in your family? How would you like important decision making to go now?
- Families often find it helpful to talk about the care they want at the end of life. Have you been able to have a conversation about this? I wonder if I might be able to help you start this conversation.
- Do you have any cultural beliefs, rituals, or traditions around illness and end of life that I should be aware of?
- What have you found most helpful or useful to you as a family at this time?
- What do you most need to manage well?
- What has not been helpful?
- What sustains you in challenging times?
- What is going well?
- What do you most want to be doing at this time? What brings you joy (or helps you get out of bed in the morning)?
- If your loved one were to die tonight, is there anything you have not said or done that you would regret? If so, how can I help you do or say what you need to do? (Ask this of the patient as well [i.e., If you were to die suddenly, is there anything you would regret not doing or saying?])
- In families, often many things are happening apart from the illness that we do not know about. Is there anything going on that is adding to what you are already coping with?

---

to then enter into the humor with them, but it may be more difficult for the nurse to initiate humor. The use of humor can provide respite from thinking about the illness, relieve tension, and demonstrate respect for the patient and family members as people if it fits with their way of being. Some strategies that nurses can use to make a connection between themselves and patients and families are provided in Box 10-5.

Relieving the Patient's Suffering

What do dying people want? They want adequate pain and symptom control, to prepare for death and to avoid inappropriate prolongation of dying, to achieve a sense of control, to live a meaningful life, to relieve burdens for their loved ones, and to strengthen relationships with loved ones (Kastbom, Milberg, & Karlsson, 2017; Milberg et al., 2014; Singer, Martin, &

BOX 10-5

Establishing and Sustaining Connections With Families

To establish and sustain connections with families, do the following:

- Patients and families need to know who you are; when you meet a patient and family for the first time, make them feel welcome, introduce yourself by name, then find out who they are and learn about them as people as well. Ask them how they would like to be called (e.g., by full name or first name). Ask them about their relationship to one another (e.g., to find out whether they are partners, sisters, friends). This is a good time to begin a genogram, which can be supplemented over time.

- Begin any interaction by clarifying your role and telling the patient and family about your "professional" self so you establish your credentials. For example, "Hello, Mr. Li. My name is Rose Steele. I'm a third-year student nurse. Sandyha Singh, the registered nurse supervising me, and I are taking care of your wife today. I'm working until 3:30 p.m. today and also will be here tomorrow, so I'll be her nurse then too. I have worked on this unit for the past 3 weeks, so I am pretty familiar with all the routines, but I'm really interested in finding out how we can fit in with what you and Mrs. Li want."

- The best approach is not "This is how we do it here," but rather "How do you like to do this?" and "How can we find a way to do that in this context?" Sometimes we cannot do it exactly the way the patient and/or family would like, so then we need to ask about what the most important pieces are so that we can come as close as possible to the desired result.

- Ensure a comfortable physical environment; let patients and families know the routines and how they can get help as needed, to provide a sense of familiarity and help you begin to make the connection.

- Privacy is often an issue and it is critical to some of the sensitive discussions that occur in palliative and end-of-life care. Try to find a private location before broaching sensitive issues.

- Describe who other team members are and what their roles are so families understand the context. Family members often do not know who to ask for what.

- Attend to the patient's and family's immediate state of well-being; it is impossible to connect with someone when you have not attended to their basic needs first. If a patient is lying in a wet bed or is in pain, family members will not be open to a "connecting" conversation with the nurse. When you demonstrate good assessment and intervention skills that result in enhanced comfort, your practice invites trust.

- Be sensitive to an individual's particular characteristics such as cultural or gender differences; making eye contact is a useful strategy for connecting in many cases, but a First Nations person, for instance, may be uncomfortable with direct eye contact. Touch is often welcome but is not universally experienced as supportive. You may need to ask about what provides comfort to the patient and family members.

- Do not let your observations of particular characteristics limit your perception by stereotyping the person; be aware of your own assumptions and biases, guarding against "operationalizing" your biases—for example, do not assume that an elderly person is deaf.

- Be sensitive to a person's way of being. Some people are outgoing and talkative; others are more withdrawn. It is a good idea to check out your observations rather than simply assuming that your interpretation of what you are seeing is correct. For example, some people become very quiet and stoic when in pain. This approach may be their way of managing pain, and not their usual "way of being." Humor may be appropriate for some people or situations, but not for others. Responding to people in ways that match their style enhances their comfort level. Another useful habit is to use the family's language. If you need to use medical terms, be sure to explain them. Sometimes family members use incorrect words (e.g., *prostrate* instead of *prostate*). Generally, the best way to handle it is to use the correct word in a matter-of-fact way and say something similar to, "Oh yes, I understand that the problem is prostate cancer."

- Not all people will want the same level of connection; you need to respect where the person is coming from and not try to force a deeper relationship. Families dealing with prolonged, life-threatening illness often have negative health care encounters that lead them to be wary of new health care providers and make them careful in how much, and in whom, they trust. Sometimes it takes time and the repeated demonstration of trustworthy behaviors before they are willing to begin to trust a new health care provider.

- Patients and families differ in their expectations of what health care providers should provide; some only want information, some expect only physical care, and still others expect more of a supportive relationship. The key here is in asking for expectations. This does not mean that you can meet the expectations and you may want to preface the request with a statement such as, "To be most helpful to you, I need to know what you

(continued)

BOX 10-5

Establishing and Sustaining Connections With Families *(cont.)*

would like. I may not be able to do things exactly as you prefer, but we can work together to get as close as possible."

- Many times you will find that when you simply meet the patient's and family's expectations without imposing your own, further opportunities for connecting may evolve.
- Once the connection has been made, it is important to pay attention to nurturing it so that it is sustained over time.
- Sustaining the connection allows you to learn even more about the patient and family so you can continually adapt your care according to their needs; it is also a way of demonstrating your trustworthiness by inviting the patient and family to get to know and trust you. When you are well connected, you are more likely to offer useful interventions that the family will accept.
- Ways of sustaining the connection include spending time with the patient and family, asking good questions, noticing what they are doing that is positive or helpful, and being available. Sometimes the only thing we can do is to stay with patients and families as a witness to their suffering.
- Making and sustaining the connection is a two-way process that has to do with sharing parts of yourself with patients and families as you seek a common bond. This process may mean revealing some personal details about your life. There are a few circumstances when it is appropriate, for example, when the patient or family ask you a direct question about yourself or when you have had an experience that helps you understand what the family may be experiencing. Revealing personal details can be helpful in inviting trust, but they should be brief and should not take the focus away from the patient and family.
- Continuity of care, such as having the same nurse be in contact with the same patient during some period of time, is important. It is critical that team members effectively communicate with one another to support continuity of care.

- It is not just the quantity but also the quality of time we spend with a family that makes the difference. For example, if you clear your mind before coming into the room, come to the bedside, and are calmly attentive to the patient rather than doing multiple tasks while also talking, the encounter will seem longer and be more satisfying to the patient.
- The "best" nurses are those who give the impression of "having all the time in the world," even when they are really busy. One way of doing this is to come into the room and sit or stand by the bedside, even if only briefly.
- Taking the time to "be there" for patients and families instead of being in a rush maintains the connection. This requires you to be mindful and to let go momentarily of all the demands that compete for your attention.
- Even when you are not actually with patients and families, it is important that they feel as if you will be available when they need you; simple things such as saying hello and good-bye at the beginning and end of shifts, and also at break times, help them know your availability. Let the patient and family know how long you are available and when you will be back (e.g., "I'm just popping in to see how your pain is and won't be able to stay long, but I'll be back in about half an hour and will be able to spend more time with you then").
- Informing patients and families so they know what to expect and keeping your word, such as being there when you say you will be, also sustain the connection.
- Instead of having your routine set for the day, adapt your routine to what the patient and family need at the time.
- Be flexible because you are always working under constraints; share these constraints with patients and families, and tell them if you need to change the plan you have made with them.
- Changing plans often requires the support of colleagues who can take over for you or help out as needed.

Kelner, 1999). Concern about becoming a burden to their family may keep dying people from talking to family members about their fears and about dying (Kuhl, 2002). At the same time, family members are worried about burdening the dying person. These worries, coupled with health care providers' avoidance of difficult discussions because of fear of disrupting hope (Robinson, 2012), can create a conspiracy of silence that contributes to a sense of isolation and aloneness for dying people and their loved ones. One of the ways nurses can be helpful is to assess who is talking to whom, who knows what, and what is holding people back from having conversations that nurture and strengthen the relationships that are often deeply desired within the family. Suffering can be alleviated by inviting and assisting families to come closer together and to engage in meaningful conversations (Wright & Leahey, 2012).

Meaningful conversations, however, are not possible unless the dying person is physically comfortable. Adequate pain and symptom control is the first priority of dying people. It is also the first priority for family caregivers, who need to become skilled palliative care providers (Mehta et al., 2014; Robinson et al., 2012). Witnessing the suffering of their dying family member when there is uncontrolled pain and symptoms is traumatic for family members. Therefore, foundational to good family palliative and end-of-life care is vigilant application of knowledge and skills in pain and symptom management (Cronin, Arnstein, & Flanagan, 2015). Nurses need to understand the variety of symptoms common to patients at the end of life so they can anticipate, prevent when possible, recognize, assess, and effectively manage pain and symptoms with both traditional and complementary therapies (see chapter Web sites later on Davis*Plus* for resources). Key to this is regular, systematic assessment using standardized assessment tools, such as the revised Edmonton Symptom Assessment System (ESAS-R; Alberta Health Services, 2010). Involving the dying person, as much as possible, in planning and treatment decisions supports the need for achieving a sense of control as more and more of their life feels out of control.

Relieving suffering yields improved quality of life, but no single definition exists for the most important factors that contribute to a good quality of life (Johansson, Axelsson, & Danielson, 2006; Norris et al., 2007). This is because only the individual and family know what constitutes quality of life for them. Individual needs must be assessed. Norris and colleagues (2007) found higher patient quality of life ratings associated with a variety of activities, such as playing music that was meaningful to the patient, attending a place of worship, having a familiar health care team available (for patients at home), and having individual preferences respected. Predictably, other components contributing to better quality of life include valuing everyday activities, maintaining a positive attitude, having symptoms relieved, feeling in control, and feeling connected to and needed by family, friends, and health care providers (Aspinal et al., 2006; Johansson et al., 2006).

Empowering Families

Family palliative and end-of-life care is a strengths-based approach. It is about building and nurturing family strengths to ensure that quality of life, as defined by the family, can be achieved as closely as possible. Rather than solely focusing on deficits or areas that the nurse perceives as problematic, palliative care emphasizes empowering families to manage this challenging time in their own unique way by noticing and building on strengths, while at the same time effectively addressing problems. All the empowering strategies require good communication skills. The focus should be on maximizing the patient's and family's capacity to use their own resources to meet their needs and respecting their ability to do so. Nurses empower patients and families by creating an environment in which their strengths and abilities are recognized, by encouraging them to consider various options, by assisting them in fulfilling their needs and desires through the provision of information and resources, and by supporting their choices. Several specific interventions that empower families are commending families, educating families about clinical options and constraints, and helping families to help themselves. The Carer Support Needs Assessment Tool (Aoun et al., 2015) is both an assessment and intervention resource that has been shown to effectively engage family caregivers in conversations about their needs, priorities, and solutions.

Family members appreciate recognition for their knowledge of the patient, their competencies, and their caring (Davies et al., 2013). Nurses can facilitate this appreciation by commending the work of the caregiver in the presence of the ill person. Commending families and family members is a very powerful intervention (Wright & Leahey, 2012), especially in the presence of the ill person. Caregivers may be better able to cope with caregiving when the ill person recognizes and appreciates their role (Hunstad & Svindseth, 2011; Stajduhar et al., 2008). Effective commendations involve making specific observations of patterns of family strengths that occur across time (Wright & Leahey, 2012). Similarly, parents appreciate recognition of their parenting role and skills. Nurses' commendations may help to strengthen parents' relationships with their child and their view of their parental role (Hinds et al., 2009).

Empowering also is about making patients and families aware of options and constraints about clinical care and available resources so they can make choices that are most appropriate for them (Davies et al., 2017; Robinson, Bottorff, McFee, Bissell, & Fyles, 2017). For example, home death is often the

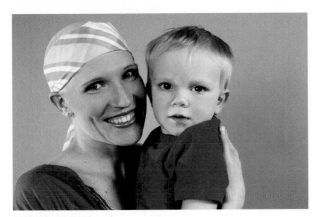

© iStock.com/120b_rock

patient's desire and, typically, family caregivers are deeply committed to doing whatever it takes to honor this preference (Robinson et al., 2012). Yet there is growing evidence that family caregivers are unprepared to take on the job of providing care and they lack the necessary education and support along the journey (Henriksson & Årestedt, 2013; Mehta et al., 2014; Robinson et al., 2012; Topf, Robinson, & Bottorff, 2013). Under these circumstances, family caregivers can suffer negative health consequences and are at risk for complicated bereavement (Topf et al., 2013). Engaging both the patient and involved family members in discussion about preferences for care, preferences for place of death, and available resources may assist negotiations regarding decisions that can be simply taken for granted when family members automatically step forward to take up the role of caregiver. Choice empowers families.

Strain on families may be reduced when families feel more capable in their ability to provide and manage the patient's end-of-life care and better able to attend to their own self-care needs and difficult emotions or interactions (Merluzzi, Philip, Vachon, & Heitzmann, 2011). Nurses need to assess families for their knowledge, skills, and concerns, and then offer appropriate interventions. Some interventions include providing information about the illness, its treatment, and its prognosis; teaching family members how to provide adequate care to their loved one; and encouraging family members to share their fears and other emotions, and then providing the needed support (e.g., in discussions, or referring to appropriate resources such as a social worker who can arrange for respite care). Facilitating hope for a longer life or for a peaceful death and providing adequate information and emotional and instrumental

support also may help reduce the burden (Hunstad & Svindseth, 2011; Shirado et al., 2013).

Empowering patients and families may include helping them to do what they themselves want and need to do, rather than health care providers taking over and doing it for them (Davies et al., 2017). For example, although it may appear quicker and easier for the nurse to assist a patient out of bed, it may be important that the patient moves by herself or that a family member is taught to assist. Sometimes the nurse will need to be creative in finding ways to empower patients and families. Consulting and collaborating with other team members can help identify creative ways to empower family members across diverse environments and situations.

It is important to assess the capacity of patients and families to do for themselves, and then find ways of supporting them when hopes and expectations exceed capability. Careful assessment of the situation is central to knowing when to act on behalf of patients and families, and when to encourage them to manage themselves, because if the nurse "does for" patients and families when they can care for themselves, their sense of competency may be diminished, which can be disempowering. On the other hand, if the nurse expects family members to do everything on their own, they may feel isolated and unsupported (Stajduhar, Funk, Jakobsson, et al., 2010).

Providing Information

Families often have a need for information, but may not know what questions to ask. A lack of knowledge and feeling uninformed can leave people feeling isolated, frustrated, and distressed (Andershed, 2006; Hunstad & Svindseth, 2011). Some families want a great deal of detailed information, whereas others feel overwhelmed with too much information and find that it interferes with their ability to live as normal a life as possible. Therefore, ongoing assessment of how much and what types of information families want is important (Allen, 2014; Davies et al., 2017). This assessment also needs to include how much information should be offered directly to the patient, especially a child (Hays et al., 2006; Hsiao, Evan, & Zeltzer, 2007; Yoshida et al., 2013). A wide variation exists in the age at which parents believe a child is old enough to be included in illness discussions (Mack et al., 2005). Even when the patient is an adult, some families may believe that not all information should be shared with the patient (Royak-Schaler et al., 2006). These beliefs may be based on cultural norms and fear of taking away hope or needlessly increasing fear. Nurses need to be aware of their legal responsibilities and ensure that they do not withhold information inappropriately. They also must convey their responsibilities to the family and initiate an open dialogue about the importance of communication. As previously alluded to, some families may hold a culturally based belief that an adult patient should not be told a life-limiting diagnosis (Yoshida et al., 2013). One way of approaching this is to ask the patient whether she wants information about her medical condition, and, if not, who in the family should be given information, and whether this person should be considered her chosen substitute decision maker.

As a family nurse, it is important to know what information can be offered that is likely to make a positive difference for family caregivers. Nurses are in one of the best positions to understand and appreciate the challenges for family members to take up the job of caregiving. Most family members do not have a medical background and do not know what to expect when they take on the role of caregiver (Stajduhar, Funk, & Outcalt, 2013). They do not know how to provide basic care effectively, such as assisting the ill person in activities of daily living, such as toileting and bathing; assisting the ill person to move without causing more pain; managing symptoms such as nausea and breathlessness; or even safely working with equipment such as an oxygen tank. They need knowledge and skills that they do not even know they need until they are alone in the midst of providing care (Stajduhar et al., 2013). Noticing what the ill family member needs, anticipating future needs, listening to both the ill person and the family caregiver, assisting them to negotiate how care will be done at home, working directly with the family caregiver to provide knowledge and model essential skills, and determining available resources and gaps in services are some examples of interventions that may prove supportive.

Timing is important—information and teaching need to come before crises, and at a time that is meaningful to the family (Stajduhar et al., 2013). The key is listening carefully to both the ill person and the family caregiver and bringing knowledge forward to support them in their mutual goals. At the same time, it is important to recognize and assist with strategies to maintain "normal" roles within

a family, such as parent or spouse (Price, Jordan, Prior, & Parkes, 2011; Rodriguez & King, 2014; Stajduhar, Funk, Jakobsson, et al., 2010; Weidner et al., 2011). Family caregivers have reported that interventions aimed at separating them from their dying family member, such as exhortations to leave the bedside and get some sleep, are often not helpful and can be experienced as disrespectful (Robinson et al., 2012). Family caregivers may see these interventions as evidence that nurses really do not understand their commitment to the dying person and to providing care, regardless of the personal consequences. As previously mentioned, one intervention that is very powerful is offering situation-specific commendations.

When patients and family members are empowered with the amount and kind of information they want, and at the time they need it, the result is more effective partnerships with health care providers. Nurses are in a key position to act as a liaison between the health care team members and the family. Patients and families should be encouraged to ask questions, and these questions should be answered with full explanations and support. There is some evidence that family caregivers may be reluctant to reveal difficulties providing care because they are afraid that care will be taken away from them (Topf et al., 2013). Therefore, nurses need to create an environment that allows family members to speak openly and without fear.

Nurses are sometimes reluctant to invite questions from families because they are concerned they may not have an answer. Simply knowing the questions that the family would like answered is valuable information, and many times the questions do not have clear answers. For example, the question of "When will my family member die?" cannot be easily answered. Nurses may not know the answer, and that is all right. If possible, however, nurses can show their trustworthiness by seeking the information and providing it in a timely fashion.

Overall, families need to have honest and understandable information about a variety of areas, including the following:

- The patient's condition
- The illness trajectory
- Prognosis (keeping in mind that prognosis is inherently uncertain because we cannot predict when death will occur)
- Symptoms to expect and treatment options

- How to provide physical care
- What to expect (including signs of impending death, which allows family members the opportunity to say final good-byes)
- Ways of coping (including helping families become aware of possible strategies, such as respite and mental pauses)
- The dying process
- How to access additional support
- What aids (e.g., wheelchairs, beds, lifts) may be helpful and where to get them
- The care system in which this all occurs

Provision of this type of information is linked to reduced caregiver burden, improved coping, self-efficacy, increased hope, reduced anxiety, and enhanced quality of life (Henriksson & Årestedt, 2013; Northouse et al., 2010).

The way in which information is shared is as important as the content of the information. Critical components of the process of sharing information include timing, pacing, and both verbal and nonverbal conveyance of respect, empathy, and compassion (Davies et al., 2017; Gutierrez, 2012). The timing and pacing, in particular, are important to allow families to absorb the reality of the situation and to make informed decisions (Davies et al., 2017; Meert et al., 2007). Not rushing families to make decisions is important; however, giving information as early as possible to allow for ongoing discussions and decision making with a clearer mind rather than waiting for a crisis that may be fraught with emotion results in better outcomes (Allen, 2014; Macdonald, Liben, & Cohen, 2006). The use of simple, jargon-free language is also helpful. In emotionally intense situations, little information is absorbed and it must be repeated over time, so nurses should be willing to clarify repeatedly for family members without becoming impatient. Asking clarifying questions of all family members to ensure that information is being understood is also important (Davies et al., 2017). Nurses also need to attend to their own and family members' nonverbal language (Henry, Fuhrel-Forbis, Rogers, & Eggly, 2012). For instance, watching the person's face to determine if she looks confused, upset, or comprehending can help assure information is being understood and welcomed. Moreover, the nurse's body language can aide communication. For example, standing close to a family member when talking about care rather than standing in the doorway of a patient's room gives the impression of having time to talk and listen rather than being in a hurry to move on. Moderation of the tone of voice can change a statement from sounding annoyed or without compassion to respectful and empathetic (Davies et al., 2017).

Through learning about other families' experiences, patients and family members can better understand their own experience. Nurses can share insights gained from other families both from practice and research. For example, a nurse may share: "Other families have told me that talking about what their child's death might be like was one of the hardest things they ever had to do, but once they knew there was a plan in place for how to handle the possible symptoms or issues that may happen, they were able to stop worrying about all the 'what-ifs' and just focus on having the best time possible with their child." Having information about other families going through similar experiences enables patients and family members to connect better with health care providers, which in turn enhances decision making and planning for the future.

Balancing Hope and Preparation

A fair amount of ambiguity always exists when working with families at the end of life, regardless of whether the situation is acute or chronic. Nurses need to become comfortable with the inherent uncertainty and help families live well within an uncertain context. One common ambiguity surrounds prognostic uncertainty. Given that we cannot predict when death will occur, families need to be encouraged to attend to what they view as important and to take advantage of the moment. When a patient or family member asks, "How long?" the nurse might reply by asking, "What would you be doing differently now if you knew that the time was very short?" In response to their answer, suggesting that they do whatever "it" is, and if they get to do "it" again next week or next month or even next year then that would be a bonus, may help family members achieve what matters most in the difficult circumstance of advanced illness.

As a patient's condition changes and deteriorates, the hopes and expectations of the patient and family may change as well. Hope often shifts from a more global perspective—such as hope for a cure—to a more focused or specific perspective, such as a hope to live long enough to see her grandchild who is due in a few months. Nurses can help facilitate this change in hope by asking powerful questions, such as, "If your loved one were to die tonight, is there anything you have not said or done that you would regret?" or "If you were to die suddenly, is there anything you would regret not doing or saying?" Such questions encourage patients and families to consider what is most meaningful to them and allow them to shift their hope to areas that may be more attainable. Nurses who participate in these discussions can help maintain hope for some things while not providing false hope. They also can offer to help patients and families do or say what they need to do.

For some families and in some cultures, a need is present to keep fighting for every chance at life, hoping for a miracle, until the last possible moment, even when they may know this is considered medically unrealistic (Robinson, 2012). As a nurse, it is important to find the balance between supporting families in their hopes and still being comfortable talking about death and preparing the patient and family for what is to come, including advance care planning (Hsiao et al., 2007; Jackson et al., 2012; Rini & Loriz, 2007; Robinson, 2012; Robinson et al., 2006). Therefore, when preparing the family for what is to come, the information must be provided in a sensitive manner that acknowledges hope (Robinson, 2012; Shirado et al., 2013). One way of doing this is to use a hypothetical question (Wright & Leahey, 2012), such as, "If things don't go as we hope, what is most important for you to have happen?" Another phrase that is sometimes helpful is suggesting that a family "hope for the best and plan for the worst."

Parents of dying children identify a need to balance hope and despair (Konrad, 2008; Moro et al., 2011) and appreciate when health care providers support hope without offering false hopes (Gordon et al., 2009; Monterosso & Kristjanson, 2008). Lack of discussions about the possibility of death are closely linked to parents' belief that health care providers sometimes give false hope that the child will survive the illness (Gordon et al., 2009; Monterosso & Kristjanson, 2008). False hope may be detrimental to parents' ability to prepare for the child's death, so nurses need to be mindful of what they say and how they say it. Honest acknowledgment of the severity of the situation is important.

Facilitating Choices

A major role for nurses is to be an advocate for patients and families and facilitate their choices. But to do so, nurses need to know what the patient and family want. One specific intervention is to encourage advance care planning so that everyone is clear about the patient's preferences regarding end-of-life care (Reinhardt et al., 2014). Other interventions include assessing the extent of both the patient's and family members' desire for involvement in decision making, and then respecting that desire; assessing their awareness about the possibility of death, and opening lines of communication; and identifying and then building on the patient's and family's strengths in order to optimize choices (Gallagher et al., 2015; Jackson et al., 2012).

Advance Care Planning

At the end of life, patients may be unable to participate in making decisions about their care, leaving family members to make decisions based on their understanding of what the patient would want if he were able to participate. One way in which families can prevent misunderstandings and can promote facilitation of choices is by discussing wishes and desires in advance. Advance care planning is a process that involves reflection and communication. It is a way of letting others know personal future health and care preferences, so that if the individual becomes incapable of consenting to or refusing treatment, others—especially a designated substitute decision maker or the person who will speak for a person when that person cannot—will make decisions for that person that reflect his values and wishes, regardless of their own desires. Advance care planning often involves not only discussions with family and friends, but also writing down end-of-life wishes; it may even involve talking with health care providers and financial and legal professionals. The Canadian Hospice Palliative Care Association (n.d.), in collaboration with the National Advance Care Planning Task Group, provides several valuable online resources about advance care planning, including a workbook to guide writing the plan.

An *advance directive* specifies the medical treatments an individual does or does not want at the end of life; for example, resuscitation if her heart stops. It is usually a legally binding document, but nurses must be aware of the legal requirements within their own workplace jurisdiction (e.g., state or province). Fewer than 30% of adults have an advance directive, and even for those adults who do have them, they may not be available when needed or be specific enough (Dunn, Tolle, Moss, & Black, 2007). If someone has written an advance directive, her substitute decision maker should have a copy. It is important that health care providers are made aware of a patient's advance directives (Jackson et al., 2012) and, preferably, have a copy in the patient's chart. Nurses need to make themselves familiar with such advance directives so they can advocate for the patient as needed when decisions are being made.

Advance care planning is a process that is best initiated early in the illness experience and revisited as the illness progresses because preferences can change over time (Robinson, 2011, 2012). These types of conversations are difficult to have among family members, and families may appreciate assistance to initiate and facilitate the conversation. Nurses can facilitate the process and empower both patients and families by encouraging them to talk about end-of-life issues and preferences long before they are faced with the situation. By initiating discussions about substitute decision making, choosing a substitute decision maker, and the legalities of representing the patient's wishes, decisions can be well thought out rather than crisis oriented. The process of substitute decision making can be a very demanding one for families, particularly if they have not had discussions about the patient's preferences (Jackson et al., 2012). Having a written advance care plan, and/or an advance directive, assists family members by helping them understand the patient's wishes, which can then inform decision making (Robinson, 2011, 2012). Documentation of wishes and preferences is also helpful when there are differences among family members about what they think is best for the ill person. In addition, when faced with actually making decisions, family members often appreciate acknowledgment of the difficulty of their role, and the nurse's attentive, respectful support throughout the process will be very helpful (Jackson et al., 2012).

Physician-Assisted Suicide and Medical Assistance in Dying

One aspect of advance planning may include a patient determining when and how she or he will die, within specific legal contexts. Globally, several countries legally allow for people who are suffering to arrange for their own death as a medical intervention. In the United States, the state of Oregon enacted the Death with Dignity Act in 1997, which allows individuals with a terminal illness to end their lives through the voluntary self-administration of lethal medications that are expressly prescribed by a physician for that purpose. Since then, physician-assisted suicide (PAS)

is now permitted in California, Colorado, Oregon, Vermont, and Washington. Physician-assisted dying (PAD) is also legal in Montana because of a 2009 State Supreme Court ruling. To legally qualify for a prescription under PAS/D legislation, individuals must be a resident of the applicable state, be at least 18 years of age, be mentally competent to make and communicate their own health care decisions, and be diagnosed with a terminal illness that, if allowed to take its natural course, will lead to death within 6 months (Oregon Health Authority, 2016). In addition, individuals must be able to self-administer and ingest the prescribed medication.

The American Nurses Association (ANA, 2013) prohibits nurses' participation in assisted suicide or euthanasia. However, the ANA also acknowledges that in some states nurses may be involved when a patient makes a choice to end his or her life. The ANA refers nurses to their statutory body (e.g., the Oregon Nurses Association) for guidance on how to proceed. Nurses are not obliged to participate in PAS/D, but they are required to not abandon their patient and so must make sure that someone else will provide care if the nurse chooses to not deliver care.

On June 17, 2016, the federal government of Canada received formal approval for amendments to the Criminal Code so that medical assistance in dying (MAID), under certain circumstances, would no longer be considered a criminal offense. Nurses in Canada must now be familiar with the wording of Bill C-14, *An Act to amend the Criminal Code and to make related amendments to other Acts (medical assistance in dying)*, and must work within both this legislation and their relevant regulatory standards. An important limitation to the nursing role expressly requires that only a physician or nurse practitioner administer the substance that will bring about death. Therefore, most nurses may assist (e.g., by preparing medication), but must not actually administer the medication. Similarly, if a patient is given a prescription to self-administer the medication, then nurses should not assist with the administration of the medication (see the Canadian Nurses Protective Society Web site at https://www.cnps.ca/ for further information). Nurses must ensure that their practice is consistent with not only the law and the guidelines from their regulatory bodies but also their employer's position on whether or not MAID is permitted within the setting and, if so, the policies and procedures that outline how and by whom MAID may be undertaken. It is also important to note that the amendments to the Criminal Code do not impose an obligation for nurses to participate in MAID. However, nurses continue to have a legal duty of care to patients and must not abandon them. Therefore, it may be necessary to refer to or involve other health care providers in certain circumstances.

Regardless of where a nurse is practicing, it is critical that nurses understand and practice within all appropriate laws, rules, and standards. If something is not clear then nurses should seek advice, including legal as necessary, to ensure that they understand the consequences of the actions they are contemplating—whether choosing or refusing to participate in MAID or PAS/D.

Involvement in Decision Making

Families may be facing their first experience with death and dying, and they often depend on nurses to help them in their process. Families may not know what they need or what might be possible (Selman et al., 2007); they may expect health care providers to bring up issues when appropriate—that is, the family members may feel it is not their place to raise issues first (Robinson, 2011), so nurses need to open the conversation. It is important first to assess and then respect the patient's and family's desired level of involvement in discussions about the end of life and in decision making. Nurses should ask questions such as, "How are important decisions made in your family?" and "How would you like important decision making to go now?" so they understand the family's approach and can facilitate appropriate interactions that respect family choice.

Some patients and families may want full responsibility for decisions; some may want to be involved but not make final decisions; some may want the physician to take the initiative and make all decisions (Selman et al., 2007); and some patients want their family members to make decisions (You et al., 2014). Some parents feel that making decisions for the child is inherently a parental role, but not all want to have complete responsibility for final decisions (Brosig, Pierucci, Kupst, & Leuthner, 2007; Hays et al., 2006; Meyer et al., 2006; Rodriguez & King, 2014). Again, assessment of preferences about decision making is important. Nurses can use questions such as, "I understand that different family members will have different talents or strengths; how do you most want to be involved?" to uncover family members' preferences so they can work with the family in ways that facilitate choice.

Regardless of their actual role in the decision-making process, parents want to be recognized as the experts on their child and as the central, consistent figures in their child's life (Rodriguez & King, 2014; Sullivan, Monagle, & Gillam, 2014). As such, they want health care providers to seek out and respect their knowledge, opinions, observations, and concerns about their child (Davies et al., 2017; Hsiao et al., 2007; Kars, Grypdonck, & van Delden, 2011; Meyer et al., 2006; Weidner et al., 2011; Widger & Picot, 2008; Woodgate, 2006). Therefore, nurses should verbally acknowledge that the parent's input is critical and they should be mindful of paying attention to facilitating the parent's choices, regardless of their own beliefs.

The involvement of family members in decision making can have a lifelong effect on the well-being of family members (Surkan et al., 2006; You et al., 2014). Nurses, therefore, must foster good communication to ensure that the patient's and family's needs and wishes are understood and supported within a caring relationship that is built on partnership between professionals and families (Robinson, 2011). Many times health care providers block families from participating because they feel they know what is best or because they are trying to protect families. But effective end-of-life care is not possible unless open and mutual communication occurs between families and professionals, and families participate in shared decision making to the extent they desire (Robinson, 2011). Questions such as, "If you were to think ahead a bit, how do you see things going in the next few weeks?" and "Families often find it helpful to talk about the care they want at end of life. Have you been able to have a conversation about this? I wonder if I might be able to help you start this conversation," can be used to learn what a patient and family want. See Box 10-4 for other questions that may help nurses become cognizant of a family's choices.

Awareness of Possibility of Death

Lack of early information about the possibility of death makes it difficult for family members to come to terms with decisions such as the withdrawal of life-sustaining therapy or the use of cardiopulmonary resuscitation (CPR) (Heyland, Frank, et al., 2006). Families faced with these types of decisions usually place great value on open, honest, and timely information, but they also need to be listened to in terms of their intimate knowledge of the patient rather than just spoken to (Allen, 2014; Hunstad & Svindseth, 2011; Seccareccia et al., 2015). Moreover, it is crucial to prepare the family for what to expect when life-sustaining therapy is withdrawn. For example, families need to be aware that death may occur very quickly, or may take hours or days (Wiegand, 2006). When decisions are made, such as withdrawal of life-sustaining therapy, any delays past the agreed-on time for implementing the decision may greatly increase the family's anxiety (Wiegand, 2006). Therefore, it is important for nurses to keep the family informed about the reasons for any changes to the plan and to be available to talk with family members when needed.

Building on Strengths

Nurses need to recognize the dying person's and family members' rights and abilities to make their own decisions and then make an effort to find out what is important to them. It is important to focus on what patients and families *can* do, rather than on what they *cannot* do. Nurses can reinforce those aspects of the self that remain intact, and assist patients and families to recognize their own strengths and abilities. Individual and family strengths can be built on, which can smooth the way for patients and families to meet their own needs. Nurses can work with patients and families by making suggestions, providing options, and planning strategies that will allow them to achieve their goals. Professional knowledge may be invaluable in guiding families to consider options and possible routes of action that they would not have thought of without input; for example, the use of special equipment that allows a patient to have the bath that he thought was not possible because of his weakness. Furthermore, the nurse may have a clearer sense of the consequences of certain choices, which again is extremely valuable information. At the very least, the nurse can seek out answers to families' questions and be a resource for families.

Facilitating choices also means identifying and accepting a patient's and family's limitations, and finding ways to work with them so they can achieve an outcome that is both positive and satisfactory to them; for example, suggesting new activities that are appropriate for the patient's current capabilities. It is important that relationships remain mutual and reciprocal, and patients in particular need to experience their positive contribution to their family members. Thus, as patients get sicker, their contribution will look different and may focus on such things as words of wisdom rather than concrete actions.

Offering Resources

One nurse cannot be all things to every patient and family. It is important to be aware of other team members, such as spiritual or pastoral care providers (Wall, Engelberg, Gries, Glavan, & Curtis, 2007), social workers, and others who may be available to provide support to the family. Furthermore, the nurse should be knowledgeable about hospital- and community-based services, such as hospice, that may be available to support families both before and after the death (Price et al., 2013). Nurses can offer these other resources and services to families, but each family will decide what will actually be helpful for them. For some families, using inpatient respite services during the last year of life may help relieve their burden, if only for a short time, whereas other caregivers may experience feelings of guilt and increased stress caused by worrying about the quality of care provided during respite (Robinson et al., 2017). Caregivers may be supported in their role simply by knowing there are other resources and support readily available, even if they do not make use of them (Stajduhar et al., 2008).

Encouraging Patients and Families

Patients and family members often seek approval and encouragement from professionals as they make decisions about how to meet their needs. Encouraging is an important strategy in empowering patients and families to do for themselves. This means verbally and nonverbally supporting patients and families in their choices, providing reinforcement for each individual's ideas, and demonstrating support by finding ways to facilitate their choices. Encouraging does not necessarily mean that the nurse *agrees* with the choice, merely that the nurse supports the patient or family member in finding ways to enact the choice. At the same time, encouraging does not mean the nurse abandons her expertise, which is complementary to the expertise of the family. Sharing professional knowledge and perspective contributes to fully informed decision making.

Nurses can sometimes think that they know what is "best" for patients and their families. As caring professionals, nurses have families' best interests at heart and want to protect them as much as possible. Even as nurses value each person as a worthwhile individual who has the right and ability to make his or her own choices and decisions, they may find that the patient's and family's desires conflict with what they believe is "best" based on their professional experience and knowledge (Price et al., 2013). Times such as these can cause moral distress as nurses struggle with supporting the patient and family, while remaining "true" to professional knowledge and ethics. Negotiation skills may be severely tested in such situations, and sometimes the nurse will be tempted to override a patient's wishes. Some nurses describe their bottom line as "ensuring patient safety," and unless the patient's physical safety is compromised they will support the patient's choice, even when they disagree with it. An example of a possible disagreement might be when a patient and family decide to continue caring at home and the nurse thinks admission to hospice or a hospital is the best option. Encouraging supports families to figure out ways to do what is important for them in the best way possible.

Managing Negative Feelings

End-of-life care is not all encouragement and positive feelings. Many patients and family members also have negative feelings that influence their experiences. Talking with patients and family members (often individually) about those negative feelings gives them permission to have, experience, and deal with them. For many people, negative feelings, such as guilt or anger, are suppressed or internalized. Others openly express their anger but displace it onto someone else, often the nurse or other family members. The ability to diffuse a situation effectively requires nurses to learn how to accept someone else's negative feelings in an open and non-defensive manner. It means not taking their words as a personal attack, but realizing that patients and family members simply need a safe outlet for their frustrations and negative feelings. The nurse's role is to listen in an accepting way and allow them to ventilate. It can be hard to face an angry tirade, but most people will calm down once they have said what they need to say and they realize that the listener values their feelings even if they are negative ones. Questions that are often useful include "How can I help?" or "What needs to be different?"

Sometimes, however, people will remain angry or guilty despite best efforts; diffusing will not always be successful. Some people are so angry about what is happening to their loved one and their family that they cannot move to any other emotional state. During these instances, it is best to accept that this is their reality and find ways to work with them. This is often a time when nurses need the support of colleagues, and a team approach may help to lessen the effects of working with these patients and families (Anderson et al., 2015; Hendricks-Ferguson et al., 2015). Other interventions that may be helpful include referral to resources such as social work, pastoral care, psychology, and support groups.

Facilitating Healing Between Family Members

Negative feelings and misunderstandings can cause or expand rifts in families. If a nurse can facilitate healing between family members that unifies the family, the family can function better as a team and members are better equipped to move through the dying process. The nurse can help mend relationships by interpreting family members' behaviors to one another and helping them to see each other's point of view. Sometimes an outsider can bring clarity to a situation that is impossible for those members who are enmeshed in it. An assessment question that may be useful is this: "Is there anything that is unsaid or undone in the family that needs your attention?" Be careful, though, that questions are not aimed at "fixing broken families." Many families that you might think are dysfunctional do not see themselves as having difficulties or needing to change. They will not accept attempts to "fix them" and, indeed, may find concerns about the family intrusive. Furthermore, relationships develop over many years and yet interventions occur in a relatively short period. Large changes in family dynamics cannot often be expected during the short time a family works with the nurse. Rather, seeds are often planted, and when the family is motivated to make changes, improvements in family function will occur. Sometimes all that can be done is to acknowledge that certain things cannot be altered and often genuine and empathetic presence is the best intervention that can be offered. Level of family functioning will need to be attended to carefully, and the expectation that a family will pull together to cope with the process of dying may be unrealistic. Noticing the family members' love for the ill member and acknowledging their mutual desire for the best for their ill member (even though there may be quite different ideas about what is best) is sometimes helpful.

Family Meetings

Family meetings typically involve the patient, those family members desired by the patient, and the relevant health care providers (Hudson, Quinn, O'Hanlon, & Aranda, 2008). They should routinely be offered on admission to a setting and further meetings be called by the patient/family or health care provider on an as-needed basis. Family caregivers often have difficulty with the transition of providing care at home to transferring care to others when the patient is admitted to a hospital or hospice (Harrington, Mitchell, Jones, Swetenham, & Currow, 2012). This is a good time for a family meeting. Family meetings should be considered a proactive approach and not be held in reserve only for crisis situations. Family meetings are beneficial to facilitate consistency in everyone's understanding of the situation and the expected course for the illness (Hudson et al., 2008; Wiegand, 2006), as well as for negotiation of care. They enable patients, family members, and health care providers to meet together to discuss any issue, but they are not family therapy (Fineberg, 2005, 2010).

Nurses are ideal partners to lead these end-of-life family conferences. In all settings, the nurse can assist families in preparing for the meetings by helping them to write down questions that they want to raise at the meeting and informing the family about what to expect during the conference. Family satisfaction can be enhanced when clinicians allow time for family members to speak about what they have been experiencing, facilitate shared decision making, and express support for the family's decisions (Sullivan, da Rosa Silva, & Meeker, 2015). It is helpful to begin by eliciting the family's understanding of the situation, as well as pressing concerns, before moving to the health care providers' perspectives. Different family members and providers will have different ideas, so it is useful to request different perspectives. Afterward, discussing with the family how the conference went, the changes in the patient's plan of care and what they mean, and how the family feels about the conference as well as the changed plan of care helps to solidify decisions made during the family meeting (Hudson et al., 2008; Sullivan et al., 2015). Summarizing decisions that were made and then supporting the family in these decisions can help strengthen the family's trust in the care plan.

More than one family meeting may be necessary as the patient's condition changes or if the family needs time to think or further discuss issues before decisions are made (Hudson et al., 2008; Wiegand, 2006). The proportion of time the family spends talking during these conferences is more important than the total length of the conference in increasing family satisfaction and decreasing conflict between families and health professionals (McDonagh et al., 2004). Yet, on average, typical family conferences involve the health care provider speaking for 70% of the time and listening for only 30% of the time (McDonagh et al., 2004). It is important to ensure that families do the majority of talking during family meetings. In addition, be mindful of nonverbal communication, because it is often the main method of communication, and is particularly powerful when the topics are emotional. For example, arms wrapped tightly around the body may indicate anxiety, whereas interrupting may be a sign of impatience.

Finding Meaning

When recovery is impossible, nurses must consider their role in helping patients and families find meaning in the experience as they care for and assist families. Patients and families often struggle to understand why the patient is dying. They try to make sense of the experience, and they search for ways to make the patient's life and inevitable death meaningful. Their search for meaning may involve examining relationships within the family or with a higher power (Hexem, Mollen, Carroll, Lanctot, & Feudtner, 2011). Some people will be more successful at finding meaning than others or the process may not occur until long after the death (Widger et al., 2009).

As a nurse, you can assist in this process of finding meaning by truly listening and hearing what family members have to say. Engaging in a relationship and dialogue will be empowering and can help families create meaning even in a difficult situation (Davies et al., 2017). There are many different ways of finding meaning, and not all individuals will overtly search for meaning. However, part of the nursing role is to accompany people as they try to make sense of their situation. No one can find meaning for someone else (Robinson et al., 2006). Each individual will seek his own meaning in his own unique way. Some may be very articulate about their philosophical and spiritual beliefs and how they influence meaning for them (Hexem et al., 2011; Knapp et al., 2011). Others may talk about these issues in more concrete terms, perhaps rarely having articulated their thoughts and feelings. Still others may "talk" through their actions. Finding meaning gives strength to people; therefore, you will find that it is empowering for families. Nurses who examine the concepts of meaning of illness and dying with patients may gain a deepened understanding of the patients' experiences, which may lead to changes and improvements in the way care is provided (Cadell et al., 2014). One way to begin this examination is by asking the patient: "Can you tell me what it is like to be at this point in your life?"

Care at the Time of Actively Dying

Patients who are dying are often most concerned about how they will die rather than that they are dying (Kuhl, 2002). Excellent pain and symptom management is critical as uncontrolled pain or symptoms such as nausea and breathlessness create suffering for *all* family members. A "good death" may contribute to family members feeling more at peace with the death (Martz, 2015), as well as having a sense of satisfaction and accomplishment (Witkamp, van Zuylen, Borsboom, van der Rijt, & van der Heide, 2015). Thus, facilitating a good death is an imperative for nurses (Gagnon & Duggleby, 2014). What constitutes a good death, however, is not well understood (Cipolletta & Oprandi, 2014). For nurses, a good death is possible when "patients and families: (a) were included in decision making, (b) were kept informed, (c) accepted that death was imminent, and (d) were in an appropriate environment" (Gagnon & Duggleby, 2014, p. 403). Ideally, the death was peaceful and pain free. A bad death has been defined by a "lack of opportunity to plan ahead, arrange personal affairs, decrease family burden, or say good-bye" (Steinhauser et al., 2000, p. 829).

In the context of a palliative care approach, the language of care, quality of life, relief of suffering, and

the principles of palliative care become important in helping families attain a "good death." When a cure is not possible, families often react to the news with a blanket statement: "We want everything done." But that may not be what they mean literally. Families may just believe that if they agree to palliative care, treatment will be withheld, and they will be abandoned because death is the expected outcome (Gillis, 2008). Delaying palliative care compromises the ability to achieve a good death. Clear discussions are needed about the continued provision of active care with a shift in emphasis to quality of life instead of prolongation of life. Such discussions will reassure families that, indeed, everything is being done and they are not being abandoned.

No matter the setting, family members are often afraid of the actual death event and have little or no understanding of what dying entails (Seccareccia et al., 2015). There are four dimensions to preparation: (1) Medical, which relates to receiving clear prognostic information as well as information about the physical and psychological changes that signal death is approaching; (2) Psychosocial, which entails saying good-bye, sharing intimate time, and resolving conflicts; (3) Spiritual, which may involve a religious aspect as well as time to reflect on the meaning of life and death; and, (4) Practical, which focuses on completing unfinished business (Loke, Li, & Man, 2013). Nurses can help alleviate families' fears by finding out what they know and what they need. You can then prepare families for the death (Kehl, 2014), acting as a coach during the dying process (Martz, 2015) to help them recognize the signs of imminent death so they are aware of what will likely happen when the signs appear (see Box 10-6). This preparation may be even more crucial for families in the home, who may be alone at the time. It also is important in the ICU and emergency department to tailor your information to the situation (Peden-McAlpine, Liaschenko, Traudt, & Gilmore-Szott, 2015). For example, a patient's breathing will not change if he is on a ventilator. Creating a sacred space to facilitate saying good-bye may be a very helpful intervention (Peden-McAlpine et al., 2015).

Generally, an illness begins to weaken the body when a person is nearing death. Some health conditions affect vital body systems, such as the brain and nervous system, lungs, heart and blood vessels, or the digestive system, including the liver and bowels. As illness progresses, the body becomes unable to use the nutrients in food, resulting in weight loss and a decline in appetite, energy, and strength. More time is spent resting, and in the final few days before death people usually sleep most of the time. If families are aware of this natural progression, they may be less distressed, for example, when their loved one stops eating. One common end-of-life phenomenon, delirium, poses unique relational challenges and can be distressing for family members (Wright, Brajtman, & Macdonald, 2014). Sedation at the end of life may be necessary to control severe symptoms, such as terminal restlessness that accompanies delirium. Box 10-6 lists signs of imminent death that should be shared with families.

Communication and relationships continue to be important as death approaches (Munn & Zimmerman, 2006). Nurses can encourage family members to continue talking to their loved ones even if they are nonresponsive, because they may still be able to hear (Brajtman, 2005). You can model this type of interaction by continuing to speak to the patient and treating him with dignity throughout the dying process and even after the patient has died (Forster & Windsor, 2014). You can demonstrate respect for the family and its intimate knowledge of the patient by seeking its advice on things that were soothing or calming to the patient in the past, such as particular music, foot rubs and back rubs, or a particular way of arranging the pillows, and then following these

---

BOX 10-6

Signs of Imminent Death

Signs of imminent death include the following:

- Decline in physical capabilities
- Decreased alertness and social interaction
- Decreased intake of food and fluids
- Difficulty swallowing medications, food, and fluids
- Visual and auditory hallucinations
- Confusion, restlessness, and agitation

Physical changes as death nears include the following:

- Circulation gradually shuts down; hands and feet feel cool, and a patchy, purplish color called *mottling* appears on the skin; heart speeds up, but also weakens, so pulse is rapid but hard to feel.
- Bowel movements and urine production decrease as less food and fluid are taken in; may be no urine output in last day or two of life; constipation is not usually an issue to be managed in the last week of life; loss of bladder or bowel control can be managed with frequent skin care and the use of adult incontinence products, or even a urinary catheter if needed.

Changes in breathing often provide clues about how close someone is to death. As the automatic centers in the brain take over the regulation of breathing, changes generally occur in the following ways:

- The rate of breathing tends to be more rapid.
- The pattern or regularity in breathing becomes irregular, almost mechanical.
- The depth of breaths (may be shallow, deep, or normal) tends to become more shallow. There may be periods of apnea where breathing pauses for a while. When the pauses in breathing appear, a noticeable

pattern often develops: clusters of fairly rapid breathing that start with shallow breaths that become deeper and deeper, and then fade off, becoming shallower and shallower; may be 5 to 10 breaths in each cluster, and each cluster is separated by a pause that may last a few seconds or perhaps up to 30 seconds; called the Cheyne-Stokes pattern of breathing and is occasionally seen in healthy older adults as well, especially during sleep.

- The kinds of muscles used in breathing may change; the person may start to use the neck muscles and the shoulders, but though it may look as if the person is struggling, unless he or she is agitated it is simply "automatic pilot."
- The amount of mucus or secretions that build up because the person is unable to cough can be noisy (rattling or gurgling) and sometimes upsets people at the bedside even though it is unlikely to be distressing to the dying person, who is usually unconscious; some people call it the "death rattle," and it can be treated by medication to dry up the secretions. Because the term *death rattle* may cause strong emotional reactions, the term *respiratory congestion* is now recommended.
- The pattern of breathing in the final minutes or perhaps hours of life: the breathing takes on an irregular pattern in which there is a breath, then a pause, then another breath or two, then another pause, and so forth. There may be periods of 15 to 30 seconds or so between final breaths.
- After the last breath very slight motions of breathing may happen irregularly for a few minutes. These are reflex actions and are not signs of distress.

suggestions or encouraging the family to do so (Brajtman, 2005).

Many family members want to be present when their loved one is imminently dying; it is often important that they have an opportunity to say good-bye (Andershed, 2006). Thus, you need to be aware ahead of time about a family's wishes and ensure that members are called if there is a change in the patient's condition so they can be present, if possible, at the time of death if that is what they want. The days, hours, and minutes leading up to a child's death are often seen by parents as their last opportunity to be a "good parent" to the child. Their ability to be physically present, emotionally supportive, and an effective advocate for their child is often key to viewing themselves as good parents in the years after their child's death (Rini & Loriz, 2007; Woodgate, 2006). "Normal" parent activities such as bathing, feeding, or holding the child, even in the midst of technology that is being used to support the child's life, allow parents to develop or continue their bond with their child and sometimes to be able to say good-bye to their child (Brosig et al., 2007; Meyer et al., 2006; Rini & Loriz, 2007; Robinson et al., 2006). Nurses facilitate parents' wishes at this time and provide an environment that allows for parents to fulfill their parental role.

We cannot know when a patient will die, and despite our best efforts, sometimes this happens when family members are not present. Sometimes the patient dies when the family member has nodded off to sleep or stepped out of the room for a cup of tea. When family members wish to be present, it is important to talk about the possibility that this may not happen.

Bereavement Care

Once the patient dies, the work of the nurse does not end (O'Connor, Peters, Lee, & Webster, 2005). Several family members may be present for the death, all of whom may need support, advice, information, and time to begin the grieving and healing process. Family members may wish to stay by the bedside and say whatever words seem appropriate. For some cultures, rituals may need to be conducted (O'Connor et al., 2005; Sousa & Alves, 2015). Some families may want active involvement in caring for the patient's body or at least to know the body will be cared for

in a respectful manner (Forster & Windsor, 2014; Widger & Picot, 2008). There is no harm in touching the person's body, and there should be no rush to move the person until everyone has had a chance to say their final good-byes.

Family members who were not present for the death may need to be contacted and may wish to see the patient before he or she is taken to the morgue or a funeral home. Family members can be encouraged to be together if they wish and to take as much time as needed after the death. The nurse's presence as family members express their emotions may help them to create meaningful final memories and begin to process their experience (Rini & Loriz, 2007; Wisten & Zingmark, 2007). Additional team members, such as pastoral care, may need to be contacted to assist in supporting the family. Some families will appreciate assistance with or information on arranging funerals (de Jong-Berg & Kane, 2006; Rini & Loriz, 2007).

Particularly when the patient who has died is a child, families may appreciate receiving a collection of mementos such as pictures, locks of hair, and handprints or footprints (de Jong-Berg & Kane, 2006; Rini & Loriz, 2007; Tan, Docherty, Barfield, & Brandon, 2012; Widger & Picot, 2008). Some families later regret not taking mementos, but others may be distressed if mementos are taken, especially pictures, against their wishes (Blood & Cacciatore, 2014; de Jong-Berg & Kane, 2006); therefore, determining what each family wants and needs requires sensitivity and a careful approach.

In some cases, autopsy and organ or tissue donation may be possible. Nurses and other health care providers sometimes view such discussions as an intrusion and, thus, because of their own discomfort, they do not approach families. Parents in particular may have lingering regrets, however, if they miss an opportunity to help another child or to receive answers to some questions about their own child's death (Macdonald et al., 2006; Widger & Picot, 2008). Therefore, these conversations can be very beneficial should they be indicated. It is also important to make sure that when autopsies are done, families are given the results in a timely and compassionate manner (Macdonald et al., 2006; Meert et al., 2007; Rini & Loriz, 2007; Wisten & Zingmark, 2007). Families may want to meet with health care providers to discuss autopsy results, clarify the events leading to and the circumstances of the death, and be reassured that everything possible was done and the right decisions were made (Macdonald et al., 2006; Milberg, Olsson, Jakobsson, Olsson, & Friedrichsen, 2008; Wisten & Zingmark, 2007; Woodgate, 2006).

It was previously thought that healing meant a person got over the loss and severed ties with the deceased. It is now known that one does not "get over" the loss of a loved one; rather, families will forever have links with the person who has died (Moules, Simonson, Fleiszer, Prins, & Glasgow, 2007). The ways in which continuing bonds exist for different types of loss and their associations with positive and negative outcomes for bereaved individuals is only beginning to be explored (Foster et al., 2011). Nurses can do much to facilitate a healthy start to their grieving journey and to help them find meaning in death; nurses' actions at the actual death event are critical. Family members vividly remember the moment of their loved one's death. They often remember who was present, what was said, what was done that was helpful, and what was not so helpful. Many remember that it was the nurse who was with them at the moment of death, or that the nurse was the first to respond to the family's call about a change in their loved one's condition. More often than not, families clearly recall the nurse's words and actions. What is done for and with family members at the time of their loved one's death can have a profound and long-lasting impact on them. It is important to remember that, although the death may be one of many for the nurse, it may be the first and only for the family; therefore, a person's death should never be treated as "just a job" on the part of the nurse. Be cognizant too that clichés such as "this was meant to be," "he is in a better place," or referring to the deceased person as an angel may make families feel that the death is minimized, as is the impact of the death on the family. Simple expressions, such as "I am sorry for your loss" (Bloomer et al., 2013, p. 26), are more often appreciated.

Nurses should have an understanding of loss, know how to support families in grief, and be able to provide quality bereavement care. Beginning nurses often worry about showing emotion, such as crying, in the presence of family members. Family members are often deeply touched when they see a nurse's genuine emotional response (Butler et al., 2015), but it is critical that the family not be put in the position of caring for the nurse.

Provision of bereavement care by the nurse offers the opportunity for continued contact with the family and signifies the importance of the family to the nurse (Collins-Tracey et al., 2009; Davies et al., 2007; de Cinque et al., 2006; de Jong-Berg & Kane, 2006; Meert et al., 2007; Rodger, Sherwood, O'Connor, & Leslie, 2007). Follow-up activities that many families appreciate include calls, cards, attendance at the funeral, and offers to make referrals to additional sources of support (Butler et al., 2015). Families may appreciate written information on practical issues, such as what to do next, and about grief or other sources of support (D'Agostino et al., 2008; de Cinque et al., 2006; de Jong-Berg & Kane, 2006; Rini & Loriz, 2007; Rodger et al., 2007), as well as information to share with extended family and friends on how to offer effective support. Depending on the setting, bereavement care may continue for a period of time in the community and helps family caregivers "move on" in their lives (Cronin, Hynes, et al., 2015). Sometimes health care providers call or send a card to families on the first anniversary of the patient's death, especially if it was a child who died. This simple contact acknowledges that the grieving process takes time and can make families feel really cared for, once again highlighting the importance of the patient and family to the health care provider (Collins-Tracey et al., 2009).

Special Situations

There are some situations that can be challenging for nurses to consider and deserve additional attention. More specific assessment and intervention tools may be required in order to offer optimal care.

Children's Developmental Levels and Facilitating Grieving

Children tend to express some common behaviors and emotions depending on their developmental level. However, it is still important to recognize that everyone grieves differently. Generally, children aged 2 to 4 years do not yet completely understand that death happens to everyone and that it is permanent. They may use play to work out their thoughts and may ask questions such as, "Daddy died? When will he come home?" Regression in behavior, crying, general anxiety, and temper tantrums are all common responses. Children of this age need consistent routines and short, honest answers to help them feel safe and to ensure that they do not develop incorrect ideas about death. It is important to not use euphemisms because, for example, a child who is told that she has lost her father may start searching for the lost person and not learn that death is permanent (The Dougy Center, 2017).

Children aged 5 to 8 years are concrete thinkers who may use magical thinking. They often still see death as reversible, and they can feel responsible that their thoughts or wishes caused the person's death. They typically ask repetitive questions and worry about abandonment and safety. These children may also regress and may show somatic signs of grieving (e.g., headaches, stomachaches). Honest explanations and avoidance of euphemisms are needed with this age group, and the children need to be allowed to talk about their experiences and ask questions (The Dougy Center, 2017).

As children mature, they begin to understand abstract ideas such as death and grief and they realize that death is permanent. Children aged 8 to 12 years may still have some concrete thinking, but they also start to think about how the loss will affect them. Some children may feel regret and guilt, believing that their thoughts or actions led to the person's death. These children need to have safety and predictability re-established in their lives and they should be offered various ways to express themselves (The Dougy Center, 2017).

Teenagers, 13 to 18 years old, understand that death is permanent, but they sometimes struggle with more existential questions about the meaning of life and death. Withdrawing from family is common as children in this age group tend to rely more on peers. Safety and security continue to be issues for some, yet teenagers may also increase their own risk taking (e.g., drug and alcohol use), and thoughts of suicide or self-harm may appear. Some teenagers may feel responsible for caring for younger siblings or other adults, whereas others may push themselves to be perfect. Patience, reassurance, and nonjudgmental listening are all important (The Dougy Center, 2017). See Chapters 12 and 13 for further information about family nursing when children are part of a family.

Facilitating Connections for Children When a Family Member Is Critically Ill

When a family member is critically ill, families and health care providers may have a concern about the importance and impact of bringing children to visit, whether at home, in the ICU, or in any other setting. Yet, these visits may reduce feelings of separation, guilt, abandonment, fear, loneliness, and worry for the child (Karlsson, Andersson, & Ahlström, 2013). Children can generally decide for themselves if they wish to visit and, where possible, families and health care providers should respect their decision. Those younger than 10 years old visiting a relative may be most interested in the equipment, whereas older children may spend more time focused on the person they are visiting (Knutsson & Bergbom, 2007). The visit can also benefit the patient by acting as a diversion, offering hope, and bringing a sense of normalcy (Karlsson et al., 2013). Thus, nurses should offer families the option of bringing children in to visit loved ones.

Talking with the patient and family about previous experiences with children visiting can be helpful, for example, "Sometimes family members are afraid that a child will be very upset to see grandpa looking so sick. Are you worried about that possibility?" and "In my experience, children are very curious, as well as resilient. They often suspect that something bad is happening and they imagine terrible scenarios. Being truthful and also letting them see for themselves what is happening can be very beneficial." You can assist families to prepare children beforehand about what they will see and what to expect; you also can be present during the visit to support family members in answering questions and to make the child feel welcome and an important part of the family (Karlsson et al., 2013; Knutsson & Bergbom, 2007). It is important that everyone realizes a child's reactions are somewhat unpredictable; one child may seem unaffected, whereas another may be upset and crying. Nurses should acknowledge that every reaction is "normal" and work with the child in a way that meets his needs at the time. Though it may be difficult for a critically ill patient when a child chooses not to visit, you can help the patient understand by sharing your knowledge about how children need to make their own decisions and you can offer ways to assist in maintaining connections between the child and the ill family member through cards, calls, and frequent updates about how the patient is doing.

When Death Is Sudden or Traumatic

Unlike with chronic illness, a sudden or traumatic death leaves little time for families to come to terms with the situation. Further, the nature of a frequently chaotic environment when death is traumatic or sudden may contribute to a lack of communication between health care providers and families. It is important that the information given to families includes the big picture; otherwise, families often receive different pieces of information from each health care provider and may have trouble putting it all together to understand that it actually means the patient is dying. This may be more of an issue in situations when there is a sudden illness or injury because the family did not know what to expect and may be unprepared for what is happening (Hinkle, Bosslet, & Torke, 2015; Rini & Loriz, 2007). Please refer to Chapter 14 for more detailed discussion about supporting families when the death of their loved one is sudden or traumatic and occurs in an acute care setting.

Dying at Home

Families need professional support, particularly in the area of symptom control, to make a home death "happen" (Mehta et al., 2014; Morris et al., 2015). Caring for a dying family member at home can be extremely demanding work—physically, emotionally, psychologically, and spiritually. The primary caregivers require support and resources to be successful. First and foremost, the family and the nurse need to discuss the dying process, existing resources, and present and future needs. Then together they can develop a plan that anticipates changes. For example,

symptom crises, such as escalating pain, need to be anticipated and addressed in advance. When the family is committed to supporting death at home, it can be devastating when a symptom crisis results in death in the middle of a busy emergency department. Box 10-7 provides some practical suggestions about what you need to consider and perhaps facilitate when someone is dying at home.

PALLIATIVE CARE AND END-OF-LIFE FAMILY CASE STUDIES

Three family case studies are presented in this section to demonstrate the art and science of family nursing in palliative and end-of-life care. The Jones family was introduced in Chapter 2 and is reintroduced here to demonstrate family care when the person who is dying is the mother. Please return to Chapter 2 and reacquaint yourself with the family and familiarize yourself with the Jones family genogram in Figure 10-1. The Garcia family case study illustrates how a student nurse working with a preceptor assists a young family during and following the death of an infant. The Wall family case study illustrates the importance of involving extended family and traditions in the care of a Native American family when they experience the death of an elder.

BOX 10-7

Practical Considerations When Someone Is Dying at Home

The following are considerations for in-home care of the dying person:

- Involvement of expert resources, such as hospice, and an interprofessional team, including volunteers
- Symptom management plan, including anticipating changes such as inability to swallow and the need for parenteral medications, as well as management of breathlessness and agitation
- Advance care planning, including the presence of a DNR order if necessary
- Equipment such as a hospital bed and commode
- Identification of willing informal support persons (friends, church, extended family)

- Development of a list of things that willing people can do, for example, a calendar for preparation of meals, house cleaning, someone to visit so the caregiver can get out for a walk
- Respite for the caregiver(s), which may be planned hospice admissions or the overnight placement of a paid professional
- Financial implications and available support, for example, compassionate benefits program
- Contact numbers of resources
- Discussion of unfinished business to enable a peaceful death
- Discussion of alternatives should dying and death at home become impossible for any reason

Case Study: Jones Family

Linda, the mother in the Jones family, has been living with multiple sclerosis (MS) for 13 years. (See Figure 10-1 for the family genogram.) Early in the illness, Linda experienced relapses where her symptoms worsened, but these were followed by periods of remission where she recovered back to "normal." Since Travis's birth, her relapses have become more frequent, and although her symptoms sometimes improved a little, her condition steadily worsened.

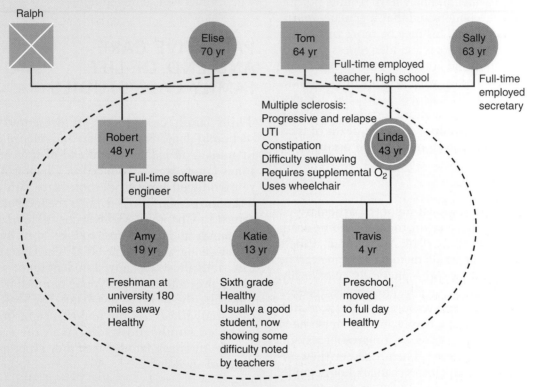

FIGURE 10-1 Jones Family Genogram

Before Linda's discharge from the hospital where she was treated with antibiotics for pneumonia after aspiration, the primary nurse, Catherine, initiated a family meeting with Linda, Robert, and Linda's physician. Catherine had noticed Robert's fatigue and his repeated questions about whether Linda was really ready to come home. Catherine had also noticed Linda's reluctance to take medications (particularly for pain), her determination to walk with her cane despite serious unsteadiness, and the deepening silence between the husband and wife.

Catherine began the conversation by asking Linda and Robert about their understanding of the MS at this point. Linda quickly responded, saying that the pneumonia was really an unusual "one-time" problem, and although it had set her back, it would not be long before she was back on her feet. Robert worried out loud that it seemed things were getting progressively worse. He was concerned about how Linda would manage at home alone in the mornings and with Travis in the afternoon when he returned from preschool. Noticing the difference in perspective, Catherine acknowledged she could see how there might be differences because MS is, indeed, a "tricky" illness that is difficult to predict. She asked Linda and Robert to think back to how things were a year ago and to what had happened during the last year. Both noticed that the hospitalizations had become more frequent, the recoveries were more difficult, and, overall, Linda was not doing as well. The physician, Dr. Brooks, who had been listening quietly, remarked that, although MS was often an unpredictable disease, it seemed that Linda's MS had changed into a different kind of illness than it had been at first. He agreed that now the MS was more steadily progressing, and that it seemed things were getting worse more quickly. Linda said she could see this but kept hoping that the situation would turn around.

Case Study: Jones Family (*cont.*)

Catherine then asked what the family's goals for care were. Linda was quick to answer, "Remission—I want full remission." Robert was slower to reply. He said, "I am so tired, and it hurts me so much to see you suffer. I want you to be comfortable, to be free of pain, to enjoy the kids rather than snapping at them. . . ." Linda said, "I'm just trying so hard to get back to normal. I always thought that a wheelchair would be the end for me. And I'm just so tired." Catherine acknowledged that MS often creates profound fatigue in many family members and wondered which of the children might be most affected. Both Linda and Robert agreed that, of the children, Katie was suffering the most from tiredness. She picked up a lot of the pieces of Linda's work in the home, beginning supper preparations and looking after Travis. Often, she would be up late at night working on homework, but her grades had been slipping and she had been crying more. Linda worried that Amy was also tired as she spent a great deal of time driving home on weekends to care for the family.

Dr. Brooks interjected at this point saying that their primary goal for care during this hospitalization had been to cure the pneumonia. He noted that, although they were successful, they had not been able to assist Linda toward a remission of her MS. He remarked that with the change in the MS, it seemed that the hope for remission might not be possible. He then asked, "If things continue the way they are going, where do you think you will be in 6 months?" Linda began to cry and said she was thinking she might not be alive. The pneumonia scared her, and she was frightened about aspirating again, so she had been decreasing what she ate and drank. Robert was worried about how he could continue to work full time supporting the family and also care for Linda at home, especially as it seemed there was so little he did that was "right" for Linda.

Catherine replied that the "new" MS was clearly creating challenges for the family and wondered if it was time to shift the focus of care more toward comfort and quality of life for all family members, while at the same time working to prevent problems such as aspiration. She explained that as illness gets more demanding, additional supports are needed. She also explained that as illness gets intrusive, attention needs to be paid to what is most important to living well for all family members. Linda was getting tired at this point and having a lot of difficulty holding her head up, so Catherine asked if they could schedule another meeting. Robert and Linda readily agreed, saying they knew they needed to talk about these things but just did not know how. Catherine asked them to do some homework: to each identify their biggest concern, as well as what was most important to living well at this time. They were asked to find this out from the children too, and a meeting was scheduled for the next day. Dr. Brooks let them know that he wanted to speak with them about Linda's preferences for care should she have another experience with pneumonia.

The next day, Linda, Robert, Catherine, and Dr. Brooks all met again. Linda began the conversation, saying she had done a great deal of soul searching and was most worried about suffering from unmanageable pain and being a burden to her family. She was wondering if perhaps she should not go home but should be admitted into a care facility. Robert was most worried about burning out and not being able to support Linda and the children as he wanted. They had had a three-way conversation with each of the children last evening. Amy was most worried that her mother was going to die, and she let her parents know that she was planning on leaving university to move back home. Katie was most troubled by her lack of friends as her friends were no longer including her in their activities. Travis missed his mother, and wanted her to be able to read stories to him and play with him more.

The things that were most important to Linda's quality of life were reducing her pain, having Amy continue at university, being more involved in Katie's and Travis's everyday lives, being able to attend a service at her church on a weekly basis, and reconnecting with Robert. She said her greatest hope was to be at home as long as possible. Robert wanted to be able to sleep, to go to work without constantly worrying about Linda, and to reconnect with Linda. He too wanted her at home as long as possible. Both Linda and Robert agreed that for them to live well, they needed more help in their home. Options were discussed, including the possibility of Elise (Robert's mother) moving in to be of assistance, and preplanned, short stays in hospice for respite. Linda did not want Elise doing her personal care, so again, they discussed their options. Dr. Brooks and the family developed a systematic plan for pain management. During the assessment process, he learned that Linda was refusing her medications because she was concerned they were contributing to her irritability with Robert and the children. He was able to reassure her that this was not the case; in fact, her unmanaged pain was more likely a major negative influence. They devised a plan for long-acting pain medication so that Robert would be able to sleep through the night. They consulted a dietitian regarding ways to manage swallowing problems, and scheduled a home assessment by the team physiotherapist so as to safely maximize Linda's mobility.

(continued)

Case Study: Jones Family *(cont.)*

Both Catherine and Dr. Brooks commended Linda and Robert on the deep love they saw within the couple and how effective they were at problem solving, systematically working their issues through until achieving a mutually satisfying outcome. Finally, Dr. Brooks raised the topic of what Linda's preferences for care would be if she should experience development of pneumonia again. He explained that this was a real possibility because Linda's respiratory muscles were weakening. Dr. Brooks understood that both Linda and Robert wanted her home as long as possible, so he was curious about whether she would want to come to the hospital to be treated with intravenous antibiotics as she had during this hospitalization. Linda stated this would be her preference, especially if she was likely to be able to go home again after the treatment. Dr. Brooks explained that as her muscles become weaker, she might need the assistance of a breathing machine (ventilator) to give the antibiotics time to work against the infection, and asked whether she would want that. Linda was not sure what her preference would be in this situation, but she was very clear that she did not want to be "kept alive on a machine." She and Robert wanted more time to discuss this question, and they wanted to consult with their pastor, so they agreed to continue the conversation at the next doctor's appointment. Robert and Linda agreed to visit the local hospice to explore respite opportunities, as well as end-of-life care, should staying at home prove too difficult.

Three weeks later at the scheduled appointment with Dr. Brooks, Linda let him know that many things were going better with Elise in the house and home visits from Catherine, as well as a personal care aide. Amy agreed to stay in college with the promise from her parents that she would be told immediately if Linda's health changed. All family members were feeling less tired. Linda stated that she was not ready to leave Robert and the children, but was in a dilemma about the use of a ventilator if she developed pneumonia. She continued to worry that she might be kept alive on the machine, which to her would not be considered living. Dr. Brooks explained that, if necessary, one possibility was a time-limited trial of a ventilator to determine whether the antibiotics would work. Both Linda and Robert agreed. This was a difficult discussion, and Linda expressed distress about her loss of independence and her deep sorrow about the possibility of leaving her children. She admitted to swinging between despair and anger, and that both made it hard for her to enjoy her days. This was new information to Robert, who had noticed her struggling but thought things would work out over time. Through assessment, it became apparent that Linda was experiencing depression. She agreed to try an antidepressant medication and to join a local MS support group.

Eight Months Later:

Linda experienced fever, congestion, and shortness of breath after aspiration. The health team initiated antibiotics and managed symptoms to relieve pain, breathlessness, fever, and constipation. Linda occasionally had periods of acute shortness of breath where she worried that she might not be able to take her next breath. The fear served to make the breathlessness worse, so the visiting nurse showed both Linda and the family how to slow and deepen breathing by consciously breathing together. Dr. Brooks made a home visit and asked Linda about admission to the hospital. When he could not assure her that she would get off the ventilator, Linda declined, saying she wanted to stay with her family. Robert agreed. A family meeting with Catherine and Dr. Brooks was held at Linda's bedside to discuss what the family would experience if the pneumonia progressed. They developed a family ecomap (Figure 10-2) and they increased support services with more frequent visits from the nurse, care aide, and friends (particularly from Linda's support group). They discussed a move to hospice, but all agreed that home was the best place for Linda, and that death at home was their preference.

Linda engaged in one-on-one time with each of her children. They talked about their best memories together, what they most loved about each other, and their hopes and dreams for the future as the children grow up. Robert participated by videotaping the conversations. Each child was given a journal, and together with Linda, they drew pictures, wrote notes, and gathered mementos to capture these conversations. She organized gifts for their birthdays and for Christmas in the upcoming year. It was not that she knew she was dying, but she had been encouraged to plan for the worst and hope for the best, to do the things that needed doing. The family received the same encouragement so they were all able to have special time with Linda during the last few months. Linda died surrounded by her family.

Case Study: Jones Family *(cont.)*

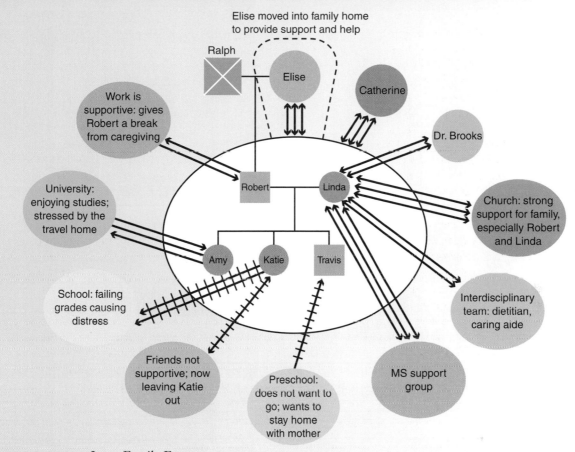

FIGURE 10-2 Jones Family Ecomap

Six Weeks Later:

Catherine visited the family 6 weeks after Linda's death and found them managing well. Pictures of Linda were everywhere. Elise continued to live with the family, and they thought this was the best plan for the time being. Robert had taken some time off work to be with the children after Linda's death, but shortly afterward all went back to work and school. Amy still came home on some weekends. Robert, Amy, and Katie talked of their sense of having done the very best they could to honor Linda's preferences. They took comfort in the fact that she died at home. They marked the 1-month anniversary of Linda's death with a visit to her grave site, taking flowers and a picture Travis had drawn of his mother. Family members drew support from different sources: each other, friends, their pastor, and some of the people from the MS support group who continued to visit. The children continued to read and reread the letters Linda had written; for Travis, this was part of his bedtime ritual. They were sad, and some days were better than others; they had a sense that the weight of their grief was lifting.

Case Study: Garcia Family

You are a nursing student in your final clinical placement. I am your preceptor, a clinical nurse specialist (CNS) on the palliative care team in a children's hospital. You asked for this placement as a final-year nursing student because you have come across several situations during your student experiences where you wished you knew how to talk and be with a patient and her family when the patient was dying. You realize that all nurses, from novice to expert and in all areas of nursing practice, need to develop skills in the area of death and dying. Please acquaint yourself with the Garcia family genogram in Figure 10-3. Consider what it would be like if you were the student working with this family.

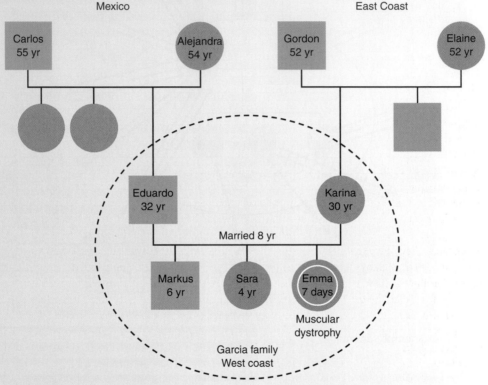

FIGURE 10-3 Garcia Family Genogram

We have received a new consultation to meet with Emma and her parents, Eduardo and Karina Garcia. We learn that Emma is 7 days old and is a beautiful little baby with a perfect little face, big dark eyes, and lots of dark hair. Emma is on a ventilator because she has severe congenital muscular dystrophy and is unable to breathe on her own. Babies with severe disease, such as Emma, have a very limited life expectancy, typically only a few weeks. Her severe muscle weakness means she is not able to breathe on her own for any length of time. We have been asked to meet with Emma and her family because they have decided, in consultation with their health care team, to withdraw ventilator support. As part of the palliative care team, we have been invited to assist Eduardo and Karina to decide how, when, and where the withdrawal might occur.

Before meeting with this family for the first time, we realize how important it is to prepare ourselves. We know that we need to pause for a moment and consider how we might begin this conversation with Eduardo and Karina. We also want to ensure that we have in place whatever we might need to facilitate this first meeting.

We make arrangements to meet with Eduardo and Karina in a quiet, private room where we will not be interrupted. Pagers are turned off and other staff are covering for us so that we will have time to sit with the parents and really listen to what they have to say. Given that there will be several challenging things to discuss, we invite the neonatal intensive care unit (NICU) social worker, who already has a relationship with the family, to join us for this meeting.

Case Study: Garcia Family *(cont.)*

Before meeting the family we spend some time talking about different ways to begin the conversation with the parents. There are as many ways to start this conversation as there are clinicians. This is the beginning of what we hope will be a therapeutic relationship during one of the most difficult times a family can experience. Eduardo and Karina need to know who we are. It is often hard for parents to keep track of health care providers—who we are, what we do, and how we can be helpful. This is especially true in highly emotionally charged situations. So, we typically start with brief introductions. Sometimes, rather than starting the conversation by saying why we are here, it is helpful to gain an understanding of why the parents think we are meeting and then continue from there.

We start the meeting by each introducing ourselves. Then one of us says, "Tell us your understanding of why we are meeting today." To facilitate our connection with this family, we also ask Eduardo and Karina to tell us about Emma—*not* her medical condition, but what they have noticed about her or experienced in their relationship with her as parents. In answer to our query, one of the things Karina tells us is that she thinks Emma has Eduardo's eyes. Eduardo has noticed that she follows Karina with her eyes and he says, "She really knows her mom."

We learn that after talking with both sets of grandparents (mostly by telephone as Eduardo's family is in Mexico where he and Karina met and Karina's parents live across the country), the health care team, and their priest, Karina and Eduardo have indeed come to the decision that the most loving thing they can do as parents is to withdraw Emma's ventilator and allow natural death. We encourage them to discuss their concerns, fears, and hopes for the time they have now with Emma. There is much silence and tears as the parents try to put into words all the thoughts swirling in their heads. They tell us that their focus is on having Emma experience as much of normal newborn life as she can. And they want to touch her and care for her. They want her to spend time with her 4-year-old sister, Sara, and 6-year-old brother, Markus; to be in her car seat; to be bathed, cuddled, and have her diaper changed by both her mom and dad; to be baptized; and most of all to see the sun. We learn that it was the middle of the night when Emma was born, after which she was immediately transferred from her small community to our tertiary urban hospital 3 hours away, so she had seen the moon but not the sun. Eduardo is a forestry worker and the family loves to be outdoors. They cannot believe that one of their children will never spend any time outdoors. Neither Karina nor Eduardo had been able to hold Emma before she was whisked away. Karina has held her in the NICU, but Eduardo has been reluctant because of all the tubes. He is feeling sad that her pervasive muscle weakness means she cannot grab onto his finger the way Sara and Markus did as babies and he is searching to find another way to connect with Emma. Both parents express worry about how to help Sara and Markus understand what is happening in a way that does not frighten them. Although both Karina and Eduardo are committed to their decision, they are afraid that Emma may suffer when the ventilator is withdrawn. They are worried about watching her struggle for breath. The parents ask us for a week to have these experiences with Emma; they also want time for additional family members to visit and to plan for withdrawal of the ventilator.

Following our meeting with Eduardo and Karina, we meet with the involved NICU staff members, who are quite concerned with the proposal that we wait a week to discontinue the ventilator. This is not the way it usually happens and they worry the family will only become more attached to Emma, finding it harder and harder to let her go, or that something will change in Emma's health status that may lead to an earlier death than what the parents expect. We provide further explanation and facilitate a meeting between the parents, Eduardo and Karina, and the NICU staff. At the meeting, NICU staff members are able to express their concerns and the family is able to respond, as well as talk about their wishes. Hearing each other's fears and hopes is helpful and there is now agreement and support for the parents' request. Eduardo and Karina understand that it is possible something could happen unexpectedly with Emma and, although everything possible will be done to ensure that she is comfortable, the staff will not provide CPR if her heart stops.

Emma and her parents move into one of the private family rooms in the NICU. Karina's parents, Elaine and Gordon, who came to care for Sara and Markus in the family home, bring them to stay in a nearby hotel. This proximity enables them to visit often and to get to know the newest member of their family. Before their first visit, we spend time talking with Eduardo and Karina about how to prepare the siblings for seeing Emma, as well as explaining similarities and differences in how Sara and Markus may understand what is happening. Another member of the team, a child life therapist, spends time with Sara and Markus individually and together to assess and support their understanding and coping with Emma's illness. Eduardo and Karina join some of the discussions and have some of their own time with the child life therapist. They learn how young children come to understand serious illness and death and that Sara and Markus will likely have questions about Emma for many years. They are happy about the picture books and other resources on how to support their children over time.

(continued)

Case Study: Garcia Family *(cont.)*

During the week, even in the midst of the technology that is still needed to keep Emma breathing, Eduardo, Karina, Grandma Elaine, Grandpa Gordon, Sara, and Markus do all the things that families with newborns usually do. The family is given the opportunity to say hello and good-bye to their new family member all at the same time. Eduardo holds Emma for the first time and they take many, many pictures and videos. They give Emma her first haircut and each saves a tiny lock of hair tied with a ribbon. Sara and Markus each create a memory box with drawings, the locks of hair, Emma's hand- and footprints, and copies of the photos. They also help the child life therapist make molds of Emma's hands and feet, as well as their own. Eduardo's parents arrive from Mexico and several close family members and friends come to meet Emma and witness her baptism in the hospital chapel. The list of hopes and dreams for this time gets ticked off. Eduardo and Karina also use this time to contact a funeral home in their home community and make arrangements with their priest for Emma's wake and funeral.

One day we take Emma, her parents, her siblings, and her grandparents outside to the hospital's play garden where it is beautifully clear and sunny with a gentle breeze blowing. Hospital security has closed the garden to other families and staff so it is intimate and peaceful. Emma is able to feel the sun on her face for the first time. The child life therapist is there to support Sara and Markus. They both seem to enjoy this family outing; they run over to see Emma, give her a kiss, and then head off to explore the sandbox and the swings before coming back again for a hug from their parents. Eduardo and Karina ask if we think that Sara and Markus really don't understand the situation and that is why they keep running off to play. The child life therapist reassures them that this is a typical way for children to cope and essentially they are just taking in what they can handle at their own pace. The child life therapist continues to follow the children's lead in supporting whatever they want to do and wherever they want to be in the garden. A nurse from the NICU stays close to Emma to assist her to breathe while she is being held by her parents and grandparents. Everyone relaxes and shares stories about Karina's pregnancy, the labor and delivery, and the things they have learned about Emma the last few days. We take more family pictures and video to send to the rest of the extended family that night. To our surprise, the parents feel so comfortable in the garden that they ask if the ventilator can be discontinued in the garden. We set about making this request happen.

Eduardo, Karina, and Elaine meet with us, the neonatologist, the NICU CNS, and the NICU social worker; we explain how we will keep Emma comfortable when the ventilator is withdrawn. The family is reassured to learn that there are medications that will ensure that Emma does not struggle for breath and that we will not allow her to suffer. Eduardo asks what it will be like when the ventilator is taken away. We are able to help them understand that we do not know how long Emma will be able to breathe without assistance, but it could be minutes to hours; her breathing will slow, become irregular, and then stop. Her color will change and she will feel cool. Eduardo and Karina decide that they would like to be by themselves with Emma when she dies. Sara and Markus will stay at the hotel with their grandparents and then may come back to see Emma before she is taken to the funeral home.

Both parents seem to be coping fairly well with the situation, with Eduardo taking on the role of the "strong one" and Karina appearing more fragile. On the day of Emma's death, however, we are surprised at the reversal of roles, as Eduardo looks disheveled and distressed whereas Karina has done her hair and makeup; she's wearing a special outfit and seems "in control." We had hoped for sun, but somehow the weather seems more in keeping with the mood. You comment to her parents that Emma has seen the moon and the sun and now she is experiencing a true West Coast day—foggy and gloomy! Emma is given some medications so she won't experience any pain or distress and is settled with her parents in a secluded corner of the garden. The priest performs last rites. The nurse removes all the tape and then the endotracheal tube while Emma remains peaceful in her parent's arms. We give the family private space to be together but, along with other members of the team (the priest, the NICU social worker, and the NICU nurse with additional medications ready in case Emma experiences any distress), are available in the play garden if needed.

The play garden is on a busy street and we are concerned that the level of traffic noise might be disturbing to the family. Our concerns are heightened when the siren starts at the nearby fire hall and the fire truck roars past; Emma's dad simply walks over to the fence and lifts her up to see her first fire truck. Emma and her parents walk the paths of the garden. Although there is still bustle and noise around them, it is clear that Emma and her family are in their own little world. Although they had opportunities to do "normal" family things during the last week, this is the first time Emma and her parents experience each other without interference from machines, tubes, wires, or other people.

Emma lives for another 2 hours. After she dies, her parents continue to hold her for another hour. Both sets of grandparents return with Sara and Markus to say good-bye to Emma. Although the children were both told how Emma would look and

Case Study: Garcia Family *(cont.)*

feel after she died, Markus in particular has many questions about whether or not she is hungry, why she is cold, and if she is just sleeping. Karina responds gently to all their questions to help them understand what has happened. When the family is ready, Sara and Markus spend some time with the child life therapist while a senior nurse, Patrick, partners with you to help Karina and Eduardo prepare Emma's body. Patrick asks the parents if they have any special rituals they would like to do and he also explains about what needs to be done to meet the hospital rules. Everyone works together and though it is sad there is also a peacefulness as Karina and Eduardo talk about how happy they are to have done things the way they wanted to. They thank you and Patrick and say how grateful they are that the staff made it possible for Emma to die in peace in such a beautiful setting; Karina and Eduardo say that they will never forget what the staff did. With one last kiss on Emma's forehead, they leave for home with the rest of their family.

Patrick assists you to complete all the charting and necessary paperwork related to Emma's death. As Eduardo and Karina decided against having an autopsy, Emma does not need to go to the hospital morgue. Patrick calls the funeral home and accompanies you as you carry Emma's body in a special softly colored and patterned bag to meet the funeral home director at the staff entrance to the hospital. You return to the unit and spend some time talking with Patrick and me. We make sure that you have a way home and a friend available to spend the evening with you. I also contact your clinical coordinator to let her know about the day's events to make sure that you have some ongoing support from the faculty. A few days later I invite you to attend a special debriefing session to be held with NICU staff.

As the funeral is held 3 hours away, you are unable to attend. I suggest that you may want to send a note to the family and offer to review it if needed (Box 10-8).

One Month Later:

That was not the end of our relationship with this family. We make a home visit a month after Emma's death where we learn about the funeral. Karina and Eduardo remark that they were very happy when two of their favorite NICU nurses came to Emma's funeral. They tell us about how moved they were when they received notes from you and some of the other nurses, as well as a card from the NICU staff. They tell us that it helps them to know she touched the hearts of those who looked after her. We discuss how Karina and Eduardo are managing as a couple and as parents. Eduardo is back at work; Sara and Markus are back at preschool and school. Both sets of grandparents have gone home. At this point we draw an ecomap (Figure 10-4) of the family's community connections, discuss their experiences of grief, and work together to map out avenues of support available locally. We let Karina and Eduardo know that they will receive a letter with an appointment to see a geneticist in about 6 months. Because there was a genetic component to Emma's diagnosis, they may want to explore genetic testing and understand any possible risks for future pregnancies. A follow-up visit with the NICU neonatologist, CNS, and social worker will be coordinated to occur on the same day to respond to any questions the parents may have about Emma's illness and death, as well as to see how they are all coping. They are invited to bring Sara and Markus at that time to meet with the child life therapist.

BOX 10-8

Example Note to Family From Student Nurse

Dear Eduardo, Karina, Markus, and Sara,

It was my privilege to get to know all of you and to meet Emma. She had the most beautiful expressive eyes and so clearly looked at each of you when you spoke to her. It was amazing to watch all of you together and to see Emma experience so much life in such a short time. Your love for her and for each other was evident in everything that you did.

I learned so many things about how families can be together and live life to the fullest even in the midst of such difficult circumstances. I know my experience with your family will make me a better nurse with other families in the future. Emma and all of you will forever remain in my thoughts.

All my best,
_____, Student Nurse

(continued)

Case Study: Garcia Family (*cont.*)

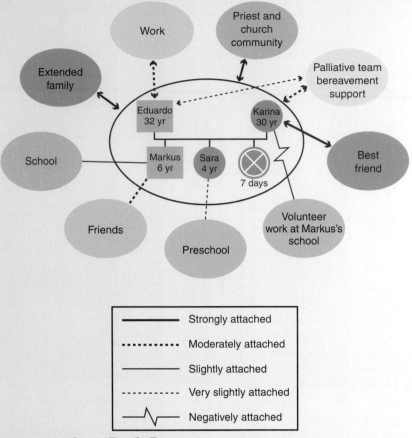

FIGURE 10-4 Garcia Family Ecomap

We also let them know that the NICU has a formal program where, with the parents' permission, staff nurses are supported to contact families at regular intervals in the first year after the death and then send a plant on the 1-year anniversary. Karina and Eduardo express their appreciation for such a program and say they can only imagine how hard it will be on the anniversary of Emma's death; to know that the NICU staff who looked after her will be thinking of them gives them great comfort.

Case Study: Wall Family

Robert Wall was a 78-year-old divorced man. He lived in rural Montana and was a member of the Confederated Salish & Kootenai Tribes. He lived alone in his home in the small town where he was born and raised. He was recently taken to the hospital after he suffered a fall in his home. In the local emergency room, bone fractures and other musculoskeletal injuries were ruled out. During his examination, he was diagnosed with severe weakness, difficulty breathing, recent weight loss, and severe dehydration. For many years he had been using various inhalers for his breathing and has reported more difficulty with his breathing lately. An initial reading of the chest x-ray showed a mass in his right lung. He refused hospital admission for further work-up of his symptoms but agreed to follow-up at the tribal health clinic the next day.

Case Study: Wall Family *(cont.)*

Tribal Health Clinic Visit:

Mr. Wall presented to the tribal health clinic a couple of days later after the tribal health nurse called to ask if he needed a ride to the clinic. She had reviewed his records from the emergency room visit, including the chest x-ray report and his refusal for hospital admission. On the phone, he mentioned that he had not yet come to the clinic because he was not feeling well enough to leave the house. His brother gave him a ride and provided him with assistance to walk into the clinic where he was treated by the tribal health nurse and physician.

Medical and Social History:

Upon assessment, Mr. Wall was a vague historian about his medical and social history. His tribal health record confirmed chronic asthma and emphysema, hypertension, and alcoholism. His lung condition was exacerbated by decades of smoking one pack or more of cigarettes per day. He reported that he drank several beers each day "when I feel good enough" and he denied illicit drug use. Approximately 30 years ago, he was involved in a near-fatal car crash and had "hardware" in both hips that caused significant pain in his legs and lower back. He had multiple surgeries following his accident. He reported taking pain pills from time to time and an occasional sleeping pill to manage his symptoms although he had no current prescriptions. He was not currently taking any medications or supplements regularly except a Tylenol "every so often."

Mr. Wall was one of three remaining (five total) male siblings in his family. He had been married and divorced "too many times" and had two daughters who lived locally, a son and a daughter who lived in another state, several grandchildren, multiple nieces and nephews, and several extended family members and friends in the community. (See Figure 10-5 for the Wall family genogram.) He spent several decades living in California but returned to his home community approximately 15 years ago. He was an avid antique gun collector and enjoyed traveling to gun shows across the state.

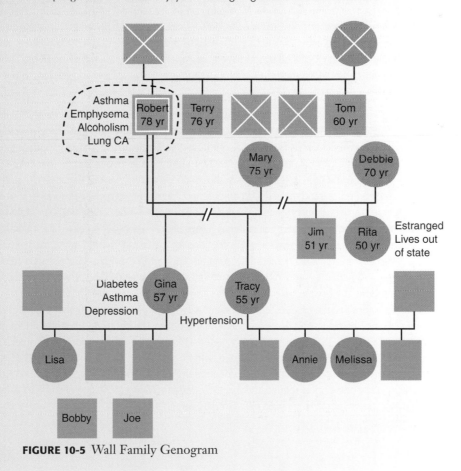

FIGURE 10-5 Wall Family Genogram

(continued)

Case Study: Wall Family *(cont.)*

Condition, Health Beliefs, and Trajectory of Illness:

Mr. Wall admitted to the tribal health physician that he had not been feeling well for several weeks. He reported that it had been months since he had been able to attend a gun show or go out for his daily lunch with friends at the local Veterans of Foreign Wars bar. He was hoping to get some medicine that might make him feel better so he could go home. Again, he declined admission to the hospital, stating that it was not something he would ever want. After some discussion, he was willing to accept home health visits from the tribal health nurse. He was prescribed hydrocodone/acetaminophen for pain and lorazepam for anxiety and/or sleep. The nurse provided him with a written plan for the medications and for possible symptoms of alcohol withdrawal. He agreed to have the nurse visit on Monday following the weekend. He agreed that his brother would check on him throughout the weekend.

On the morning of the home visit, Mr. Wall had declined significantly. When the nurse arrived, she observed that he was much weaker, less communicative, and more dyspneic. He was now confined to the couch in his living room and had been incontinent of urine. He was no longer able to perform activities of daily living or get himself to the bathroom. His oral intake was poor and it was not clear that he understood how to take his medications. After confirming his wishes to not go to the hospital, the nurse called the tribal health physician to report his condition and discuss a referral to hospice. Mr. Wall was agreeable to this approach and asked the nurse to call his brother and his daughters.

Admission to Hospice:

By the afternoon, the family had gathered at Mr. Wall's home to meet with the hospice nurse. The tribal health nurse also attended the admission visit in order to continue to provide support for the patient and family in a collaborative manner with the hospice team. It was also important to continue support from the tribal health team because of the trust the team had developed with Mr. Wall. A primary goal for the visit was to engage in communication with the patient and family about the patient's terminal condition and his choices for care. Because the conversations between palliative care clinicians, patients, and families that focus on transitions to hospice and palliative care often signal the beginning of the dying process, it was important to have in the home those family members identified by the patient as important for decision making (Kirby, Broom, Good, Wootton, & Adams, 2014). A family-centered approach to the hospice admission was utilized and addressed the following priorities:

1. *Decision making:* It was important to discuss with the family what was currently known about Mr. Wall's condition in order to clarify his choices for care. He was considered appropriate for admission to hospice because of the physician's certification of terminal illness and his preference for comfort care rather than curative treatment. It was important to consider his personal cultural beliefs when discussing his illness with the family. The hospice team secured the patient's signature for a DNR (Do Not Resuscitate) or a Comfort One [Montana] order that documented his wishes. Family discussion centered on ensuring that his wishes were carried out and making sure other family members were given accurate information.
2. *Comfort care/pain and symptom management:* A complete pain and symptom assessment was completed to understand the patient's current condition and potential sources of suffering. Medication reconciliation helped the nurse identify the patient's needs for medication refills and additional recommendations for the primary provider.
3. *Family support:* Mr. Wall lived alone and would need to rely on family support to provide personal and comfort care in his home. As his disease progressed, he would require bathing, medication administration, and other personal care needs. His daughters, brothers, and granddaughters were willing to provide care so that he would not be alone.
4. *Home safety:* A safety assessment included making an agreement with the patient and family that the guns would be locked away during the period of home visiting to ensure safety of the patient, family, and staff. Assessment of fire hazards in the home and education on oxygen precautions were completed. Durable medical equipment was ordered to support safe care for the patient (e.g., hospital bed, wheelchair, bedside commode).
5. *Culture and traditional practices:* An assessment of the patient and family's traditional practices was an important priority. The patient declined chaplain support but did request that his extended family and friends be allowed to visit the home and support his family. His daughters requested a Catholic priest to pray with them.

(See Figure 10-6 for the Wall Family ecomap.)

Case Study: Wall Family *(cont.)*

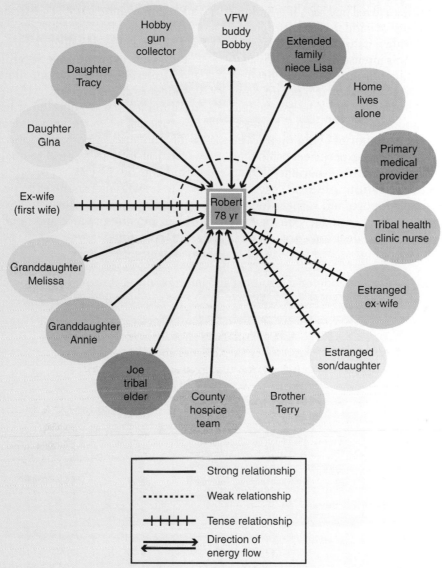

FIGURE 10-6 Wall Family Ecomap

Outcomes and Family Functioning:

Once Mr. Wall was admitted to the hospice program, his condition progressed rapidly. His decline was difficult for his family, particularly his daughters who had spent the majority of their lives estranged from their father. During this time, they provided loving care and shared close communication with their father. The hospice team and the tribal health team worked collaboratively with the family to care for Mr. Wall in his home until his peaceful death. At the time of his death, he was surrounded by his family. Each family member felt they had been able to share special moments with him and to say good-bye.

SUMMARY

Nurses are in a unique position to help families manage their lives when a loved one has a life-limiting illness or faces an acute or sudden death. Providing palliative and end-of-life nursing care as you accompany a family during this intense period is a privilege that should not be taken lightly. The importance of the nurse-family relationship in affecting and effecting positive outcomes cannot be overstated; this relationship can make the difference between a family who has good memories about their loved one's death and a family who experiences prolonged suffering because of a negative experience. Open and trusting communication; physical, psychological, and spiritual support; and respect for the families' right to make their own decisions, as well as support to facilitate these decisions, are essential components of quality palliative and end-of-life care. The following points highlight the concepts that are addressed in this chapter:

- Palliative and end-of-life care are inherently family-focused.
- The principles of palliative care can be enacted effectively in any setting, regardless of whether death results from a chronic illness or a sudden/traumatic event.
- All nurses need to develop at least basic competencies in the area of death and dying.
- Therapeutic nurse-patient and nurse-family relationships are central to quality palliative and end-of-life care.
- Nurses who incorporate the principles of palliative care are more effective in tailoring their nursing practice and family interventions.

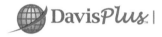 Davis*Plus* | For additional resources and information, visit **http://davisplus.fadavis.com**. References and Suggested Web sites can be found on Davis*Plus*.

Chapter 11

Trauma and Family Nursing

Deborah Padgett Coehlo, PhD, C-PNP, PMHS, CFLE

Henny Breen, PhD, RN, CNE, COI

Critical Concepts

- Trauma is a key experience affecting the family system.

- Trauma-informed care (TIC) is an important part of nursing care for all clients, including families, to improve outcomes, avoid biased and inaccurate assessments and interventions, and to prevent unethical decision-making processes.

- Adaptive responses to trauma are more likely to become problematic when resiliency traits are underdeveloped.

- Post-traumatic stress disorder (PTSD), a medical diagnosis, is based on a cluster of symptoms in response to trauma that can be acute or chronic and can occur months, or even years, after a disaster or traumatic event such as war.

- The Ecological Systems Theory can guide nurses in applying TIC.

- When one or more family members are traumatized, all family members and family relationships can be affected.

- Perpetrators of trauma can experience trauma themselves. Nurses who focus on TIC can address the dilemmas of caring for perpetrators through mandatory reporting and family-focused care.

- Secondary trauma can occur whenever a family member or caring provider is exposed to victims of trauma and is impacted by their response to the traumatic event(s).

- The family response to trauma of one or more of its members cannot be understood or treated by focusing on individual family members alone. Family members can provide key contextual information about past traumatic events and experiences that help explain current responses.

- Dysregulation is the abnormality or impairment in the regulation of a metabolic, physiological, or psychological process.

- Community systems can prevent, treat, and measure negative outcomes to traumatic events. If community agencies are not well trained and prepared, communities will suffer.

- Larger political and social systems can influence and be influenced by individual, family, and community trauma in a positive or negative way.

- Nursing focuses on the individual, family, community, and societal reactions to trauma in order to optimize positive outcomes and prevent or treat problematic stress responses. Nurses are key in supporting health rather than focusing on the pathology of a trauma response.

Trauma has been an increasing area of attention across the field of mental health for the past two decades. Between the advanced understanding of brain function and general physiology, as well as the mind and body response to severe and/or prolonged stress, and the increase in traumatic stress experienced by families through war, natural disasters, and family violence, the need to understand, prevent, treat, and monitor the effects of trauma on individuals and families has never been more vital. Further, the effects of trauma transcend individuals and families, but also affect communities and the broader society. Trauma influences future generations as the effects influence individual family genetics, community, and societal cultures. The negative effects of trauma are most profound during early childhood development, touching every domain of growth, with the potential of negative outcomes in adulthood, such as higher rates of mental illness, unemployment, substance abuse, and failed relationships.

The care by nurses of families experiencing traumatic stress revolves around preventing trauma when possible, supporting the development of resiliency, and, when not preventable, working toward positive outcomes. This chapter focuses on the current knowledge about trauma and nurses' key role in the field of TIC. This care emphasizes the importance of preventing, treating early, and encouraging resilience and the ability to make meaning out of negative events. This chapter also stresses an understanding of secondary trauma, or the negative effects of witnessing trauma of others, whether that other person is a stranger, family, or fellow professional. This discussion is particularly salient for nurses, because they are some of the most likely health care providers to encounter traumatized victims in their everyday practice. Nurses are among the highest professional groups to experience vicarious or secondary trauma, as a consequence to their exposure to traumatized clients (Best Start Resource Center, 2012).

POST-TRAUMATIC STRESS DISORDER

The diagnosis of post-traumatic stress disorder (PTSD) has grown significantly during the past two decades, as well as the understanding of differences in symptoms across developmental ages and stages. Whereas the key symptoms of re-experiencing the

trauma through painful memories and nightmares, hypervigilance, and emotional instability are common to adults, children are more likely to react with withdrawal and mood dysregulation. These symptoms cross ethnic groups and time. The number of individuals with PTSD in turn affects communities. Larger cultures and societies shift as the number of trauma victims grows, adding other negative consequences that include poor health, higher rates of other mental health disorders, and an increase in family violence.

The American Psychological Association first recognized PTSD as a diagnosis and began to categorize symptoms of it in 1980. Since that time, researchers and clinicians have identified the complexity of this disorder and the lifelong, intergenerational impact of repeated and prolonged trauma experienced by individuals, families, communities, and societies. Since this publication in 1980, researchers have attempted to clarify and expand the diagnosis to cover different categories of trauma, such as combat, horrific accidents, and child abuse; different content such as domestic violence, natural disasters, and war; and different cultures such as genocide victims and victims of natural disasters across cultures and across time. The *DSM-IV* and *DSM-IV-TR* included PTSD as a subcategory under anxiety disorders, including three categories of symptoms (APA, 2000; McNally, 2004; National Center for PTSD, 2016).

1. Re-experiencing the trauma
2. Avoidance and numbing
3. Increased arousal

The *DSM-5* has taken PTSD out of the category of anxiety and developed a separate category titled Trauma and Stressor Related Disorders (Friedman et al., 2011; Schmid, Petermann, & Fegert, 2013). The scope has been expanded to include both experiencing a traumatic event and witnessing or repeatedly hearing about a traumatic event. Further, the *DSM-5* has included four categories of symptoms (APA, 2013):

1. Intrusion of thoughts about the trauma
2. Avoidance of discussion or other stimulus reminding the person of the trauma
3. Increased arousal or sensory sensitivity
4. Negative cognitions and moods

Today, it is estimated that up to 10% of the general population across the world meets the criteria for a diagnosis of PTSD, with areas experiencing war or severe natural disasters experiencing the highest rates. When further divided between geographical areas, ages, and genders, the prevalence rates vary, with risks higher for women and adolescents and lower risks in Asian countries (U.S. Department of Veterans Affairs, 2007). When considering children and adolescents, it is important to note that most PTSD is caused by (1) abuse and neglect across time, (2) witnessing violence within the home and/or neighborhood, and (3) experiencing single incident traumatic events such as motor vehicle accidents and natural disasters (Salmond et al., 2011).

The number of studies on individual trauma and outcomes has increased in the past decade, as has awareness that PTSD is not limited to individuals, but rather affects individuals, families, communities, and societies. The understanding of the political and societal influences on the diagnosis, treatment, and continued research in this area explains in part the continued need to explore trauma and the relationship to family health. The extent of damage to physical and mental health caused by trauma has now been realized. This chapter uses the Ecological Systems Model (Bronfenbrenner, 2005) to explore current understanding of risk and protective factors of PTSD, and uses that knowledge to further understand the multidisciplinary approach to TIC that goes beyond the medical model of diagnosis and treatment. Family nurses are in a key position to understand, recognize, prevent, and treat trauma at multiple levels. Case studies throughout this chapter illustrate the complexities of trauma and its effect on all family members, and the strong influence nursing care can have on short- and long-term outcomes.

THEORIES APPLIED TO TRAUMA

Trauma care has progressed significantly during the past two decades, with a plethora of studies published to clarify evidence-based practice across cultural groups, ages and genders, geographic areas, and types of trauma experienced. Historically, health care providers considered trauma to be a form of hysteria, meriting ineffective treatments as severe as hysterectomies. Currently, the treatment approaches recognize the modern understanding of trauma as a complex stress disorder with several applicable underlying theories. For purposes of this book, we delve into trauma understanding and care using the Substance Abuse and Mental Health Services Administration (SAMHSA)'s guide to TIC (2015), the Ecological Systems Model (Bronfenbrenner, 1984, 1995: Bronfenbrenner & Lerner, 2004), and the Family Systems Theory (Bowen, 1978) as the underlying models to guide practice.

Trauma-Informed Care

TIC has emerged as a leading guideline for those health care providers, including nurses, who care for and are affected by trauma in their clients. SAMHSA (2015) has been a leader in identifying key principles guiding TIC, including:

1. *"Realizing* the widespread impact of trauma and understanding potential paths for recovery;
2. *Recognizing* the signs and symptoms of trauma in clients, families, staff, and others involved with the system;
3. *Responding* by fully integrating knowledge about trauma into policies, procedures, and practices; and
4. Seeking to actively resist *re-traumatization."* (SAMHSA, 2015, paragraph 2)

Further, nurses applying TIC provide safety for their clients by building safety, trust, peer support, collaboration, and empowerment, while attending to historical, cultural, and gender issues using evidence-based practices. Hobfoll et al. (2007), following a review of literature investigating interventions that worked with trauma survivors across cultures, identified five essential elements of TIC immediate and long-term interventions, including:

1. Promoting a sense of safety, including building positive social support
2. Promoting calming skills
3. Promoting a sense of self-efficacy and collective efficacy for families
4. Promoting "connectiveness" between family members
5. Instilling hope: "To see a future that is better than the trauma present" (Evans & Coccoma, 2014, p. 47)

The TIC approach is consistent with the foundational principles of the nurse-client relationship. By using these guiding principles, it is believed that victims of trauma who suffer from mental health issues, such as substance abuse, depression, anxiety, eating disorders, and social isolation, will be better served when there is understanding of how the trauma has an impact on the trajectory of a person's life. By working with individuals, families, and communities that have experienced trauma, health care providers can build a more collaborative approach to care. Several evidence-based approaches to working with victims of trauma include strategies for individual therapy (e.g., Eye Movement Desensitization and Reprocessing [EMDR]) and group therapy (e.g.,≈Trauma, Addiction, Mental Health, and Recovery [TAMAR]). Other approaches include changes to the treatment environment to prevent retraumatization (i.e., elimination of the use of restraints and isolation as punishments for individuals struggling with emotional dysregulation; SAMSHA, 2015). TIC is a shift away from pathology of trauma to recognition of the physical, relational, and emotional changes that occur in response to trauma. The questions for clients shift from "What is wrong with you?" to "What happened to you and how is it affecting your life?" (Evans & Coccoma, 2014; SAMHSA, 2014). TIC is also one of the few models that embraces working with survivors of trauma and their families (SAMHSA, 2014).

Ecological Systems Model

Bronfenbrenner (1996) identifies four systems that interact together in the Ecological Systems Model: the *microsystem, mesosystem, macrosystem,* and *exosystem*. He later added the system of time, or the *chronosystem,* to describe the impact of history and time on individuals, families, communities, and societies. Time is integrated as a concept within each of the four other ecological systems. The understanding of the impact of trauma on a micro- to exosystem level helps health care providers and policy makers understand the interconnections between trauma and abuse to individuals, families, communities, and societies, and the impact of that trauma across time, generations, and geographical and cultural systems. Trauma tends to be repeated if nothing intervenes to stop the pattern. Interventions intended to stop and/or alter these patterns are much more effective when chosen and implemented with the complexity and interconnections between systems in mind. See Figure 11-1 for a visual portrayal of Bronfenbrenner's Ecological Systems Model.

Microsystem

The *microsystem* involves the individual and the systems within that individual, including physiological (i.e., respiratory, cardiovascular), developmental, and psychological (i.e., sensory perceptions, memory). The role of trauma in violating and damaging physical and mental well-being and negatively affecting development of children and adults is no longer questioned. The negative impact of trauma on individuals ranges from interference with healthy development of attachment to physical and mental illness across the life span (Afifi, Boman, Fleisher, & Sareen, 2009). Although understanding the impact of trauma on individuals is important to understanding family trauma, care of these individuals in isolation is less effective than providing care within the context of the family. The *microsystem* provides a beginning knowledge to family trauma, but the *mesosystem* adds a deeper understanding.

Mesosystem

The effect of trauma on any one individual within the family has a significant impact on family development and family functioning. The stress response from trauma is felt from experiencing, witnessing, or being informed about an act of violence against others. Younger children and those with intellectual disabilities who do not have the ability to process or understand the traumatic events are more vulnerable to developing problematic stress responses. This is also the case when the trauma is repeated and unpredictable (APA, 2013). This traumatic stress response is experienced by family members directly or witnessed by other family members, expanding the experience beyond the *micro* level to the *meso* level of reaction. For example, children's reactions to trauma and their resiliency skills are shaped in part by family experiences and reactions as well as cultural experiences. The act of witnessing trauma includes direct observation as well as hearing about traumatic events repeatedly from family members. Further, how family members react to a traumatic event will have a direct impact on how other family members will respond. For example, if parents cannot regulate their own reactions and cannot support the child because of their own physical, mental, or emotional difficulties, then their child is at higher risk for developing mood dysregulation and an inability to develop healthy attachments.

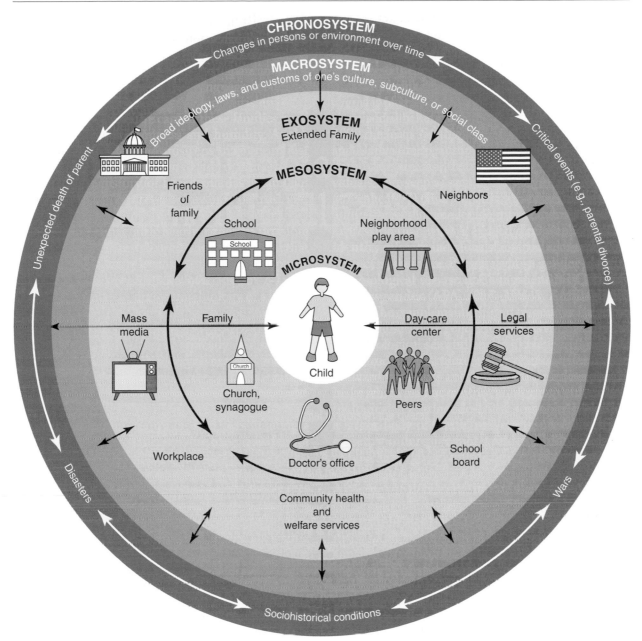

FIGURE 11-1 Bronfenbrenner's Ecological Systems Model

Likewise, if parents lack support and positive coping strategies, they are less likely to be able to provide support to their child.

Macrosystem

Trauma at the macro level includes all trauma within a community. This level of trauma not only influences individuals (micro) and families (meso), but has an impact on how a community reacts and recovers from trauma. During the past two decades, the growing disparity between mental health and access to mental health services within a community has been well documented (Friedman, 2016). Traumatic events within schools, for example, have increased the awareness of the need for more in-depth and comprehensive mental health services to prevent these events and to be available to treat the victims and perpetrators (i.e., bullies) following these events.

Schools have been identified as key community systems that can provide both prevention and treatment services. More than 60% of schools already attempt to address trauma at a community, or *macrosystem*, level through prevention services, community preparedness such as town meetings and educational programs, provision of temporary food and shelter following a disaster, counseling services, and/or behavioral programs (Taylor, Weist, & DeLoach, 2012). Using TIC when working with schools experiencing trauma improves outcomes, especially for traumatized youth (i.e., school bullying, school shootings, or school suicides) (Cohen et al., 2009).

Exosystem

The exosystem includes the larger culture and government or laws and justice within a culture. The exosystem is touched by and touches on individuals, families, and communities. For example, the cultural reactions and legal responses to a natural disaster have grave implications for individuals, families, and communities. Consider the response by the government to Hurricane Katrina in 2005, with the delays and the disorganization during and after the disaster. These gaps in services were believed to be a contributing factor to the high rates of severe trauma reactions in survivors (Mills, Edmondson, & Park, 2007). Researchers have explored the dysregulation and hyperarousal of individuals during this time, and have found that similar processes can and do occur at a larger, systemic level. Judith Warner, in a 2010 *New York Times* article (Warner, 2010), observed that the large-scale dysfunction of federal regulatory systems, including the banking meltdown, collapse of the housing market, and failure of levees during Hurricane Katrina, resulted in the United States as a *country* struggling with symptoms of PTSD for several years after the hurricane hit the shores of Louisiana. Likewise, 16 years after the nightmare of the 9/11/2001 terrorist attacks, the United States is still engaged in war across many boundaries. The incidence of diagnosed PTSD for veterans has increased significantly during this time, from 0.7% of all military personnel diagnosed with PTSD in 2004 to 8% of all military personnel diagnosed with PTSD in 2012 IOM, 2014).

Family Systems Theory

The Family Systems Theory focuses on the interaction between family members and the impact of an individual's health and behavioral responses on other family members, as well as other family members' reactions and health impact on individuals. The metaphor of a wind chime is commonly used to describe the Family Systems Theory, with one chime, or individual family member, being struck by other chimes, or other family members, to make music or cacophony. The wind flowing through the wind chimes represents the stressors that flow through every family. The wind can be a gentle breeze, or low stress level, or higher winds, similar to high stress and less controlled stress levels. The Family Systems Theory, when considered through an ecological looking glass, can help explain the impact of trauma within and surrounding families.

The remainder of the chapter examines the types of trauma that individuals, families, communities, and societies at large currently face, along with implications for nurses.

EARLY TRAUMA

Early trauma shapes early attachment, developmental progress, and early brain development, which can be understood through the lens of the Ecological Systems Model.

Attachment

Because early trauma has been shown to interfere with healthy development of attachment, attachment theories are used as a basis of research and understanding. Failure to develop healthy attachments during childhood are commonly linked to later issues with developmental growth and physical and mental well-being. Bowlby (1973), an early researcher and theorist in the area of attachment, identified the importance of early attachment for healthy development. During healthy attachment, an infant learns to trust his or her caregivers and develops the ability to compartmentalize isolated threats or fears. When severe abuse or neglect occurs, an infant learns to mistrust his or her caregivers and views the environment as unsafe and threatening. This process destroys the infant's ability to compartmentalize threats, leading to the inability to self-regulate emotions, behaviors, and physiological processes (i.e., sleep and elimination) (Evans & Coccoma, 2014).

Developmental Trauma Theory

Heller and LaPierre (2012), in describing their Developmental Trauma Theory, categorized this early traumatic interference with attachment by describing five core areas of concern: (1) interference with connection to others, (2) lack of attunement or ability to recognize physical and emotional needs, (3) lack of trust in caregivers and the environment, (4) difficulty with boundaries between self and others, and (5) difficulty developing a sense of love and healthy sexuality. Table 11-1 illustrates the Neuroaffective Relational Model Five Core Needs developed by Heller and LaPierre (2012). More specific symptoms of failure to develop healthy attachments related to experiencing trauma include the following:

■ Absence of self-regulation—inconsistent and unpredictable patterns of eating and sleeping, and mood regulation.
■ Lack of response to caregivers—poor eye contact, lack of response to consoling measures, withdrawal, and isolation.
■ Lack of response to the environment—inability to pretend play, interact with toys, and/or experience shared pleasure with others (Heller & LaPierre, 2012; Joubert, Webster, & Hackett, 2012).

If untreated, children experiencing trauma struggle in cognitive, emotional, and social development (Evans & Coccoma, 2014; Heller & LaPierre, 2012; Joubert et al., 2012; Perry & Pollard, 1998). The Developmental Trauma Theory proposed by Heller and LaPierre (2012) also describes the survival strategies individuals (micro level) learn in order to cope with traumatic experiences, thereby expanding the understanding of the negative impact of trauma on attachment. These coping strategies interfere with healthy development. For example, whenever an individual experiences a severe threat, the sympathetic-adrenal-medullary (SAM) axis is triggered. This reaction is followed by a release of catecholamines, norepinephrine, and epinephrine, which in turn trigger the hypothalamic-pituitary adrenal (HPA) axis. The hypothalamus in the brain works during this process to regulate heart rate, respiratory rate, and blood flow, and stimulates the amygdala to store the memory and the response for quick reaction to future threats. The adrenal gland then releases cortisol, our stress hormone, that eventually allows activation of the fear extinction process, or eventual recovery from the stress (Evans & Coccoma, 2014). Refer to Figure 11-1 for an illustration of this typical physiological reaction to stress or threats. When repeated trauma occurs, a state of constant fear develops, causing distinct physiological and psychological changes.

Research during the past 50 years has explored why prolonged or repeated trauma results in a different response in individuals compared with a typical stress response from isolated threats. Three areas of the brain have been identified as key factors in altering a healthy stress response that saves lives to a trauma-related response that causes chronic physical and mental disorders (Evans & Coccoma, 2014):

■ *Amygdala:* With prolonged trauma, the amygdala becomes hyperactive, which interferes with the ability to appropriately process trauma memories, and decreases the function of the prefrontal cortex, causing a decreased ability to think about the response to present traumas and problem solve appropriate reactions.
■ *Hippocampus:* The hippocampus is responsible for changing explicit memories, or new

Table 11-1 Neuroaffective Relational Model Five Core Needs	
Core Need	**Description**
Connection	Lack of ability to form healthy connection with caregivers or significant support people
Attunement	Lack of ability to recognize physical and emotional needs
Trust	Lack of ability to trust others
Boundaries	Difficulty setting healthy boundaries
Deep sense of love and sexuality	Inability to form deep loving relationships, and, as adults, connect deep love with healthy sexuality

Source: Heller & LaPierre, 2012.

memories, into implicit memories, or patterns (i.e., driving a car, riding a bike, or skiing change from an awkward new skill to an automatic skill that takes little conscious thought). Severe or prolonged trauma interferes with this process, resulting in feelings of inadequacy and doubt. Further, the hippocampus is responsible for differentiating past experiences from present experiences. With severe and prolonged trauma, this differentiation is damaged, causing an individual to respond to a memory, or a similar sensory trigger (i.e., vision or sound), as if the trauma were repeating itself in the present. Finally, the hippocampus is responsible for repeated memories retrieved for a variety of cognitive, physical, and emotional functions. In the context of severe and repeated trauma, however, this process results in intrusive memories interfering with function.

■ *Prefrontal cortex:* This part of our brain is responsible for cognitive processing of traumatic memories. Without prefrontal cortex functioning, *fear extinction,* or the resolution of the SAM axis response, cannot occur. With hyperactive activity in the amygdala, the prefrontal cortex cannot be fully functional, resulting in unresolved traumatic memories.

These three areas, when affected by severe and repeated trauma, have an impact on an individual's ability to process, store, and appropriately retrieve memories. In turn, the neurological system, in response, alerts the brain to stay in survival mode. Because this system is activated continuously when repeated trauma occurs, the individual's ability to feel safe is threatened, resulting in a state of constant hyperarousal. This constant state of arousal causes an individual to become overwhelmed, leading to an abrupt shift to the parasympathetic system, and the individual shuts down, withdraws, becomes numb, disassociates, or falls into sleep. Sleep, eating, and digestive patterns are affected, and excitable behavior builds again with the next remembered or experienced trauma. Emotions range from hyperstimulated (i.e., hysteria or excessive, inconsolable crying) to numbness (no reaction to the environment). Without resolution, the individual develops a state of fear and gradually loses the ability to regulate emotional and autonomic reactions.

If uninterrupted, the young child will develop secondary complications, including anxiety, shame, isolation, mood dysregulation, and uncontrolled anger or explosive outbursts (Alisic, Jongmans, Van Wesel, & Kleber, 2011; Evans & Coccoma, 2014; Salmond et al., 2011).

As a child develops into adulthood, he may try to adapt to those feelings by abusing substances or avoiding emotions (Evans & Coccoma, 2014; Heller & LaPierre, 2012). The underlying fear remains; the threat to self and to the ability to survive is not over. Symptoms emerge over time, including the following (Heller & LaPierre, 2012).

■ Lack of affect
■ Feelings of shame
■ Separation from others
■ Avoidance of emotionally disturbing situations or people
■ Overintellectualizing and avoiding of emotions
■ Lack of attunement or awareness of bodily and related needs
■ Fear of being alone while at the same time feeling overwhelmed by others
■ Fear of death and illness
■ Fear of their own anger
■ Fear of intimacy
■ Strong need to control
■ Desire for altered states and disassociation
■ Cognitive impairments, including difficulty with auditory processing, memory, and attention
■ Feelings of helplessness
■ Hypovigilance or hypervigilance

Physical symptoms of prolonged and repeated trauma in childhood include the following:

■ Disrupted sleep
■ Eating disorders
■ Panic disorders
■ Obsessive-compulsive disorders
■ Rage
■ Depression
■ Addiction
■ Cardiovascular disorders
■ Autoimmune disorders

A pattern emerges across time. Figure 11-2 illustrates the developmental pattern of maladaptation to early trauma.

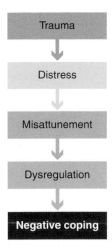

FIGURE 11-2 Developmental Pattern of Maladaptation to Early Trauma

Environmental Trauma

Studies on the impact of war, terror, and unexpected natural disasters on children have resulted in the identification of the term *disaster syndrome*. Smith (2013) described this syndrome as a combination of symptoms of PTSD, including anxiety, dissociation, and depression. The loss of people, support, routines, and assumptions regarding safety and regularity, as well as parental response, all affect the severity of a child's response. Parental response is influenced by parents' prior diagnosis of mental illness, prior coping strategies, and number of past traumatic experiences. Children respond to their family members' emotional and physical changes related to trauma. When an individual (micro level) experiences trauma over time, his interaction with others (meso level) and his ability to interact in a functional manner with his community (macro level) are altered. One distinct difference between children and adults experiencing trauma through environmental events is that adults tend to have less PTSD because of the support of the community and decreased feelings of isolation, whereas children feel more isolated during these events because of profound fear of losing their supportive loved ones (Evans & Coccoma, 2014).

The human desire for regulation of the autonomic nervous system, with a return to balance, is strong. Individuals are highly motivated to find this balance, and will pursue strategies to achieve this goal through either positive measures (e.g., healthy patterns of sleep, eating, exercise, meditation, yoga, and spiritual connection) or negative measures (e.g., drug-seeking behavior, obsessive thinking patterns, or avoidance patterns) (Evans & Coccoma, 2014). These negative patterns interfere with every stage of development, primarily altering cognitive, emotional, communication, and social domains. Although young infants cannot consciously think about their reactions to trauma, their emotions and related autonomic reactions are affected in a measurable way (Evans & Coccoma, 2014; Heller & LaPierre, 2012). Infants have bottom-up responses, or responses starting with brainstem or autonomic reactions to external threat, moving up toward emotional responses. Adults, in contrast, experience trauma initially from thought, or the cortex of the brain, and move down to emotional response, and finally autonomic or brainstem reaction. This is considered top-down reaction. Another important differentiation between infants and adults is that infants tend to have a broad interpretation of experiences, whereas adults are able to separate experiences and feelings between experiences. The difference in reaction is caused by the difference in development of pathways from the frontal cortex to the brainstem as the brain develops across time. The pathways are reinforced by experiences and interactions in the environment (Heller & LaPierre, 2012). Figure 11-3 illustrates bottom-up and top-down responses to trauma.

This variance in response to trauma is important to understand: Adults who experience trauma can make a distinction between different experiences in their lives, and therefore *feel* badly about a specific experience; infants and young children cannot differentiate between experiences and therefore, when they experience trauma, they tend to think *they are* bad (Heller & LaPierre, 2012). Young children and adults, however, if left untreated following a trauma, can regress back to thinking and feeling they are bad as a global response to trauma.

Early Trauma and Brain Development

The understanding of the impact of early trauma on brain development has led to detailed study of the impact on brain development and plasticity, or the ability of the brain to recover from injury. When considering trauma or major stress, the body is governed by two main systems: the neurological system and the endocrine system. These two systems ensure

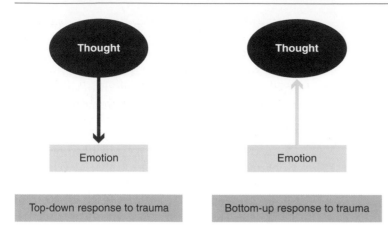

FIGURE 11-3 Top-down and Bottom-up Reaction

survival of the individual through stimulation of the sympathetic nervous system when the individual is threatened, and the parasympathetic nervous system when the individual is safe and relaxed. Hans Selye (1976), a renowned theorist on stress, identified the connection between the hypothalamus, the pituitary gland, and the adrenal glands, now commonly referred to as the HPA axis. To summarize this process, the hypothalamus links the nervous system to the pituitary system, which secretes hormones that regulate homeostasis. If homeostasis is not reached, the adrenal glands secrete the stress hormones, epinephrine and norepinephrine. These hormones stimulate the sympathetic nervous system, and the result is increased heart rate, dilation of pupils, relaxation of bronchial tubes, increased tension and circulation of blood to large muscles, and initial stimulation of the prefrontal cortex through a surge of dopamine, followed by bypassing the prefrontal cortex to the amygdala.

This bypass process encourages rapid action based on the previous experience of threats, and the assumption that the same threat has occurred and the same action for survival is needed. When this process is stimulated repeatedly and without resolution, the connection between the limbic system (where automatic actions based on emotions and repeated actions rather than thought occur) and the cortex (or the thinking part of the brain that includes judgment, creativity, and prediction of action on future consequences) is pruned (i.e., cut). When the connection is pruned, sensory perception becomes scattered and disorganized. By bypassing the prefrontal cortex, the individual exchanges accuracy, judgment, and the ability to learn for speed. The

bypassed prefrontal cortex provides the individual with the executive functions of detailed assessment, regulation of emotion or thought, inhibition of inappropriate responses, expressive speech, and problem-solving skills. Over time, an individual constantly facing threat through trauma develops a fearful identity, avoids relationships because of previous threats, has uncontrolled emotional outbursts or withdrawal, disassociates from the present, and/or experiences depression.

The hippocampus, which is key in neuroplasticity or the ability to generate new neurons and new neuron pathways (known as neurogenesis), is impaired. This process explains why many who experience prolonged and repeated trauma struggle with cognitive impairments, such as poor short-term memory, difficulty with concentration, difficulty learning new skills, and poor sensory integration, especially auditory processing (Sherwin & Nemeroff, 2011). This process has been found to be more severe in both children and adults experiencing relational trauma, or trauma inflicted by people in a position of trust (meso level), than those experiencing trauma from inanimate objects (e.g., motor vehicle accidents) or environmental trauma (i.e., natural disasters) (Evans & Coccoma, 2014; Heller & LaPierre, 2012). This process is most damaging when the trauma experienced occurs early in life, and continues throughout childhood, causing an initial and prolonged damage to normal brain development (Alisic et al., 2011; Evans & Coccoma, 2014). For family nurses, it is important to assess the start and duration of any family trauma occurring to a child or young adult.

Early Childhood Trauma

The impact of early trauma and the negative long-term outcomes has led to further study of the effect of childhood trauma on adult health. The Adverse Childhood Experiences Study was conducted between 1995 and 1997 (CDC, 2016) provided landmark evidence that early trauma does indeed have negative consequences for adult health. The study was conducted as a collaboration between Kaiser Permanente and the Centers for Disease Control and Prevention (CDC), and entailed surveying 11,000 individuals across a decade, linking adverse childhood experiences with adult physical and mental health variables. The results revealed a relationship between the number of adverse childhood experiences and the number of comorbid outcomes, including adulthood depression, panic disorder, substance abuse, sexual promiscuity, relationship problems, and domestic violence (Mersky, Topitzes, & Reynolds, 2013). Figure 11-4 illustrates the relationship between adverse childhood experiences and adult comorbid conditions. The findings of this hallmark study led to a more in-depth understanding of the cumulative effect of repeated and numerous traumas experienced during childhood, and the effect on brain development. More recent studies to confirm these findings continue to support the negative impact of multiple adverse events in childhood on the occurrence and

outcome of chronic illnesses in adults. Gilbert et al. (2015) analyzed 53,998 surveys from adults from 10 states and the District of Columbia using the Adverse Childhood Experiences questionnaire to measure the number of adverse effects in childhood, and the Behavioral Risk Factor Surveillance System to measure the number of chronic conditions in adulthood. The results confirmed increased risk of mental and physical chronic conditions in adulthood for those experiencing adverse childhood experiences, with increased risk as the number of adverse events increased. This study also noted that minority groups, those living in poverty, those with lower education, and women were at higher risk for adverse childhood experiences. This study validates the need to prevent adverse childhood experiences as a key measure in improving health in adults.

Clearly, understanding early trauma and the negative impact on children and development allows health care providers to grasp better the effect of traumatic events on adults. Studies have found that resiliency is one factor that determines which adults will continue to suffer from childhood trauma versus which adults will thrive following trauma. Of interest is that the number of traumatic events is found to be consistently higher in men, but women have a higher incidence of PTSD following trauma. This is consistently true for civilian populations across geographical locations (Kilpatrick et al., 2013). One theory is that women experience sexual assault and traumatic abuse from male partners, supporting the idea that relational trauma is more traumatic and more difficult to cope with than inanimate or nonrelational trauma (Brown, Burnette, & Cerulli, 2014). Further, sexual assault is often accompanied by shame and self-blame, which increases the risk of PTSD (La Bash & Papa, 2014). More recent studies have looked at the complexity of childhood trauma leading to continued re-exposure in adults in the forms of intimate partner violence and adult sexual assault. This too is more common in women. Brown et al. (2014) studied 162 women who were seeking court-ordered restraining orders for protection against abusive intimate partners. Of these 162 women, 103 (64%) exhibited symptoms of PTSD. The authors also found a significant correlation between the incidence of childhood trauma and the severity of PTSD in adulthood among these women.

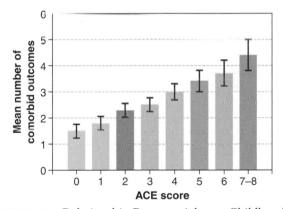

FIGURE 11-4 Relationship Between Adverse Childhood Experiences and Comorbid Conditions. Adverse Childhood Experiences Include Verbal, Physical, or Sexual Abuse, As Well As Family Dysfunction (e.g., an incarcerated, mentally ill, or substance-abusing family member; domestic violence; or absence of a parent because of divorce or separation) (*Anda, Felitti, Bremner, Walker, Whitfield, Perry, Dube, & Giles, 2006*)

Resiliency

Through the improved understanding of childhood trauma and related reactions, the concept of resiliency is more fully understood, or why some who experience the same or similar event will adapt without any measure of physical or emotional damage or even report growth, whereas others become severely and chronically disabled. "Most contemporary researchers now agree that resilience refers to positive outcomes, adaptation or the attainment of developmental milestones or competencies in the face of significant risk, adversity, or stress" (Naglieri, LeBuffe, & Ross, 2012, p. 242). Research has focused on identifying factors or characteristics that are consistently found in those individuals found to be resilient. The factors most commonly cited as resiliency qualities include the following (Afifi & MacMillan, 2011; Overland, 2011):

- Social connectedness and positive supportive relationships
- Competent parenting
- Absence of mental illness in caregiver(s)
- Easy to moderate temperament
- High intelligence
- Ego-resiliency, or the acquisition of a strong sense of self across the life span with or without trauma (Philippe, Laventure, Beaulieu-Pelletier, LeCours, & Lekes, 2011)
- Compassion
- Optimism
- Gratitude
- Determination
- Meaning and purpose in life
- Caring for self and attuning to own needs
- Trusting others to help
- Internal locus of control
- High self-esteem
- Strong self-efficacy
- Vicarious resiliency (Hernβndez, Gangsei, & Engstrom, 2007)

Research on resiliency continues. For example, Philippe et al. (2011) investigated 118 clients from an outpatient clinic in Canada and found that if ego-resiliency traits were present before a traumatic event, then negative outcomes, including anxiety, depression, and self-harm, decreased by as much as 30%. Although resiliency characteristics often precede the traumatic experience, this is not always the case. Deblinger, Runyon, and Steer (2014) studied 250 youth in an inpatient treatment program for children who had experienced sexual and physical abuse. They confirmed that those individuals with the highest vulnerability scores and the lowest resiliency scores had the highest scores for depression. Resiliency traits, therefore, should be assessed by family nurses to determine those that were present before the trauma and reinforced, versus those that are lacking and need to be taught and supported. Resiliency can buffer the negative impacts of trauma on the individual's brain development.

Recent studies have shifted from individual traits of resiliency to family traits of resiliency, recognizing that close family support has a significant influence on both the genetic influence on resiliency as well as the environmental influence on learning and using resiliency traits (Walsh, 2016). This emphasizes the strength of using Bronfenbrenner's Ecological Systems Model when assessing and treating not only trauma, but family resiliency as well.

Resiliency has moved beyond just preventing negative outcomes following a traumatic event, but understanding why some individuals and families report growth or positive meaning after a traumatic event or events. This phenomenon was first described by Antonovsky (1987) following his research on Holocaust survivors. He identified three characteristics of those that were healthy following prolonged trauma:

1. Finding solutions to problems (engaging cognitive functioning in the prefrontal cortex)
2. Identifying supportive resources
3. Identifying capacity (engaging motivation)

Later research by Antonovsky (1993) included the development of the Sense of Coherence Scale, now commonly used to assess survivors of trauma translated into several languages. This scale measures well-being or health following trauma, rather than pathology. Shakespeare-Finch and Armstrong (2010) used this research to guide their research on post-traumatic growth (PTG). They studied survivors of motor vehicle accidents, bereavement, and sexual assault, and found that those sexually assaulted had the lowest scores for PTG compared with the other two groups. They proposed that personal trauma, such as sexual assault, is experienced in isolation and surrounded by shame, whereas other types of trauma are often accompanied by societal support and are without social stigma. Others have confirmed this idea, with sexual assault across the life span having higher levels of PTSD when compared with natural disasters, accidents, or other types of physical abuse (Evans & Coccoma, 2014). Resiliency in war victims offers further understanding into who will develop PTSD versus who will not. Studies have shown that women and children, and those vulnerable within a population, often suffer more in a war than soldiers. Evans and Coccoma (2014), after their review of literature, felt that part of this pattern is the increased isolation and lack of support of women and children; also part of this pattern is the praise and acknowledgment of soldiers, with honorary rituals for their service, while women and children remain silent victims. Children respond differently than women. The degree that children survive trauma without negative consequences depends on the nature of the threat, the stage of development, and the degree of cognitive awareness of the event, previous trauma experience, cultural beliefs, the quality of support, the proximity to the event, and individual resiliency traits (Evans & Coccoma, 2014; Masten, 2011). These studies help nurses realize the importance of making sure that trauma survivors are not left alone and isolated, but rather supported and respected, and that care is developmentally appropriate. Masten (2011), following a review of four decades of research on resiliency, concluded that interventions that were strengths-based and competence-focused, as well as interdisciplinary and developmentally appropriate, were the most successful. For example, a multidisciplinary parenting class that addresses individual challenges (i.e., emotional regulation) to global challenges (i.e., finding appropriate child care) can build resiliency traits and boost protective factors in parents and children. Research is continuing on a molecular to global level and involving diverse disciplines to identify preventive factors for individuals and communities across time.

FAMILY TRAUMA

Families experience trauma as a family and through individual members. This section discusses both (1) family trauma through disasters and war, and (2) individual experiences of trauma and their effect on family members. Each member of the family experiences trauma differently, with different symptoms, reactions, and needs for recovery. For example, both parents and children experience similar symptoms of PTSD, but adults are more likely to experience re-experiencing the event through nightmares and flashbacks, whereas children are more likely to avoid similar experiences (e.g., avoiding riding in a car after a car accident) or avoid talking about the event. Both children and adults experience hyperarousal, or the HPA axis response to stress (Evans & Coccoma, 2014; Heller & LaPierre, 2012). When this occurs, parenting often becomes overwhelming as children overreact to environmental stimuli and parents overreact to the stressors of parenting. Each family member in turn can easily be misdiagnosed as depressed, anxious, or having attention deficit-hyperactivity disorder (ADHD) and the opportunity for effective and comprehensive treatment is therefore lost. The National Center for PTSD (2016) has identified 10 key areas that affect family functioning when one or more members are diagnosed with PTSD:

1. Increased sympathy by family members, which may provide support for the family member with PTSD or prolong feelings of victimization.
2. Increased negative feelings about the person with PTSD. These feelings are often triggered by changes in the person with PTSD, from changes in mood regulation, to depression, to explosive outbursts. The person is no longer the same as the person they knew before.
3. Avoidance is a common reaction by individuals with PTSD and by family members. Family members often circumvent talking about anything related to the trauma, and may dodge other topics hoping to avoid angry outbursts. Individuals with PTSD tend to avoid social situations because of fear of not fitting in or being questioned about the trauma. This, in turn, leads to social isolation of all family members as they try to support the individual with PTSD.
4. Depression is common among individuals with PTSD and their family members. The longer the symptoms of PTSD last, the more likely family members may lose hope that their family member will ever get back to normal.

5. Anger is common among family members as they struggle to cope with changes in the person with PTSD and anger that expectations are not being met.

6. Guilt and shame are common for family members as they feel helpless to change negative family functioning and find themselves feeling angry about the individual's illness.

7. Health problems increase in individuals with PTSD and their family members, including substance abuse, reduction in healthy immune response, and negative effects of poor eating habits, poor sleep, smoking, and lack of healthy exercise.

8. Fear and worry develop as their worldview changes given the intimate knowledge that terrible things can happen. Family members may also worry about symptoms of anger and unpredictable behavior that is manifested by the person experiencing PTSD.

9. Drug and alcohol abuse occurs as a way to escape their negative feelings.

10. Sleep problems develop, especially when it is a problem for the trauma survivor.

These outcomes can leave parents feeling inadequate and spouses feeling angry, guilty, and disillusioned. Nurses are often at the forefront of trauma care, as they encounter family members during traumatic events from war, natural disasters, family violence and abuse, and severe illness or unanticipated accidents. The nurses' role with families facing PTSD in a loved one include education of the outcomes of PTSD, support for all family members, advocacy for families, and referral for appropriate counseling and support resources for both the individual experiencing PTSD and the family members.

Families Affected by War

Since the turn of the century, the nature of war has changed dramatically. Warfare in the 21st century rarely involves confrontations between professional armies. Instead, wars typically are fought as grinding struggles between military personnel and civilians, or groups of armed civilians in a city environment rather than in distant battlefields. Thus, civilian fatalities from battles fought in towns and cities have increased to 90% of the casualties of war in the 21st century, as compared with only 5% in the early 1900s. Worldwide, the caseload of refugee children has grown from 2.4 million in 1974 to 7.2 million in the past decade (Bridging Refugee Youth and Children's Services, 2013). In Uganda alone, an estimated 20,000 children were forced into soldier labor during a 20-year period, with related physical abuse and witnessing of severe abuse and killing of other abducted children, including siblings (Beard, 2011). In the United States, the impact of war on families, other than for refugees, is limited to wartime separation and reunion. Over time, serving in one of the branches of the U.S. military has become far less common. Since 2001, only 1.6 million veterans (or less than 0.05% of the population) have served in Afghanistan or Iraq, compared with the 16 million or 12% of the population that served in World War II (Meagher, 2007). Still, the consequences for family members of military personnel are often dire and long lasting. Death, injury, and short- and long-term disability of the veteran are stressors that can make life difficult for families, especially spouses who become the caregiver (Burland & Lundquist, 2012). For example, an increase in traumatic brain injury sustained during war is associated with physical neurological problems that are made worse by PTSD (Rosenfeld et al., 2013).

The risk of suicide among Veterans is 22% higher when compared to U.S. non-Veteran adults. The rates for male Veterans is 19% higher than U.S. non-Veteran men. The risk for female Veteran suicide is 2.5 times higher when compared to U.S non-Veteran women (Office of Public and Intergovernmental Affairs, 2017).

During the most recent war that affected Americans, Operation Iraqi Freedom, thousands of family members were deployed. This war brought to light the effects of the trauma of war on families. This war resulted in 6364 causalities and 48,296 wounded U.S. troops. Two million children were affected by separation from parents, changes in health status of parents, and/or loss of parents because of this war. Forty-four percent of these children were under 6 years of age, and so were particularly prone to the effects of trauma from coexperiencing family trauma (Smith, 2013). As evidence of the difficulty these families face, the telephone calls to the 24-hour helpline Military OneSource, which provides counseling to veterans and their families, numbered more than 100,000 in the first 10 months of 2005; the calls increased by 20% in 2006. More than 200,000 antidepressant prescriptions were written for military families/service members during a 14-month period in 2005 to 2006. Moreover, unidentified and untreated PTSD presented special risks for family reintegration and put the veterans and their families at higher danger for maladaptive responses to stress, such as alcoholism, depression, and family violence (Black et al., 2004; Bremner, Southwick, Darnell, & Charney, 1996; Davis & Wood, 1999). Most soldiers have transient symptoms of stress following a traumatic event. These symptoms resolve for most when stability and routine are restored. This is the same pattern for children. But the risk for trauma-related symptoms in children from their parents' traumatic experiences increases with prolonged separation from parent(s) and decreased time between recovery from one traumatic event to onset of another (i.e., repeated deployment, or repeated terror associated with war) (Smith, 2013). Because of the increased understanding of the risk of trauma to family members, the military has funded numerous studies to identify effective strategies to prevent PTSD in soldiers and their family members. One program, entitled Building Resilience And Valuing Empowered Families (BRAVE Families), employs strategies used for families experiencing effects from urban violence, Hurricane Katrina, and the World Trade Center terrorist attack. These strategies include individual and family education and support about PTSD, art and play therapy for children, parenting guidance, and group therapy and support (Smith, 2013). The goal of programs designed to reach PTSD at the meso level is to reach more families experiencing trauma early rather than waiting for families to experience pathology first.

The National Comorbidity Survey (NCS) evaluated PTSD symptoms for 5877 individuals between the ages of 15 and 54 in the United States. The results indicated that the lifetime prevalence of PTSD in the American sample was 8%, and a higher percentage of women (10%) met PTSD criteria than men (5%). Interestingly, more men (61%) reported exposure to potentially traumatic events than women (51%). These differences suggest that other factors, such as the type of trauma, may also play an important role in the development of PTSD. For example, the NCS study found that rape was the trauma most likely to cause PTSD for both men (65%) and women (46%). However, less than 1% of men reported a history of rape as compared with 9% of women. Combat-related trauma was found to be the second most common cause of PTSD in men (39%), whereas no women in this study reported exposure to combat-related trauma (Peterson, Luethcke, Borah, & Young-McCaughan, 2011).

Family Violence and Trauma

Family violence is generally divided into three categories: physical violence, emotional violence, and sexual abuse. The cause of family violence is well studied and is considered multifaceted, with influences ranging from multigenerational trauma (Hulette, Kaehler, & Freyd, 2011), social and cultural learning, mental disorders, and oppression (Abbassi & Aslinia, 2010).

Family violence is often both a cause and an outcome of PTSD in family members. Orcutt, King, and King (2003) examined the impact of early-life stressors, war-zone stressors, and PTSD symptom severity on partners' reports of recent male-perpetrated intimate partner violence among 376 Vietnam veteran couples. The results indicated that several factors are directly associated with family violence, including relationship quality among the spouses, war-zone experiences of stress, and PTSD symptom severity. Experiencing PTSD symptoms because of previous trauma appears to increase an individual's risk for perpetrating family violence. Risk for partner violence is considerably higher among veterans with PTSD when both low marital satisfaction and alcohol

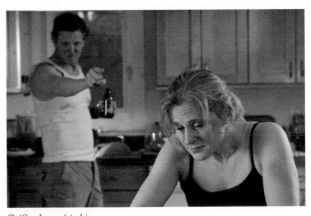

© iStock.com/ejwhite

abuse-dependence are present (Fonseca et al., 2006; Taft et al., 2005).

Domestic violence also increases the risk for PTSD and is a cause for PTSD for both the victims and witnesses of the violence. The incidence of witnessing domestic violence and related trauma continues to be a major public health problem. In 2014, it was estimated that five million children in dual-parent homes lived in a home where partner violence was present (Childhood Domestic Violence, 2014). The risk to children is great, including physical injury from getting in the "cross-fire" to psychological distress similar to children experiencing direct abuse (Kitzmann, 2012). Long-term, childhood domestic violence increases the risk for drug abuse, violent crimes, and suicide (Childhood Domestic Violence, 2014).

Other family trauma also negatively affects the individuals within the family. For example, children experiencing divorce and abuse are at particular risk for acquiring a later adult mental health illness, including PTSD and depression. In a study of 5877 individuals ages 15 to 54 years from the National Co-Morbidity Study, Affi et al. (2009) found that children exposed to both divorce and abuse had the highest rates of mental health illnesses as adults, particularly PTSD. A meta-analysis of 124 articles on long-term outcomes of children experiencing physical abuse or neglect found more depression, suicide risks, family violence, and substance abuse when compared with those not exposed to abuse and neglect (Norman et al., 2012).

The experience of trauma, especially repeated traumas, increases the risk of long-term negative outcomes for children and adults. Each family member exposed to abuse, neglect, and major transitions and loss, such as divorce, is at risk for PTSD, as well as continuing the cycle of violence within families, with repeated events increasing that risk (Hulette, Kaehler, & Freyd, 2011). As noted earlier, family resiliency traits can alter these outcomes significantly, with the result that, for most individuals who experience negative and traumatic events and have strong personal and family resiliency traits, these families do not develop negative health outcomes or repeat the family pattern of PTSD (Walsh, 2016). These findings clearly support the need for trauma-focused family care and interventions by nurses and other health care providers to prevent family-centered trauma.

Families Affected by Disasters

Disasters are events that cause widespread destruction of property, dislocation of people, and immediate suffering through death or injury. Disasters interrupt basic daily needs, such as obtaining food and shelter, for an extended period, making recovery difficult.

During the past three decades there were a total of 372,634 deaths, 995,219 injuries, and more than 61 million people negatively affected by earthquakes. The majority of deaths were related to collapsing buildings and other structures. The most vulnerable citizens were the very young and the very old, or those not able to escape without assistance from others. Earthquakes occurring in low-income countries have had the highest mortality rate largely because of the lack of protective infrastructure, as well as poor recovery following the disasters (Doocy, Daniels, Murray, & Kirsch, 2013).

Disasters are classified as either natural or human caused. Natural disasters include weather and seismic events such as floods, hurricanes, and earthquakes. Human-caused disasters include events such as fires, building collapse, explosions, acts of terrorism, or war.

Natural disasters are the most frequently occurring type of disaster. In the last 10 years, the International Red Cross reported that 1.1 million people across the world were killed by natural disasters (e.g. hurricanes, tornadoes, earthquakes, storms, tsunamis, and volcanic eruptions) (International Federation of Red Cross and Red Crescent Societies, 2012; UNISDR, 2012). An additional 100,000 people were killed worldwide from technological disasters, ranging from industrial accidents to transportation

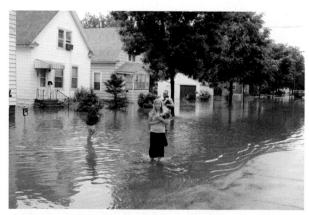

© iStock.com/PickStock

accidents (International Federation of Red Cross and Red Crescent Societies, 2016). During the years 2004 to 2005, natural disasters killed 336,540 people in the world and more than 300 million people were directly or indirectly affected by those disasters (International Strategy for Disaster Reduction, 2006). In the United States alone during 2007, tornadoes killed 80 people, and thunderstorms and accompanying floods, lightning, winds, and hail caused another 157 deaths (National Severe Storms Laboratory, 2007). In 2011 the Disaster Relief Fund requested $1.95 billion in aid for families and individuals affected by such disasters (U.S. Department of Homeland Security, 2011).

Regardless of the type of event, families are affected in multiple ways when disasters strike. Some of the many stressors that occur include loss of significant others, injuries to self or family, separation from family, or extensive loss of property. These losses result in heightened feelings of stress, with many families experiencing symptoms of PTSD. The most vulnerable suffer the most. For example, children often display sleep disturbances, depression, and anxiety, with symptoms increasing the closer the child is to the disaster and the perceived threat to self and loved ones (Evans & Coccoma, 2014).

Family Functioning and Post-Traumatic Stress Disorder

Trauma-related reactions have a negative impact on family functioning. In a study of current relationship functioning among World War II ex-prisoners of war, more than 30% of those with PTSD reported relationship problems compared with only 11% of those without PTSD (Cook, Riggs, Thompson, Coyne, & Sheikh, 2004). In Vietnam veterans, PTSD symptoms have been significantly associated with poor family functioning (Evans, McHugh, Hopwood, & Watt, 2003) and problems with marital adjustment, parenting satisfaction, and psychological abuse (Gold et al., 2007). In a review of literature related to family relationships and PTSD, Blow, Curtis, Wittenborn, and Gorman (2015) reported a similar pattern for veterans returning from Iraq and Afghanistan, with the added negative effects of traumatic brain injuries and multiple deployments. The PTSD symptoms of avoidance and emotional numbing in particular have deleterious effects on

parent-child relationships (Samper, Taft, King, & King, 2004). Among Iraq and Afghanistan veterans, trauma symptoms such as sleep problems, dissociation, and severe sexual problems predicted lower marital satisfaction for both the veteran and his partner (Blow et al., 2015; Goff, Crow, Reisbig, & Hamilton, 2007).

Gorman, Eide, and Hisle-Gorman (2010) determined that parental wartime deployments affect the children of deployed parents in multiple ways, but the clinical significance of those effects is still unknown. They concluded that there was an 11% increase in mental and behavioral health services sought during a parent's deployment. In addition, services for behavioral disorders grew by 19% and services for stress disorders grew by 18%. Although the need for mental and behavioral health increased, the need for other outpatient services decreased. Furthermore, incident rates for children were particularly higher when they were older than 8, both parents were on active duty and married, or when the male parent was deployed.

Secondary Traumatization

The impact of trauma is not limited to the traumatized persons themselves. Spouses of the injured persons seem particularly susceptible to a phenomenon called *secondary traumatization* (Dirkzwager, Bramsen, Ader, & Van der Ploeg, 2005). Secondary traumatization has only recently been described and is not yet a diagnostic category in the *DSM-V* (APA, 2013). In a study of Dutch peacekeeping soldiers and their families (Dirkzwager et al., 2005), it was found that partners of peacekeepers with PTSD symptoms reported more sleeping and somatic problems, more negative social support, and judged the marital relationship as less favorable when compared with the general population. Another study in Israel found that spouses of veterans with PTSD suffered from higher levels of emotional distress and a lower level of marital adjustment than the general population (Dekel, Solomon, & Bleich, 2005). In a qualitative study of wives of Israeli veterans with PTSD, Dekel et al. (2005) noted that the wives were carrying a heavy burden supporting and caring for their husbands and families; all of them identified personal symptoms of PTSD from hearing about their partner's trauma and experiencing the negative effects on their partner's health. Partners of veterans with combat-related PTSD experience significant levels of emotional distress (Manguno-Mire et al., 2007).

This pattern is not limited to family members caring for veterans with PTSD (Devilly, Wright, & Varker, 2009). Other studies have looked at non-family members. Thomas and Wilson (2004) reported that 7% of health care providers working with traumatized victims experience symptoms consistent with PTSD. Other researchers have attempted to define this phenomenon, using terms including *compassion fatigue, professional burnout,* and *secondary traumatic stress* (Meadors, Lamson, Swanson, White, & Sira, 2009; Newell & MacNeil, 2010). Each definition describes the psychological and physical response to caring for victims but not directly experiencing trauma. Meadors et al. (2009) studied 167 health care providers working in pediatric intensive care units. They found a significant correlation between compassion fatigue, or secondary traumatization, and symptoms of PTSD. Nurses, physicians, social workers, and chaplains described the difficulty of caring for families who had a child severely ill, injured, or dying. These professionals not only heard about the traumatic event repeatedly from families, but witnessed the traumatic events over and over as they cared for families across time. This witnessing of trauma led to secondary traumatization.

COMMUNITY AND TRAUMA

The community response to trauma can have a major impact on the degree of traumatic stress-experienced by individuals, families, and the community as a whole.

The community has a key role in the prevention and treatment of trauma. Child welfare services often respond to threats of trauma from abuse and neglect, and police services often respond to threats of domestic or community violence. Nurses as a professional group are mandatory reporters. Every state in the United States and province in Canada has enacted legislation governing the reporting of child abuse and elder abuse. Reporting requirements across countries can differ, and each health care provider is responsible for knowing which conditions require reporting to appropriate authorities. Coohey, Renner, Hua, Zhang, and Whitney (2011) identified mandatory reporting as an intervention that facilitates engagement with services that can promote resilience.

It is incumbent on all agencies that work with victims of trauma to become well versed in TIC. Agencies that work with trauma victims have a responsibility to be trained for their role in trauma care. For example, if child welfare workers are not properly trained on trauma, they may not support foster parents in appropriate reactions to children with trauma-related behaviors. This lack of support may lead to placement failure and result in children being retraumatized by multiple interruptions in attachment, initiating a dangerous cycle (Richardson, Coryn, Henry, Black-Pond, & Unrau, 2012). Box 11-1 presents responses to questions regarding exposure to trauma as a training guide for health care providers.

Consider the following scenario: A 13-year-old child, who has been sexually abused by her father, is placed into foster care. During counseling, she is encouraged to retreat to a quiet place when chaos from the crowded foster care becomes too much. Because of lack of training and poor

---

BOX 11-1

Responses to Questions Regarding Exposure to Western Trauma Discourse

Have you ever attended workshops or trainings about how people are affected by extremely frightening or traumatic events?	Have you ever listened to radio programs/read literature about how people are affected by extremely frightening or violent events?
Never: 85.9% <1 day: 7.7% <2 days: 1.3% 2 days: 1.3% 2+ days: 3.8%	Never: 19.2% 1–2 times: 16.7% 3–4 times: 39.7% 4–7 times: 15.4% 7+ times: 9.0%

communication with the counselor, her foster mother scolds her for "being too isolated." When she goes to school, she becomes overwhelmed by fear and retreats to the library to regain her homeostasis. Because her teachers are untrained and unaware of her needs, she is again punished. She begins to distrust her counselor, foster parent, and teachers, and relapses into fear, disconnection, and dysregulation. She retreats into rigid boundaries. This short vignette illustrates the importance of educating community-based service providers to understand TIC and to integrate and collaborate services to promote positive rather than dangerous and negative outcomes.

SYSTEMIC TRAUMA

The symptoms of post-traumatic stress (PTS) cross individual, family, and community boundaries. Many argue that the United States of America is suffering from PTS from repeated traumatic events such as wars, natural disasters, and economic traumas across time without resolution or intervention. This has resulted in a nation with trauma symptoms, including depression, intrusion of unwanted and negative thinking patterns, hyperarousal especially to perceived threats from others, and related health decline. One clear symptom of this premise is the decline in the general health of U.S. citizens, not unlike the health of individuals suffering from PTSD. Americans possess the shortest life span of any industrialized nation, with almost half of American adults struggling with hypertension, high cholesterol, diabetes, or all three. Further, more than one-third of adults and children are obese (U.S. Department of Health and Human Services, 2012). An increasing number suffer from stress-related illnesses, stemming from or causing mental illness, substance abuse, and domestic violence, as well as several different physical illnesses. Infant mortality is dismally high, with the United States ranking highest among the top seven industrialized countries of the world (U.S. Department of Health and Human Services, 2012). Child abuse rates are equally high when compared with other nations (U.S. Department of Health and Human Services, 2012). One-quarter of our nation's children take prescription medications. One-fifth of our nation's children have been diagnosed with a mental health illness (Hensley, 2010). Twenty-six percent of all children in the United States will experience or witness a traumatic event before they reach age 4 years (SAMSHA, 2011). These statistics show symptoms of a country experiencing dysregulation from systemic trauma.

The high obesity rate in the United States is a clear example of a nation experiencing dysregulation and fear. Obesity is growing the fastest in our poor and crowded neighborhoods. The lack of healthy foods, safe neighborhoods that support outdoor activity, high levels of stress, and presence of early and repeated trauma are key factors in causing obesity and related chronic health conditions (Karr-Morse & Wiley, 2012). Yet, the response to obesity is not centered on trauma-focused interventions, but instead on unsuccessful dieting and major surgeries.

Another indicator that the United States as a nation is struggling with high levels of trauma and related stress symptoms is the increasing rate of substance abuse. Although nicotine addiction is at an all-time low, addiction to other substances, such as alcohol and opiates, is increasing at an alarming rate (National Institute on Drug Abuse, 2012). Researchers have found that those struggling with food cravings leading to obesity and those struggling with drug addiction both exhibit decreased dopamine levels. Overeating and drug use temporarily raise dopamine levels. A lack of dopamine, particularly in the frontal cortex, is caused by early trauma more often than genetics (Karr-Morse & Wiley, 2012). A country experiencing repeated trauma without resolution quickly fills with individuals, families, and communities that are highly stressed and traumatized, with resulting increase in stress-related illnesses.

Chronic stress is toxic stress. *Toxic stress*, as defined by the Center on the Developing Child at Harvard University, is when an individual experiences strong, frequent, and prolonged stress such as chronic child abuse or neglect without adequate support (Center on the Developing Child, 2012). Toxic stress interferes with the ability to learn, be creative, stay healthy, and have joy. Countries that experience toxic stress through natural disasters, war, or dysregulation of major systems also experience a drop in the ability to learn, be creative, have healthy citizens, and have joyous outcomes. Robin Karr-Morse and Meredith Wiley, the authors of *Scared Sick: The Roles of Childhood Trauma in Adult Disease* (2012), compared our body's response to stress with the U.S. Department of Homeland Security.

Both systems are aimed at a complex and integrated system that maintains safety. When part of that system is overtaxed or disconnected, safety is threatened. Threats to the larger system, whether real or imagined, can further overwhelm the system and lead to disease.

The greater culture and societal laws and policies can influence the incidence and the treatment of trauma. Countries riddled with war, poverty, and disease have higher incidents of stress-related symptoms, whereas countries that support policies that decrease violent solutions to problems, provide broad access to preventive and primary health care, and decrease poverty have lower incidences of stress-related symptoms. For example, the incidence of PTSD in New Zealand is estimated to be 6.1% of the population (U.S. Department of Veterans Affairs, 2007), whereas the incidence of PTSD in the Gaza Strip was found to be 77% of 9- to 18-year-olds exposed to the ongoing Israeli-Palestinian conflict (Fasfous, Peralta-Ramírez, & Pérez-García, 2013). The extent that countries can prevent and/or treat the causes of post-traumatic stress early clearly influences the health of the citizens in every country.

Many argue that the traumatic events experienced over the course of the last two decades in the United States were too rapid to resolve and caused a chronic state of fear in the country. For example, in 2005 the United States experienced Hurricane Katrina, continued involvement in the Iraq war, economic collapse, raging wildfires in California, a severe snowstorm in New England, and a school shooting. U.S. citizens watched these disasters unfold with little support or education on how to process these events to avoid post-traumatic stress symptoms. Today, many individuals talk about feeling numb to the disasters watched on television, and have increased fear related to travel, economics, and routine activities, such as attending school. The management of trauma symptoms need to expand beyond individuals, families, and communities, and include national and international traumas and the impact on a nation as a whole.

NURSES AND TRAUMA

Nurses are key to helping with the diagnosis and treatment of trauma-related illnesses in individuals and families. Their presence at the forefront of emergency care of victims of trauma and their help throughout the healing process renders nurses important members of the interdisciplinary team that prevents, treats, and evaluates care for individuals and families affected by trauma-related illnesses. This section outlines the nurse's role in the prevention, identification, and treatment of these conditions as part of an interdisciplinary team.

Trauma-Informed Nursing Assessment and Intervention

Trauma-related illnesses, including PTSD, can develop after a traumatic event or events at any age. To be diagnosed with PTSD, certain conditions must exist. The person has to have been exposed to a traumatic event; experience intense feelings of fear, helplessness, or horror (for preverbal children, the feelings of helplessness are commonly seen as withdrawal, and feelings of fear are commonly seen as intense emotional arousal); re-experience the event through flashbacks, dreams, or disturbing memories; avoid any stimuli associated with the event; avoid any reminders, thoughts, or feelings about the event; be hypervigilant; have difficulty falling or staying asleep; possess an exaggerated startle response; and have symptoms that last longer than 1 month and cause significant distress or impairment in functioning (APA, 2013; National Center for PTSD, 2010).

It is the role of nurses to assess for symptoms of PTSD. There are simple methods to screen patients who may have undetected PTSD. One easy to use tool is the Primary Care PTSD Screen (Prins et al., 2016), which consists of five questions preceded by an introductory question (referenced below).

Sometimes things happen to people that are unusually or especially frightening, horrible, or traumatic. For example:

- A serious accident or fire
- A physical or sexual assault or abuse
- An earthquake or flood
- A war
- Seeing someone be killed or seriously injured
- Having a loved one die through homicide or suicide

Have you ever experienced this kind of event? YES/NO
If no, screen total = 0. Please stop here.
If yes, please answer the following questions.

In the past month, have you. . . .

1. Had nightmares about the event(s) or thought about the event(s) when you did not want to?
   YES/NO
2. Tried hard not to think about the event(s) or went out of your way to avoid situations that reminded you of the event(s)?
   YES/NO
3. Been constantly on guard, watchful, or easily startled?
   YES/NO
4. Felt numb or detached from people, activities, or your surroundings?
   YES/NO
5. Felt guilty or unable to stop blaming yourself or others for the event(s) or any problems the event(s) may have caused?
   YES/NO

(Prins, A., Bovin, M. J., Kimerling, R., Kaloupek, D. G., Marx, B. P., Pless Kaiser, A., & Schnurr, P. P. (2016). *The Primary Care PTSD Screen for DSM-5 (PC-PTSD-5)*. [Measurement instrument]).

The screen is positive if the patient answers *yes* to any three items.

It is also important for nurses to assess risk factors and provide families with protector factors or positive coping strategies and enhancement of resiliency characteristics (Friedman, 2006; Warner, 2010). See Box 11-2 on vicarious trauma.

Risks Associated With Trauma

There are several risks and risk factors associated with both adults and children exposed to traumatic events of which nurses should be aware:

- *Suicidal risk*: because of feelings of numbness, disconnection from support people, chronic fear and anxiety, and feelings of hopelessness and helplessness.
- *Danger to others*: ask about firearms or weapons, aggressive intentions, feelings of persecution.
- *Ongoing stressors*: such as changes that have occurred at home, marital discord, problems at work.
- *Risky behaviors*: such as risky sexual adventures, nonadherence to medical treatment, substance use and misuse.
- *Personal characteristics*: past trauma history, coping skills, relationship attachment.
- *Limited social support*: the individual's lack of willingness to accept help and inclination to isolate.
- *Comorbidity*: coexisting psychiatric or medical problems such as depression and chronic widespread pain (CWP).

BOX 11-2
Vicarious Trauma

Trauma clearly transcends individuals, families, communities, and greater societies across time and across cultures. Nurses are often the front-line health care providers to identify and intervene when acute and chronic trauma occurs.

A real risk for nurses is the development of the attunement survival style described by Heller and LaPierre (2012). This style of coping is characterized by attuning to others' needs and neglecting one's own needs, which is an apt description of the lived experiences of many nurses. If nurses identify themselves as givers, yet neglect their own needs, they are at a high risk for vicarious trauma, or the development of PTSD symptoms from caring for or witnessing trauma in others. This condition is also referred to as *compassion fatigue* and *secondary trauma* in the literature (Afifi et al., 2009).

This term has evolved as helping health care providers were identified as being at high risk for negative psychological reactions to their job, with early descriptions of burnout. Symptoms of burnout include feeling overwhelmed, hopeless, helpless, and unappreciated. Motivation is lost, and if unrecognized and untreated, it may lead to depression, loss of job, and, in the long term, early death (Smith, Segal, & Segal, 2012). Although burnout can be caused by repetitious and uninspiring work, it can also be caused by vicarious trauma. Prevention of vicarious trauma is possible through education, avoiding professional burnout, and professional and peer support during and after caring for traumatized patients (Pearson, 2012).

Child risks associated with PTSD include the following:

- *Dysregulation*: unpredictable or irregular sleep and eating patterns, and difficulty regulating moods and emotional responses.
- *Poor connection*: difficulty forming or maintaining relationships, with a tendency to be alone, have poor eye contact, and resist connection with others.
- *Poor cognitive development*: difficulty with attention, short-term memory, problem solving, creativity, and play. High incidence of learning disabilities, particularly auditory processing disability.
- *Poor attunement skills*: difficulty recognizing and asking for needs.
- *Inability to trust*: difficulty forming relationships, oppositional behavior, sleep problems.
- *Hyperarousal*: increased response to environmental stressors or memories, with rage, anger, or severe anxiety.

The best evidence-based nursing treatments for the individual with PTSD include both psychotherapeutic interventions—such as cognitive-behavioral therapy (CBT) and family therapy—and education and monitoring of medications, primarily SSRIs (Friedman, 2006; Herbert & Sageman, 2004; Sautter et al., 2006; U.S. Department of Veterans Affairs, 2016). CBT is one type of counseling. Research shows it is the most effective type of counseling for PTSD. The U.S. Department of Veterans Affairs (VA) is providing two forms of CBT to veterans with PTSD: cognitive processing therapy (CPT) and prolonged exposure (PE) therapy. Prevention is the goal with primary treatment of potential post-traumatic stress response; several programs start interventions at the time of the traumatic event rather than waiting for symptoms to develop. Sufficient evidence for psychological first aid is widely supported by available objective observations and expert opinion and best fits the category of "evidence informed" but without proof of effectiveness. An intervention provided by volunteers without professional mental health training for people who have experienced a traumatic event offers an acceptable option. Further outcome research is recommended (Fox et al., 2012).

Once symptoms develop, outcomes improve with a combination of individual and family therapy, along with appropriate medication management of symptoms when needed. For example, in a study of seven children following a bus accident, the combination of individual and family therapy with selective serotonin reuptake inhibitors (SSRIs) resulted in a remission of PTSD symptoms, whereas the control group that only received medication without family therapy still had symptoms 3 months later (Stankovi et al., 2013). In the cases where medication and family therapy were used, researchers used systematic family therapy (SFT), a structured family therapy protocol, to facilitate family involvement and family-directed interventions. It proved effective in preventing chronic PTSD in victims.

Secondary Family Traumatization Assessment and Intervention

To help the traumatized family, the nurse should first realize that traumatized families rarely seek family-focused intervention. Instead, they often present with problems that are not immediately related to the traumatic events they have experienced (Figley & Barnes, 2005). Nurses should learn the parallel processes of individual and systemic stress reactions that follow a traumatic event. Figley and Barnes (2005) offer suggestions to help clinicians recognize family responses to traumatic events and offer some interventions to help patients and families affected by these events. For example, families are affected by the individual's symptoms of PTSD. They know the story of the trauma, witness the symptoms, and want to help in some way. Therefore, the family spends more and more time caring for the traumatized member. Moreover, while the traumatic event is being persistently re-experienced by the exposed family member, the other family members are responding to this individual's expressed need for support. As the primary affected family member tries to avoid stimuli and reminders of the trauma, the other family members must devote increased time, energy, and problem solving to avoid conversations, people, places, and things that might stimulate memories. They have to cope with withdrawal and numbing that goes along with the primary affected family member's diminished interest in usual activities, refusals to see friends, and inability to express love and caring. The family becomes increasingly more isolated. Family members have to manage problems with sleep, outbursts of anger and rage, exaggerated startle responses, and hypervigilance about safety. These factors increase the risk of secondary traumatization or symptoms of trauma reaction in family members from witnessing the traumatic stories and the negative impact on the primary family member.

Nurses applying TIC using the Ecological Systems Theory Approach to Trauma Treatment begin the treatment by correcting interrupted trust and attachment (Heller & LaPierre, 2012). Infants and young children who experience rejection and abuse early in life often expect that same experience from present and future caregivers. A trusting and therapeutic relationship must form. This process is slow, as the child or adult who has learned to avoid feelings and relationships will first resist, and then struggle with moderating those feelings and relationships, and then, if successful, learn to trust. The initial steps of treatment are as follows:

1. Move slowly: building connections can be terrifying to a traumatized individual.
2. Build trust: building a therapeutic relationship depends on being predictable and trustworthy.
3. Be empathetic: you may be the first kind person in their lives.
4. Help children and adults listen to and explore their new skills at identifying emotions, organizing thoughts and emotions, and learning different reactions and responses to their emotions.
5. Help build self-esteem through teaching top-down thinking. For example, if an adult has always felt he was bad because of traumatic events in his life, help him rethink about the events being bad instead.
6. Gradually support and encourage connection with their own feelings, then their body responses and reactions, and finally connection to other people. The connection to other people should also be gradual, starting with close caregivers or family members, and advancing as tolerated to outside peers and associates.

7. Be available to help the child or adult explore feelings of rejection, anger, abandonment, and fear. Many individuals who have experienced trauma have survived by becoming numb. As this numbness fades, survival feels threatened. During this transition from numbness to feeling, many may withdraw for varying periods of time. A therapeutic nurse will recognize this pattern and avoid judging the traumatized individual during these phases.
8. Help children and adults connect with others, as support has been found to be a key factor in successful treatment of trauma (Evans & Coccoma, 2014).

The nurse working with a traumatized family needs to explore each family member's perception of what happened both before and after the event. The family may block the telling of trauma if the family was the cause of that trauma. Listening to individuals and observing for signs of secondary trauma can be critical to getting help for all family members. The nurse needs to recognize that the family's worldview will have been altered by the traumatizing events and that its attitudes and beliefs may shift from safety to suspicious, distrustful attribution regarding the motivations of others, including helping health care providers. Hypervigilance and controlling behaviors may actually interfere with the family getting the help it needs. In addition, if the stressors impinging on the family go unattended, a pattern of poor communication and blaming may become the central family dynamic. Also, the roles in the family may shift, with some members becoming more enmeshed with the traumatized member and others withdrawing from the family system. Children may have to take on the role of emotional caretaker for the parents and thus be compelled to hide their own feelings and fears, while other siblings act out to express anger, leading to more parenting stress. Most emerging trauma treatment has as its main shortcoming the focus on the individual rather than the family system. Careful implementation of interviewing techniques and the exploration of the family life experience through ecomaps will assist nurses in accessing the complex relationships and characteristics of families living with trauma or post-traumatic complications. Nurses are also key in finding resources for families that use a family approach to trauma care.

The nursing role also includes looking at community actions and societal responses to trauma at a personal, family, community, and societal level, and how that trauma affects health. Becoming involved with prevention strategies, such as community preparedness for disaster, can lead to improved community health. Working with national organizations to provide organized community-based interventions for traumas can be an important step to preventing negative long-term consequences.

Participating in research and implementing research findings that demonstrate the impact of trauma on all ecological levels can help improve treatment plans and outcomes. Finally, shaping policies at the national level that support families in need, by decreasing poverty, improving access to health care, supporting parents with improved child-care options and improved parenting education and support, and reducing environmental stress, can be an important step to reducing the impact of trauma in children, adults, families, communities, and nations.

Case Study: Knoll Family

This case study offers an example of a family that experienced trauma, and the impact of individual trauma and family trauma on all family members. The events that occurred within this family illustrate the complexities of prolonged and repeated trauma, as well as resiliency characteristics touching the individual, family, community, and nation.

Family Members:
- Mother: Laura (age 45)
- Father: Victor (age 46)
- Oldest daughter: Natalie (age 24 years)
- Middle daughter: Kimberly (age 23 years)
- Youngest daughter: Taylor (age 22 years)

Figure 11-5 shows the Knoll family genogram.

The Knoll family initially sought care at a multidisciplinary clinic because of increasing concerns about their youngest daughter, Taylor. They started this care when Taylor was 15 years of age, and complained that Taylor was refusing to attend school, using marijuana and alcohol on a daily basis, and was currently dating a man who was 20 years older. When they threatened to call the police, Taylor stated she would "run away and never return."

Family Development:
The mother, Laura, has a history of intimate partner violence from her husband, causing her to escape across the country when her daughters were ages 3, 4, and 6, respectively. She remarried when her daughters were ages 8, 9, and 11, respectively. All three girls did well until adolescence, with participation in sports, family activities, and school. Her youngest daughter abruptly stopped all participation in school and sports at age 13 years, and began befriending peers that were involved in drugs. Her mother sought treatment through her primary care physician, who recommended residential care. In spite of 3 months' residential treatment, the same problems continued. When Laura's oldest daughter disclosed memories of sexual abuse from her biological father when she was in preschool, Laura became overwhelmed. She had just asked her ex-husband to take care of her younger daughter as she did not know how to help her. In spite of her ex-husband being an active alcoholic with a history of physical violence and now under suspicion of sexual abuse of her oldest daughter, this decision brought more guilt and shame to Laura. However, Taylor insisted on going to live with Laura's ex-husband and did not believe he sexually abused her sister. Taylor came back after 6 months. Laura tried other resources and agonized as she watched her youngest daughter struggle through years of methamphetamine and heroin addiction. Her ex-husband moved to town when her daughters were 18, 19, and 21, respectively. This added to her stress, as he demanded participation in family activities and celebrations, and demanded rides from all family members as he did not have a driver's license. This caused strain in her current marriage. Today, Laura works full time and cares for her four grandchildren on a regular basis. She has recently started counseling because of feelings of depression and being overwhelmed with family responsibilities.

The father, Victor, lived across the country from his family from the point of divorce until 5 years ago. Divorce occurred against his will when his three daughters were ages 3, 4, and 6, respectively. Although he has had other partners, he continued

Case Study: Knoll Family *(cont.)*

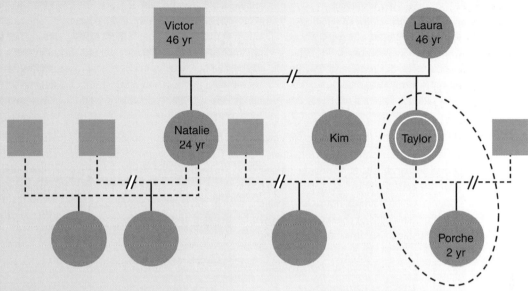

FIGURE 11-5 Knoll Family Genogram

to try to get back together with his ex-wife, trying to convince her that the domestic violence was only caused by his heavy drinking. He denied any sexual abuse of his daughter. He continued drinking alcohol in spite of being diagnosed with hepatitis C and cirrhosis of the liver. He was agreeable to having his youngest daughter come live with him when she was 14 years of age, which lasted 6 months. Taylor left her father's home because of his "constant drinking." Two years later Victor moved to the same town as his children and ex-wife. He currently joins the family for all family events and celebrations. He maintains employment off and on, and relies on his daughters for transportation to his job as he does not have a driver's license because of repeated citations for driving under the influence (DUIs).

Natalie grew up with her mother and two sisters from the time of her parents' divorce to her mother's remarriage when Natalie was 10 years old. She then lived with her mother, stepfather, and two sisters. She did well in school and participated in activities throughout her school years. When she was 17 years old, she disclosed memories of sexual abuse. She was distraught to learn that her siblings did not believe her, and her mother told her to "forgive your father; that was a long time ago." She sought counseling on her own, but now notes that she continues to pick abusive men as partners. She has two children from different fathers, and both fathers are incarcerated for drug sales. She is completing her college degree in counseling.

Kimberly, the middle daughter, grew up with her mother and sisters until her mother remarried when she was 8 years of age. She then lived with her mother, stepfather, and two sisters. She did well until high school, when she developed incapacitating panic disorder. This caused her to avoid school. She received antianxiety medications for approximately 1 year and reported feeling better. She received her general equivalency diploma (GED) when she was 20 years of age, and now works as a housecleaner. She has had the same partner for the past 4 years, and they have one daughter together. Her partner is concerned about her alcohol abuse and has threatened to leave if she does not seek treatment.

Taylor, as the identified patient, stated she did well in school and with peers until she was 13 years of age. She states she then became very depressed and lost interest in all that she previously cared about. She remembers being in residential care and being diagnosed with bipolar disorder. She was given medications, but she refused to take any of the medications once she left the treatment facility. Upon return home, she returned to using drugs as a strategy to "feel something" and "have the energy to do anything." Taylor spent 6 months with her father at age 14 years, but returned stating he "drank too much." Taylor then went back to residential care for 6 months, followed by 3 years of methamphetamine and heroin addiction.

(continued)

Case Study: Knoll Family *(cont.)*

She earned her GED, and has been fully employed in computer technical help for the past 5 years. She gave birth to her daughter, Porche, 2 years ago. Because Porche's father was trying to get custody because of Taylor's drug use, she re-entered drug treatment. During this treatment time, she experienced a flooding of memories of her father sexually abusing her during her preschool years. She stated she remembered her father getting drunk and sexually abusing her in a closet in their old home. She stated she felt shame and extreme guilt that she did not believe her sister when her sister disclosed the same abuse. She stated she did not know how to set boundaries with her father to this day, and requested help keeping her father out of her life. Currently, her father calls her almost daily, and demands help with transportation three to five times per week.

Function:

Communication within the family started out as avoidant, with each family member feeling unable to share thoughts and feelings with other family members. Boundaries were blurred and unclear (i.e., mother being unable to say no to having her daughter live with a suspected sexual abuser, and Taylor being unable to say no to seeing her father in spite of memories of sexual abuse). Through intensive counseling and parent coaching within the clinic and through home visits, the family now participates in healthier communication patterns, nonviolent problem solving, and shared positive experiences. Each family member, however, continues to show signs of chronic PTSD, caused by repeated and severe traumas within the family. When asked about traumatic events, the family summarized the following:

- Intimate partner violence
- Alcohol addiction of father
- Sexual abuse of two daughters by father; father denies this
- Drug addiction by Taylor

Laura was asked about resiliency skills for both herself and her daughters. She felt she had positive support through her parents, a strong religious affiliation including daily prayer, the absence of any substance abuse, and the ability to adapt to the many changes and traumatic events occurring across time. She noted that her daughters were her support as well as her burden. She stated that they were very adaptable at times to big changes. Resiliency areas where this family lacked included: optimism, self-efficacy, and poor ability to set healthy boundaries.

Nursing Interventions:

Microsystem: The individuals within this family needed a thorough and comprehensive assessment of symptoms of trauma-related health concerns given the history of repeated and prolonged trauma. The mechanism of prolonged stress for Taylor started in early childhood, given her symptoms of mood dysregulation, attention deficit disorder, depression, and drug addiction. Likewise, her older sister, Natalie, experienced early childhood trauma, but her symptoms and outcome were different. She struggled more with relationship struggles, choosing men who would abuse her and desert her, similar to her biological father. Taylor's middle sister, Kimberly, denied any memories of sexual abuse. She did, however, show signs of trauma through her panic disorder and alcohol dependency. Given that two out of three daughters remembered being abused, it is likely Kimberly experienced abuse, too. Laura struggled with her own abuse. She suffered from intimate partner violence, which is often accompanied by sexual assault (Evans & Coccoma, 2014). She also witnessed her daughters all struggle through adolescence and young adulthood because of their past abuse and her difficulty setting boundaries.

The understanding of each of the individual's experiences and related traumas helps the nurse identify the need for individual care for each family member. The daughters and mother started family care with individual counseling. They soon built a trusting relationship with the therapist and learned across time to become more attuned to each of their own needs, learned to ask for their needs appropriately, and discovered how to regulate their responses to emotions.

Mesosystem: Family-centered care was instituted after 3 months of individual counseling to improve family development and functioning. Family self-care strategies were initially implemented to stabilize and organize the family, followed by family meetings to address communication and problem-solving skills, as well as ways to build positive connections between and among family members. During the family meetings, the family also discussed the effects of trauma on the family, especially the difficulty all family members had in setting healthy boundaries with Victor. The family is now currently preparing to meet with Victor and enforce clear boundaries to prevent further trauma.

Case Study: Knoll Family *(cont.)*

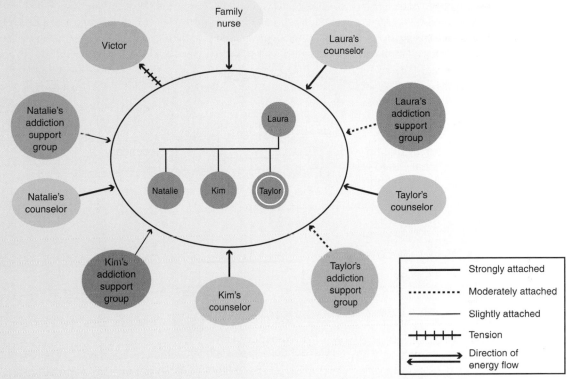

FIGURE 11-6 Knoll Family Ecomap

Macrosystem: This family struggled with finding supportive community resources. See Figure 11-6, the Knoll family ecomap, which depicts the subsystems. This family experienced trauma care at a time when addiction services were separated from TIC. Therefore, Taylor did not address her own trauma until early adulthood. Likewise, her siblings and mother did not receive TIC until almost two decades after the trauma occurred.

Exosystem: This family was affected by societal rules, culture, and policies. The availability of health care through the state allowed services to this family, but limited those services to weekly contacts with specified providers rather than the family being able to pursue professionals skilled in TIC.

Outcome Following Treatment:

Following 1 year of TIC, this family is no longer demonstrating symptoms of PTSD. Each family member is experiencing positive connections within and outside the family. During this treatment period, the family worked with the same nurse, with interventions focused on ongoing family assessments, care coordination to facilitate better relationships across the family care–provider ecology, improving family communication and closeness through the use of rituals and routines, and individually targeted development of resiliency characteristics. All family members, except the biological father, are sober, and all members report more energy, ability to express emotions, and decreased hyperarousal toward their biological father/ex-husband.

Case Study: Caldwell Family

Mr. Caldwell, a 47-year-old National Guard soldier who is in the hospital for a hernia repair, had returned home from a 12-month deployment to Iraq, where he had his first exposure to combat in his 18 years of National Guard duty. Before deployment, he worked successfully as a fireman paramedic and was a happily married father with two children. He and his wife were socially outgoing with a large circle of friends from the same rural area in which they both grew up. They have been married since high school. See a genogram and ecomap for the Caldwell family in Figures 11-7 and 11-8.

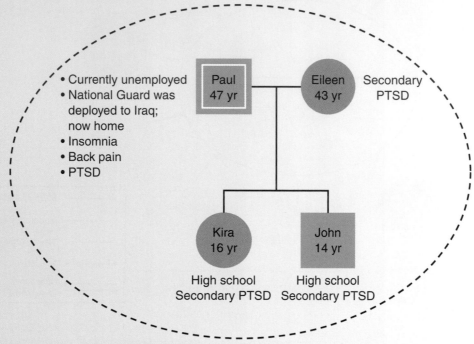

FIGURE 11-7 Caldwell Family Genogram

While in Iraq recently, Mr. Caldwell had extensive exposure to other soldiers' combat injuries as the noncommissioned officer in charge of the battlefield medical aide station. His unit treated the severe, crippling injuries of soldiers en route to the trauma hospital. The aide station was often overrun with multiple casualties. He treated soldiers from patrols and convoys in which improvised exploding devices destroyed vehicles and wounded or killed people. Although he did not have to kill enemy combatants, he agonized that he may also have been responsible for the deaths of some soldiers because he simply did not have enough men or resources to treat all the casualties adequately. When asked about the worst moment during his deployment, he readily stated it was when he was unable to intercede while a Humvee with a bleeding soldier draped over the hood and several wounded soldiers in the back drove by the aid station, because the driver's view was blocked by blood gushing on the windshield and the driver could not see him waving the Humvee to safety.

When he first returned home, things seemed to be okay. But more than 2 years after coming home, he has had more and more difficulty relating to his wife. He reports feeling angry all the time, and that no one will listen to him. Sleep has become difficult. He has to sleep on the recliner in the living room because his back hurts so badly that he cannot lay flat. When he does sleep, he has a recurring, vivid nightmare about turning a corner outside of a building in Baghdad where he encounters an insurgent with a rifle who shoots him. His daughter complains that he has become so overprotective that he will not let her go out with any friends, much less any boys. His wife reported that he has been emotionally distant since his return. His employer, who initially supported him, has reported that his work at the fire department has suffered dramatically. During a recent burning motor vehicle extradition drill, one of the car's tires exploded. The unexpected explosion rattled him so much that he became unable to go to work anymore. Mr. Caldwell says that since his deployment, he no longer has an identity—he cannot work, and he no longer feels like he can fulfill his obligations as a husband and a father. He reports that he sometimes experiences strong surges of anger, panic, guilt, and despair and that at other times he has felt emotionally dead, unable to return the love and warmth of

Case Study: Caldwell Family *(cont.)*

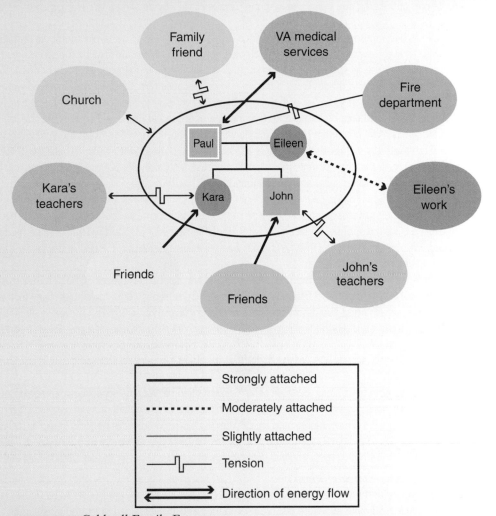

FIGURE 11-8 Caldwell Family Ecomap

family and friends. He does not want to get a divorce, but fears this will happen. Although he has not been actively suicidal, he reported that he sometimes thinks everyone would be better off if he had not survived his tour in Iraq. He is currently on several medications for back pain from his on-the-job injury at the fire department. He is complaining of a lot of postoperative pain.

This composite case illustrates several kinds of war-zone stressors. Mr. Caldwell felt helpless to prevent several deaths. In addition to that feeling of helplessness, he had to witness the horror of many people dying, and had to respond to emergencies on a very unpredictable basis. Nurses, who are taking care of patients who have had a difficult return to civilian life need to be aware of the complicated nature of readjustment. As this case illustrates, the prevalence of PTSD may increase considerably during the 2 to 6 years after veterans have returned from combat duty (Hermes, Fontana, & Rosenheck, 2015).

This family is dealing with the chronic problems that occur when a veteran returns home with significant PTSD. The care for this family, when delivered from a Family Systems Theory perspective, will need to address Mr. Caldwell's PTSD, as well as the family's ever increasing secondary traumatization from his stress responses.

Theoretical Perspective:

Using a family systems theoretical approach, the plan of care for Mr. Caldwell includes referral for his PTSD and providing the family members with education and resources about what they can do to address their own secondary trauma, as well as

(continued)

Case Study: Caldwell Family *(cont.)*

support his recovery. As part of the plan, the nurse can help the Caldwell family by drawing a family ecomap that shows resources currently being used.

Because Mr. Caldwell has been traumatized by his experience with war, ultimately all his family members and family relationships are affected. Mr. Caldwell's war experience was his alone, but his wife is being affected by the symptoms he is experiencing, symptoms that will get worse as she takes on even more of a caregiving role following his surgery. The children are baffled by the changes in their father, and do not know quite what to do. Because Mrs. Caldwell is so involved with caring for him, the children do not feel like they can go to her with their problems. In addition to their parents not being available to them emotionally, both children have had to take on family roles that their parents used to manage. For example, the daughter, Kira, now must do more of the family meal preparation and house cleaning. The son, John, has to do all the yard work, which has made it harder to spend time with his friends. Both teenagers are starting not to do as well in school because of the constant tension in the home and their fears that their parents may divorce. Because Mr. Caldwell's trauma is so severe, it is highly likely the other members of the family will suffer secondary traumatization.

This family's response to the trauma of Mr. Caldwell from war cannot be understood or treated by focusing on just his care (microsystem). His family members (mesosystem) can provide key contextual information about past traumatic events and experiences that can explain current responses. In fact, they are a central reason why Mr. Caldwell wants to get better and resume more of his leadership roles within the family. As he has been spiraling downward, the rest of the family has followed and all now report deteriorating mental health.

The boundaries or borders for this family may both be protective and act as a barrier to seeking help. It may be that Mrs. Caldwell feels it is disloyal to talk about her husband's problems with an outsider. Mr. Caldwell has many fears about admitting his difficulties and feels ashamed about how his problems have affected his wife. Mrs. Caldwell is afraid to ask for help because she does not want her husband to feel any more embarrassment than he does already. They are both suffering in silence, reluctant to talk to each other, or to anyone else. The nurse will have to create a trusting relationship to overcome this natural reluctance to share family secrets. One of the things that may help is to explain how providing this information may enhance the medical team's ability to provide quality care.

In this case, the spousal relationship has suffered because of Mr. Caldwell's trauma. Wartime separation and reunion, and then later problems with PTSD from combat, have created some marital dysfunction that was not there before. In this situation, the marital relationship as a subset within this family is the most problematic area. By helping this family improve this one area of its family functioning through appropriate referral, the nurse could have a great impact on the rest of the family subsystems. Because this is a new experience for Mr. and Mrs. Caldwell, they are not quite sure how to deal with it, plus they are reluctant to seek outside help at this time.

Assessment and Intervention Considerations:

The assessment and intervention for the Caldwell family focuses on PTSD and secondary trauma. As we can see clearly from this case, although Mr. Caldwell's traumatic exposure occurred some time ago, undiagnosed or inadequately treated PTSD could complicate his surgical recovery. PTSD is associated with more physical health problems and somatic symptom severity (Hoge, Terhakopian, Castro, Messer, & Engel, 2007). Although CWP—defined as pain in various parts of the body and fatigue that lasts for 3 months or longer—has thus far been documented only in veterans from the first Gulf War, the potential for this phenomenon to emerge in current combat veterans is high. CWP is associated with greater health care utilization and a lower quality of life (Forman-Hoffman et al., 2007). Researchers working for the Veterans Administration have documented that a substantial percentage of Iraq and Afghanistan veterans experience ongoing or new pain, of which 28% is reported to be severe (Gironda, Clark, Massengale, & Walker, 2006).

In this instance, postoperatively Mr. Caldwell may be having more problems with pain perception, pain tolerance, and other kinds of untreated chronic pain. In addition, PTSD symptoms may make it difficult for the nurse to communicate with the patient, may reduce the patient's active collaboration in evaluation and treatment, and reduce patient adherence to medical regimens.

Assessment:

Because trauma is underrecognized, patients with PTSD are not properly identified and are not offered education, counseling, or referrals for mental health evaluation. There are simple methods to screen patients who may have undetected PTSD. As noted, one easy to use tool is the Primary Care PTSD Screen (Prins et al., 2004).

Case Study: Caldwell Family (*cont.*)

Next, assess the family for possible symptoms of secondary traumatization. How are Mr. Caldwell's wife and children responding to his symptoms? What symptoms are they experiencing because of his difficulties? Identify how roles may have shifted for this family given Mr. Caldwell's current circumstances. Is the family still functioning as a strong cohesive unit? How have things changed? How open is this family to working with the nurse? What might help facilitate this?

Nursing Interventions:

Provide education about PTSD and secondary trauma. Because the family's participation is essential in identifying symptoms of PTSD and planning treatment, the nurse must create an environment that is supportive and inclusive of family members in order to work in partnership with the family. There are several sites on the Internet that can help the nurse develop educational fact sheets that can be shared with patients and families. The Veterans Affairs National Center for PTSD and the Defense Department's Walter Reed Army Medical Center collaborated to develop the Iraq War Clinician Guide https://www.ptsd.va.gov/professional/materials/manuals/iraq-war-clinician-guide.asp). The next step that the nurse should take in intervening with the Caldwell family is referring all family members for further care. Set up a plan for referring to a PTSD specialist those patients who show signs of potential PTSD and who are amenable to receiving additional evaluation or counseling. In this instance, the nurse could provide the family with a list of possible options. Many local areas have lists of returning veterans' counseling services that include counseling for couples and families. Involve the family in the plan of follow-up care.

SUMMARY

In this chapter, we discussed trauma and how TIC may be employed with patients by family nurses. Key points include the following:

- Trauma affects the entire family system.
- Trauma-related illnesses are more likely to develop when resiliency traits are lacking either before or after the trauma.
- Trauma-related illnesses can occur months, or even years, after a disaster or traumatic event such as war occurs. Trauma-related illnesses, particularly PTSD, affect both children and adults, with adults more likely to have flashbacks of the incident and children more likely to develop hypersensitivity and avoidance of similar situations (e.g., avoiding cars after a motor vehicle accident).
- The Ecological Systems Theory can guide nursing assessment and interventions to help families cope effectively with trauma.
- When one or more family members are traumatized by an experience, all family members and family relationships are affected.

- The more severe the trauma an individual family member suffers, the more likely the other members of the family are at risk for secondary trauma.
- The family response to trauma of one or more of its members cannot be understood or treated by focusing on individual family members alone. Family members can provide key contextual information about past traumatic events and experiences that help explain current responses.
- Community systems can prevent, treat, and measure negative outcomes to traumatic events. If community agencies are not well trained and prepared, the risks for undetected and untreated trauma-related illnesses increase.
- Larger political and social systems can influence and be influenced by individual, family, and community trauma. If nations experience severe trauma, they, as a whole, show signs of trauma response.
- Nursing focuses on the individual, family, community, and societal reactions to trauma in order to optimize positive outcomes and prevent or treat negative implications.

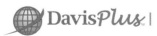 | For additional resources and information, visit **http://davisplus.fadavis.com**. References can be found on Davis*Plus*.

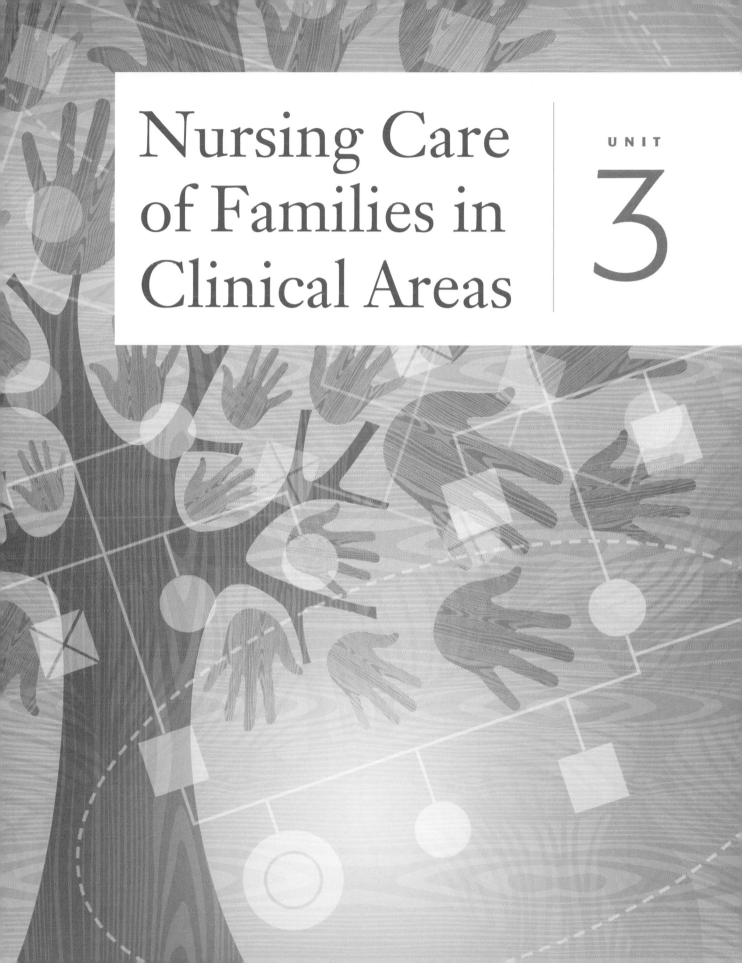

Nursing Care of Families in Clinical Areas

Chapter 12

Family Nursing With Childbearing Families

Linda Veltri, PhD, RN

Karline Wilson-Mitchell, DNP, MSN, CNM, RN, RM

Joyce M. O'Mahony, RN, PhD

Critical Concepts

- Childbearing family nursing is not synonymous with obstetrical nursing, which only considers the woman as the client and the family as the context for care. In contrast, childbearing family nursing considers the family as the client, the family as the context for the care of its members, or both. Childbearing family nursing primarily focuses on health and wellness rather than on procedures and medical treatment.

- Nurses must understand and utilize multiple theories to plan and guide nursing care for childbearing families.

- Nurses must understand the impact that social policy, available resources, and geographical location have on childbearing families.

- The holistic care of these families is best provided with an approach that acknowledges the social determinants of health and the integration of all the members of the health care team and community resources.

- Nurses need to be aware of stressors that childbearing families encounter before, during, and after reproductive events so they can anticipate, identify, and respond to needs appropriately.

- The family constellation and the definition of family depend on the culture, worldview, sexual orientation, and perspective of the family. Consequently, childbearing family nursing necessitates demonstrating respect and cultural competence.

- Nursing care for adoptive families should be provided in a manner similar to what is provided to biological families. Nurses should recognize and meet these families' special needs, regardless of the family constellation.

- Nurses caring for childbearing families experiencing infertility must consider, understand, and address the family's emotional and physical needs.

- Understanding the many ways families experience grief and loss allows nurses to advocate for practices that best facilitate childbearing as a transitional event in the life of the family.

- A process of bereavement should be anticipated with perinatal loss, adverse perinatal outcome, diagnosis of congenital or genetic disorders, palliative care, or the birth of a child with special needs.

(continued)

■ When a mother or a newborn has serious threats to health, family nurses act to maintain and promote family relationships. Threats to the health and integrity of the family become a reality when separation from family members occurs (e.g., apprehension of children because of child protection risks or incarceration of the mother).

■ Understanding the effect a new baby has on all family members allows nurses to work to help parents develop realistic expectations about themselves, each other, and their children, as well as to identify appropriate support and resources.

■ Postpartum depression is treatable and recoverable. Therefore, family nurses must work diligently to identify and refer women for appropriate treatment as early as possible to reduce the effects of maternal depression on the woman and her family.

■ Family nurses can be leaders in practice, policy development, and research related to childbearing families.

Before the onset of professional nursing in North America during the late 19th century, caregivers for childbearing families were women. Female family members, in-laws, neighbors, friends, and midwives came to the home to encourage, support, and nurture a woman during and after childbirth (Bourgeault, 2006; King et al., 2015; Linn, Wilson, & Fako, 2015). During this time, many of these women midwives were settlers who followed the European colonists and were African slaves or First Nations/Native Americans (Dawley & Walsh, 2016). Similarly, in Canada, Canadian pioneer and Aboriginal midwives also attended births up through the 1940s. It was these women caregivers who maintained family functions of the household, tended to new babies and mothers' other children, and provided postpartum physical care. Male obstetricians emerged as primary clinical providers of birth management and influenced both maternity education and health care policy in the 1860s. However, male family members, friends, and children were excluded from the childbirth experience until the 1970s. This practice was justified by the belief that nonmedical participants increased the risk of introducing infection into the perinatal setting.

Beginning in the late 1960s, families became increasingly knowledgeable about childbearing and desirous of a more satisfying birth experience as a family event. Families became savvy health care consumers who found hospital routines and policies too restrictive if they required strict adherence to newborn feeding and sleeping schedules, kept fathers and siblings out of the delivery room, or separated parents from their newborns. In response, informed families lobbied for changes in childbearing practices; they used evidence to support not separating mothers and babies immediately after delivery,

as well as other hallmark findings demonstrating improved parent-child attachment with immediate and frequent contact between mothers, fathers, and siblings and their newborns (de Chateau, 1976, 1977; Johnson, 2013; Klaus et al., 1972; Martell, 2006). Families presented compelling arguments for hospitals to support exclusive breastfeeding, kangaroo-care or "skin-to-skin" baby carrying, and delayed cord clamping (Aghdas, Talat, & Sepideh, 2014; Niermeyer, 2015; Renfrew, McCormick, Wade, Quinn, & Dowswell, 2012).

In time, nurses, hospitals, and other health care providers for women began to recognize the effect reproductive events have on all family members, as well as the reciprocal influence of the family on the parents and infants. This recognition has resulted in inclusion of family concepts into nursing care of childbearing families. With the trend for increased family education about reproductive events, increased responsibility for family members to plan for care during pregnancy and delivery, and shorter hospital stays after birth, postpartum care is returning to family care within the context of the home with nursing guidance, rather than being medically based in a hospital. This shift in focus from caring for the individual woman as the client toward consideration and inclusion of the family in care from preconception to the postpartum period is known as *childbearing family nursing*. The historical perspective is outlined in Box 12-1.

Notably, the practice of childbearing family nursing is not synonymous with obstetrical nursing. Obstetrical nursing considers the woman as the client and views the family as the context for care. Childbearing family nursing, by contrast, considers the family as the client and the family as the context for the care of its members. It is a health and wellness, rather

BOX 12-1
Historical Perspective of Childbearing Family Nursing

Historical Perspective

Late 1800s: Industrialization

- Families moved to more urban areas; household size and functions diminished.
- Traditional networks of women were not always available, and mothers needed to replace care previously carried out in the home.
- Childbearing still occurred at home for many middle-class families.
- European colonists, African slaves, and First Nations/American Indians served as midwives.

First Third of the 20th Century

- The hospital became the place for labor, birth, and early postpartum recovery for middle-class families.
- Many immigrant and working-class urban families continued to have newborns at home with their traditional care providers.
- An impetus to the development of public health nursing was concern for the health of urban mothers and babies.
- Realizing that the health needs of all the family members were intertwined, early public health nurses considered families, not individuals, as their clients.

1930s Through the "Baby Boom" of the 1950s

- In Canada, Canadian pioneer and Aboriginal midwives attended births up through the 1940s.
- With the dramatic shift of births to hospitals, family involvement with childbearing diminished.
- Concerns about infection control contributed to separation of family members.
- Family members, especially males, were forbidden to be with women in the hospital.
- Babies were segregated into nurseries and brought out to their mothers only for brief feeding sessions.
- Nurses focused on the smooth operation of postpartum wards and nurseries through the use of routine and order.

- Despite these inflexible conditions, families tolerated them because they believed that hospital births were safer for mothers and newborns.

1960s to 1970s

- Families and health care providers questioned the need for heavy sedation and analgesia for childbearing and embraced natural childbirth.
- A feature of natural childbirth was the close relationship between the laboring woman and a supportive person serving as a coach; in North America, husbands assumed this supportive role.
- Expectant parents actively sought out physicians and hospitals that would best meet their expectations for father involvement and the control over childbearing began to shift from health care providers to families.
- Some nurses were skeptical about the changes families demanded, but others were enthusiastic about increased family participation.
- Many hospital-based maternity nurses began to consider themselves to be mother-baby nurses rather than nursery or postpartum nurses, and labor and delivery nurses often collaborated with family members in helping women cope with the discomforts of labor.

1980s to the Present

- Klaus and Kennel's research (1976) served as the impetus for the growth of family-centered care (American College of Obstetricians and Gynecologists and the Interprofessional Task Force on Health Care of Women and Children, 1978).
- Today, promotion of family contact is becoming the hallmark of childbearing care.
- Many hospitals have renamed their obstetrical services, using names such as Family Birth Center to convey the importance of family members in childbearing health care even though obstetrical care is becoming more dependent on technology.

than an illness model of care. Similarly, childbearing family nurses take a holistic approach to care; they consider the woman and her family's physical, mental, emotional, spiritual, social, and cultural indicators of health. Using this family-centered approach to care requires that childbearing family nurses *assist* families to make informed choices to achieve outcomes desired versus *telling* families what is best for them (Ward, Hisley, & Kennedy, 2016).

Family nursing with childbearing families covers the period before conception, pregnancy, labor, birth, and the postpartum period. Childbearing family nursing traditionally begins with a family's decision to start having children and continues until parents have achieved a degree of relative comfort in their roles as parents of infants and/or have ceased the addition of new children to their families. Often, childbearing family nursing is expanded to include the periods between pregnancies and includes other aspects of reproductive care such as family planning, infertility, perinatal loss, sexuality, adoption, foster care, and parenting grandchildren. Decisions and changes surrounding childbearing vary for families throughout the reproductive cycle. Factors driving these decisions or changes include prevailing health policies and the family's cultural, socioeconomic, and psychological needs. Therefore, the beginning and end points of the reproductive period may be different for each family.

The focus of childbearing family nurses is centered on family relationships and the health of all family members. Therefore, nurses involved with childbearing families use family concepts and theories as part of developing the plan of nursing care. This chapter starts by presenting theoretical perspectives that guide nursing practice with childbearing families. It continues with an exploration of family nursing with childbearing families before conception through the postpartum period. The chapter concludes with implications for nursing practice, research, and policy, along with two case studies that explore family adaptations to stressors and changing roles related to childbearing.

THEORY-GUIDED, EVIDENCE-BASED CHILDBEARING NURSING

Application of theory to family health situations during childbearing can guide family nurses in making more complete assessments and planning interventions congruent with the pattern of events during childbearing. Several of the theories discussed in Chapter 2 contribute to nurses' understanding of how families grow, develop, function, and change during childbearing. Two theories in particular, Family Systems Theory and Family Developmental and Life Cycle Theory, are especially applicable to childbearing families. A brief summary of these theories and their application to childbearing families follows.

Family Systems Theory

Family Systems Theory provides a framework for viewing the family as a system: as an organized whole and/or as individuals within the family who

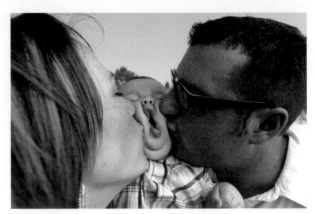

© LindaYolanda/iStock/Thinkstock

form interactive and interdependent systems. Four main concepts underlie this theory: (1) All parts of the system are interconnected, (2) the whole is more than the sum of the parts, (3) all systems have some form of boundaries or borders between the system and its environment, and (4) systems can be further organized into subsystems. Family systems are primarily designed to maintain stability, and a change in one member of the family affects all members of the family.

Becoming parents or adding a child brings stress to a family by challenging family stability, not only for the nuclear and extended family systems themselves but also for the individual members and subsystems of the family. As new subsystems are created or modified by pregnancy and childbirth, a sense of disequilibrium exists until a family adapts to its new member and re-achieves stability. For example, changes in the husband-wife subsystem occur as a response to development of the new parent-child subsystems.

Imbalance, or disequilibrium, occurs while adjustments are still needed and new roles are being learned. Families with greater flexibility in role expectations and behaviors tend to experience these periods of disequilibrium with less discomfort. The greater the range or number of coping strategies available to the family, and the greater the ability and support available to engage in various family roles, the more effective the family's response will be to both internal strains and external stress associated with childbearing. External stresses, such as concerns about outside employment, child care, and lack of health insurance, may be important in predicting family disequilibrium. These issues have emerged as significant stressors as new immigrant and refugee families settle and integrate into their new communities (Amoako & Kapiriri, 2016; Miramontes et al., 2015). Consequently, researchers and policy makers encourage health care providers to employ creative strategies, innovation, and cultural sensitivity in their role as global citizens (Miramontes et al., 2015). Internal strains such as an ill or special needs child, or unhealthy habits such as substance abuse, may tax family coping mechanisms to the breaking point. Therefore, it is imperative that nurses identify both present and potential family stressors and assess the effect of stressors on family stability.

Family Systems Theory is especially effective for use by childbearing family nurses because, following childbirth, families who are in a state of change and readjustment tend to have more permeable family boundaries. For example, families with flexible or open boundaries have varying degrees of openness to the outside environment, which stems from the need for additional resources beyond what the family can supply for itself. Consequently, a family in transition may be engaged in more interactions with systems outside the family and may become more receptive to interventions such as health teaching than it would be at other times in the family life cycle (Kaakinen & Harmon-Hanson, 2014). This openness of family boundaries allows nurses more access to the family for assessment, diagnosis, and health promotion.

On the other hand, childbearing family nurses should be aware of very closed or enmeshed families who may have nonpermeable or "closed" boundaries as they are likely to reject outside influences, including nursing care. Families can become closed because they interpret the outside environment and systems as hostile, threatening, or difficult to cope with. These families are challenging for nurses because they are less readily accessible or responsive to family nurses.

Nurses working with childbearing families from a systems perspective view the family as the client and aim to assist families to maintain and regain stability. Therefore, assessment questions should be focused on the family as a whole. At the same time, it is important to remember that family nurses also work with the individuals and the subsystems within the family. Interventions need to be directed at the various systems and levels of subsystems within the family. For example, a family ecomap will help the nurse see how individual members and the family as a whole relate to one another and to the community around them. Understanding the family process and functioning through careful assessment of the family as a whole and the individual family members allows the nurse to offer intervention strategies that will help provide stability in the family's everyday functioning.

Family Developmental and Life Cycle Theory

Duvall's (1977) Family Developmental and Life Cycle Theory described a process of developing over time that is predictable and yet individual, based on unique life circumstances and family interactions. Although the life cycle of most families around the world follows a universal sequence of family development, it is important for childbearing family nurses to recognize that wide variations exist in the timing and sequencing of family life cycle phases (Berk, 2013; Duvall, 1977). Many present-day childbearing families in North America do not fit into the classic sequence and timing of family developmental stages and tasks originally described by Duvall and Miller (1985). For example, families may be blended, with one or both partners having children from a previous relationship. Other types of nontraditional family structures include adoptive families; communal or multigenerational families; and parents who may be cohabitating, unmarried, single, of the same sex, or have children born later in life (Berk, 2013; McKinney, James, Murray, Nelson, & Ashwill, 2013; Stephens, 2013). Therefore, nontraditional and high-risk families—such as those experiencing unusual levels of stress from marital conflict and divorce, violence, substance abuse, having a child with special needs, infertility, being an adolescent parent, or stressors during refugee migration and settlement—require care that is different from that needed by traditional families (McKinney et al., 2013). In addition, families who are members of vulnerable populations may experience multiple and intersecting stressors from discrimination because of race, socioeconomic level, ethnicity, gender, and/or sexual orientation.

Despite how diverse the family is today, Family Developmental and Life Cycle Theory remains a helpful guide for childbearing family nurses because it addresses the patterns of adaptation to parenthood that are typical for many families. This theory has relevance for family nurses regardless of how families are structured, because the essential tasks families must perform to survive as healthy units are generally present to some extent in all families (Pillitteri, 2014).

According to Duvall's (1977) Family Developmental and Life Cycle Theory, family changes occur in stages during which there is upheaval while adjustments are being made. What occurs during these stages is generally referred to as a developmental task. The Childbearing Family with Infants stage is pertinent to childbearing family nursing practice because it is during this stage that childbearing families must accomplish nine specific tasks in order to grow and achieve family well-being. These nine tasks for childbearing families and nursing interventions are explained in the following subsections.

Task One: Arranging Space (Territory) for a Child

Arranging space (territory) involves families making space preparations for their infants. Families often accommodate newborns by moving to a new residence during pregnancy or the first year after birth or by modifying their living quarters and furnishings. Families may delay or avoid space preparations for a new baby for several reasons. For example, busy families, those who fear or have experienced prior fetal loss, and families involved with adoption or foster placement may delay or avoid space preparations. For some groups, such as Orthodox Jews, preparation for a baby's material needs, such as blankets and diapers during pregnancy, is not acceptable; it may mean bad luck or misfortune for the baby (Cassar, 2006; Rich, 2011). The lack of space preparation may also result from the parents not having accepted the reality of the coming baby (denial). It may also emerge from various social risks or health disparities, including expensive health care needs incurred by other family members; inadequate, unsafe housing arrangements or homelessness; underemployment or poverty; recent immigration; and incarceration. Adolescent parents may not make space arrangements because of denial of the pregnancy or fear of repercussions from their families if pregnancy is revealed.

Family Nursing Interventions

- Inquire about the safety and health of the family's home environment, food, security (including freedom from domestic violence), space arrangements made for the baby,

and other child-care resources, community resources, or other support systems.
- Refer refugee and other families who are homeless or live in inadequate or unsafe housing to appropriate resources for obtaining safer housing.
- Inquire about the families' thoughts, values, beliefs, and possible fears about making preparations for the anticipated arrival of the baby.
- Assist families to explore and manage their fear about survival or loss of the baby and then mobilize resources to help them cope so that family development can continue.
- Assist adolescents to find ways to communicate with their families and make plans for the future placement and well-being of the infant and the adolescent parents.
- Work with prisoners, interested stakeholders, and state/federal penal systems to establish units where newborns and mothers can stay together to encourage bonding and breastfeeding while the mother is incarcerated.

Task Two: Financing Childbearing and Child Rearing

Childbearing results in additional expenses and lower family income. American families, having experienced two major economic downturns since the start of the 21st century, are finding the decision to bear and the ability to raise children increasingly financially difficult (Guttmacher Institute, 2009; Oberg, 2011). Low-income families and children, especially African Americans and those of Hispanic descent, have been disproportionally burdened by these recessions and continue to struggle just to make ends meet (Bruening, MacLehose, Loth, Story, & Neumark-Sztainer, 2012; Oberg, 2011). Financial stresses can be even harder for mothers without partners, women who provide most of the income for their families, mothers who are fleeing domestic violence, or mothers experiencing unplanned pregnancy. Non-older adults, people in low-income families with at least one worker in the family, and families with precarious immigration status (including refugee claimants or migrant workers) may likewise experience severe financial stress because of lack of health insurance coverage (Kaiser Family Foundation, 2016; Simich, Hamilton, & Baya, 2006). These populations are particularly vulnerable to fiscally restrictive social policies aimed at limiting systemic health care costs. For example, the Canadian

Immigration Bill C-31 reduced accessibility to Interim Federal Health Program (IFHP) coverage and limited eligibility for immigration and refugee status, thus producing increases in uninsured newcomers as a consequence (Parliament of Canada, 2012). Though the subsequent government enacted legislation to improve the situation, challenges continue to exist.

Health care surrounding childbirth can add another layer of financial stress on a family. Health care providers may not be able to accept patients who are uninsured, insured by federal or state programs, or cannot pay out of pocket for obstetrical services, further increasing the financial strain on families. A portion of this financial stress, experienced by Canadian childbearing families, is offset by a publicly funded universal health care plan. In the United States, the Affordable Care Act (ACA; H.R. 3590) has reduced the number of uninsured Americans and, thus, helped alleviate some of the financial stressors childbearing families face (Kaiser Family Foundation, 2016). Under the ACA, most health plans are required to cover 10 essential health benefits, including maternity and newborn care (U.S. Department of Health and Human Services, 2015).

Although most employed women miss some employment during childbearing, many return to the labor force or increase the number of hours worked following childbirth (Mattingly & Smith, 2010). Others, especially those of high socioeconomic status or with a college/university education, may choose to delay re-entry into the workforce or forego possible career advancement during childbearing (Mattingly & Smith, 2010). Adolescent mothers are especially prone to financial difficulties because childbearing may disrupt their education, which increases their risk for future poverty (McKinney et al., 2013). Regardless of the reason, there are many consequences of missed employment for woman beyond loss of earnings during the childbearing years. Other consequences are detailed in Box 12-2.

Family Nursing Interventions

- Assist families to find high-quality resources, such as nutrition programs, food banks, family shelters, counseling or settlement services, and government-funded prenatal clinics, including midwifery clinics, community health centers, or public health clinics that support families with limited socioeconomic resources.
- Identify barriers to prenatal care, such as cultural differences, lack of transportation or insurance coverage, child care, hours of service that conflict with family employment, and difficulty obtaining or using health care benefits.
- Assist families to find safe and appropriate child care by providing culturally appropriate information and resources in their preferred language.
- Fully inform families about their health care options resulting from reform and redesign of the health care system.
- Educate families about new federal health care coverage and assist them to navigate the enrollment process.
- Advocate for expansion of Medicaid eligibility for poor adults in all U.S. states.

BOX 12-2

Consequences of Maternal Unemployment During the Childbearing Years

Consequences of maternal unemployment during the childbearing years include:

- Loss of status or identity of an employee
- Earnings lost during the times of unemployment
- Loss of on-the-job training opportunities and opportunities for advancement in career
- Depreciation of skills and experience, often followed by a loss of confidence about returning to work

- Loss of work-related benefits if job is subsequently lost
- Family medical leave taken before childbirth may reduce the leave time available postpartum
- Reinforcement of traditional roles and responsibilities in two-parent, heterosexual families where the father takes the breadwinner role

Sources: Adapted from Galtry, J., & Callister, P. (2005). Assessing the optimal length of parental leave for child and parental well-being. How can research inform policy? *Journal of Family Issues, 26*(2), 219–246; Schwartz, D. A., & Engler, C. (2015). Unravelling the mysteries of the Family and Medical Leave Act. *GP Solo, 32*(2), 30; and Weckstrom, S. (2012). Self-assessed consequences of unemployment on individual wellbeing and family relationships: A study of unemployed women and men in Finland. *International Journal of Social Welfare, 21*(4), 372–383.

Task Three: Assuming Mutual Responsibility for Child Care and Nurturing

The care and nurturing of infants bring sleep disruptions, demands on time and physical and emotional energy, additional household tasks, and personal discomfort for caretakers. New parents spend most of their time caring for children, thus decreasing both leisure and downtime, both of which are important to maintain balance in the family. Parents can experience role strain and role overload from combining the increased work within the family with employment demands, or they may face difficulty arranging and affording child care.

The first decision parents make regarding their infant's nutrition is whether to breastfeed or bottle feed. With the exception of decreased feeding costs, the benefits of breastfeeding have traditionally been viewed in North America as being primarily for the child. For example, breastfed babies are less likely to develop diarrhea, ear, or other infections and have a reduced rate of sudden infant death syndrome (SIDS; Anatolitou, 2012). Evidence also suggests "breastfeeding may be associated with a small but measurable advantage in cognitive development that persists into adulthood" (Anatolitou, 2012, p. 13). Worldwide, the consensus is that exclusive breastfeeding for around 6 months is best for both mother and child and that "the duration of breast-feeding that is best must be individualized to the family unit" (Godfrey & Lawrence, 2010, p. 1598). Sufficient evidence confirms that mothers who breastfeed for 1 year or longer experience multiple physiological and emotional benefits. These benefits include reduced risk for breast and ovarian cancer, osteoporosis, type 2 diabetes, cardiovascular disease, rheumatoid arthritis, and postpartum depression (Anatolitou, 2012; Godfrey & Lawrence, 2010). Nurses must be aware that the father or partner's role in the newborn feeding decision and the level of support and encouragement are important factors in the success of the breastfeeding relationship (Datta, Graham, & Wellings, 2012).

In both the United States and Canada, the rate at which women initiate breastfeeding is very high. The rate at which women in North America are exclusively breastfeeding at 6 months following birth falls dramatically (Chalmers et al., 2009; Godfrey & Lawrence, 2010). Although the rate

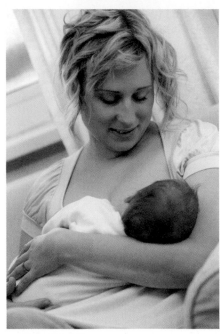

© iStock.com/Dean Mitchell

of breastfeeding has increased in all demographic groups, certain populations are less likely to breast-feed, including lower-income women; first-time mothers; African Americans; women participating in the Special Supplemental Nutrition Program for Women, Infants, and Children (WIC); those with high-school education or less; and those employed full-time outside the home (Godfrey & Lawrence, 2010; Johnston & Esposito, 2007).

Additionally, an increasing number of clients identifying as mothers, women, or transgender men report concerns surrounding postpartum hypogalactia following breast reduction surgery. These parents derive a more satisfying postpartum experience and their newborns benefit when their lactation efforts are respected and supported, for example with lactation aids, pumping, and formula supplementation (Thibaudeau, Sinno, & Williams, 2015; Wolfe-Roubatis, & Spatz, 2015). It is crucial for childbearing family nurses to understand the relationship between maternal employment and breastfeeding practices, including the phenomenon of infant feeding with breast milk that has been pumped while the mother is away from the home. Furthermore, nurses should strive to provide a culturally safe environment for families by keeping abreast of the changing landscape of evidence-based strategies and concerns of a culturally diverse clientele (Zamora, Lutter, & Peña-Rosas, 2015).

For both mothers and fathers, one of the benefits of having a period of time off from work following childbirth is the increased ability for parents and their newborn to establish a relationship through the process of bonding and attachment. A vast body of research on bonding and attachment, beginning with Bowlby (1952), continued by Ainsworth (1967), and popularized by Klaus and Kennel (1976), supports the premise that optimum child development and well-being is achieved through early and ongoing contact between mothers, fathers, and their newborn. Mothers may automatically bond with their newborns throughout pregnancy and early contact within minutes of the child's birth. By contrast, fathers must work to establish a bond by being involved in the delivery, as well as being available to the infant to strengthen paternal attachment through early contact with the infant in the months following birth (Klaus, Kennell, & Klaus, 1995).

If an infant must be separated from the parents because of prematurity or for medical or surgical interventions, interruptions in bonding may occur. To promote optimal bonding in these special circumstances, the nurse must allow parents early and frequent access to the baby, encourage parents to be involved in the care of their infant, practice skin-to-skin contact, and speak to and hold their newborn (Fegran, Helseth, & Fagermoen, 2008). If these actions are not possible, photographs of the infant should be sent to parents as soon as possible and they should be updated frequently with information about the newborn's status. The affectionate bond (or attachment) that develops between parents and their children may be one of the motivational driving forces for engaging in infant care and nurturing even under difficult circumstances.

Family Nursing Interventions

- Educate parents about the realities of parenting, such as interrupted sleep and changes in time management and family roles.
- Teach the family to alternate who responds to the baby's needs, including feeding, changing, and comforting.
- Assist parents to develop new skills in caregiving and ways of interacting with their babies, such as baby carrying, smiling, talking to their infant, or making eye contact.
- Observe for signs of attachment by listening to what parents say about their babies and by observing parent behaviors. Box 12-3 outlines parental behaviors that facilitate attachment.
- Refer families who do not demonstrate nurturing behaviors to other professionals, such as local counselors, psychologists, social workers, or childhood development experts, who can provide more intensive intervention.
- Promote culturally competent perceptions of parenting behavior in minority cultures by building partnerships in the ethnic community of the families in care. Respected elders,

---

BOX 12-3

Parental Behaviors That Facilitate Attachment

Selected parental behaviors that facilitate attachment between infant and parent include:

- Arranges self or the newborn so as to have face-to-face and eye-to-eye contact with infant.
- Directs attention to the infant; maintains contact with infant physically and emotionally.
- Identifies infant as a separate, unique individual with independent needs.
- Identifies characteristics of family members in infant.

- Names infant; calls infant by name.
- Smiles, coos, talks to, or sings to infant.
- Verbalizes pride in the infant.
- Responds to sounds made by the infant, such as crying, sneezing, or grunting.
- Assigns meaning to the infant's actions; interprets infant's needs sensitively.
- Has a positive view of infant's behaviors and appearance.

Sources: Adapted from Alden, K. R., Lowdermilk, D. L., Cashion, M. C., & Perry, S. E. (2012). *Maternity and women's health care* (10th ed.). St. Louis, MO: Mosby; Davidson, M. R., London, M. L., & Ladewig, P. A. (2016). *Olds' maternal-newborn nursing and women's health across the lifespan* (10th ed.). Upper Saddle River, NJ: Pearson Prentice Hall; and Schenk, L. K., Kelley, J. H., & Schenk, M. P. (2005). Models of maternal-infant attachment: A role for nurses. *Pediatric Nursing, 31*(6), 514–517.

doulas, or community members may act as translators and cultural brokers for the health care team (Wilson-Mitchell, 2008).

■ Provide information about and support for breastfeeding, including how to manage lactation problems, feeding expressed breast milk when appropriate, and referral for lactation consultation as necessary (Lawrence, 2010; Newman & Pitman, 2009).

■ Participate in active listening and respect for mothers who decline breastfeeding or "chest-feeding," possibly because of a past history of trauma, body image concerns, or postoperative sequelae of breast reconstruction.

■ Promote maternal and paternal early and frequent contact with their newborn; encourage involvement in newborn care activities.

Task Four: Facilitating Role Learning of Family Members

Learning roles is particularly important for childbearing families, including those families that depart from traditional heterosexual structures. For many couples, taking on the role of parents is a dramatic shift in their lives. Difficulty with adaptation to parenthood may be related to the stress of learning new roles. Role learning involves coming to understand the expectations about the role, developing the ability to assume the role, and taking on the role. Another important demand that children create, which affects women in particular, is increased housework. Household chores associated with children (laundry, cleaning, cooking, child care, etc.) can lead to increased levels of distress for women and can affect relationships between partners. The relationship between gay men or women is also affected when the couple takes on the parenting role. For example, parenting can result in differing energy levels between partners, especially if one partner has assumed primary responsibility for child rearing. The toll parenting has on their ability to be good partners to each other influences their relationship (Giesler, 2012).

The stress of parenting depends in large part on marital status, race and ethnicity, identification as heterosexual or gay, or the presence of a child with chronic illness. For example, Nam, Wikoff, and Sherraden (2015) found higher average parenting stress among Hispanics followed by African Americans,

Native Americans, and whites. Gay couples who decided to become parents revealed that sacrificing lifestyle goals and desires—such as travel and changes to the quality of their sex life—was a source of stress in their partner relationship (Giesler, 2012). Cousino and Hazen's (2013) meta-analysis revealed that generic aspects of caregiving, unrelated to a child's chronic illness, increased stress for parents of children with chronic illness. Parents also experience stress related to frequent health care appointments and demanding treatment regimes.

Family Nursing Interventions

■ Encourage expectant women to bring their partners into the experience by sharing their physical sensations and emotions of being pregnant and restating the value of their role as parents.

■ Assist and encourage pregnant couples to explore their attitudes and expectations about the role(s) of their partner within the household and family after the baby arrives.

■ Encourage contact with others who are in the process of taking on the parenting role, especially if the parents are isolated, adolescent, same sex, or culturally diverse and living apart from traditional networks. Respect culturally prescribed roles that resist (or require) change from the prevailing Western cultural worldview.

■ Provide opportunities for fathers and other partners or significant others in the family to become skilled infant caregivers.

■ Empower parents by assisting them to recognize their own strengths.

■ Moderate parenting stress by assisting new mothers, especially mothers from minority or racialized groups, to reduce their depression symptoms and develop strong social support networks (Nam et al., 2015).

Task Five: Adjusting to Changed Communication Patterns

Childbearing families experience changes in their overall communication patterns in order for the family to accommodate newborn and young children. The role of new parents also requires changes in communication patterns. As parents and infants learn to interpret and respond to each other's communication cues, they develop effective, reciprocal communication patterns. Nurses can assist parents in correctly interpreting and responding to their infant's communicative cues. For example, many babies respond to being held by cuddling and nuzzling, but others respond by back arching and stiffening. Parents may interpret the latter as rejecting and unloving responses, and these negative interpretations may adversely affect the parent-infant relationship. Positive parenting practices, self-esteem, and parenting efficacy have been found to increase with accurate interpretation and response to infants' communicative cues (DiCarlo, Onwujuba, & Baumgartner, 2014; Paris, Bolton, & Spielman, 2011).

Abusive head trauma, which includes shaken baby syndrome, is an extreme example of an inability to adapt to changed communication patterns with an infant. Whether intentional or unintentional, shaking a baby as a form of communication in response to anger and frustration with crying, or in an attempt to accomplish discipline, will result in traumatic brain injury. Infants age 2 to 4 months are at the greatest risk for shaken baby syndrome, a form of physical child abuse that occurs among families of any ethnicity, income range, or family composition. Males, mothers, and other female caregivers alike have been found to have shaken babies. However, infants suffer worse injuries from male perpetrators who are more likely than females to be convicted of this crime (Centers for Disease Control and Prevention, 2016; Cleveland Clinic Children's, 2011).

Communication between parents also changes with the transition to parenthood. During the years of childbearing, many couples devote considerable time to career development. The time demands of work coupled with parenting may affect a couple's relationship. Along with taking on the everyday aspects of rearing children, communication can then either fall to the wayside or be the key way of making the new family structure function effectively.

Family Nursing Interventions

- Educate parents about different infant temperaments so they are able to interpret their baby's unique style of communication.
- Teach parents how to recognize and respond to their baby's cues.
- Encourage parents to talk to and engage in eye contact with their baby.
- Educate parents on the various reasons for crying and methods of comforting a crying baby.

- Educate parents and infant caretakers that it is never appropriate or safe to shake a baby.
- Support paid family leave workplace policies that would allow working parents to be with their infants between 4 and 20 weeks of age, a period of increased infant crying (Centers for Disease Control and Prevention, 2016).
- Incorporate couple communication techniques into education of expectant parents.
- Promote effective couple communication by encouraging the partners to listen to each other actively using "I" phrases instead of blaming one another.
- Encourage couples to set aside a regular time to talk and to enjoy each other as loving partners.

Task Six: Planning for Subsequent Children

After the birth, some couples will have definite, mutually agreed-on plans with each other for additional children, whereas others may have decided against future children or be ambivalent about family plans. The nurse should be aware that many couples resume sexual intimacy before the routine 6-week postpartum checkup and, therefore, pregnancy may occur even if the mother is breastfeeding. Therefore, postpartum teaching should include information about when it is safe to resume intercourse after childbirth and reliable methods of birth control. Childbearing family nurses are a valuable resource for those desiring information or demonstrating a willingness to discuss family planning options.

Family Nursing Interventions

- Identify the power structure and locus of decision-making control in the family when discussing reproductive matters.
- Consider a family's cultural and religious background before initiating a discussion about contraceptive choices because these factors often dictate whether the discussion is appropriate.
- Explore previously used methods of contraception for appropriateness after childbirth.
- Provide current, evidence-based information about family planning options either during pregnancy or in the immediate postpartum period.
- Debunk myths about breastfeeding as a method of family planning.

Task Seven: Realigning Intergenerational Patterns

The first baby adds a new generation in the family lineage that carries the family into the future. Expectant parents change roles from being their parents' children to becoming parents themselves. Childbearing may signify the onset of taking on an adult role for adolescent parents and for some cultural groups. Childbearing changes relationships within extended families as parents' siblings become aunts and uncles, children from previous relationships become stepsiblings, and parents become grandparents.

Siblings typically experience many emotional changes with the arrival of a new family member. Feelings of confusion, hurt, anger, resentment, jealousy, and sibling rivalry are common among younger siblings, as is behavioral regression. Parents should be prepared for these emotional upheavals with strategies that will help the sibling(s) adjust to and accept the new baby.

Grandparents often provide the greatest amount of support to families when a child is born. The degree of their involvement may be linked to cultural expectations. Research has shown that Hispanics, Asians (Zhao, Esposito, & Wang, 2010), Africans, and many other cultures traditionally value the extended family. The nurse should be aware that in these cultures grandparents are a strong influence on child-rearing practices and are often intimately involved in daily family dynamics (Lewallen, 2011).

Family Nursing Interventions

- Assist new parents to seek support from friends, family members, organized parent groups, and work colleagues as a way to cope with the demands of parenting.
- Work with families to develop strategies that maintain their couple activities, adult interests, and friendships.
- Facilitate partner discussions about perceptions of extended family involvement in care of the new child.
- Facilitate new parents' participation in the decision-making process when health care decisions are required for their child, such as infant nutrition decisions.
- Provide learning opportunities to help move new parents from dependence to independence and self-reliance.
- Offer sibling classes during childbirth education for young children (2 to 8 years) and

provide parents with information on how to help ease the transition.
- Offer classes for grandparents during childbirth education with topics varying from assistance with household management to current recommendations on infant positioning, feeding, and clothing, as well as positive strategies to help them assume a supportive (non-parenting) role.

Task Eight: Maintaining Family Members' Motivation and Morale

After the initial excitement that often surrounds the arrival of a new baby, families must learn to adjust to and cope with the demands that caring for the baby will have on their time, energy, sexual relationship, and personal resources. Many new mothers experience postpartum fatigue, which is a feeling of exhaustion and decreased ability to engage in physical and mental work (Davidson, London, & Ladewig, 2016). Women may be fatigued because of many interrelated factors, including the blood loss associated with birth, breastfeeding, sleep difficulties, and depression. In addition, a relationship exists between maternal fatigue and postpartum depression (PPD), both of which affect family processes (Davidson et al., 2016). Female gender roles often require women to be accountable for a disproportionate amount of domestic work, rearing of other children, demands of new infant care, and employment outside the home (O'Mahony & Donnelly, 2013). The first 3 months after childbirth are recognized as the most vulnerable emotional period for mothers (Dennis & Dowswell, 2013; Ward et al., 2016) and, by extension, for their families. During this time and extending past the first year postpartum, mothers' depressive symptoms can continue; therefore, nurses must be alert for cues of depression from the new mother and other family members (Dennis, Heaman, & Vigod, 2012).

In the months following childbirth, families must be realistic about infant sleep patterns and crying behaviors, the potential to experience loneliness, and changes in their sexual relationship. For example, many young families, especially single mothers, experience loneliness in the postpartum period because they live in communities far from their extended families. Some families have recently moved into a new neighborhood and may not have established friendships or a sense of community. Many ethnically diverse groups had special support and recognition of the postpartum period in their countries of origin. For example, by not taking part in traditional childbirth rituals such as the practice of "doing the month" (laying-in period of 40 days), new immigrant mothers may be more prone to depression. Traditional practices have been recognized as protective factors and have implications in the prevention and treatment of PPD (Morrow, Smith, Lai, & Jaswal, 2008).

Family Nursing Interventions

- Inform family members about ways to promote comfort, rest, and sleep, which will make it easier for them to cope with fatigue.
- Promote parental rest while a baby needs nighttime feedings by encouraging parents to alternate who responds to the baby.
- Teach parents ways to cope with a crying infant, which will boost family morale, increase confidence, and allow family members to get additional sleep.
- Provide information on ways parents can reduce isolation and loneliness by seeking support from friends, family members, organized parent groups, work colleagues, and community support groups such as La Leche League.
- Encourage parents to articulate their needs and to find help in ways that support their self-esteem as new parents.
- Counsel couples about changes in sexuality after birth and help them develop mutually satisfying sexual expression.
- Help families to develop strategies that maintain their couple activities, adult interests, and friendships.
- Take a proactive approach to prepare and educate women and their families about signs of PPD.

Task Nine: Establishing Family Rituals and Routines

Family rituals and routines consist of activities that the family performs and teaches its members for continuity and stability (Ward et al., 2016). The predictability of rituals helps babies develop trust. Family rituals have been described as celebrations, traditions, religious observances, and other symbolic events. Family rituals include the observance of celebrations such as birthdays, whereas family routines center on meal, bedtime, and bathing; greeting and dismissal routines (a kiss goodbye or goodnight); children's special possessions such as a treasured blanket; and nicknames for body functions. For some families, rituals have special cultural meanings that nurses should respect. When families are disrupted or separated during childbearing, nurses can help them deal with stress by encouraging them to carry out their usual routines and established rituals related to their babies and other children.

Family Nursing Interventions

- Determine the special cultural meaning each ritual has for the family and respect those meanings.
- Assess through observation and/or questioning, or as guided by an assessment survey tool, how families observe or acknowledge important days.
- Encourage families to carry out their usual routines and established rituals related to their babies and other children.
- Create a supportive environment that encourages parental knowledge and confidence in caring for themselves and their infants.
- Facilitate couple discussion of bedtime and bathing routines, a baby's special possessions such as a treasured blanket, nicknames, language for body functions, and welcoming rituals such as announcements, baptisms, circumcision, or other celebrations.

Family Transitions

Though it is not another task, transition is a major concept in the Family Developmental and Life Cycle Theory (Duvall, 1977). Inherent in transition from one developmental stage to the next is a period of upheaval as the family moves from one state to another. Historically, "transition to parenthood" was thought by early family researchers to be a crisis (LeMasters, 1957; Steffensmeier, 1982). The idea of transition to parenthood as a crisis is being abandoned. More recent work focuses on the transition processes associated with a change in families. Current discourse on family development is tempered by acknowledgement that the definition of family is dynamic, with intersections of race, class, and poverty influencing how families address challenges such as disabled children, disparity, discrimination, and illness (Conger et al., 2012).

Life transitions, including entering pregnancy or parenthood, are peak times for change (Rasmussen,

Dunning, Hendrieckx, Botti, & Speight, 2013). Nurse researchers have mostly focused on the transition to motherhood. Even though other family members experience the transition when a newborn joins the family, concepts related to motherhood give nurses insight into family transition. For example, opening of self relates to making a commitment to mothering, experiencing the presence of a child, and caring for the child. The notion of family transition gives a foundation for nursing interventions that promote parenting because opening of self involves the real experience of being with and caring for the child. Nurses who understand the stressors that families experience as they transition from one state to another can use this theoretical concept to realize that a mother or father may be frustrated over not being able to cope in old ways.

Just as no one theory covers all aspects of nursing, no single theory will work for every situation involving childbearing families. Therefore, nurses must understand and utilize multiple theories to plan and guide nursing care for childbearing families. Major concepts from Family Systems Theory and Family Developmental and Life Cycle Theory help nurses organize assessments and manage the predictable and unpredictable experiences childbearing families encounter.

CHILDBEARING FAMILY STRESSORS

Childbearing family nursing begins when a couple anticipates and plans for pregnancy, has already conceived, or is planning to adopt a child. Any pregnancy-related event such as infertility, adoption, pregnancy loss, or an unplanned pregnancy may be enough to disrupt the delicately formed bonds of the family in this stage. Nurses need to be aware of problems childbearing families might encounter before, during, and after reproductive events so that they can anticipate, identify, and respond to needs appropriately.

Infertility

The ability to conceive is a major milestone in a couple's life (Wong, Pang, Tan, Soh, & Lim, 2012). Both men and women perceive fertility to be a sign of competence as reproductive human beings. Therefore, the experience of infertility can be a life crisis that disrupts a couple's marital and/or sexual relationship. Infertility is "a disease defined by failure to achieve a successful pregnancy after 12 months or more of appropriate, timed unprotected intercourse or therapeutic donor insemination" (American Society for Reproductive Medicine, 2012, para 1). Infertility is a medical and social problem that is of concern to childbearing family nurses, especially in cultures where the expectation of motherhood is strong and because of the increasing trend of delayed childbearing in all industrialized countries (Gossett, Nayak, Bhatt, & Bailey, 2013; Wong et al., 2012).

Nurses should anticipate that infertile couples will experience several different physical, emotional, and psychological symptoms. Couples dealing with infertility struggle between feelings of hope and hopelessness, and they report feelings of sadness, fatigue, anxiety, and urgency; changes in sleeping patterns (e.g., oversleeping, night waking, insomnia); and headaches (Braverman, Domar, Brisman, & Webb, 2015; Eggertson, 2011; Wilson & Leese, 2013). Their level of success with advanced reproductive technology and the level of empathetic responses they receive from caregivers often influences their perceptions of satisfaction and well-being (Wilson & Leese, 2013). Problems with infertility change a couple's social relationships and support, which may result in increased levels of depression and psychological distress (Box 12-4).

The experience of infertility is stressful for both men and women. Yet the way in which men and women respond varies (Galhardo, Moura-Ramos, Cunha, & Pinto-Gouveia, 2016). For example, many men believe their central role during fertility treatment is to be a source of strength and support for their partner (Malik & Coulson, 2008). In contrast, women typically experience a higher risk for emotional distress than men. Feelings of anger, anxiety, shame, loss of self-esteem, grief, and depression are just some emotions that infertile woman report experiencing (Wong et al., 2012). Women want to spend time talking about their infertility experience, whereas men report that talking about it only increases their anxiety. Therefore, men dealing with infertility tend to talk, communicate, and listen less than do women. Men also cope with infertility through avoidance and by disguising their feelings to protect themselves, their partners, or both (Sherrod, 2006; Wong et al., 2012). More recently, men-only online discussion boards have provided opportunities via forum posts for men to

BOX 12-4

Common Symptoms and Stressors Infertile Couples May Experience

Some common symptoms and stressors
experienced by infertile couples are:

- Irritability
- Insomnia
- Tension
- Depression

- Increased anxiety
- Anger toward each other, God, friends,
  and other fertile women
- Feelings of rejection, alienation, stigmatization,
  isolation, and estrangement

Sources: Braverman, A. M., Domar, A. D., Brisman, M. B., & Webb, K. J. (2015). ART nurses as the patient's partner in care: Targeting depression, stress, and other barriers. *Contemporary OB/GYN, 60*(6), S1–S12; Peterson, B. D., Sejbaek, C. S., Pirritano, M., & Schmidt, L. (2014). Are severe depressive symptoms associated with infertility-related distress in individuals and their partners? *Human Reproduction, 29*(1), 76–82; and Sherrod, R. A. (2004). Understanding the emotional aspects of infertility. Implications for nursing practice. *Journal of Psychosocial Nursing, 42*(3), 42–47.

emote in relation to infertility. In this venue, men "talk" to each other about the emotional burdens of infertility, personal coping strategies, and their relationships with others (Hanna & Gough, 2016).

Testing and treatment for infertility is expensive. Assisted reproductive therapy services provided in the United States and Canada, for the most part, are not covered under most health insurance plans or by provincial health insurance. Two Canadian provinces, Quebec and Ontario, have made provision for in vitro fertilization, a type of advanced assisted reproductive therapy, to be a covered treatment only under certain conditions.

Infertility testing and treatment is also painful, time consuming, and inconvenient. It can lead to a loss of spontaneity and privacy in sexual activities, which only compounds the stress and strain couples are experiencing. Although every test or treatment is another painful reminder of the inability to reproduce, it is nurses' lack of knowledge and understanding of the emotional aspects of infertility that really frustrates infertile couples. Therefore, couples interpret nursing care to be insensitive and uncompassionate when nurses focus primarily on physiological or technical aspects of infertility rather than on emotional needs (Lutter, 2008; Sherrod, 2004). Therefore, it is vital that nurses caring for childbearing families experiencing infertility understand, consider, and address the emotional needs of couples undergoing assessment, diagnosis, and treatment for infertility. Families experiencing the crisis of infertility are in as much need of a personal touch as they are of technical competence and accurate, evidence-based information about testing and treatment options. See Box 12-5 for specific nursing interventions to help couples deal with infertility.

Adoption

Adoption is one of the many ways women, alternative couples, and those experiencing infertility or other issues may become parents (Giesler, 2012; Sherrod, 2004). Many different types of families adopt (U.S. Department of Health and Human Services, n.d.), including single parents, families formed by second parents or with stepparents, transracial, transcultural, relative, and lesbian, gay, bisexual, queer, or transgender (LGBTQ) families. Although adoptive mothers and families may not experience the physical context of pregnancy, they may have many of the same feelings and fears as biological families (Cao, Roger Mills-Koonce, Wood, & Fine, 2016; Fontenot, 2007). Childbearing family nurses must be aware that all parents react to the strong intense feelings and emotions, ranging from happiness to distress, in the first moments they meet their child, regardless of the way in which a family is formed. Even though the child is not biological or the parental relationship may not be established immediately at birth, bonding can be just as strong and immediate for adoptive parents and children (Hockenberry & Wilson, 2015; Rykkje, 2007). Therefore, nurses caring for women in the preadoptive and early postadoptive period must recognize and provide care that is respectful and family-centered according to the needs of the individual family. Although many of the clinical assessment and physical needs might differ, educational, parenting, and feeding concerns may be similar to those of biological mothers in the prenatal and postpartum periods (Cao et al., 2016; Fontenot, 2007)

Once families decide to adopt a child, they may pursue several routes, such as international adoption (also known as intercountry), public domestic adoption, or private domestic adoption. In the United States,

BOX 12-5

Nursing Interventions That Are Helpful to Couples Dealing With Infertility

Helpful nursing interventions for couples with infertility include the following:

■ Avoid assigning blame to one partner or the other.
■ Encourage social support from friends, spouse, or significant other.
■ Assess couples' coping strategies, encourage open discussion between couples, suggest different coping strategies.
■ Facilitate communication between couples in order to give men, in particular, the opportunity to acknowledge

and express their feelings and process their response to the infertility experience.

■ Provide information related to cost and insurance coverage for treatment.
■ Suggest appropriate stress-relieving activities, such as acupuncture.
■ Refer to support groups and/or other professionals for counseling.

Sources: Adapted from Grant, L.-E., & Cochrane, S. (2014). Acupuncture for the mental and emotional health of women undergoing IVF treatment. A comprehensive review. *Australian Journal of Acupuncture and Chinese Medicine, 9*(1), 5–12; Sherrod, R. A. (2004). Understanding the emotional aspects of infertility. Implications for nursing practice. *Journal of Psychosocial Nursing, 42*(3), 42–47; Sherrod, R. A. (2006). Male infertility: The element of disguise. *Journal of Psychosocial Nursing, 44*(10), 31–37; and Wong, C., Pang, J., Tan, G., Soh, W., & Lim, J. (2012). The impact of fertility on women's psychological health: A literature review. *Singapore Nursing Journal, 39*(3), 11–17.

BOX 12-6

International and Transracial Adoption: Issues and Challenges

Issues and Challenges to Families Before International and Transracial Adoption

■ Ability to travel on short notice to pick up a child
■ Changing political conditions, which may stop the adoption process at any time
■ Ways family will maintain the adopted child's natural heritage
■ Ways family will deal with racial and other types of prejudice
■ The many rules and conditions that sometimes prevent families from adopting a child from a particular country

Issues and Challenges to Families After International Adoption

■ Limited postadoption resources are available, such as pediatricians trained in international adoption or

international adoption clinics for families seeking help for a child's developmental and behavioral problems.

■ The child's emotional and developmental issues can be exhausting and financially tax the family
■ Limited or no information about the child's maternal or paternal medical history can be a source of uncertainty and adoptive parental stress.

Issues and Challenges to Families After Transracial Adoption

■ There is a need to redefine the family as multiracial and multiethnic when white families adopt nonwhite children.
■ Extra attention and comments about the child's looks may occur from strangers in public places.
■ Neighbors, family members, and others may express prejudice toward the child.

Sources: Adapted from Gunnar, M., & Pollak, S. D. (2007). Supporting parents so that they can support their internationally adopted children: The larger challenge lurking behind the fatality statistics. *Child Maltreatment, 12*(4), 381–382; Pillitteri, A. (2014). *Maternal and child health nursing: Care of the childbearing and childbearing family* (7th ed.). Philadelphia, PA: Lippincott Williams & Wilkins; Rykkje, L. (2007). Intercountry adoption and nursing care. *Scandinavian Journal of Caring Sciences, 21*(4), 507–514; and Smit, E. (2010). International adoption families: A unique health care journey. *Pediatric Nursing, 36*(5), 253–258.

domestic adoption can be a difficult, lengthy, bureaucratic, and costly process that takes anywhere from 2 to 7 years for a healthy infant (National Adoption Center, n.d.). The laws favoring birth mothers also complicate domestic adoption. This long waiting period, and fear of the court system, results in many families turning

to intercountry adoptions, which generally take 1 to 4 years before a child can enter the United States. The length of time it takes to complete intercountry adoptions is dependent on many factors including: the child's country of origin's procedures, the adoption service provider's process, the U.S. immigration process, and the specific circumstance of the adoption (Intercountry Adoption, 2013). One drawback to an international adoption is that little to no information about the child's birth parents' background, prenatal health care, or medical history may be available to the adopting family (Gunnar & Pollak, 2007; Smit, 2010). The lack of birth history places families at risk for adopting a child who may have experienced a significant number of threats to physical health as well as brain and behavioral development, which can contribute to future struggles as families cope with the consequences of these problems (Gunnar & Pollak, 2007; Smit, 2010). Box 12-6 lists other issues and challenges related to international and transracial adoption.

In Canada, approximately 20% of families are affected by adoption, either through the public child welfare (foster care) system or private adoption agencies. A prerequisite for all Canadian adoption is successful completion of the Parent Resource for Information Development and Education (PRIDE) course. In addition, private Canadian adoption agencies are required to provide birth parents with counseling before the birth, to offer emotional support for adoptive parents, and to organize the court and legal services involved.

Private adoption is another alternative for families considering adoption. Private adoptions can range from being strictly anonymous to very open, where the adopting couple and birth mother get to know each other extremely well. Often, the Internet is a place where women wanting to place babies for adoption and families seeking to adopt connect. Canadian families wishing to adopt should be aware that some provinces do not allow for direct advertising on the Internet or in newspaper classifieds (Canada Adopts!, 2014). Regardless of how North American families connect or interact with the birth mother, it is paramount that families pursuing private adoption retain professional legal advice and counsel to ensure that everyone involved, including the birth father, understands the legal ramifications and to work out all aspects related to the adoption before the baby's birth. In Canada, adoption falls under provincial jurisdiction and, therefore, laws are highly variable between provinces. For example, some provinces allow families themselves to find a child to adopt rather than having an agency choose one for them. Nurses should encourage Canadian families working with private agencies to understand any adoption restrictions or limitations set by the province in which they reside (Canada Adopts!, 2014).

Nurses should be aware that when a private adoption has been negotiated, one of the important points is whether the adopting family will be present at the child's birth. Nurses must also be prepared and ready to intervene should a birth mother reverse her decision to give the baby up for adoption, or a birth father who has not relinquished his legal right to the baby asserts his rights (McKinney et al., 2013; Pillitteri, 2014). See Box 12-7 for appropriate nursing interventions when caring for adoptive families.

BOX 12-7
Nursing Interventions for Adoptive Families

Following are selected nursing interventions for adoptive families:

- Encourage families to seek help from adoption experts and agencies.
- Encourage families to understand and follow any legal and provincial limitations or restrictions related to adoption.
- Refer families to adoption specialists, such as social workers, counselors, and lawyers.
- Recommend families speak with and secure pediatric providers during the preadoptive process.
- Recommend adoptive parents attend parenting classes and include them in prenatal and infant care classes.

- Incorporate adoptive-sensitive material into classes and other educational resources.
- Keep lines of communication open between nurses and adoptive families as a way to alleviate fears about being judged or undermined.
- Address other siblings' response to the adopted child because a biological child's feelings of inferiority or superiority to an adopted child can interfere with relationships within the family.
- Address family concerns about attachment issues.

Sources: Adapted from Canada Adopts! (2014). Adopting in Canada. Retrieved from www.canadaadopts.com/canada/domestic_private. shtml; Fontenot, H. (2007). Transition and adaptation to adoptive motherhood. *Journal of Obstetrics, Gynecologic and Neonatal Nursing, 36*(2), 175–182; Pillitteri, A. (2014). *Maternal and child health nursing: Care of the childbearing and childbearing family* (7th ed.). Philadelphia, PA: Lippincott Williams & Wilkins; and Smit, E. (2010). International adoption families: A unique health care journey. *Pediatric Nursing, 36*(5), 253–258.

Perinatal Loss

Perinatal loss is not uncommon and it is a traumatic event for families around the globe (Armstrong, Hutti, & Myers, 2009; Callister, 2014; Umphrey & Cacciatore, 2014). Losing a child during pregnancy, after birth, or in the early postpartum period is one of the hardest things a family can experience. The loss may be anticipated and voluntary, such as with abortion or relinquishing parental rights for adoption, or unanticipated, such as death or loss of custody to the state. An adoptive family may lose their intended child if a birth mother changes her mind about giving up a baby for adoption. Box 12-8 lists other types of perinatal loss that families may experience.

Loss of a child is a unique and profound experience for parents. When parents lose a child, they lose a part of their hoped-for identity, including all hopes and dreams held for the child they anticipated and loved; they also often experience a lack of social recognition regarding the significance of their loss (Armstrong et al., 2009; Heazell et al., 2016; Umphrey & Cacciatore, 2014). Societal invisibility of infant loss contributes to parental frustration, especially when they are denied time to mourn or are asked why they are not yet over their loss (Umphrey & Cacciatore, 2014). One mother put it this way when describing her loss experience, "Oh God, please help me. I need someone to help me pass through this pain" (Callister, 2014, p. 207). Therefore, nurses caring for childbearing families must engage in ongoing assessment and interventions related to potential, previous, or current loss.

Grief and a process of bereavement should also be anticipated secondary to perinatal loss, an adverse perinatal outcome, diagnosis of congenital or genetic disorders, palliative care, or the birth of a child with special needs.

Nurses providing care to childbearing families should anticipate that each family member will experience loss differently. For example, research shows that mothers are more apt to grieve visibly by emotional expression, sharing of feelings, and participation in grief support groups. Fathers, in contrast, tend to feel a sense of loneliness and isolation and have feelings of helplessness. Fathers, who often see their role as primarily supportive of their partner, may feel the need to "act as men" by being strong and may hold back their own feelings of grief and pain (Koopmans, Wilson, Cacciatore, & Flenady, 2013; Umphrey & Cacciatore, 2014). Siblings may describe their grief experience as "hurting inside" as a way to express feelings of sadness, frustration, loneliness, fear, and anger (Heazell et al., 2016). Grandparents experience a triple measure of grief and sorrow when a grandchild dies: their own personal grief as a human being suffering the death of a loved one; the pain over the loss of a grandchild, which carries with it the loss of their dreams and expectations for their relationship with that child; and seeing their own children suffer (Heazell et al., 2016).

Considering the effect of perinatal loss on all family members, nurses must work to support and strengthen the familial bond in the face of such loss (Heazell et al., 2016; Koopmans et al., 2013). Nurses can support families' experience of perinatal loss by being present and listening attentively, expressing

---

BOX 12-8

Types of Perinatal Loss Families May Experience

Families may experience the following types of perinatal loss:

- Miscarriage
- Elective abortion
- Ectopic pregnancy
- Selective reduction after in vitro implantation of multiple fertilized eggs
- Stillbirth

- Death of a child after a live birth
- Recurrent pregnancy loss
- Death of a twin during pregnancy, labor, birth, or after birth
- Termination of pregnancy for identified fetal anomalies, which is increasing because of technological advances in prenatal diagnosis of such anomalies
- Loss of the anticipated "perfect" child because of anomalies or malformations

Source: Adapted from Callister, L. C. (2006). Perinatal loss: A family perspective. *Journal of Perinatal Neonatal Nursing, 20*(3), 227–234.

emotions, gathering memorabilia, and helping the family make meaning of the experience. Referral to support groups or provision of a list of available resources may be helpful depending on the needs of the grieving couple or family (Koopmans et al., 2013; McKinney et al., 2013). Compassionate Friends is one of many groups to which nurses might refer grieving parents, siblings, and grandparents for support.

Culture influences how families respond to perinatal loss. Therefore, it is essential for nurses to understand several different culturally diverse practices and rituals associated with loss, as well as provide culturally competent care. In Western cultures, holding, touching, and mementos are commonly used support strategies. However, mothers from certain countries may avoid touching and holding their stillborn babies because these behaviors are considered unacceptable in their countries of origin (Callister, 2014; Heazell et al., 2016). Patients may also have specific burial requirements, depending on culture or religion. Families from Indigenous and Muslim cultures may request early burial and accommodation in the hospital room for respected religious elders to perform rituals (Cacciatore, 2009; Cacciatore & Flint, 2012). Nurses demonstrate cultural sensitivity when they validate what families perceive to be the "right way" to grieve (Callister, 2006; Chichester,

2005). Box 12-9 lists cultural perinatal loss practices and rituals of select cultural groups.

Pregnancy Following Perinatal Loss

Psychological distress is higher in parents who have experienced a prior perinatal loss, with maternal anxiety about a child's well-being extending a year or more after the birth of another child (Armstrong et al., 2009). Women may not perceive pregnancy as normal after experiencing perinatal loss but rather may be plagued with a sense of anxiety, insecurity, ambivalence, doubt, and concern that another loss may occur (Davidson et al., 2016; Umphrey & Cacciatore, 2014; Wool, 2013). They also experience higher levels of anxiety than fathers (Armstrong et al., 2009). Fathers may shut down their feelings when pregnancy occurs after loss because of unresolved feelings related to prior pregnancy loss. They may even be too frightened to share or may not be conscious of their feelings. Nurses caring for childbearing families during pregnancy after perinatal loss are in a prime position to help mothers and fathers open doors of communication that may have been closed because of fear. One strategy nurses could use to encourage communication is to ask fathers "How are you doing?" in front of the mothers, which provides an

---

BOX 12-9
Perinatal Loss: Cultural Practices and Rituals

Cultural practices and rituals following perinatal loss include the following:

- Hmong families may request the placenta following birth because of their belief that burying it prevents problems of the soul.
- Jewish families may request to remain with the body at all times out of respect. Newborns may be named and circumcised at burial so they can be included in family records.
- Muslim babies born after more than 4 months' gestation may be named, bathed, wrapped in a seamless white sheet, and buried within 24 hours.

Bodies are traditionally buried intact, so taking locks of hair may not be permitted.
- Puerto Rican families may call on faith healers and spiritualists to assist the baby on his or her journey into the next life.
- Roma families may want to avoid any association with death and bad luck/impurity (mahrime), so they may leave the hospital suddenly and shift responsibility for burial to the hospital.
- American Indians/Alaskan Natives may request to remain with the baby until death to pray.

Sources: Adapted from Callister, L. C. (2006). Perinatal loss: A family perspective. *Journal of Perinatal Neonatal Nursing, 20*(3), 227–234; Chichester, M. (2005). Multicultural issues in perinatal loss. *Lifelines, 9*(4), 314–320; Palacios, J., Butterfly, R., & Strickland, C. J. (2005). American Indians/Alaskan Natives. In J. G. Lipson & S. L. Dibble (Eds.), *Cultural and clinical care* (pp. 27–41). San Francisco, CA: The Regents University of California; and Sutherland, A. H. (2005). Roma (Gypsies). In J. G. Lipson & S. L. Dibble (Eds.), *Cultural and clinical care* (pp. 404–414). San Francisco, CA: The Regents University of California.

opportunity to share what they are feeling (Davidson et al., 2016; Koopmans et al., 2013; Umphrey & Cacciatore, 2015). Additionally, nurses need to be caring, sensitive, and patient. They need to offer clear specific information about prenatal care and opportunities for both parents to ask questions. If anxiety or unresolved grief issues are present, a referral to a grief counselor may be supportive and beneficial for the parents (Davidson et al., 2016; Wool, 2013).

THREATS TO HEALTH DURING CHILDBEARING

For the majority of families, childbearing is a physically healthy experience. For some families, however, health during childbearing is threatened and the childbearing experience becomes an illness experience. In such cases, concern for the physical health of the mother and the fetus tends to outweigh other aspects of pregnancy; rather than eagerly anticipating the birth and baby, family members experience fear and apprehension. Moreover, the family's functioning and developmental tasks are disrupted as the family focuses its attention on the health of the mother and survival of the fetus or baby. Childbearing nurses must be aware that families with threats to health have additional needs for maintaining and preserving family health.

Acute and Chronic Illness During Childbearing

This chapter defines *acute* as health threats that arise suddenly and may have life-threatening implications. Examples of acute health threats childbearing families may encounter are fetal distress during labor and pulmonary embolism for postpartum women. In contrast, *chronic* comprises conditions occurring during pregnancy that persist, linger, need control, or have no cure and that require careful monitoring and treatment to avoid becoming an acute threat to maternal or infant health. Gestational hypertension, preexisting and gestational diabetes, and postpartum depression are some examples of chronic health threats. Some threats to health during childbearing vacillate between acute and chronic. For example, preterm labor can be an acute health threat that results in a preterm birth. If preterm labor contractions are suppressed, it becomes a chronic health threat requiring adherence to prescribed regimens to keep contractions from recurring.

Effect of Threats to Health on Childbearing Families

Chronic threats to childbearing health are disruptive to childbearing families. Knowledge of the family as a dynamic system explains why the effects of these chronic conditions extend to the entire family and result in the upset of family functioning, communication, and roles (Arestedt, Persson, & Benzein, 2014). When childbearing health is threatened, all family members experience stress as families strive to regain balance. For example, three sources of stress that alter family processes when the mother or infant experiences a chronic health threat are (1) assuming household tasks, (2) managing changes in income and resources, and (3) facing uncertainty and separation.

Assuming Household Tasks

When women experience chronic threats to childbearing health, other members of the family must assume responsibility for household tasks and functioning, regardless of whether the condition is managed at the hospital or at home. Assumption of household tasks by others creates family stress, especially for partners who must take on the role of caring for the family, as well as caring for the expectant mother and/or infant (Maloni, 2010). Expectant fathers especially may find that all their time and energy are consumed by employment and household management, tasks that previously were shared or done solely by their partners. Children's lives change when mothers have to limit activities. Toddlers do not understand why their mothers cannot pick them up or run after them. The resulting frustration for children can manifest itself in behavioral changes, such as tantrums and regression in developmental tasks (e.g., toilet training).

Managing Changes in Income and Resources

An at-risk pregnancy is stressful in terms of the family's finances and other resources. For example, if a mother is placed on bedrest to manage antepartum bleeding from a placenta previa she may miss time away from paid employment. Or a mother may not have the ability to seek employment, which also results in loss of income. At the same time, medical expenses may increase because of the need for increased care, including possible neonatal intensive care and maintaining multiple health care provider visits or hospital stays. Personal expenses associated with the cost of specialized diets, medications, and hiring personnel to assist with household tasks may also increase; such costs are not usually covered by health care systems in Canada or the United States. For families already in debt or struggling with unemployment or other financial challenges, these threats to health serve to increase the burden of debt.

Although resources, such as energy and social networks, cannot be measured as easily as money, family nurses are in a position to help families consider and manage changes in their nonmonetary resources. Some of the nonmonetary changes that family nurses should anticipate families will encounter include the following: that others outside of the nuclear family may need to assume various household tasks such as meal preparation, laundry, and cleaning; that all families may not have social networks or extended families in the immediate vicinity; that changes in employment may cause separation from persons and activities that were stimulating; and that isolation, regardless of the cause, can increase a family's burden.

Facing Uncertainty and Separation or Loss

The unpredictable nature of high-risk childbearing makes planning for the future difficult for childbearing families because it leaves them facing uncertainty and possible separation. For example, expectant parents, especially employed women, face uncertainty with pending preterm birth because they may not

---

BOX 12-10

Family Nursing Interventions for Childbearing Families Experiencing Chronic Threats to Health

Assuming Household Tasks

- Help families find ways to streamline and prioritize household tasks to reduce stress and increase adherence to medical regimens.
- Assist adults to list household management tasks and determine who does what when so that the family can be more efficient and effective in managing these tasks.
- Educate families about the impact of parents' health difficulties on children.
- Provide practical, age-appropriate suggestions for managing children, such as hiring a teenager after school for active play with young children.
- Encourage parents to provide ways for young children to have some quiet one-on-one time with their mothers as a way to reduce stress for both mothers and children.

Managing Changes in Income and Resources

- Refer families to an appropriate counselor who can explore with family members ways to manage financial problems.
- Assist families to identify others outside of the nuclear family who can assume various household tasks, such as meal preparation, laundry, and cleaning.
- Help families identify and use resources, such as home-health agencies and parents' groups in the community, to assist with household management.
- Encourage families with necessary resources to use a computer to connect with each other, friends, coworkers, and other at-risk families to prevent or decrease feelings of isolation.

- Direct families to appropriate Internet sites, such as the ones listed in the Suggested Web sites section on DavisPlus.

Facing Uncertainty and Separation and Loss

- Acknowledge the difficulties of uncertainties associated with difficult perinatal situations.
- Be honest and informative about the condition and prognosis of both the mother and fetus.
- Use terms understood by all family members to provide accurate and thorough explanations tailored to families' anxiety levels.
- Assist families to cope with basic tasks of living in high-tech settings such as the neonatal intensive care unit.
- Investigate and reduce the barriers families may encounter at a distant perinatal center, such as lack of transportation, employment, and the threatening environment of a strange setting.
- Provide families with information on where to stay, how to find reasonably priced meals, how to obtain transportation, and where to park a car.
- Encourage use of electronic communication, such as e-mail, to facilitate contact between family members and health care professionals.
- Encourage calling families about their members' progress and sending photographs as a way to help families cope with uncertainty and enhance relationships of physically separated family members.
- Encourage family members to participate in care of their infants to promote development of parenting skills.

be able to determine accurately when to begin and end parental leave because of the need to cope with sudden hospitalization. Separation can occur when mothers are suddenly hospitalized or when families living in remote rural areas are transferred to a distant perinatal center for days or weeks. When families are separated, it becomes difficult for them to maintain and develop family relationships. Separation from the family and concerns about family status are two of the greatest stressors experienced by women hospitalized for chronic threats to childbearing health (Maloni, Margevicius, & Damato, 2006). In addition, small children experience extreme anxiety over the sudden departure of their mother, especially if they are unprepared or unable to comprehend what is happening to their mother and the new baby.

Even if the logistical problems related to separation are solved and a family can be together, coping with basic tasks of living is challenging in new settings. For instance, a family may not know where to stay, how to find reasonably priced meals, how to obtain transportation, or where to park a car. Box 12-10 presents nursing interventions related to childbearing families who are experiencing chronic threats to health.

FAMILY NURSING OF POSTPARTUM FAMILIES

All family members experience household upheaval during the first few days and weeks a newborn is in the home. Throughout the childbearing cycle, nurses assist families to understand, prepare, and respond to the effect of a new baby on the family. Assisting parents to be realistic in their expectations about themselves, each other, and their children helps them to plan ahead by identifying appropriate support and resources. This section discusses appropriate nursing assessments and interventions family nurses should incorporate into their practice when caring for families during the postpartum period.

Feeding Management

Success in feeding their babies induces feelings of competency in mothers. A family's comfort with its infant feeding method is as crucial for physical, emotional, and social well-being of the infant as is the food itself. Regardless of the parents' choice of feeding method, nurses' instructions need to emphasize the development of relationships between infant and parent through feeding. Being held during feeding enhances social development whether a baby is being breastfed or bottle fed. Parents should take the time during feedings to enjoy interacting with their babies. When the infant is adopted, social interaction with feeding is a special opportunity for developing attachment.

Even though the act of breastfeeding is associated with the mother, fathers and partners need not be excluded from the feeding experience. Nurses can promote parent-infant attachment by encouraging fathers and partners to be involved with feeding. For example, the father can burp the baby during or after feedings, hold and comfort the infant once feeding has been completed, and feed the baby a bottle of expressed breast milk once breastfeeding is well established (McKinney et al., 2013). Early involvement of fathers and partners in feeding is beneficial later when infants are being weaned from the breast or mothers are preparing to return to employment.

Many people assume that breastfeeding is "natural" and so should not present any difficulties. Nevertheless, many women initially may experience breastfeeding difficulties, especially if the baby has difficulty latching or milk takes longer than expected to come in. It is important that nurses assess a mother's breastfeeding technique early and provide hands-on teaching so mothers can learn how to breastfeed successfully. Referral to a lactation consultant may be necessary before the new family leaves the hospital. Most hospitals have lactation specialists in the hospital and some also provide postdischarge services in the community. Nurses should also ensure that the family is given resource information about breastfeeding, including how to obtain assistance at post-discharge clinics when breastfeeding challenges arise.

Attachment

Positive parent-infant attachment must take place to foster optimal growth and development of infants, as well as to encourage the parent-infant love relationship. The attachment process requires early involvement and physical contact between parents and their infant for a strong link to develop (Barlow, Bennett, Midgley, Larkin, & Wei, 2015). Extreme stress, health risk factors, and illness can interfere with the physical contact and early parent-infant involvement needed for the development of attachment. Stressful conditions that pull parents' energies and attention away from their newborns can be detrimental to attachment. Adoption can be another factor influencing attachment, especially if the child had multiple caretakers or frequently changed living location. Children who were adopted from more stable environments may also have attachment difficulties if they struggle to transfer their attachment from a previous caretaker to their adoptive parents (Smit, 2010).

Nurses should be alert for families who are likely to have difficulty with attachment, especially if family history indicates a parent has suffered abuse, neglect, or abandonment during childhood. In addition, nurses may identify families at risk for poor attachment through listening to what parents say about their babies and by observing parent behaviors. Families at risk for poor attachment may have misconceptions about infant behavior, such as believing that infants cry just to annoy their parents. Hence, family nurses must address verbal expressions of dissatisfaction with the infant, comparison of the infant with disliked family members, failure to respond to the infant's crying, lack of spontaneity in touching the infant, and stiffness or discomfort in holding the infant after the first week. Although isolated incidences of these behaviors are probably not detrimental to attachment, persistent trends and patterns could be an indicator of future relationship difficulties.

Another signal of attachment difficulty is inconsistent maternal behaviors, such as a mother who exhibits intense concern at times interspersed with apathy at other times without any predictable cause or pattern. Therefore, an important step when assessing attachment behaviors is to evaluate whether the parent-infant relationship is progressing positively and if the enjoyment and love of the child is growing over time. If the parents' enjoyment of the baby as a unique individual and their commitment to the baby are not progressing, the nurse needs to help the family understand what attachment is and also needs to identify factors that might be interfering with attachment to the infant. For example, mothers struggling with PPD need treatment for their depression before they can address attachment to the infant. Nurses can assess, support, and positively affect mothers and their families through postpartum home visits (Aston et al., 2015). Childbearing family nurses may need to refer families who do not demonstrate nurturing behaviors to other professionals such as social workers, psychotherapists, and developmental specialists who can provide more intensive interventions that will help parents care for and nurture their children.

Siblings

No matter what age siblings are, the addition of a new baby affects the position, role, and power of older children, thereby creating stress for both parents and children. Teaching parents to emphasize the positive aspects of adding a family member helps them focus on sibling relationships rather than rivalry. Parents need help to address *all* the children's needs, not just those of the new baby. Parents may be concerned about whether they have enough energy, time, and love for additional children. Practical ideas for time and task management can alleviate some of their concerns, as can helping parents delegate nonparenting tasks, such as housecleaning and meal preparation, to friends and relatives when possible.

Postpartum Depression

The period after childbirth can be a stressful time for women because of their need to face the new tasks of the maternal role. Changes in relationships, economic demands, and social support also take place during this time and can result in postpartum stress (O'Mahony & Donnelly, 2013). PPD has also been described as a "thief that steals motherhood," that is, it robs women of happiness during the first several weeks to months of the postpartum period (Beck, 2006, p. 40).

The "postpartum or baby blues" are a common postpartum experience, with up to 80% of mothers experiencing this temporary emotional distress during the first 3 to 5 days after delivery. These changes in mood may be caused by the quick hormonal changes after delivery, fatigue, emotional let-down, and the stresses of being a new mother. Depressive symptoms that persist during the first year are of concern to family nurses because they can adversely affect maternal health and the ability of mothers to function in their new role (Beck, 2006; O'Mahony, Donnelly, Raffin Bouchal, & Este, 2013). PPD is a treatable disorder; prompt intervention improves long-term outcomes. The optimal treatment plan for a woman with PPD involves a coordinated interdisciplinary team and a holistic, family-centered approach.

BOX 12-11

Signs of Postpartum Depression

The following are signs of postpartum depression:

- Sadness
- Frequent crying
- Insomnia or excessive sleeping
- Lack of interest or pleasure in usual activities, including sexual relations
- Difficulty thinking, concentrating, or making decisions

- Lack of concern about personal appearance
- Feelings of worthlessness
- Fatigue or loss of energy
- Depressed mood
- Thoughts of death: suicidal ideation without a plan; suicide plan or attempt

---

Sources: Adapted from Davidson, M. R., London, M. L., & Ladewig, P. A. (2016). *Olds' maternal-newborn nursing and women's health across the lifespan* (10th ed.). Upper Saddle River, NJ: Pearson Prentice Hall; and Driscoll, J. W. (2006). Postpartum depression: How nurses can identify and care for women grappling with this disorder. *Lifelines, 10*(5), 399–409.

Left unidentified and untreated, PPD leads to serious consequences for families, such as maternal suicide, poor attachment to the infant, altered family dynamics, and lowered cognitive development in children. Considering these consequences, it becomes imperative that all health care providers educate woman and their families about potential causes and symptoms of PPD, as well as immediately identify and appropriately refer women experiencing this mood disorder so that early treatment can begin (Ballantyne, Benzies, & Trute, 2013; O'Mahony, 2017; Vigod, Sultana, Fung, Hussain-Shamsy, & Dennis, 2016). Box 12-11 lists signs of PPD.

Usually women do not volunteer information about their depression out of shame, fear, lack of understanding about the seriousness of their illness, or lack of available access to appropriate health care services (O'Mahony et al., 2013; Vigod et al., 2016). Therefore, it is incumbent on nurses to identify its existence by understanding and recognizing the signs and symptoms, even if they are subtle. If the new mother is making negative comments about herself, the baby, or her partner; if she is ignoring her other children's needs; if her physical appearance shows signs of neglect; or if family members report a change in the woman's mood or behavior, it is time to screen for PPD. Childbearing family nurses might consider incorporating the two-question screening measure that Jesse and Graham (2005) developed as a rapid way to begin the identification of women at risk for PPD. Use of this scale simply involves nurses asking women two questions: "Are you sad or depressed?" and "Have you experienced a loss in pleasurable activities?" Women who answer yes to both of these questions should be referred to a mental health care provider (Driscoll, 2006).

Family nurses caring for childbearing families might also consider using one of many readily available and easy-to-use depression scales, such as the Edinburgh Postnatal Depression Scale or the Postpartum Depression Predictors Inventory—Revised, as a routine screening tool for PPD (Davidson et al., 2016; McKinney et al., 2013). In particular, the Edinburgh Postnatal Depression Scale has been found to be valid for several cultures, has been translated into several different languages, and has been used with men (Driscoll, 2006; Schumacher, Zubaran, Roxo, & White, 2010; Small, Lumley, Yelland, & Brown, 2007). Regardless of which screening tool is used to identify women at risk for PPD, childbearing family nurses have a professional responsibility to assess for the disorder, recommend women be referred for treatment, and provide self-care strategies and support to the woman and her family (Driscoll, 2006; England & Sim, 2009; Horowitz, Murphy, Gregory, & Wojcik, 2011).

Although much attention has been given to maternal PPD, shifting gender roles and paternal involvement in child care require adjustments for men as well, which puts them at risk for experiencing depression after the birth of a child, especially if the mother is depressed. This consequence makes sense to nurses who understand Family Systems Theory because anything that affects one family member directly or indirectly affects other family members. Viewed from this theoretical perspective, it is easy to see how maternal or paternal depression affects all family members and relationships within the family and results in serious implications for family health and well-being. Therefore, family nurses must recognize PPD in fathers or other partners just as in mothers, because when both parents are depressed, the risk

BOX 12-12

Nursing Interventions for Postpartum Depression

Nursing interventions for postpartum depression include the following:

- Help women differentiate between myths of the mother role—which imply that at 6 weeks after birth, women are ready to resume all their previous activities—and the reality of motherhood.
- Assist women to recreate, restructure, and integrate changes that new motherhood brings into their daily lives.
- Encourage women with postpartum depression to share feelings as they grieve the loss of who they were and begin to build on who they are becoming.
- Solicit input from family members about changes in mood or behavior.
- Offer information about PPD at various times to perinatal women through outreach support.

- Encourage women to seek help with symptoms of anxiety, anger, obsessive thinking, fear, guilt, and/or suicidal thoughts.
- Ensure that regular PPD screening is a shared responsibility between obstetrics, primary/community health, and family health care providers.
- Develop standard protocols for screening men whose partners are depressed after childbirth.
- Ensure that education for PPD extends to include family members.
- Work with women to establish connections within community-based services for new mothers and their families.

Sources: Adapted from Driscoll, J. W. (2006). Postpartum depression: How nurses can identify and care for women grappling with this disorder. *Lifelines, 10*(5), 399–409; O'Mahony, J. M., Donnelly, T. T., Este, D., & Raffin Bouchal, S. (2012). Using critical ethnography to explore issues among immigrant and refugee women seeking help for postpartum depression. *Issues in Mental Health Nursing, 33*(11), 735–742; and Sethna, V., Murray, L., Netsi, E., Psychogiou, L., & Ramchandani, P.G. (2015). Paternal depression in the postnatal period and early father–infant interactions. *Journal of Parenting, Science and Practice, 15*(1), 1–8.

to infants and children increases. As with mothers, recommendation of a referral for fathers to mental health care providers should be made in an effort to initiate early treatment and reduce negative effects on the family system (Habel, Feeley, Hayton, Bell, & Zelkowitz, 2015; Sethna, Murray, Netsi, Psychogiou, & Ramchandani, 2015). Box 12-12 lists additional nursing interventions for PPD.

POLICY IMPLICATIONS FOR FAMILY NURSING

The concerns of childbearing family nursing go beyond care of the individual family. Nurses are participants in understanding, developing, and implementing policy as it relates to childbearing families. Much of Chapter 4 addresses important social policy issues relevant for childbearing families. The legal definitions of family, official recognition of the diversity of families, access to health care, alternatives to traditional childbearing such as cross-cultural adoption, and growing needs of poverty-stricken and other disenfranchised families are just a few of the policy areas vital to childbearing family nursing.

Nurses need to be aware of the effect of legislation on childbearing families. One example is family

leave for childbirth, which can profoundly affect the health and development of childbearing families. In the United States, the Family and Medical Leave Act (FMLA), a federal law enacted in 1993, entitles family members to take up to 12 weeks of *unpaid* time away from employment for certain medical or family reasons and ensures employees return to their same position. Birth, adoption, foster placement of a child, and caring for a child or spouse with a serious condition are permissible reasons for mothers and fathers to take leave under the FMLA. Unfortunately, many families cannot take advantage of FMLA benefits because the act only applies to those who worked for their current employer for a certain number of months and hours, for certain size businesses, and for a covered employer (Schwartz & Engler, 2015). Unlike the citizens of many developed nations, parents in the United States are not entitled to government benefits for childbearing except for tax deductions and other incentives. Many European countries, by contrast, offer paid parental leave.

In Canada, some social policies have been put into place in an effort to assist both parents to balance work-life issues and manage the care of newborns. All families in every Canadian province and territory are entitled to maternity leave or parental leave following childbirth and adoption.

A federally funded Employment Insurance (EI) program, except in Quebec, provides 15 weeks of paid maternity/parental leave at 55% of the mother's usual salary (to a maximum amount, which in 2016 was $537) providing she worked 600 hours in the 52 weeks before the onset of maternity leave. In the event of a premature birth, this benefit may be extended anywhere from 17 to 52 weeks. Families residing in the province of Quebec receive maternity, paternity, parental, and adoption benefits under the Quebec Parental Insurance Program (Government of Canada, 2016).

All types of policies affect family nursing every day. Health policy has far-reaching ethical and practical implications for childbearing family nursing. For instance, certain genetic screening during pregnancy and hearing screens for the newborn have become compulsory for health care providers in some Canadian provinces. Moreover, cystic fibrosis screening in pregnancy and newborn screening for metabolic and genetic diseases are mandatory for maternity providers in many American states. The informed decision-making models that are the impetus for these policies are not replicated in European health care systems; by contrast, they often are negatively viewed as eugenic solutions (i.e., with the goal of producing genetically improved offspring) to reduce the incidence of disability. European systems, unlike in North America, heavily fund services for disabled children and their families.

Hospitals also have policies affecting families that should be of concern to family nurses, especially considering how varied the family of today is. For example, increasing numbers of nontraditional families, such as lesbian couples, are having children through donor insemination or adoption (Roberts, 2006). Yet policies that guide perinatal practices—from the visual images hanging on the wall to if or how well partners are welcomed in prenatal groups, the delivery room, or other hospital environments—may be a barrier to these particular families' welfare and relationships (Goldberg, 2005; Roberts, 2006). In these situations, family nurses have an obligation to speak out on behalf of families. Often, nurses think of policies as entities beyond their control. In actuality, nurses have a voice and power in forming and changing policies. Beginning steps include close scrutiny of their practice settings for issues related to the welfare of families and their members.

FAMILY CASE STUDIES

This section illustrates the art and science of nursing with childbearing families. The Sanders family demonstrates family nursing care when unexpected health problems occur during pregnancy. The Housah-Ibrahim family case study reveals how a nurse provides culturally sensitive care to young parents who are quite new in the country.

Case Study: Sanders Family

Tom and Mary Sanders have been married to each other for 6 years. Tom, age 28, and Mary, age 28, have one child named Jenny who was born at full term 2 years ago. Mary did not experience any health problems with her first pregnancy. At that time, the Sanders lived in a large city in the western part of the United States, near their parents, siblings, and childhood friends. Two years later, the Sanders had moved to a small town 500 miles away from their friends and families to find better professional opportunities for Tom, a software engineer, and more affordable housing. A month after the move, they discovered that Mary was about 3 months pregnant. Although Tom's new job provided medical insurance for the family, Mary was concerned about finding and obtaining obstetrical care in their new community. Even though it would strain family finances, Mary decided to postpone seeking employment as a secretary until after the birth and to concentrate instead on fixing up the older two-story house they had bought.

Unexpectedly, Mary had health problems with this pregnancy. At 27 weeks' gestation, her obstetrician diagnosed gestational diabetes, which required Mary to modify her diet to keep her blood glucose under control. Following an anxiety-provoking episode of painless vaginal bleeding at 29 weeks, she was diagnosed with a complete placenta previa. Mary's physician insisted she stay on bedrest except for a very brief daily shower and use of the bathroom. Tom had to take over meal preparation, house cleaning, and caring for Jenny. He arranged the living room so Mary could lie on the couch and Jenny could play near her mother while he was at work. Because he had not yet accrued vacation or sick time, Tom could not take time off from his job to help Mary and take care of Jenny without sacrificing pay. Mary found it difficult to follow her diet and stay on bedrest.

Case Study: Sanders Family *(cont.)*

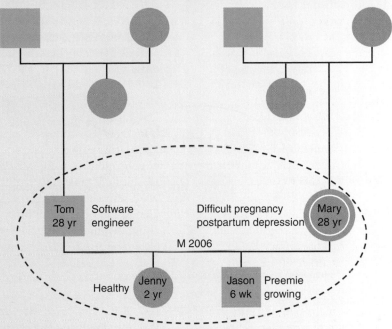

FIGURE 12-1 Sanders Family Genogram

She was frustrated because she had to stop her house renovation, and Tom's cooking and housecleaning were not up to her standards. She was tempted to run the vacuum cleaner, wash dishes, and eat sweets while Tom was at work. After a few days, Mary quickly tired of doing crafts, sewing, or puzzles. She was lonely for her mother and the support of friends who were 500 miles away; she longed for companionship, but found herself complaining and nagging Tom when he was home. Jenny frequently had tantrums because she could not play outside with her mother and began to have lapses in toilet training.

At 32 weeks of pregnancy, Mary experienced a large vaginal bleed that continued over a 4-hour period. Her physician sent her to a perinatal center 100 miles away from home because it had better facilities to perform a cesarean section delivery and care for preterm babies. Jenny went with her parents to the perinatal center to wait until one of her grandmothers could come and take care of her. Jason was born 2 hours after the Sanders arrived at the perinatal center hospital. Figure 12-1 presents a Sanders family genogram.

Mary was discharged from the perinatal center within 72 hours after Jason's birth. Her hemoglobin was 100 mg/dL following a transfusion of 2 units of blood. At home, she felt extremely weak, experienced significant incisional pain, and was overwhelmed by household tasks and caring for Jenny. She was disappointed that she was unable to breastfeed the baby because of his undeveloped sucking reflex and immature lungs. Despite her use of herbs and the breast pump, only 3 ml of milk were expressed every 2 hours, which she dutifully froze for transport to the hospital. Two weeks later, she was weeping frequently, felt very sad, had no appetite, and had difficulty sleeping. Being with their new son was difficult because each visit required a 200-mile round trip. Tom had a full-time job and Mary cared for Jenny during the day. Jason, the new baby, remained at the perinatal center in the special care nursery until he was mature and stable enough to go home 4 weeks later. At her 6-week postpartum checkup, Mary told the office nurse that she did not enjoy caring for her new baby and she had difficulty with her sleep. Based on this information, the office nurse asked Mary to complete the Edinburgh Postnatal Depression Scale. Figure 12-2 presents the Sanders family ecomap and how the nurse mobilized resources to help this family.

(continued)

Case Study: Sanders Family *(cont.)*

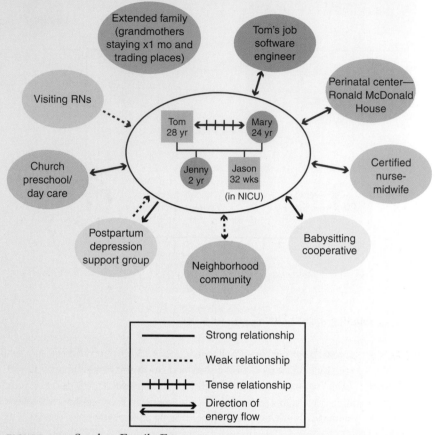

FIGURE 12-2 Sanders Family Ecomap

Case Study: Housah-Ibrahim Family

Fatima Housah, age 21, and Abdi Ibrahim, age 28, have been married for 3 years and are excited that Fatima is expecting their first baby. Abdi grew up in Somalia and was trained as an engineer in South Africa. He currently works as a taxicab driver in a large urban city in Canada while attending night school to obtain credentials in engineering. Abdi's mother and father live and work 1 hour away in an adjacent city. Following a wait of 3 years, Abdi was relieved when Fatima's application for permanent residence was finally accepted so that she could remain in Canada. She had arrived 1 year earlier as a refugee claimant who had experienced much hardship and ethnic persecution in Somalia and then in the refugee camp in Uganda. Her experience of frequent moving between refugee camps and fleeing rebel-led violence has left her with post-traumatic stress disorder. She is receiving emotional support from the women at the local mosque. Fatima has two sisters, a brother, and an aunt who reside in another Canadian province and she feels lonely for them at times. Talking by computer on Skype only causes her to miss them more. Fortunately, many of the women from the local Muslim Community Centre have offered her friendship. They are teaching her how to take the bus and subway and how to find ethnic foods in the local markets. She is grateful that they taught her how to use the kitchen appliances safely. She had never used a stove before coming to Canada. Figure 12-3 presents a family genogram for Fatima and Abdi's family.

Case Study: Housah-Ibrahim Family *(cont.)*

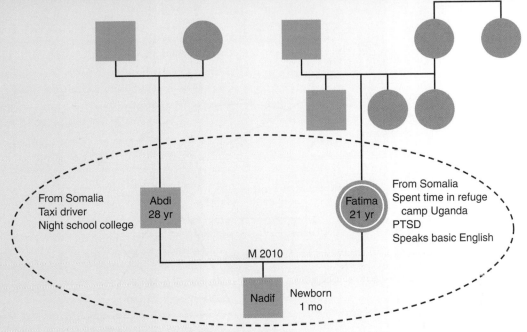

From Somalia
Taxi driver
Night school college

Abdi
28 yr

M 2010

Fatima
21 yr

From Somalia
Spent time in refuge
camp Uganda
PTSD
Speaks basic English

Nadif   Newborn
1 mo

FIGURE 12-3 Housah-Ibrahim Family Genogram

Fatima is concerned about her prenatal care. Even though the imam at the mosque says that a male physician could provide emergency care for her, she believes that a female provider might be more understanding. Finding a female maternity care provider has been a challenge in this community despite being insured by Canada's universal health care plan. To date, Fatima has had sporadic prenatal care at the walk-in center. By 32 weeks, however, she was able to find a female midwife with whom she has had five prenatal visits so far. At one of these visits Fatima reveals that she is worried about how her first-degree circumcision as an infant (which involved only a clitorectomy, thus leaving the labia and urethra intact) will affect the birth.

At 41 weeks' gestation, Fatima starts to feel lower abdominal cramps that continue for more than 2 hours and proceed to include lower back pain. The couple does not own an automobile, so they rush to the closest hospital by ambulance. Fatima notes that the nurse who greets them in the Labor Floor Triage room is a female; she is very kind and speaks slowly and gently. This approach is helpful because Fatima's English is still fairly basic. She defers to Abdi, who answers all the medical history questions. Further assessment reveals that her cervix has not started to change and that she is contracting regularly. Fatima is admitted to the hospital after 22 hours of prodromal labor and her female midwife consults the attending obstetrician regarding the need for oxytocin augmentation. A Somali interpreter is called to the bedside so the midwife and female consulting obstetrician can obtain consent to start medication to augment labor. Because of her past experiences, Fatima is resistant to medication and distrustful of medical authorities. In halting English, Fatima asks why the midwife wants to interfere with the natural processes of labor. Although she is not crying, her face appears to be drawn and frightened under her hijab (head scarf).

Twenty-four hours following vaginal delivery of a healthy baby boy named Nadif, Fatima is discharged home. Abdi is eager to participate in infant care although this is not the traditional father's role in Somali culture. He has learned how to change Nadif's diapers and to bathe him. Abdi stays up late surfing the Internet to learn more about fatherhood and about how to cook iron-rich foods for Fatima because she is too exhausted most evenings to cook. Abdi's parents are able to visit on weekends to help with the baby and thus provide much-needed support for this family. In addition, this couple has several community supports in place, as well as a follow-up appointment with a pediatrician at the public health center for the baby. Figure 12-4 presents Fatima and Abdi's family and how the nurse mobilized resources to help this family.

(continued)

Case Study: Housah-Ibrahim Family *(cont.)*

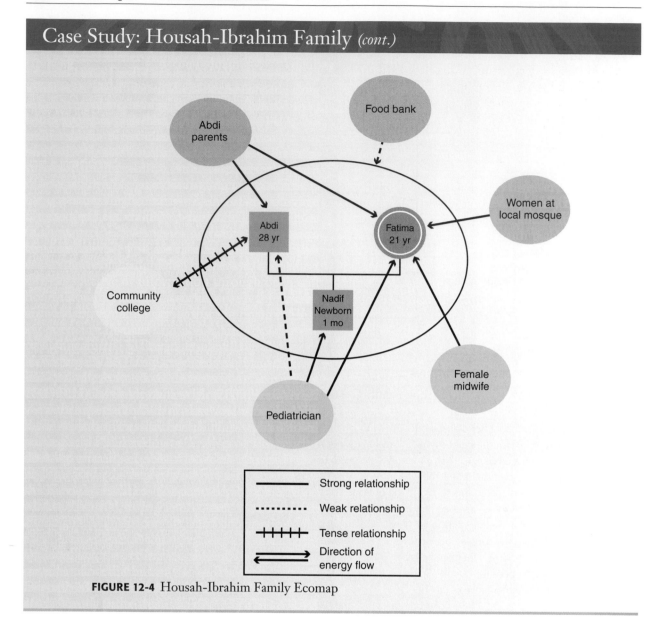

FIGURE 12-4 Housah-Ibrahim Family Ecomap

SUMMARY

Childbearing family nursing focuses on family relationships and the health of all members of the childbearing family, even during times of extreme threats to maternal health. Several different theories available to nurses encountering families during childbearing can help guide their assessment of the family, their plan of care, and interventions for the family. Nurses are also in a position to have a powerful influence on the development of family-friendly policies at both the federal and practice setting levels.

- Several theories, including Family Systems Theory and Family Developmental and Life Cycle Theory, are helpful to guide nurses' understanding of childbearing families and to structure nursing care.
- Stress-producing pregnancy-related events disrupt family functioning regardless of how the family is structured (traditional or nontraditional).
- While giving direct physical care, teaching patients, or performing other traditional modes of childbearing nursing, family nurses

focus on family relationships and the health of all members of the childbearing family.

■ Acute and chronic health conditions can develop during pregnancy and, thus, disrupt family functioning, development, and structure. When health threats arise, all family members experience stress as they strive to regain balance.

■ Childbearing family nurses can assist families to understand, prepare for, and respond to the effect each newborn has on the family.

■ Nurses must participate in policy development and implementation as it relates to childbearing families.

■ Nurses need to be aware of the effect of legislation on childbearing families.

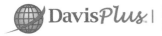 | For additional resources and information, visit **http://davisplus.fadavis.com**. References and Suggested Resources can be found on Davis*Plus*.

Chapter 13

Family Child Health Nursing

Deborah Padgett Coehlo, PhD, C-PNP, PMHS, CFLE

Critical Concepts

- A major task of families is to nurture children to become healthy, responsible, creative adults.

- Families are the major determinant of children's health and well-being.

- Most parents learn the parenting role "on the job," relying on experiences from their own childhood in their families of origin to guide them.

- Parents are charged with keeping children healthy, as well as caring for them during illness.

- Common health promotion challenges of children and their families are experienced during transitions as individual members and their families grow and change.

- Because the leading causes of morbidity and mortality among youth are substance use, sexual activity, and violence (both suicidal and homicidal), there is a need for increased attention to health promotion and prevention in these areas.

- Abuse and neglect may be defined differently across cultures, but nurses must be alert to helping families understand when child-rearing practices harm rather than nurture children.

- Families with children will experience challenges and stressors related to congenital and chronic health conditions, and related stressors to acute, chronic, and end-of-life transitions.

- The family-centered care model can be used by family child health nurses to facilitate and teach healthful activities for growth, prevention of injury and disease, and management of illness conditions in families.

- The aim of nurses is to help families develop appropriate ways to carry out family tasks necessary to promote health and to prevent or positively cope with illness and disease.

- Although most child-rearing families experience acute illnesses and become familiar with managing these crises, families do not anticipate that their children may have chronic illness.

- With their knowledge of family and child development, nurses can collaborate with families with chronically ill children to help them strive toward developmental landmarks.

- Family child health nursing must be practiced in collaboration and cooperation with families, as well as other health care providers, according to principles of family-centered care.

A major task of families is to nurture children to become healthy, responsible, creative adults who can develop meaningful relationships across the life span. An important job of all parents is to keep children healthy and care for them during illness. Yet most mothers and fathers have little formal education for health care of children. In fact, most parents learn the role "on the job," relying on their childhood experiences in their families of origin to help guide them. Advice from other parents and professionals augments information from families of origin, but this advice is generally implemented only when questions or problems arise.

Family nurses help families promote health, prevent disease, and cope with illness. The importance of family life for children's health and illness care is often invisible, because families' everyday routines are commonplace and lie below the level of awareness of health care providers. Family daily life, however, influences many aspects of children's health, including the promotion of health and the experience of illness in children. In turn, family daily life is influenced by the children's health and illness.

Families are groups with unique characteristics, including specific family experiences, memories, and related intergenerational relationships; structure and membership; family rules and routines; aspirations and achievements; and ethnic or cultural patterns (Burr, Herrin, Beutler, & Leigh, 1988). Family structure and function interact with and are influenced by these family characteristics. Healthy outcomes for children—such as tripling their birth weight by 1 year of age, or successfully completing high school—are partially attributable to the intangible, invisible daily interactions among family members. Nurses, in partnership with families, examine how the characteristics of families influence health.

Family child health nursing entails employing nursing actions that consider the relationship between family tasks and health care and their effects on family well-being and children's health. Nurses care for children within the context of their family, and they care for children by treating the family as a whole. Nurses keep in mind that families affect their children's health, whereas children's health affects their families. Family child nurses care for children in a variety of clinical settings and care situations.

This chapter provides a brief history of family-centered care of children and then presents foundational concepts that will guide nursing practice with families with children. The chapter goes on to describe nursing care of well children and families with an emphasis on health promotion, nursing care of children and families in acute care settings, nursing care of children with chronic illness and their families, and nursing care of children and their families during end of life. The case study illustrates the application of family-centered care across settings.

ELEMENTS OF FAMILY-CENTERED CARE

Family-centered care is a system-wide approach to child health care. It is based on the assumption that families are children's primary source of nurturance, education, and health care. Family-centered care has emerged, in part, in response to increasing family responsibilities for health care. The general principles of family-centered care include the following:

1. Recognizing families as the "constants" in children's lives, whereas the personnel in other systems, including the health care system, fluctuate
2. Openly sharing information about alternative treatments, ethical concerns, and uncertainties with families to guide decision-making processes
3. Forming partnerships between families and health care providers to decide jointly what is important for families
4. Respecting the racial, ethnic, cultural, and socioeconomic diversity of families and their ways of coping
5. Supporting and strengthening families' abilities to grow and develop (Lewandowski & Tesler, 2003)

See Table 13-1 for more details on the elements of family-centered care.

Families are the key health care providers for children. Families determine the culture of health care, including establishing healthy living patterns, care for acute illnesses, and care for chronic illnesses. Health care providers have recently acknowledged the importance of families in developing a comprehensive and holistic treatment plan for those children who need health care services. Families acknowledge the uncertainty that surrounds their

Table 13-1   Elements of Family-Centered Care

Elements	Definition
1. The Family Is at the Center	The family is the constant in the child's life.
2. Family-Professional Collaboration	Collaboration includes the care of the individual child, program development, policy formation at all levels of care—hospital, home, and community.
3. Family-Professional Communication	Information exchange is complete, unbiased, and occurs in a supportive manner at all times.
4. Cultural Diversity of Families	Honors diversity (ethnic, racial, spiritual, social, economic, educational, and geographical), strengths, and individuality within and across all families.
5. Coping Differences and Support	Recognizes and respects family coping, supporting families with developmental, educational, emotional, spiritual, environmental, and financial resources to meet diverse needs.
6. Family-Centered Peer Support	Families are encouraged to network and support each other.
7. Specialized Service and Support Systems	Support systems for children with special health and developmental needs in the hospital, home, and community are accessible, flexible, and comprehensive.
8. Holistic Perspective of Family-Centered Care	Families are viewed as families, and children are viewed as children, recognizing their strengths, concerns, emotions, and aspirations beyond their specific health needs.

Source: Lewandowski, L., & Tesler, M. (Eds.). (2003). *Family-centered care: Putting it into action. The SPN/ANA guide to family-centered care.* Washington, DC: Society of Pediatric Nurses/American Nurses Association.

child's health, and they want to be informed partners of the health care team's decision making, as well as valued collaborators in the care of their child (Griffin, 2003). Hummelinck and Pollock (2006) qualitatively studied eight families who were caring for a child with a chronic condition and found that, although each family had diverse needs, all parents wanted to be included in knowing the diagnosis, treatment plan with information on possible side effects, and prognosis. Additionally, all parents expressed that having information about the care of their child helped them communicate treatment needs to their child, increasing adherence to care. In societies that respect diverse opinions, a health care team that includes the family is preferable to a hierarchical team with physicians at the top, nurses in between, and families at the bottom. Family-centered care attends to the importance of families in health care.

Starting in 1987, Surgeon General Koop began the initiative to include families on the team that provided care for children with special needs. Although the ideas presented were initiated with children with special health care needs (CSHCN), the elements apply to all families with children, and to both well-child care and care for children with diagnosed illnesses. The Association for the Care of Children's Health further defined the specific key elements to family-centered care in 1994. These elements are now widely accepted and used by health care providers and families with children with health care needs (Conway et al., 2006):

1. Recognize that the family is the constant in the child's life, whereas the service systems and personnel within those systems fluctuate.
2. Share complete and unbiased information with parents about their child's health on an ongoing basis. Understand that information may need to be repeated, especially during times of stress (i.e., at the time of diagnosis of an illness or chronic condition).
3. Recognize family strengths and individuality. Respect different methods of coping.
4. Encourage and make referrals for parent-to-parent support, such as parent support groups.
5. Facilitate parent/professional collaboration at all levels of health care—care of an individual child, family care, program development, implementation of child and family policies, and evaluation of policies.

6. Ensure that the design of health care delivery systems is flexible, accessible, and responsive to diverse families.
7. Implement appropriate policies and programs that provide physical, emotional, spiritual, and financial support to children and their families.
8. Understand and incorporate the developmental needs of children and families into the health care delivery systems.

Although family-centered care is recognized as being key in the care of children, the term itself is not consistently defined (Shields, Pratt, & Hunter, 2006) or practiced (Corlett & Twycross, 2006; Power & Franck, 2008). There have been conflicting assumptions between nurses and parents about the degree of parent participation during hospitalization, for instance. Rather than a direct discussion about what caregiving parents wanted and could do, nurses and parents indirectly worked out their roles during their interactions surrounding the care of the child (Corlett & Twycross, 2006). In an integrative review of 11 qualitative studies about family-centered care, Shields et al. (2006) found that care was a negotiation between families and staff; some parents felt imposed on when nurses made the assumption that they would do their children's basic care while in the hospital without discussing it with them first, whereas other parents appreciated the opportunity to provide care for their child.

CONCEPTS OF FAMILY CHILD HEALTH NURSING

Several foundational concepts guide nursing care of families with children: family development or career, including tasks, communication, development of support, transitions, and understanding and working together with family routines; individual development; and transitions (e.g., developmental, situational, and health/illness). Family developmental theories assume that families and individuals change over time. Not only do families experience the various developmental stages of each member, but they also progress through a series of family developmental stages. Nurses, by comparing their observations of particular families to expected family and individual developmental stages, can plan appropriate care (Table 13-2).

Family Career

Family career is the dynamic process of change that occurs during the life span of the unique group called the family. Family career incorporates stages, tasks, and transitions, and is similar to family development theory in that it takes into account family tasks and raising children. These two concepts differ, however, in that family development theory views the family in standard sequential steps, progressing from the birth of the first child, to raising and launching that child, to experiencing the death of a parent figure in old age (Duvall & Miller, 1985). By contrast, family career takes into account the diverse experiences of American families (Aldous, 1996). The family career includes both the expected developmental changes of the family life cycle and the unexpected changes of situational crises, such as divorce, remarriage, and death.

The notion of family career involves the many paths that families can take during their life span. Changes do not necessarily occur in a linear fashion. For example, family career takes into account the possibility that a person without children may marry a partner who already has adolescent children, resulting in starting parenting with adolescent children. This new parent does not build on parenting skills experienced across time, but rather starts his career at the end of his child's childhood career. Family career is a useful concept because it reminds us that families are dynamic. Table 13-3 summarizes the definitions of family career, individual development, and patterns of health/disease/illness in families. Nurses working with child-rearing families need to know that family careers are inclusive of family development stages, transitions, and diversity because these dynamics affect family health.

Family Stages

Duvall's eight stages of family development, derived from information about the oldest child, describes expected developmental changes in families that are raising children (Duvall & Miller, 1985). According to Duvall, family careers start with (1) marriage without children, then proceed to (2) childbearing, (3) preschool children, (4) school children, (5) adolescents, (6) the launching of young adults (i.e., first child gone to last child leaving home), (7) middle age of parents (i.e., empty nest to retirement), and (8) aging of family members (i.e., retirement to death

Table 13-2 Social-Emotional, Cognitive, and Physical Dimensions of Individual Development

Period	Social-Emotional Stages/ Significant Relationships	Stage-Sensitive Family Development Tasks	Values Orientation	Cognitive Stages of Development	Developmental Landmarks	Physical Maturation	Developmental Steps
Infancy Birth–1 year	Trust vs. mistrust (I am what I am given.) Primary parent	Having, adjusting to, and encouraging the development of infants. Establishing a satisfying home for both parents and infant(s). Establishing well-child health care.	Undifferentiated	*Sensory-Motor Ages— Birth–2 years* Infants move from neonatal reflex level of complete self world undifferentiation to relatively coherent organization of sensory-motor actions. They learn that certain actions have specific effects on the environment.	Gazes at complete patterns Social smile (2 mo) 180° visual pursuit (2 mo) Rolls over (5 mo) Ranking grasp (7 mo) Crude purposeful release (9 mo) Inferior pincer grasp Walks unassisted (10–14 mo)	*Rapid (Skeletal)* Transitory reflexes present (3 mo) (i.e., Moro reflex, sucking, grasp, tonic neck reflex) Muscle constitutes 25% of total body weight Birth weight doubles (6 mo) Eruption of deciduous central incisors (5–10 mo) Birth weight triples (1 yr) Anterior fontanel closes (10–14 mo) Transitory reflexes disappear (10 mo) Eruption of deciduous first molars (11–18 mo)	Anticipation of feeding Symbiosis (4–18 mo) Stranger anxiety (6–10 mo) Separation anxiety (8–24 mo) Self-feeding
Toddlerhood 1–3 years	Autonomy vs. shame or doubt (I am what I "will.") Parental persons	Parenting role development. Learning to parent toddler. Developing approaches to discipline. Understanding child's increasing autonomy. Family planning. Providing safe environment. Maintaining well-child health care.	Punishment and obedience	Recognition of the constancy of external objects and primitive internal representation of the world begins. Uses memory to act. Can solve basic problems.	Words: 3–4 (13 mo) Builds tower of 2 cubes (15 mo) Scribbles with crayon (18 mo) Words: 10 (18 mo) Builds tower of 5–6 cubes (21 mo) Uses 3-word sentences (24 mo) Names 6 body parts (30 mo) Uses appropriate personal pronouns, i.e., I, you, me (30 mo) Rides tricycle (36 mo) Copies circle (36 mo) Matches 4 colors (36 mo) Talks to self and others (42 mo) Takes turns (42 mo)	Babinski reflex extinguished (18 mo) Bowel and bladder nerves myelinated (18 mo) Increase in lymphoid tissue Weight gain 2 kg per year (12–36 mo)	Oppositional behavior Messiness Exploratory behavior Parallel play Pleasure in looking at or being looked at Beginning self-concept Orderliness Curiosity

(continued)

Table 13-2   Social-Emotional, Cognitive, and Physical Dimensions of Individual Development (cont.)

Period	Social-Emotional Stages/Significant Relationships	Stage-Sensitive Family Development Tasks	Values Orientation	Cognitive Stages of Development	Developmental Landmarks	Physical Maturation	Developmental Steps
Pre–school-age 3–5 years	Initiative vs. guilt (I am what I imagine I can be.) Basic family	Adapting to the critical needs and interests of preschool children in stimulating, growth-promoting ways. Monitoring child development. Seek developmental screening as needed. Coping with energy depletion and lack of privacy as parents. Socializing children. Providing safe environment/ accident prevention. Maintenance of couple relationship. Fostering sibling relationships.	Punishment and obedience moves to meeting own needs and doing for others if that person will do something for the child.	*Preoperational Thought (Prelogical)—Ages 2–7 years* Begins to use symbols. Thinking tends to be egocentric and intuitive. Conclusions are based on what they feel or what they would like to believe.	Uses 4-word sentences (48 mo) Copies cross (48 mo) Throws ball overhand (48 mo) Copies square (54 mo) Copies triangle (60 mo) Prints name Rides two-wheel bike	Weight gain 2 kg per year (4–6 yr) Eruption of permanent teeth (5.5–8 yr) Body image solidifying	Cooperative play Fantasy play Imaginary companions Masturbation Task completion Rivalry with parents of same sex Games and rules Problem solving Achievement Voluntary hygiene Competes with partners Hobbies Ritualistic play Rational attitudes about food Companionship (same sex) Invests in community leaders, teachers, impersonal ideals
School-Age 6–12 years	Industry vs. inferiority (I am what I learn.) Neighborhood and school	Fitting into the community of school-age families in constructive ways. Letting children go, as they become increasingly independent. Encouraging child's education achievement. Balancing parental needs with children's needs.	Moves from instrumental exchange: "If you scratch my back, I'll scratch yours" into wanting to follow rules to be "good." Then to rule orientation for maintenance of social order.	Concrete Operational Thought—Ages 7–12 years Conceptual organization increasingly stable. Children begin to seem rational and well organized. Increasingly systematic in approach to the world. Weight and volume are now viewed as constant, despite changes in shape and size.	As child moves through stage: Copies diamond, knows simple opposite analogies, names days of the week, repeats 5 digits forward, defines "brave" and "nonsense," knows seasons of the year, able to rhyme words, repeats 5 digits in reverse, understands pity, grief, surprise, knows where sun sets, can define "nitrogen" and "microscope"	Weight gain 2–4 kg per year (7–11 yr) Uterus begins to grow Budding of nipples in girls Increased vascularity of penis and scrotum Pubic hair appears in girls Menarche (9–11 yr)	Task completion Rivalry with parents of the same sex Games and rules Problem solving Achievement Voluntary hygiene Competes with partners Has hobbies Ritualistic play Rational attitudes about food Values companionship Invest in community leaders, teachers, impersonal ideals

Stage	Psychosocial	Family Developmental Tasks	Moral/Ethical	Cognitive (Formal Operational Thought)	Cognitive Milestones	Physical	Developmental Tasks
Adolescence 13–20 years	Identity vs. role confusion (I know who I am.) Peer in-groups and out-groups Adult models of leadership	Balancing freedom with responsibility as teenagers mature and emancipate themselves. Maintaining communication with teen. Establishing post-parental interests and careers as growing parents.	Increasing internalization of ethical standards; can use to make decisions.	*Formal Operational Thought.* Abstract thought and awareness of the world of possibility develop. Adolescents use deductive reasoning and can evaluate the logic and quality of their own thinking. Increased abstract power allows them to work with laws and principles.	Knows why oil floats on water. Can divide 72 by 4 without pencil or paper. Understands "espionage." Can repeat 6 digits forward and 5 digits in reverse.	*Spurt (Skeletal)* Girls 1.5 years ahead of boys. Pubic hair appears in boys. Rapid growth of testes and penis. Axillary hair starts to grow. Down on upper lip appears. Voice changes. Mature spermatozoa (11–17 yr). Acne may appear.	"Revolt" Loosens tie to family Cliques Responsible independence Work habits solidifying heterosexual interests Recreational activities
Early Adulthood	Intimacy vs. isolation Partners in friendship, sex, completion	Releasing young adults into work, military service, college, marriage, and so on, with appropriate rituals and assistance. Maintaining a supportive home base.	Principled social contract			Cessation of skeletal growth Involution of lymphoid tissue Muscle constitutes 43% total body weight Permanent teeth calcified Eruption of permanent third molars (17–30 years)	Preparation for occupational choice Occupational commitment Elaboration of recreational outlets Marriage readiness Parenthood readiness
Middle Adulthood	Generativity vs. self-absorption or stagnation Divided labor and shared household	Refocusing on the marriage relationship. Maintaining kin ties with older and younger generations.	Self-actualization—doing what one is capable of.				
Late Adulthood	Integrity vs. despair, disgust "Humankind" "My kind"	Coping with bereavement and living alone. Closing the family home in adapting to aging. Adjusting to retirement.	Universal ethical principles				

Source: Adapted from Duvall, E. M., & Miller, B. C. (1985). Developmental tasks: Individual and family. In E. M. Duvall & B. C. Miller (Eds.), *Marriage and family development* (6th ed., p. 62). New York, NY: Harper & Row; Prugh, D. (1983). *The psychological aspects of pediatrics.* Philadelphia, PA: Lea & Febiger; Thomas, R. M. (2005). *Comparing theories of child development* (6th ed.). Belmont, CA: Wadsworth.

Table 13-3	Definitions of Family Career, Individual Development, and Patterns of Health/Disease/Illness
Term	**Definition**
Family career	The dynamic process of change that occurs during the life span of the unique group called the family. Whereas family development views the family in standard sequential steps or stages, family career takes into account the diverse experiences of American families that do not occur in anticipated stages.
Individual development	Physical and maturational change of the individual over time. Some theories perceive change as stages, and others as interactional change.
Health and illness	Health is behavior that promotes optimal dimensions of well-being. Family and individual health are multidimensional; therefore, a family and/or member can have a disease and be "healthy" in another dimension of health.
Families and their members experience dimensions of health while managing illness among members.	Illness is a disease (and family management of the disease) that may be acute (time-limited), chronic (live with over time), or terminal (end-of-life).

of both parents). This theory has been challenged with the understanding that families experience several developmental stages at one time as they care for multiple children of different ages and stages, as well as accommodate changes and transitions in family structure through separation, divorce, remarriage, adoption, death of a family member, and families living together across multiple generations. Knowledge of family stages helps nurses anticipate the reorganization necessary to accommodate the expected growth and development of family members. For example, families with school-age children expect children to be able to take care of their own hygiene, whereas families with infants expect to do all the hygiene care. Likewise, family activities shift with the developmental needs of the individual family members. Families with preschoolers may enjoy a day at the playground, whereas families with adolescents would likely not choose this outing. Nurses can serve families better if they understand and work with families at different stages of family development. Nurses can also help families understand competing developmental tasks and transitions across family members and across time.

Family Tasks

Across all family stages, there are basic family functions and tasks essential to survival and continuity (Duvall & Miller, 1985): (1) to secure shelter, food, and clothing; (2) to develop emotionally healthy individuals who can manage crisis and experience nonmonetary achievement; (3) to ensure each individual's socialization in school, work, spiritual, and community life; (4) to contribute to the next generation by giving birth, adopting a child, or fostering a child; and (5) to promote the health of family members and care for them during illness. The aim of nurses is to help families develop appropriate ways to carry out the tasks necessary to prevent or handle illness and disease, and to promote health.

Transitions

Transitions are central to nursing practice because they have profound health-related effects on families and family members (Meleis, Sawyer, Im, Hilfinger Messias, & Schumacher, 2000). Family transitions are events that signal a reorganization of family roles and tasks. The literature supports the idea that how families transition early in their family careers strongly influences future transitions (Meleis et al., 2000). Further, support from health care providers and other sources has a positive impact on transitions through time, from early infancy to transition to adulthood (Rous, Myers, & Stricklin, 2007). The transitions can be developmental, situational, or related to health and illness. Developmental transitions are predictable changes that occur in an expected timeline congruent with movement through the eight family stages (e.g., the addition of a family member by birth). Because they are typical and expected, developmental transitions are also called normative transitions. Thus, family members expect and learn to interact differently as children grow.

Sometimes families may not make the transition to an expected family stage. For example, families with children who have disabilities and are not capable of independent living have difficulty launching their children because of lack of residential living facilities and caregivers.

Situational transitions include changes in personal relationships, roles and status, the environment, physical and mental capabilities, and the loss of possessions (Rankin, 1989; Rankin & Weekes, 2000). Situational transitions are also called non-normative transitions. Not all families experience each situational transition and they can occur irrespective of time. For example, changes occur in personal relationships when a stepchild is integrated into the family group, or when one becomes a new stepparent after divorce and remarriage. Changes in role and status also happen when an only child becomes a sibling after the family adopts another child or when stepsiblings or half-siblings are added to the family structure. This is different than the normative process of having a second child through birth, as the preparation during pregnancy is absent and the adopted or step/half child is often older than an infant; he or she can even be older than the biological only child. Changes in the environment occur when working parents move to a new job and family members adjust to a new house, school, friends, and community. Even greater changes occur when families immigrate to a new country, learn a new language and a new culture, and perhaps have to work at a lower-status job.

A natural disaster can destroy family possessions and heirlooms, resulting in stress, fear, a sense of loss, and problems with family members' ways of being and interacting (Schumacher & Meleis, 1994).

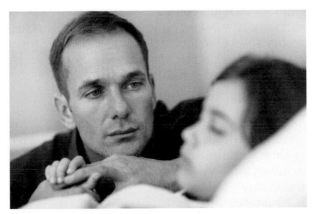

© iStock.com/kupicoo

Cohan and Cole (2002) conducted an important longitudinal study following families for 23 years to evaluate the impact of Hurricane Hugo in 1989 on marriage, birth, and divorce rates. Attachment theory (Bowlby, 1969) was the underlying theory for their work. They hypothesized that family members would become closer following a disaster as a review of literature suggested that children and adults seek close proximity and increase communication when faced with separation. Attachment theory proved true for both marriage and birth rates, as both increased significantly for the year following Hurricane Hugo, which suggested drawing closer together. On the other hand, divorce rates also increased significantly during the year following the disaster. The authors proposed that divorce may be better explained by stress theory, noting couples that are facing major stress, such as a natural disaster, have higher levels of mental illnesses including post-traumatic stress disorder (PTSD), anxiety, and depression. The diagnosis of mental illness in one or both of the spouses has been shown to decrease marital satisfaction. Further, Cohan and Cole (2002) proposed that any natural disaster may motivate families toward change, whether that change is positive (i.e., marriage or birth) or negative (i.e., divorce). The findings from the study show the importance of proximity of children to their parents during natural disasters, and the importance of nurses helping families through transitions following the natural disaster. For further information on nursing care of families dealing with trauma, see Chapter 11.

Health-illness transitions are changes in the meaning and behavior of families as they experience an illness over time. Even though there are different diseases and conditions, the illness experience follows a pattern of prediagnosis with signs and symptoms, crisis of the diagnosis, daily management of the condition called the "long haul," and a resolved or terminal phase (Rolland, 2005). Knowing the trajectory of a condition helps nurses and families recognize transition points and learn new ways of coping. For example, a family that has learned to manage its child's asthma requires new coping strategies when hospitalization occurs after the child's asthma symptoms are complicated by an upper respiratory illness and become too severe to manage at home. The family will need to reorganize itself to deal with the child's hospitalization and possibly learn to implement different asthma management approaches after hospitalization.

Transition events are signals to nurses that families may be at risk for health problems. Although families work to create and implement strategies to keep their children safe, these safety measures often fall behind during times of transition as parents find themselves coping with the stress of transition while continuing to cope with parenting stress. A developmental example is placing a crawling infant in a playpen or other enclosed space temporarily to decrease the risk of falling while the parent is temporarily busy. When the infant transitions from crawling to pulling up to standing and walking, the family needs to allow the child to expand her environment by allowing her out of the security of the playpen and by modifying the environment to make it safe for her. A situational example occurs when a married family transitions to a divorced family. Parents will need to think about new routines for caring for the children. In a two-parent family, one parent may have gotten breakfast ready while the other parent attended to the child. Now one parent will be doing both. An example of a health and illness transition would be when a child is diagnosed with type 1 diabetes mellitus. The family will make major changes in family tasks to accommodate the nutrition and medication needs of one member. Nurses, by assessing families for anticipated changes related to family and child developmental transitions, as well as situational and health-illness transitions, can help families plan for changes.

Individual Development

The individual development of all the family members in nursing care of families with children is important to consider. Child-raising families are complex groups of adults and children at different stages of development. A schematic overview of human development highlights the stages of individual experiences over time. Adult developmental needs may complement or conflict with children's developmental needs.

When nurses review with families the individual family member's developmental stages that are occurring concurrently among children and adults, they validate the complexity of family interactions. Through this review process, nurses can assist families to accommodate to children's and adults' changing needs, abilities, and thought processes across time. Table 13-2 presents three dimensions of individual development: social-emotional, cognitive,

and physical. The table is meant to be a guide and is not all-inclusive; it may not be representative of all cultures or socioeconomic statuses. Nurses can use these dimensions to identify expected developmental progression and potential areas of concern for families. This table can also be used to help understand when parents of children with developmental disabilities may feel recurrent sorrow, as they watch their child miss expected milestones (Blaska, 1998).

NURSING INTERVENTIONS TO SUPPORT CARE OF WELL CHILDREN AND FAMILIES

Families are the context for health promotion and illness care for all family members, including children. Family beliefs, rituals, and routines affect the health of all family members, including, for instance, traditional health practices around food, eating, and types of food served at meals; physical activity and rest; use of alcohol and other substances; and providing care and connection for family members (Novilla, Barnes, De La Cruz, Williams, & Rogers, 2006). Christensen (2004) concluded that the role of families in health promotion of children goes beyond protecting their health, well-being, development, and decreasing risk behavior, to teaching children to be "health promoting actors" by encouraging their active participation in health care, providing information about health care practices, and having the children make their own healthy life choices. Families are, of course, linked to and interact with their larger environments. See Chapter 2 for a discussion on the bioecological theory (Bronfenbrenner, 1997).

In well-child care, families are considered the care environment for their children. Proposed nursing outcomes of current well-child care focus on family functioning and capacity and the ability to care and nurture children while providing a safe and developmentally stimulating environment. Specific outcomes include that parents: (1) are knowledgeable about their children's physical health status and needs; (2) feel valued and supported as their children's primary caregiver and teacher, and function in partnership with their children's health care providers and teachers; (3) are screened for maternal depression, family violence, and family substance abuse and referred to specialists when needed; (4) understand and are able to use well-child care services; (5) understand and can implement developmental monitoring, stimulation, and regulation such as reading regularly to their children; (6) are skilled in anticipating and meeting their children's developmental needs; and (7) have access to consistent sources of emotional support and are linked to appropriate community services (Schor, 2007). Further, parents strongly influence childrens' healthy lifestyle choices through modeling healthy lifestyle behaviors. For example, Allen et al. (2016) discussed in their study of 57 adolescents that the eating patterns of adults had more influence on the adolescent eating patterns than any punitive approaches (i.e., restricting unhealthy foods within the environment). In promoting child and family well-being, nurses support families in care of their children using the following skills and interventions:

- Communicating with families
- Supporting development of parenting skills and healthy family functioning
- Understanding and working with family routines
- Identifying health risks and teaching prevention strategies
- Supporting health promotion in families with children

Communication With Families

Therapeutic communication with family groups is the foundation of nursing care of families with children. One important feature of communication with families with children is including all the family members in a discussion or interaction (Wright & Leahey, 1999). In initial communication, Cooklin (2001) recommends that each family member be asked to introduce himself or herself, beginning with the parent or adults of the family and proceeding with each family member in order of age from oldest to youngest. North American children, in particular, are often valued as autonomous beings. Research supports that children want to be consulted about decisions concerning their education and health care and want their opinions to be respected (Coyne, 2006). This trend is not only considered ethically correct, but also improves childrens' adherence to recommended interventions in both the health and educational

arenas (Hall, 2010; Hamill & Boyd, 2002; Kennedy, 2015; Michael & Frederickson, 2013; Prunty, Dupont, & McDaid, 2012). Nurses can assure children that they have a "real voice" by inviting them to speak, conveying that their opinion really matters, and demonstrating genuine interest in their point of view. Because the role of children in social situations is influenced by family culture, it is important to confirm that the children feel that they have permission to choose how they want to participate and that the parents confirm that they will allow the children to participate freely in the discussion (Cooklin, 2001; Kennedy, 2015).

Another important feature of communication with families is considering and adjusting communication style, content of message, and vocabulary for developmental appropriateness for each family member (Barnes et al., 2002; Cooklin, 2001; Kennedy, 2015; McKinney, James, Murray, & Ashwill, 2005). Engaging children in a casual conversation initiates a beginning relationship. Coyne's study (2006) found that children wanted to "chat" with the nurse, to know a little about the nurse as a person, and wanted the nurse to know about them. Instead of starting the conversation with the reasons behind the hospital visit, children wanted to start the conversation with questions they were familiar with and were used to answering, such as their age, grade, and where they live. Asking children what they are good at, followed by asking about personal experiences, can enhance the start of a therapeutic relationship. Playfulness may assist in establishing communication with children. Children's temperament influences how they engage with new experiences and new people. A quiet, shy child, for example, often wants to watch and see what others are doing before interacting with new people. Instead of asking questions, a nurse may elicit more conversation by inviting the child to color together, or to play together with preferred toys and chat during an activity, instead of putting the focus on what the child is saying. "Draw and tell" or "Play and tell" helps nurses learn what children are thinking and feeling through their actions rather than relying only on words (Driessnack, 2005). Asking children to draw their family and then to tell the nurse about the picture starts a meaningful conversation. As a child becomes more comfortable with the nurse, the nurse can ask the child to draw the clinic or hospital and tell about the picture.

Cognitively, children developmentally move from concrete to abstract thought. Careful explanation of abstract concepts using real objects or age-appropriate stories is especially important when working with children younger than middle-school age. If explaining surgery, for example, children will understand more if shown how the incision and bandage will appear on a doll or stuffed animal with a drawn

incision and bandage on the appropriate body part rather than just explaining the process verbally (Li & Lopez, 2008). Likewise, telling a story about a child going to surgery helps the child understand the event more easily than just telling about the procedure. See Box 13-1 for examples of discussing surgery with children. It is important to validate or confirm with all family members that the message

---

BOX 13-1

Preparing Children and Their Families for Surgery Using Hospital Play

Children learn by doing and playing. Using dolls and real equipment helps children know what to expect and act out their fears. Having parents observe helps them learn how to help their child using play.

Before starting, consult with the physician and parent to learn what information the child has been given. Decide the appropriate explanation for the child's age and emotional maturity. For young children, use neutral words such as *opening, drainage,* and *oozing* instead of *cut* and *bleed.* Gather the visual aids (e.g., pictures, doll) and equipment to be used. Do not give too much information because the child may be overwhelmed. Plan for three sessions: why she needs surgery, what to expect in the operating room, and what she will feel and do after surgery.

If a child has never been in the hospital, have toys familiar to the child such as blocks, doll houses, and stuffed animals available along with "real" equipment such as a doll with bandages similar to what the child will have, operating room masks, scrubs that nurses and doctors wear, and intravenous poles. The child may play with the familiar toys. As the child observes the nurse, tell the story of what will happen to the doll using the "real" equipment on the doll, and the child will learn that the equipment is safe.

Session 1: How Will the Surgery Make You Better?

- Ask the child what she thinks is going to happen. A child may be silent or say, "I do not know," when talking to a stranger. You can repeat a simple explanation reinforcing what she knows.
- Reassure the child that no one is to blame for her condition; make it clear that nothing she did is responsible.
- Using the doll, show where the surgery will take place and what the surgery will do to make her better.

Session 2: What Should the Patient Expect in the Operating Room and What Will Happen Before the Surgery?

- Review why surgery will make the child better.

- Talk about the steps of getting ready for surgery, such as not eating or drinking the night before and how the operation room will smell (alcohol), feel (cold), and look (big lights, a clock, people in special clothes).
- Indicate the child will wear special clothes (hospital gown). *Note:* Toddlers' body image includes keeping on their underwear, because they have just finished learning toilet training.
- Put a mask on the face and talk about a "funny smell." Use a real anesthesia mask on the doll and have the child do this too. This gives the child some control.
- Play with the thermometer, blood pressure cuff, and stethoscope for taking temperatures and listening to heartbeats and breathing on the doll, nurse, and parent.
- Show pictures of an operating room. Point out the "big lights," the clock, the nurses, and doctors dressed in blue (or whatever color your hospital personnel wear in the operating room suites) clothes and wearing "masks." Talk about the ride on a bed with wheels and doors that open in a similar way as grocery store doors. These are things the child is familiar with and will notice.
- Reaffirm that parents will walk with the child to the operating room and be with him or her when the child wakes up from the surgery. Play with a mommy doll walking with the toy doll going to the operating room. The child needs to know that his or her parents know where the child is and will be there for him or her.

Session 3: Postoperative Expectations

Using dolls, act out what will happen after surgery:

- Soreness at the site of surgery
- Pain and medication
- Positioning (how to turn after surgery, deep breathe, and cough)
- Bandages (the word "dressing" may be understood as "turkey dressing" at Thanksgiving, or playing "dress-up")
- No eating and drinking right away

conveyed is understood and to explain medical words fully. Use of clichés, such as "This won't hurt" or "It will be over before you know it," or "We just need to put a tiny stick in your arm" are rarely appropriate when communicating with children and adolescents. The amount of information given also varies across cultures and across individuals. Nurses should be careful not to overwhelm family members, including children, with information they do not want or understand. Many cultures rely and trust health care providers to make health decisions, and when too much information is given, they question that trust. Other cultures and individuals, in contrast, want as much information as possible, and feel uncomfortable when they perceive information is not being shared. Each culture tends to have an identified adult that accepts and conveys information to other family members. These differences should be considered during all teaching opportunities.

Supporting Development of Parenting Skills and Healthy Family Functioning

Providing support for the development of parenting skills is an important nursing intervention. Beginning at birth, children have a need for warm, affectionate relationships with parents. One of the earliest parenting skills found to establish healthy caregiving behavior is a parent's responsiveness to the infant's cues. Responsiveness is noticing and interpreting the infant's cues, then acting promptly in response to those cues. For example, if an infant looks away from a parent, a responsive parent will decrease stimulation until the infant turns back and re-establishes eye contact. An integrative research review about responsive parenting concluded that in developed countries maternal responsiveness in early childhood was positively correlated with long-term positive outcomes that have an impact on lifetime events, including increased intelligence quotient (IQ), improved social relationships, and improved health, whereas unresponsiveness was associated with lower IQs, poorer quality social relationships, and higher incidence of childhood behavior problems (Ermisch, Jantti, & Smeeding, 2012). In low-income countries, maternal responsiveness was associated with increased IQ, as well as with increased survival and growth, which was thought to be related to improved nutrition through positive

interaction during meal times (Eshel, Daelmans, de Mello, & Martines, 2006). Likewise, a study of 40 European American mothers revealed a strong relationship between a mother's interaction with toddlers and preschoolers and the child's rate of development (Bornstein, Tamis-LeMonda, Hahn, & Haynes, 2008). In a study focused on preventing disruption of early attachment and nurturing, Spieker, Oxford, Kelly, Nelson, & Flaming, (2012) used an evidence-based curriculum to teach nurturing and attachment skills to foster mothers caring for toddlers in the child welfare system. After 6 months, the sensitivity of the foster mothers and the developmental and self-regulation skills of the toddlers showed a modest improvement. This study emphasizes the importance of nurses teaching and supporting foster parents as they learn important parenting skills.

Parenting Styles

After the infancy period, parents begin to develop a "style" of nurturing and caring for their children. Parenting style tends to be learned from families of origin through modeling, and therefore tends to be passed down from generation to generation (Ermisch et al., 2012). The parenting style of either two-parent or one-parent families influences outcomes in children, including health, academic achievement, and social development (Baumrind, 1991, 2005; Ermisch et al., 2012; Richaud de Minzi, 2006).

Authoritative Parenting Style

An authoritative parenting style is characterized by reciprocity, mutual understanding, shared decision making, and flexibility (Sorkhabi, 2005). Although parents using this style convey clear expectations and "demands" of their children, those expectations take into consideration their children's developmental level and individual strengths, weaknesses, and personality traits, and parents provide rationale for and support to meet those characteristics, as well as warmth in their relationship with the children (Baumrind, 2005). This parenting style promotes feelings of competence in the children. The ultimate goal is to promote positive self-esteem and autonomy in their children. Authoritative parenting styles influence health by providing the ongoing message that the children have some control over good health and healthy lifestyle choices and have a positive responsibility to care for their own health through these life choices (Luther, 2007). The outcomes of this parenting style are positive across time and across cultures. Although behaviors may be more difficult during preschool years as children are given more chances to negotiate with parents than with other parenting styles, long-term outcomes tend to be better (Underwood, Beron, & Rosen, 2009). Variables studied include self-reliance, self-competence, academic performance, socially accepted behavior, and social acceptance. Williams, Ciarrochi, and Heaven (2012) illustrated that authoritative parenting styles increased flexible problem-solving skills of adolescents across 6 years compared with other parenting styles. Other family characteristics associated with healthy authoritative parenting and well-child health outcomes include parental engagement, closeness, communication, positive discipline techniques, and healthy role modeling. These positive qualities have correlated with increased social competence and self-esteem, health-promoting behaviors, and less substance abuse, as well as fewer externalizing (e.g., aggression and anger) and internalizing behaviors (e.g., depression).

Authoritarian Parenting Style

Authoritarian parenting style, in contrast, is an inflexible and unilateral style in which parents have clear expectations and demands of their children, but insist on compliance with the parental perception of what is best for their children, with limited explanation and rationale or acceptance of their children's perceptions (Sorkhabi, 2005). The authoritarian style promotes the belief that children should not control their own behavior and cannot contribute to decisions about their own health care because they do not have the knowledge or experience needed to make good decisions (Luther, 2007). Several studies have shown short- and long-term negative effects of authoritarian parenting styles across ethnic groups and cultures. For example, children raised by authoritarian parents tend to be less socially accepted and less self-reliant and have poorer academic outcomes across the United States, India, and China (Chen, Dong, & Zhou, 1997; Rao, McHale, & Pearson, 2003; Steinberg, Dornbusch, & Brown, 1992; Steinberg, Lamborn, Dornbusch, & Darling, 1992). When asking adults to recall parenting styles used by their parents, those who recalled authoritarian parents have a higher rate of depressive symptoms and poor psychological adjustment across time (Rothrauff, Cooney, & An, 2009). Family aggression and parental aggravation commonly found in authoritarian parenting were associated with less social competence, less health-

promoting behavior, and lower self-esteem scores (Youngblade et al., 2007). The long-held consensus is that children fare better when praised than when criticized or punished (Schmittmann, Visser, & Raijmakers, 2006).

Permissive Parenting Style

Permissive parenting style allows children to pursue child-determined goals with little guidance from the parents. Parents using this style tend to ignore behavior problems and may not provide the organizational support needed to assist children in reaching goals (Sorkhabi, 2005). Children raised in the permissive style are less assertive and achievement oriented, and are more likely to develop ineffective and possibly dangerous coping strategies such as using drugs, compared with authoritative and authoritarian parenting styles (Baumrind, 1991; Washington & Dunham, 2011). Permissive parents can be nurturing and warm, but too passive to establish healthy boundaries. Or they may be rejecting or neglecting in their parenting style, in which case, along with having limited expectations and responsiveness, these parents can also be punitive and have a negative reaction to parent-child interactions, as well as a lack of parental involvement with the children. This passive, but negative, parenting style is also associated with generally poor academic and social-emotional outcomes (Baumrind, 1991; Williams et al., 2012).

Uninvolved Parenting Style

The fourth parenting style studied is the uninvolved parent. This parenting style is similar to the permissive parenting style, except the parent(s) not only lacks clear boundaries and expectations, but also lacks any nurturing, warmth, and responsiveness (Maccoby & Martin, 1983). The outcomes of these children are considered far worse than the first three parenting styles, with children being at risk for negative coping strategies, including poor academic performance, drug abuse, criminal behavior, and poor social acceptance across time (Steinberg, 2001).

The findings regarding parenting style and childhood outcomes span cultures and geographical locations. One review paper, for example, concluded that in collectivist or interdependent cultures, authoritarian and authoritative styles had similar outcomes as found in individualist cultures (Sorkhabi, 2005). The effects not only cross cultures, but also cross time, as studies showing similar outcomes across cultures have been consistent from the early studies in the 1980s to more recent studies into the 2000s (Ermisch et al., 2012; Rao et al., 2003).

Specific Nursing Interventions Regarding Parenting Styles

Nurses can teach about parenting styles and help parents adopt authoritative parenting strategies when doing health promotion and illness care with child-raising families (Bond & Burns, 2006). Numerous studies have revealed that increasing knowledge about parenting increases authoritative parenting practices. Likewise, authoritative parents often seek out parenting knowledge from the moment they discover they will be parents (Washington & Dunham, 2011). Early interest in parenting leads to early positive attachment practices, and later warm and involved parenting strategies. Differing parenting styles between the two parents in one family can cause conflict in both stable and divorced families. Using counseling and education with parents can help them recognize and reflect on their differences, which can lead to a united change toward more authoritative practices.

Nursing interventions for family-focused well-child care include identification of teachable moments to discuss child development, explore parental feelings, model positive interactions with children, and reframe parents' negative attributions about their children's behavior. For example, a nurse may help a parent to see that a child's temper tantrum may be a sign of independence and a need to communicate new thoughts, opinions, and feelings without having the language or emotional regulation skills to do so, rather than the child deliberately attempting to embarrass or disobey the parent. The positive health outcomes from parents learning more appropriate parenting include the use of less physical and harsh discipline approaches, increased use of safety strategies such as placing newborns on their backs to sleep, increased likelihood that children will have up-to-date vaccines, and increased family time spent in pleasurable interactions and shared experiences. Nursing actions to reduce negative outcomes in child-raising families are to identify parental risk factors associated with abuse/neglect such as depression, family violence, poverty, high stress, lack of support, drug and alcohol use, and cigarette smoking (Zuckerman, Parker, Kaplan-Sanoff, Augustyn, & Barth, 2004). In contrast, children's readiness for school has been found to be related to identifying and supporting parental strengths, promoting strong parent-child relationships, teaching parents about child development, and involving parents in activities that encourage learning (Zigler, Pfannenstiel, & Seitz, 2008).

Understanding and Working With Family Routines

Establishing daily routines and family rituals is an important health promotion strategy. These predictable patterns influence the physical, mental, and social health of children, as well as the health of the family itself (Denham, 2002). Nurses help families integrate physical, social-emotional, and cognitive health promotion into family routines; in doing so, they affirm positive patterns of health or provide alternative ones (Greening, Stoppelbein, Konishi, Jordan, & Moll, 2007). Discussing or observing family routines and rituals offers the potential, in a nonthreatening way, to gain entry and understand family dynamics to a greater depth (Denham, 2003). Routines are important to all families in all settings. For instance, predictable and familiar routines were used by parents in homeless shelters to preserve family bonds and their connection with their community (Schultz-Krohn, 2004). Conversely, because routines and rituals have great meaning and stability for families, it is important to recognize that they are potential threats and barriers when implementing new prevention or treatment interventions, as these changes will change the stability and predictability of a family's routines and rituals (Segal, 2004). Nurses can help families understand the importance of maintaining healthy routines, especially during times of transition such as divorce or hospitalization.

Child Care, After-School Activities, and Children's Health Promotion

Child-raising families nurture children through partnerships with siblings, extended family members, nonrelated child-care providers, teachers, and other adults within the community. These relationships help to establish and maintain the family routines that are so important to health and child development. An important trend of American families today is the increasing number of mothers in the workforce requiring assistance with child care. This trend is partly caused by economic changes, increases in family instability and divorce, and the continued increase in the number of single-headed households, primarily headed by women. In 1975, 47% of women with children under age 18 years were in the labor force; by 1990, that figure was 52% (Bianchi, 1995). In 2015, close to 71% of mothers were in the labor force, with three out of four working full time (U.S. Department of Labor, Bureau of Labor Statistics,

2016). Sixty-four percent of working mothers had children under the age of 6 years (U.S. Department of Labor, Bureau of Labor Statistics, 2016).

Another important trend is the speed at which mothers return to work after the birth of their babies. In 1960, only 10% of mothers worked within 3 months of giving birth. In 2009, that percentage rose to 42% (Bianchi, 1995), and by 2010 that percentage rose to 57% (U.S. Department of Labor, Bureau of Labor Statistics, 2016). This trend continues to grow in spite of mounting evidence that children fare better when parents provide care for the first year of life (Offer & Schneider, 2011). Another important trend is the decreased birth rate for women with higher education levels. This trend is international, and highest among Japanese women. The societal impact is a growing number of low-educated mothers raising a majority of children. Meanwhile, low-educated men are choosing not to marry or have children. This trend has caused, in part, the growing number of low-educated single women raising children, whereas highly educated professional couples are choosing to have fewer children or no children at all. Family care policies are changing internationally to address this trend, with increased paid time off, increased support of early childhood education, increased support for fathers caring for young children to allow mothers to return to work, and increased pressure on employers to secure parents' jobs and job opportunities regardless of family leave.

Many families search for the best routines to balance family and work. Care for children while mothers are at work is divided between fathers, grandparents, other relatives, friends, neighbors, other nonpaid care, lay professional care (e.g., nannies and unlicensed providers), licensed home care providers, or licensed and certified center care providers. In 2011, the trend for care while parent(s) worked continued to be split between relatives and paid nonrelative employees. Twenty-one percent of the 10.8 million children younger than 5 years whose mothers were employed were cared for by a grandparent during their mother's working hours. A slightly lower percentage was cared for in a home-based or center-based child-care facility or preschool (19%). Fathers cared for 21% of children, whereas siblings cared for 1%, and other relatives cared for 5% during mothers' working hours (U.S. Census Bureau, 2013). Today, that trend continues with 51% of children being cared for by their parents up until age 3, and 31% being cared for in formal child-care centers (Offer & Schneider, 2011). Some parents strive to work nontraditional hours, work flexible hours, and work while caring for their children to avoid the risks and costs of formal child care. Studies reveal, however, that parents working either nontraditional hours or trying to work while caring for their infant spend less quality time with their infant than other mothers, and struggle to find consistent and high-quality care for their children during nontraditional hours (Moss, 2009). Moss (2009) found, in a qualitative study of parents in New Zealand, that when given a choice most parents would choose to work fewer hours when caring for young children, but feel they cannot make that choice because of the effect on family finances and job opportunities. Although studies have not been done in recent years, similar results have been found in past studies in the United States across socioeconomic classes (Hertz & Ferguson, 1996).

The quality of early childhood education and support for children is an ongoing concern for parents and societies. Multiple studies have documented the importance of education and training of early childhood teachers, developmentally appropriate environments, activities and equipment, and a recommended safe and effective teacher. Things to consider include child/teacher ratio, culturally appropriate learning strategies, family involvement, and nurturing and caring interactions between the teacher and the children. Nevertheless, most families are forced to choose child care based on cost rather than quality. Not surprisingly, families in poverty who paid for child care in 2010 spent a greater proportion of their monthly income on child care than did families at or above the poverty level (i.e., 30% compared with 7%) (U.S. Census Bureau, 2013). The cost of child care ranges by age of the child and geographic area of the family. Annual child care cost in 2016 ranged from a low of $5045 in Mississippi to a high of $17,082 in Massachusetts (Child Care Aware of America, 2016). Nurses can assist with this concern by educating families about employers providing stipends or pretax payments of child care, or about use of government stipends and tax credits for child care, by referring families to Child Care Resource and Referral Services (Child Care Resource and Referral Network, 2017) and by discussing with them the possibility of flex hours to share child-care responsibilities between mothers and fathers. Families composed of minority groups and families with children with disabilities require special consideration when choosing child-care and after-school options (U.S. Census Bureau, 2013).

School-age children often attend before- and after-school care programs. Some children care for themselves and that number increases with the age of the child. The number of children spending time home alone has dropped from 20% in 1997 to 11% in 2010 (U.S. Census Bureau, 2013). It is important that families whose children care for themselves understand safety measures, such as having a contact person the child can call in an emergency; concealing the house key during the school day so that it is not readily apparent that the child will be going home alone; and setting rules about safety, allowing friends in the house when parents are not present, and screen time (e.g., television, video games, and computer). Nurses can educate parents on the risks for children being alone at home during afternoon and early evening hours, including loneliness, increased fears, increased criminal activity, and increased adolescent sexual activity and teen pregnancy. Nurses need to be aware of state and local laws governing when a child can be left home alone without adult supervision.

Nurses, parents, teachers, governmental agencies, and other invested community members must work together to continue to develop before- and after-school programs at schools, homework telephone services with teachers and teachers' aides during the school year, and community center programs during the summer months, holidays, and other times when school is not in session and parents have to continue to work. Nurses can help families review the types of child care and after-school options available and examine the site for health protection features. They can also participate on community boards that advocate for and regulate these facilities.

By supporting working parents and care of children during working hours, healthy and predictable family routines are better maintained. Lack of reliable, predictable, and safe care for children during work hours is a significant threat to family health. Studies have consistently shown that structured, quality after-school activities, including homework clubs, sports, extra-curricular involvement, and religious programs, decrease juvenile crime, improve or sustain academic achievement, reduce the risk of obesity, and improve self-esteem. Homework assistance from adults after school decreases arguments between children and parents about homework completion (Cosden, Morrison, Gutterrex, & Brown, 2004). Structure and positive adult contact are important for children throughout their childhood, including the hours between school and the end of their parents' work day.

Identifying Health Risks and Teaching Prevention Strategies

Because of the relationship between health behaviors and illness or death, increased attention to unhealthy social-emotional behaviors is an important part of nursing practice in families with children. Specifically, nurses assess for, identify, and provide interventions to reduce risk factors associated with morbidity (sickness) and mortality (death). Specific risk factors include:

- Safety concerns for unintentional and intentional injuries and death
- Patterns leading to overweight and obese children and adolescents
- Lack of parenting knowledge and support associated with family violence and child maltreatment
- Health concerns more common to families living in poverty, including higher rates of violence, drug use, and teen pregnancy

Unintentional and Intentional Injuries

The leading cause of death among children and youth from age 1 to 24 years is unintentional injuries from accidents. In 2015, more than 12,000 children, ages 1 to 24 years, died from unintentional injuries (Center for Disease Control and Prevention, 2016). The leading cause of unintentional injuries is motor vehicle crashes, which cause the death of an average of six children per day between the ages of 1 to 24 years (NHTSA.dot.gov, Center for Disease Control and Prevention, 2016). The factor that most contributes to these deaths is the failure of children and adolescents to use seat belts, or infants to use appropriate car seats (National Center for Injury Prevention and Control, 2016). The risk for motor vehicle crashes is higher among youth ages 16 to 19 years than for any other group; substance abuse, primarily alcohol and marijuana, is considered a contributing factor in a majority of these accidents (Center for Disease Control and Prevention, 2016). Nurses can teach families that children of all ages should be properly restrained for their age and body size in motor vehicles, and that all adolescents participate in traffic education classes and receive repeated information on the risks of driving while under the influence of drugs and/or alcohol. A growing concern is the number of motor vehicle accidents caused by individuals using cell phones for texting while driving. As of December 2014, a staggering 10% of adolescents, ages 15 to 19 years old, involved in a fatal crash were found to be distracted by technology immediately before the crash (U.S. Department of Transportation, 2016). Prevention is the key intervention to reduce these statistics. Nurses can emphasize to parents that they are responsible for modeling safe driving habits, including always using seat belts, refraining from talking on a cell phone or texting during driving, and never driving under the influence of alcohol or other mind-altering substances (i.e., medications).

Intentional injuries are the second highest cause of death in children, particularly adolescents. Homicide and suicide are the second and third leading cause of death for children ages 12 to 19 (Center for Disease Control and Prevention, 2016). Suicide rates increase for minority groups throughout the United States. For example, Native Alaskan and Native American youth between the ages of 10 and 18 years have a suicide rate of 16.93 per 100,000, compared with an overall rate of 12.08 per 100,000 (Suicide Prevention Resource Center, 2016). The access to firearms, especially in high-risk groups, increases this risk.

Family child health care nurses can teach and support families in the prevention of unintentional and intentional injuries. For example, nurses can teach about appropriate car seat restraints and water safety. They can educate parents on child-proofing the home to prevent poisoning from household supplies and electrical burns from uncovered electrical outlets in toddlers. Teaching the importance of bicycle helmet use and helping families locate resources when they have limited financial means for purchasing helmets can help to minimize head trauma from bike accidents. Nurses, either in an informal role as a next-door neighbor or in a formal role through working at community or clinic programs, can help parents understand the importance of using approved safety devices, such as car seats, helmets, and door/cabinet locks.

Nurses can be key educators in recognizing signs and symptoms of suicide in adolescents, and can support friends and family members in getting help when these signs and symptoms are identified. Many communities are adopting suicide prevention strategies to reduce suicide rates, including decreasing risk factors (e.g., bullying, exposure to violence) and increasing protective factors (e.g., cultural connectiveness, improved access and awareness of mental health care, support for diverse sexual and gender identity, decreasing access to firearms, increasing mental health identification and treatment, prevention and treatment for substance abuse, and development of crisis response teams for major family and community traumas) (Suicide Prevention Resource Center, 2016). Nurses are important to these efforts, from both the individual and family level of education and support to the community level of advocacy and participation in identifying and supporting needed change.

Obesity and Overweight in Families With Children

Nurses help families recognize the harm that can result from obesity and offer methods to intervene in this leading public health problem. Although obesity rates in children have reached a plateau during the past decade, the rates continue to be a major concern for children's health. Studies across the past 5 years indicate that up to 27% of all children ages 2 to 5 years were overweight (Ogden, Carroll, Kit, & Flegal, 2012). Between 1980 and 2010, the percentage of children ages 6 to 11 years who were obese increased from 7% to 32.6%; for adolescents, it increased from 5% to 33.6% (Ogden, Carroll, Kit, & Flegal, 2012). Overweight and obese family members, including children, are at increased risk for type 2 diabetes, hypertension, hyperlipidemia, cancer, asthma, joint problems, social rejection, and depression (Jeffreys, Smith, Martin, Frankel, & Gunnell, 2004; Miller, Rosenbloom, & Silverstein, 2004; Ogden et al., 2012; Urrutia-Rojas et al., 2006). Prevention and treatment are crucial to the child and family's well-being.

The causes of childhood obesity and overweight are complex, involving the environment (e.g., home and society), genetics, family attitudes and beliefs, cultural practices, nutritional practices, and family activities (Allen et al., 2016; Baughcum, Burklow, Deeks, Powers, & Whitaker, 1998; Bruss, Morris, & Dannison, 2003; Ritchie, Welk, Styne, Gerstein, & Crawford, 2005). Family beliefs, mediated by cultural and family traditions, are thought to affect family eating behaviors (Allen et al., 2016; Baughcum et al., 1998; Bruss et al., 2003). Societal and environmental changes that include decreased physical activity, perceived threats to safety resulting in children playing indoors rather than outdoors, increased screen time, and greater consumption of high-calorie fast foods in the community and schools has contributed to the rise in obesity around the world.

Research about obesity has been a focus on a state and national level for the past decade, but effective strategies to address the problem have remained elusive. Because it is difficult to lose weight, prevention of overweight—particularly in the preschool years, a time when children are prone to become overweight or obese—is seen as one important approach (Wofford, 2008). A combined approach of education for families and children and support for changes in policies, such as building safe bike trails, offering better meals at schools, and reducing fast food access while replacing access to healthier foods, will likely have the greatest influence on reducing overweight in families. Parental involvement as role models for lifestyle changes including physical activity and healthy eating has been found to be essential in the prevention and treatment of obesity in children (Floriani & Kennedy, 2007; Skiakodegard et al., 2016; Wofford, 2008).

Supporting families in use of an authoritative approach to parenting and helping them to develop sensitive but clear parental expectations regarding self-care and food and activity choices are important nursing interventions (Luther, 2007). Specifically, childhood overweight management in families includes providing children with nutrient-dense foods; reducing children's access to high-calorie, nutrient-poor beverages and food; avoiding excessive restriction of food and use of food as a reward; encouraging children to eat breakfast; finding ways to make physical activity fun; reducing children's television, computer, and video time; and teaching parents to model healthful eating practices for children (Hodges, 2003; Ritchie et al., 2005). The American Medical Association (AMA) recommends encouraging families to eat meals at home, limit meals outside the home, and avoid giving children highly sweetened beverages (i.e., soda and excess juice); the AMA also specifies that children should get 1 hour or more of physical activity per day (AMA, 2007). Nurses can influence children's health and weight not only by helping families consider their eating and exercise activities, but also by contributing to community actions that will work in concert with family health behavioral changes. Communities that provide healthy outdoor activities, safe bicycle trails and sidewalks, and community events that encourage activity and healthy eating can help prevent obesity on a community level.

Child Maltreatment

Nurses recognize situations in which children are in danger because of child maltreatment. In 2014, an estimated 702,000 cases of child abuse and neglect occurred and approximately 1580 children died from abuse or neglect (U.S. Department of Health and Human Services, Administration for Children and Families, 2016). Children ages birth to 1 year had the highest rate of victimization of maltreatment at 68.3 per 1000 cases. Physical abuse is generally defined as a nonaccidental physical injury to the child and can include striking, kicking, burning, or biting the child by a parent, sibling, child-care provider, or other adult. Physical abuse represents 17% of child maltreatment. Child neglect is defined as not providing for a child's basic physical, educational, or emotional needs and represents 75% of child maltreatment (U.S. Department of Health and Human Services, Administration for Children and Families, 2016). In 2014, almost 8.3% of all cases of child maltreatment involved sexual abuse, and psychological maltreatment accounted for 6%. Psychological maltreatment is defined as child exploitation (i.e., child prostitution), threats (i.e., threat to kill child), and isolation. Approximately 2% of the cases involved medical neglect. Some children were victims of more than one type of abuse. Children with disabilities are especially vulnerable. Nearly 9% of victims had a reported disability, a figure that is difficult to substantiate, as not all states are required to report the number of abused victims by disability. Abuse can also lead to permanent disabilities, ranging from physical injury to lifelong mental illness. Other groups who are at higher risk for maltreatment are children of unwanted pregnancies, those living in homes where substances are abused, those living with a parent with a mental health disorder, and children with difficult temperaments. Nearly 80% of perpetrators of maltreatment were parents, and most victims know their perpetrators. More than half of all reports of abuse came from professionals involved with the children and families, including health care providers and teachers (U.S. Department of Health and Human Services, Administration for Children and Families, Administration on Children, 2016).

Child maltreatment represents a problem in family behavior that demands immediate assessment and action/intervention. Nurses are mandatory reporters and are required by law to report to authorities when they suspect that a child is being maltreated. It is important for nurses who work with children and families to understand their legal and ethical responsibilities. The Child Welfare Information Gateway (2014) provides specific information about mandatory reporting laws per state.

Nurses screen families for domestic violence by asking questions regarding the safety of the home and the incidence of family violence within the home. See Box 13-2 (Gedaly-Duff, Stoeger, & Shelton, 2000) for pertinent questions regarding family violence that affects families with children. Inquiring about family violence can be uncomfortable for nurses and other health professions. Family violence occurs across social, economic, and ethnic groups. The standard of practice is to ask all families these questions so that the stigma becomes standardized. Families frequently will seek help if given the opportunity to talk about their situations (Hibbard, Desch, Committee on Child Abuse Neglect, & Council on Children With Disabilities, 2007). By screening for family violence, nurses can assess families and children for dangerous situations, teach safety, and make a referral as necessary.

Prevention is the preferred approach for intervening with families regarding child maltreatment. Nurses identify situations that might foster child maltreatment and intervene accordingly. Risk factors thought to contribute to abuse are categorized into four domains: parent or caregiver factors, family factors, child factors, and environmental factors. Parent or caregiver factors include personality characteristics (e.g., low self-esteem, depression, poor impulse control), a history of abuse in the parent's own childhood, substance abuse, attitudes about child behavior, inaccurate knowledge about child development, inappropriate expectations of the child, and younger maternal age. Family factors include marital conflict, domestic violence, single parenthood, unemployment, financial stress, and social isolation. Child factors include age, with younger children and infants being the most vulnerable; presence of disabilities or chronic illness; and difficult temperaments. Environmental factors include poverty, unemployment, and social isolation. In all cases it is important to remember that the presence of risk factors is not an indication that the parents or family members are, in fact, abusive (U.S. Department of Health and Human Services, Administration on Children, Youth and Families, 2016). Rather, when the nurse identifies the presence of various stressors and risks, it may be appropriate to evaluate and implement interventions that may decrease the potential for abuse.

Nurses should also keep in mind the following protective factors against child abuse and neglect: parental resilience, social connections, knowledge of child development, concrete support in times of need, increased social and emotional competence of children, and non-acceptance of abuse by the community and larger society (Moxley, Squires, & Lindstrom, 2012). Strategies thought to help families are those that facilitate friendships and mutual support, strengthen parenting by teaching

---

BOX 13-2
Family Violence Screening Questions

Right Now, Who Is Living at Home With You and Your Child?

- Is everyone getting along well at home or is there a lot of stress, arguing, or fighting?
- Has anybody ever been hit or hurt, pushed, or shoved in a fight or argument at your house?
- Has anybody in the family been in trouble with the police or in jail?
- Is anybody worried that your children have been disciplined too harshly?
- Is anybody worried that your children have been touched inappropriately or sexually abused?

- Is there anybody living with you or close to you who drinks a lot or uses drugs?
- Are there guns, knives, or other weapons at your house?
- Has anything major (e.g., people dying, losing jobs, disasters or accidents) happened recently in your family?
- What is the best part and the worst part of life for you right now?

and modeling appropriate behavior with children, respond to family crises, link families to services, facilitate children's social and emotional development, and value supporting parents (Horton, 2003; Moxley et al., 2012). For example, social support from peers and professionals has been shown to be positively related to health promotion efforts in adolescent mothers (Black & Ford-Gilboe, 2004). The difference between discipline and abuse may be unclear because of different cultural traditions, but nurses must be alert to helping families learn appropriate discipline measures (Stein & Perrin, 1998). Children's early nurturing experiences and attachment relationships with their caring adults affect their future relationships and well-being.

Specific Adolescent Risks

Adolescents as a group are especially vulnerable to high-risk behaviors that can lead to illness and death. Data on the prevalence of risk behaviors among adolescents are collected by the Youth Risk Behavior Surveillance System (YRBS), using a national probability sample of 9th to 12th graders, state and local school-based surveys, and a national household-based survey (CDC, 2011). Between 2010 and 2011 in the United States, 21% of all deaths among persons age 10 to 24 years resulted from four causes: unintentional injuries or accidents (39.7%), homicide (13.6%), suicide (17.4%), and cancers (6.3%) (CDC, 2016). Health behaviors that contributed to unintentional injury or to violence were the use of alcohol and other substances, nonuse of seat belts, distractions during driving such as texting, and availability of weapons. Other health behaviors that contributed to illness and death were tobacco use, poor nutrition, sedentary lifestyle, and sexual behaviors that led to pregnancies and sexually transmitted infections (STIs).

The 2011 YRBS report revealed that adolescents often engaged in behaviors associated with significant morbidity and mortality. Nationwide, 70.8% reported drinking alcohol, with 38% reporting having alcohol within 30 days of taking the survey (a decrease from 45% in 2007), 24.1% had ridden with a driver who had been drinking alcohol, 8% had rarely or never worn a seat belt, and 23.1% had used marijuana. Twenty-six percent of all adolescents in school currently used tobacco. Thirty-three percent of high school students had experienced sexual intercourse within 3 months before the survey. Among students who were sexually active, only 60.2% reported using a condom at their last intercourse (CDC, 2011).

Violence is a significant risk factor for morbidity and mortality among adolescents. In 2014, the second and third leading causes of death for young people ages 15 to 34 were homicide and suicide (CDC, 2016). In 2014, there were 322 adolescent firearm deaths (CDC, 2016). In 2011, 5% of high school students carried a gun on school property, and 7% were threatened or injured by a weapon (e.g., gun, knife, or club) on school property (National Association of School Psychologists, 2017). Child and youth access to firearms is part of the problem. A significant percentage of adults who have minor children living in their homes report their firearms are not safely stored (Johnson, Miller, Vriniotis, Azrael, & Hemenway, 2006). Children's reports often contradict parental reports about their children's access to firearms, with children reporting knowing the location of firearms and handling firearms when parents said they did not. This is true whether or not parents lock firearms and discuss firearm safety with their children (Baxley & Miller, 2006; Grossman et al., 2005).

The American Academy of Pediatrics (AAP; 2012) takes a public health position to prevent firearm injuries by removal of guns from families' homes and communities, however; it is crucial that education in gun use also occur. In 2013, the Emergency Nurses Association made a public statement that safety for children by removing firearms in the home is a crucial step in decreasing injury and death from firearms. Nurses should include screening for guns in the home and incorporate a discussion and information about gun safety with parents. Specific results from the 2011 National Youth Risk Behavior Survey follow.

Many high school students are engaged in priority health-risk behaviors associated with the leading causes of death among persons aged 10 to 24 years in the United States. During the 30 days before the survey, 32.8% of high school students nationwide had texted or e-mailed while driving, 38.7% had drunk alcohol, and 23.1% had used marijuana. During the 12 months before the survey, 32.8% of students had been in a physical fight, 20.1% had been bullied on school property, and 7.8% had attempted suicide. Many high school students nationwide are engaged in risky sexual behaviors associated with unintended pregnancies and STIs, including human immunodeficiency virus (HIV) infection. Nearly half (47.4%) of students reported that they had engaged in sexual intercourse, 33.7% had engaged in sexual intercourse during the 3 months before the survey (i.e., currently sexually active), and 15.3% had engaged in sexual intercourse with four or more partners during their life. Among currently sexually active students, 60.2% had used a condom during their last sexual intercourse. Results from the 2011 national YRBS also indicate many high school students are engaged in behaviors associated with the leading causes of death among adults aged ≥ 25 years in the United States. During the 30 days before the survey, 18.1% of high school students had smoked cigarettes and 7.7% had used smokeless tobacco (CDC, 2011, p. 1).

Family nurses in school-based health clinics are especially well placed to participate in health prevention programs directed at high-risk behaviors leading to STIs and early pregnancy, depression, injuries, substance use, suicidal ideation, and violence. In addition, nurses have a crucial role in educating parents, especially those of adolescents, how to address safety and risk behaviors.

An alternate approach to risk assessment is to support what young people need to facilitate positive development. The America's Promise Alliance program (2017) lists the assets believed to be protective for children and predictive of positive outcomes and behaviors: violence avoidance, thriving (i.e., having a special talent or interest that gives them joy), good school grades, and volunteering. The program's five "Promises," or goals for positive outcomes, are (1) presence of caring adults, (2) safe places and constructive use of time, (3) a healthy start, (4) effective education, and (5) opportunities to make a difference. One large study demonstrated that the presence of four to five Promises resulted in positive adolescent development outcomes. Still, the same study found that only a minority of youth experienced enough of the Promises that were related to positive outcomes. Furthermore, non-Hispanic white youth were much more likely to experience the Promises than were Hispanic and African American youth (Scales et al., 2008). The primary goal in 2013 of the America's Promise Alliance program is to increase the nation's high school graduation rates.

The Influence of Poverty

Socioeconomic factors, such as poverty, lack of education, little or no health insurance, and immigrant status, are strong risk factors related to poor health (Hardy, 2002). There is evidence that behavioral symptoms of child psychiatric disorders are associated with poverty and that those symptoms can be reduced as the family moves out of poverty (Costello,

Compton, Keeler, & Angold, 2003). Programs that provide families with employment, adequate income, day care, and health insurance have been shown to have positive effects on academic achievement, classroom behavior, and aspirations (Huston et al., 2001). Children from families from ethnic minority backgrounds are more likely to live below the poverty line (Annie E. Casey Foundation, 2014) and thus they are at risk for health problems.

Families with limited financial resources and those who do not have health insurance have more difficulty with health promotion than families with insurance or other methods of payment. In the United States in 2010, 22% of children (16 million) were poor, meaning that they lived in households where the income was below $22,350 for a family of two adults and two children (National Center for Children in Poverty, 2014). In the United States in 2011, 9% of all children (6.8 million) were uninsured. Thirteen percent of children who lived in families with incomes at or below 100% of the federal poverty level were uninsured (National Center for Children in Poverty, 2014). Minority families are consistently found to be less likely to have health insurance than are white non-Hispanic families. Nearly 9% of CSHCN are uninsured for all or part of a year and of those covered many do not have adequate insurance coverage (Szilagyi, 2012). The federal government has stepped up to decrease health disparities for all children, and especially CSHCN, by implementing the Children's Health Insurance Program (CHIP). These state-run programs are designed to ensure that all children have health insurance. The criteria expanded health insurance to low-income families with children who would not qualify for state-funded health insurance (e.g., MediCal or Oregon Health Plan).

The *Affordable Care Act of 2010* maintained CHIP funding and increased the percentage of federal matching dollars from a range of 50% to 65% up to an average of 93% per state, maintained until 2015. Each state designs state-funded CHIP programs, with 28 states using a combination of expanded Medicaid services with separate child health programs, 15 states using only separate child health programs, and 7 states only using Medicaid expansion plans. The differences in design determine whether all children are entitled to CHIP benefits, or only those that qualify for Medicaid. The cost of this program has been debated, with many states concerned about the increased cost based on enrollment. The cost of health care is actually reduced, however, when children have a medical home and receive routine well-child care. The number of children now getting health care is notable, as Oregon and Washington lead the nation in increasing the number of children with health insurance by more than 20% (Medicaid.gov, 2015). Although this program has had positive effects on the health of children, there are still 7.8 million children uninsured, with 5.4 million of those children living in poverty. Further, when investigating barriers to children enrolling in state and federal programs, the most likely reason given by parents is that if the parents cannot obtain insurance, they are less likely to enroll their children. Although uninsured children pose a major risk to the health of any nation, non-older adults are four times more likely not to have insurance than children. In the United States, 36 million parents are uninsured. New initiatives are being proposed to combine programs to insure children and parents rather than just children alone (Kenny & Dorn, 2009).

Strategies to Support Health Promotion in Families With Children

Families are the major determinant of children's well-being. Nurses and other health care providers collaborate with parents, and do not view parents as secondary and apart from nurses (Bruns & McCollum, 2002). Health promotion and illness prevention can occur using a variety of strategies across settings, including the following:

- Writing or providing health information for school or community newsletters, e-mail, or online messaging
- Demonstrating and teaching health promotion activities, such as games or physical activities that promote health
- Cultivating attributes of healthy families that include accountability, self-reliance, informed decision making, access to supportive social networks, and nurturing relationships
- Encouraging family councils or family nights that provide venues for communications among all the family members
- Providing anticipatory guidance about high-risk periods in child and youth development; for example, childproofing the home before the infant begins to crawl or walk or providing assistance with appropriate limit setting as an adolescent gets his driver's license. The

use of a contract for teen driving has reduced teen reports of risky behaviors such as driving under the influence of alcohol or riding with someone who has been drinking (Haggerty, Fleming, Catalano, Harachi, & Abbott, 2006; Novilla et al., 2006).

- Providing connections with school and community services; for example, children learn meanings, responses to, and values about health through their interactions in their school communities. Nurses can refer families to community resources, such as the federally funded Head Start programs that serve families of children who are economically disadvantaged and children who have disabilities (American Academy of Pediatrics, 1973). Head Start has increased high-school graduation rates and lowered rates of juvenile arrests and school dropout rates (Gray & McCormick, 2005).

CARE OF CHILDREN WITH CHRONIC ILLNESS AND THEIR FAMILIES

Although most families raising children experience acute illnesses and become familiar with managing these crises, families do not anticipate that their children may have a chronic illness. They are often unprepared for the unknowns and uncertainties of the course of the disease, the effect on their children's development and adulthood, or the effect on each family member and family life.

Defining Chronic Illness in Families With Sick Children

Families of children with chronic illness are diverse and represent all racial and ethnic groups and income levels. Chronic health problems, long-term conditions, disability, and CSHCN are phrases used to describe children with a health problem that cannot be cured. These heterogeneous conditions include, but are not limited to, the following:

- *Medical problems*: allergies, asthma, diabetes, congenital heart disease, joint problems, blood disease, spina bifida
- *Disabilities related to developmental delay and rare genetic syndromes*: Down syndrome, cerebral palsy, mental retardation, autism

■ *Health-related behavioral and educational problems*: attention deficit-hyperactivity disorder (ADHD), learning disability
■ *Social-emotional conditions*: depression and anxiety
■ *Consequences of unintended injuries or acute illness*: head trauma and paralysis

Many children have more than one problem. The term CSHCN is used for families whose children "have or are at increased risk for a chronic physical, developmental, behavioral, or emotional condition and who also require health and related services of a type or amount beyond that required by children generally" (McPherson et al., 1998, p. 139). According to the 2011 to 2012 National Survey of Children With Special Health Care Needs, approximately 14.6 million individuals between 0 and 17 years of age in the United States have a special health care need (Data Resource Center for Child and Adolescent Health, 2012). Of these children with special needs, 78.4% reported having one disorder and 41.4% reported having two or more health conditions. The most common health conditions are as follows:

■ Attention Deficit Disorder/Attention Deficit Hyperactivity Disorder (32.2%)
■ Asthma (35.3%)
■ Learning disability (27.2%)
■ Speech problem (15.6%)
■ Developmental disability (14.7)
■ Behavioral problem (13.6%)
■ Anxiety disorder (13.4%)

Of these children, 65% have complex health care needs that require treatment beyond a medication prescription. The functional impact of these special health needs is significant for the children and families. Approximately 92% of these children have at least one functional deficit, 72% have two functional deficits, and 46% have four or more functional deficits.

All families fare better when they have knowledge of the trajectory and management of the specific disease or chronic illness. The trajectory of the disease or condition, according to Rolland's model of chronic illness, includes the following categories:

1. *Sudden or gradual onset*: Sudden onset of a chronic illness can be from an acute illness, such as meningitis, or an acute accident, whereas gradual onset can be from genetic conditions such as muscular dystrophy.

2. *Prognosis of chronicity, relapse, or death*: Chronic conditions include cystic fibrosis, learning disabilities, or cerebral palsy; relapsing conditions include arthritis, certain mental health disorders such as depression, and asthma; and death or fatal disorders include certain types of cancer or genetic disorders.

3. *A stable or degenerative course over time*: A stable course over time includes disorders such as well-managed asthma, whereas a degenerative condition includes certain types of cancer and multiple sclerosis.

4. *The degree of incapacitation and amount of uncertainty*: The degree of incapacitation varies by illness and within illnesses, such as cerebral palsy ranging from mild and non-incapacitating to severely incapacitating. The amount of uncertainty also varies, such that children diagnosed with certain types of cancer can receive effective treatment, or follow a course of uncertainty and instability for many years.

These categories are helpful to review with families as the specifics of disease management (Rolland, 2005). Nurses and other health care providers tend to reteach the disease and medicine management when it is really the social-emotional and behavioral responses that are troubling families. It may be the degree of unpredictability and lack of role models that interfere with children and their families' abilities to cope, rather than the degree of severity of the illness or disease management (Rodrigues & Patterson, 2007). If nurses spend time with the family carefully assessing their knowledge versus social and emotional responses to their child's illness, the plan of care will be more appropriate and effective.

Families with children who have chronic illnesses vary greatly in their needs, ranging from families who are rarely affected by their children's condition, such as mild asthma, to those who are significantly affected, such as children who are ventilator-dependent. But to varying degrees, all families of children with chronic conditions bear the consequences of their children's conditions. A noncategorical approach, or the understanding by health care providers and parents that care across different diagnoses has similar needs and qualities, directs attention to the consequences that several different chronic conditions have on the children, their families, their communities, and health care systems (Perrin et al., 1993; Stein, Bauman, Westbrook, Coupey, & Ireys, 1993). The intent is to manage the symptoms so that the children and families can maintain their well-being and move toward each member's and the family's goals. The 2001 CSHCN survey provided questions to help nurses and families understand the impact of chronic illness on the family. To gain a family perspective, nurses can ask similar questions as the 2001 CSHCN survey (Children & Adolescent Health Measurement Initiative, 2016):

- Does the condition limit the child's ability to dress and learn self-care?
- Does the condition interfere with the child's daily activities, such as playing and going to school?
- Does the condition require special assistance or technology and/or medication management?
- Does the condition cause family members to cut back or stop working?
- Can the family access and get a referral for special services for the child, as well as family support services?
- Is health care insurance adequate for the child and other family members?
- In the case of adolescence, has the young person's health care begun to be transferred to adult providers?

Parenting a Child With Chronic Illness

Parenting is the nurturance of children to become healthy, responsible, and creative adults. The interdependencies among child, parents, and the whole family within their community can be compared with a set of nesting dolls. Children with chronic illnesses are cared for by their families, who share a household and family history, are nested in communities, and use local and national health care systems. The complex, changing interactions among child, family, and community provide the context of parenting a child with chronic illness into adulthood. Tasks specific to health care are integrated with nurturance during their caregiving. Caregiving burden involves both the amount of time spent and the degree of difficulty in caregiving activities; however, parents have objected to the word "burden" to describe the care they willingly give to their children (Wells et al.,

2002). Sullivan-Bolyai, Sadler, Knafl, and Gilliss (2003) described the parenting responsibilities as taking care of the illness, nurturing and caring for their child, maintaining family life, and taking care of oneself. A detailed presentation of children living with a chronic illness can be found in Chapter 9.

Taking Care of the Illness

Direct care of children's illness involves the time, knowledge, and skills to do technical and nontechnical management, while simultaneously caring for the child's developmental and emotional needs (Moskowitz et al., 2007). Technical care and time involves doing procedures and monitoring for changes in their children's illness. This includes specialized care, such as administering medications and cleaning indwelling tubes. It accounts for crisis care (e.g., unanticipated seizure, elevated temperature), which may involve complex first aid or emergent transportation to the hospital. Nontechnical care is the time and skills needed for feeding, bathing, dressing, grooming, bowel and bladder care, transferring from the bed to a chair, and toileting, along with the necessary extra laundry and house cleaning.

Complex illness care, such as suctioning tracheotomy tubes or diet and insulin regulation, sometimes frightens relatives (e.g., grandparents) who may normally help with child care (Nelson, 2002). Finding qualified caregivers that parents trust is more difficult than finding care for healthy children (Macdonald & Callery, 2008). Parents cut back or quit work in order to provide care (Schuster & Chung, 2014) or decide against taking a new job if the health insurance benefits will not cover their children's health care needs.

Parents also coordinate resources for their CSHCN. Illness needs involve clinic visits, specialized therapy, community pharmacy stocking medications, and medical equipment delivered to the home. CSHCN also need wellness care. The AAP recommends a "medical home" in pediatric offices in order to provide disease prevention through immunizations, promote wellness through anticipatory guidance, address illness questions, and ideally serve as a coordination center for families of CSHCN (Sadof & Nazarian, 2007; Van Cleave, Heisler, Devries, Joiner, & Davis, 2007). Not all pediatrician offices have the resources or training to provide coordination of care and specialized consideration of well-child care for CSHCN.

Besides health care, parents advocate for special educational services. The Individuals with Disabilities Education Act (IDEA), passed in 1975 and renewed by the Disabilities Educational Improvement Act of 2004 (U.S. Department of Education, 2004), requires free public education to all eligible children. For children with disabilities, this involves an individual family service plan (IFSP) for children birth to 5 years, and an individual education program (IEP) for children 5 to 21 years. The 504 Plans mandated from the Rehabilitation Act of 1973 can also be used for children with health impairments to provide appropriate accommodations and adaptations to curriculum, daily instruction and test taking, and standardized local and state level testing. Local school system budgets are challenged to meet all the educational and special needs of their students. Some families may move to another school district if a school has reduced special needs services. Families living in rural areas seem to struggle the most with finding appropriate and available special educational services for their children. Families add time to an already stretched schedule to advocate for their child's educational needs.

Nurturing the Child

The care of a child with chronic illness does not exclude nurturing the child as the foundation to care. Parents often feel overwhelmed with the tasks involved with illness care and management, and may need support and encouragement to maintain optimum nurturing. The common aspects of positive nurturing—including regular touch and rocking; encouragement of social connections, such as mutual eye contact; shared positive experiences; shared discoveries; shared communication; and response to physical, emotional, and spiritual needs—can be pushed aside as medical treatments, procedures, and appointments take precedence. While other parents are enjoying play dates, parents of children with chronic illnesses are often transporting their child to appointments with health care providers, or providing medical care and therapies at home. Nurses can play a key role in helping parents reprioritize nurturing their child by explaining the importance of nurturing activities to health and optimum brain development, as well as by modeling nurturing actions while providing medical care. Nurses can also help to alleviate parents' guilt of wanting to nurture and play with their child rather than provide medical care, and help parents delegate medical care to professionals when possible.

Maintaining Family Life

Nurturing the family as a whole and keeping each member moving toward family and individual goals are as important as illness management (Sullivan-Bolyai, Sadler, Knafl, & Gilliss, 2003). Parents, as the leaders, help the family find meaning in the situation and find ways to include caregiving into daily life. The meaning of the child's illness and the family's identity can change over time. Families may define themselves by the illness, such as a "diabetic family." Illness patterns that are chaotic challenge efforts to create family life. For example, children with ADHD can exhibit poor impulse control, learning difficulties, and hyperactivity. Families are constantly adjusting to their child's behavior. As children with ADHD mature and learn ways to be successful with the help of teachers and health care providers (National Institute of Mental Health, 2016), the family identity may become "a family" with a CSHCN rather than an "ADHD family."

Parents maintain the household and financial security (Sullivan-Bolyai et al., 2003). Mothers tend to do the immediate household activities and care of the children. Fathers continue to focus on instrumental activities, such as financial security and home repairs. Both parents grieve and worry about their children's future and struggle balancing work and time with their family (Chesler & Parry, 2001; Feudtner, 2002). Single-parent households are faced with the demands of caregiving, household management, and maintaining financial security (Ganong, Doty, & Gayer, 2003).

A common concern for parents of CSHCN is the healthy development and care of siblings. Parents want the siblings not to be forgotten or overshadowed by the child with the chronic illness (Hallstrom & Elander, 2007). Siblings may assume the responsibilities of the parent, such as the 5-year-old who shares a bedroom with the sick sibling alerting his parents that his baby sister needs suctioning (Coffey, 2006). Siblings often try to do well in school to gain parent approval and alleviate parent concern for them because they see their parents working so hard to care for their ill sibling (Hutson & Alter, 2007). They take pride in being able to help their sibling, simultaneously complaining of doing more than their share of chores and noticing differential treatment from their parents and other relatives. Sibling research has mixed findings that show increased risks for behavior and academic problems on one hand, with improved empathy and independence skills on the other (Sharpe &

Rossiter, 2002). Sibling adjustment improved when parents provided problem-solving skills, established open communication about current and future concerns, and supported resiliency characteristics; these included finding support outside the home, establishing positive experiences and interests, and supporting positive meaning to challenging experiences (Giallo & Gavidia-Payne, 2006).

A strong husband-wife relationship is important in any family, but creating opportunities for being a couple is even more challenging for families with CSHCN. A ritual such as "date night" fosters closeness and provides an opportunity for open communication and problem solving without the distractions of parenting (Imber-Black, 2005). Another challenge is deciding roles and responsibilities between parents to avoid caregiver burnout. Some parents agree to divide activities, whereas some trade, so that each can learn the other's skills. Agreement and support of each other's parenting is the anchor for the family. Also, accepting the need for time away from parenting for both parents is important. Finding safe and appropriate respite care for families with CSHCN is a barrier to partners and marital couples, especially in rural areas. Coordinated care between health clinics, specialty clinics, educational services, and social services can increase the resources for parents and increase the chances of finding appropriate respite care.

Parents also have to manage social stigma, which is most common for families of children who have visible disabilities, such as limb deformities or morbid obesity; are technology dependent; have developmental/behavioral disabilities; or have a fear-based disease, such as HIV infection. Managing stigma means finding safe environments where families can relax and participate, such as Special Olympics or organizations designed to bring similar families together (e.g., National Autism Association). Without a feeling of trust and safety, families are likely to limit social activities or split the family so that the child with the disability is cared for while other family members participate in social events (Rehm & Bradley, 2005; Sandelowski & Barroso, 2003). A major risk for families with CSHCN is social isolation and lack of social support (Wang & Barnard, 2004).

Parental Self-Care

It is difficult for parents to take care of themselves when they are balancing illness care and the ongoing demands of family life (Hallstrom & Elander, 2007; Sullivan-Bolyai et al., 2003). Mothers and fathers, each in their own way, grieve the lost dream of a healthy child. The busy-ness of daily care can distract parents from thinking that their child is not normal. The differences, however, become more evident when the condition worsens or at family events, making distraction a more difficult coping strategy to use. For example, the "first day of school" is celebrated when boarding the school bus, but using the wheelchair lift or watching other children board the regular bus while a child with special health care needs waits for the special education bus makes the child's difference visible. Validating their sadness is a nursing action that gives parents and children the opportunity to grieve what might have been and celebrate what is and has been accomplished. Their sadness, called "chronic sorrow," is a normal grief response (Gordan, 2009). Evidence-based nursing intervention strategies for families experiencing chronic sorrow (Gordan, 2009) are divided into two areas: (1) internal management methods and (2) external management methods. Internal management builds on interventions initiated by an individual such as reading literature about their child's or sibling's condition, engaging in a personal stress reduction activity, or joining a support group. Nurses can provide these individuals local, regional, and national resources; Internet resources that are vetted as evidence-based; or other credible resources. External management strategies are those provided by health care professionals, such as counseling, medications for insomnia or anxiety, pastoral or spiritual care, and referrals to an organization or resources to assist with financial concerns created by their child's health condition.

Conditions that were fatal in the past (e.g., premature birth, leukemia, cystic fibrosis) are now considered chronic and are currently managed in outpatient clinics and in the home (Eiser, 1994). Parents may struggle and not be able to care for their child, especially if needs are complex or behavior is so difficult that injury to the child or other family members is a risk. These parents may seek out-of-home placement, but feel guilty about it. They may see themselves as being a "bad parent" (Nelson, 2002; Wang & Barnard, 2004). Finding appropriate community resources for specialized care is difficult. Respite services and home care are fragmented. Parents move between hope and despair, and are at risk for caregiver burnout and depression if appropriate support is not available (Wong & Heriot, 2008). Nurses have a key role in assessing the family's ability to maintain care, the need for increased support or home care, and the need for out-of-home placement when needed.

"Living worried" was found to be part of the day-to-day parenting of children with chronic illness (Coffey, 2006). Parents worried about their judgment. When should they call the doctor or go to the emergency department? They worried about their family. Did their in-laws blame their side of the family for the illness (Seligman & Darling, 1997)? They worried that the neighbors would report them for child abuse, as their toddler screamed, "Don't do it, Mommy . . . please don't hurt me anymore!" during an insulin injection. They worried their child was parenting them, after saying, "It's alright Mommy, don't be sad. It doesn't hurt too bad." Parents continued to worry even after the child transitioned from home to an adult independent living situation, with concerns about financial stability, exploitation of the adult child by others, and general happiness (Coffey, 2006). Nurses can help families to decrease their worry by connecting parents to support groups to discuss their worries. Connecting a family with another similarly situated family is an important nursing intervention (Gallo & Knafl, 1998).

Normalization and Family Management Styles in Childhood Chronic Illness

Families are expected to take their children home, master complex treatments, and do it in such a way as to not dominate the child's life, but to integrate the care into daily family life (Knafl, Deatrick, & Kirby, 2001). Interestingly, nurses use the language of sickness or disability, such as "families of children with chronic illness" and "families of children with special health care needs." In contrast, families use the phrase, "my child is normal except for . . . [fill in the condition]." Families tend to focus on the entire child, and work continuously to normalize their child, whereas nurses continue to focus on the illness. An important stage for families, after the crisis of a chronic illness diagnosis, is to act to normalize their situation. The characteristics of normalization are as follows:

- Acknowledging the condition and its potential to threaten family life
- Adapting a normalcy lens for defining child and family
- Engaging in parenting behaviors and family routines that are consistent with normalcy

- Developing management of the condition that is consistent with normalcy (e.g., schedule preschool for afternoon session so that physical therapy and medications can be done in the morning)
- Interacting with others based on view of the child and family as normal (Knafl et al., 2001; Knafl, Deatrick, & Havill, 2012)

Striving for normalcy is not the same as denial. Parents in denial refuse to adjust schedules to meet the needs of their child's health needs in hopes of the child being viewed as normal by others, whereas parents who strive for normalcy alter schedules to allow their child to participate in as many normal activities as possible.

Families are stressed but not all are adversely affected and some report being stronger from the experience of having a child with a chronic illness (Hayes, 1997; McClellan & Cohen, 2007; Miles, 2003; Mussatto, 2006; Rodrigues & Patterson, 2007). Nurses knowledgeable about disease, illness, and family interactions can assess the complexity of a family's situation and adaptation to the chronic illness over time. Nurses can help families benefit from identifying individual and group family strengths and thinking about their goals as individuals and as a family (Tapp, 2000). Other nursing interventions to help normalize include matching support to the family's developmental stage and addressing areas assessed for individual care planning. Challenges of families whose children have disabilities and chronic conditions are listed in Table 13-4.

CONSENT IN FAMILY CHILD HEALTH NURSING

Families with children experiencing acute or chronic illness or injury may be asked to make difficult decisions regarding health care. In most instances, when young children are involved, health care providers collaborate with parents to obtain informed consent, except in emergency situations when parents are absent. As children grow and develop, it is important for them to take on more responsibility as primary guardians of personal health and decision making (American Academy of Pediatrics, 2007; American Academy of Pediatrics Committee on Bioethics, 1995). Some family members and health care providers may feel uncomfortable with the inclusion of children in

Table 13-4 **Stages, Tasks, and Situational Needs of Families of Children With Disabilities and Chronic Conditions**

Stages	Tasks	Situational Needs That Alter Transitions
Beginning family: *Married couple without children.*	Establish mutually satisfying relationship. Relate to kin network. Family planning.	Unprepared for birth of children with disabilities; prenatal testing or visible anomalies at birth begins process. In the United States, parents usually want to know their infants' diagnosis as early as possible.
Early childbearing: *First birth, up to 36 months.*	Integrate new baby into family. Reconcile conflicting needs of various family members. Parental role development. Accommodate to marital couple changes. Expand relationships with extended family, adding grandparent and aunt/uncle roles.	Learn the meaning of infants' behavior, symptoms, and treatments. Hampered nurturing and parenting, if children are not able to respond to parents' efforts to interact with them (e.g., not smiling or returning sounds in response to parental cooing). Search for adequate health care. Establish early intervention programs (speech and physical therapist, specially trained teachers).
Family with preschool children: *First child developmental age 3–5 years.*	Foster development of children. Parental privacy. Increased competence of child. Socializing children. Maintenance of couple relationship.	Formal education of disabled children starts at birth with early intervention programs. Families may not find adequate programs even into preschool years. Failure to achieve developmental milestones (toilet training, self-feeding, language) signals chronic sorrow. Families try to establish routines for themselves and their children.
Family with school-age children: *Oldest child developmental age 6–13 years.*	Letting children go. Parental needs balanced with children's needs. Promoting school achievement. Prepare for high-risk behavior related to drugs and sexual experimentation.	Move children from family care to community care; requires creating new routines and relationships. Explain to school officials and others the needs of the children. Negotiate appropriate school services and curriculum. Behavioral problems may isolate families.
Family with adolescents: *Oldest child developmental age 13 years until leaves home.*	Loosening family ties. Couple relationship. Parent-teen communication. Maintenance of family moral and ethical standards. Promote safe sexual development.	Continued dependency may mean children never achieve leaving home. Family examines how to continue family life with increasing physical growth but ongoing dependence of children. High-risk behavior related to sexual activity and drugs.
Launching center family: *First through last child to leave home.*	Promote independence of children while maintaining relationship. Couple relationship, build new life together. Midlife developmental crisis for adults.	Financial costs do not decrease because children still require dependent-type care.
Families in middle years: *Empty nest to retirement.*	Redefine activity and goals. Provide healthy environment. Maintain meaningful relationships with aging parents. Strengthen couple relationship.	Redefine relationships with grown children and CSHCN.

(continued)

Table 13-4	Stages, Tasks, and Situational Needs of Families of Children With Disabilities and Chronic Conditions *(cont.)*	
Stages	**Tasks**	**Situational Needs That Alter Transitions**
Retirement to old age: *Retirement to death of both parents.*	Deal with losses. Living place may change. Role changes. Adjust to less income. Chronic illness. Mate loss. Aware of death. Life review.	Arrangements for CSHCN.

Source: Gedaly-Duff, V., Stoeger, S., & Shelton, K. (2000). Working with families. In R. E. Nickel & L. W. Desch (Eds.), *The physician's guide to caring for children with disabilities and chronic conditions* (1st ed., pp. 31–76). Baltimore, MD: Paul H. Brookes.

health care decision making. Some authorities believe that children may not make rational decisions, and yet adults are not held to the same standard of being rational when they make personal health care decisions (Zawistowski & Frader, 2003). Each child's decision-making capacities should be assessed and given serious consideration using Piaget's cognitive developmental stages as a guide (American Academy of Pediatrics, 2007; American Academy of Pediatrics Committee on Bioethics, 1995). Children, especially adolescents, want to be involved in decision making regarding their health care. Younger children have a difficult time visualizing the future, but adolescents can and want information that will help them visualize the positive and negative consequences of their health care decisions (Ruggeri, Gummerum, & Hanock, 2014).

Laws regarding informed consent of minors vary from state to state. It is important that health care providers be knowledgeable of individual state statutes. In Virginia, for example, Abraham's Law resulted from a case where an adolescent refused to comply with physician-recommended treatment (Marques-Lopez, 2006). This 2007 law allows minors 14 years of age or older to refuse medical treatment for a life-threatening condition. Even with this law, most adolescents make these decisions in collaboration with parents and health care providers when able, and as with any informed consent, children and adolescents make better decisions when they are given developmentally appropriate explanations of risks and benefits.

Some states consider some minors "emancipated" and give these individuals the authority to make personal health care decisions. The age of minors is decided by each individual state, and varies depending on the decision being considered. For example, whereas consuming alcohol is limited to those 21 years and older, most states allow for specific medical decisions to be made by individuals older than the age of 18 years. These minors may be self-supporting, live outside of the parental home, or be married, pregnant, a parent, or in the military; they may also be declared emancipated by the courts. Some states also have statutes related to "mature minors." These persons are not emancipated but still have the authority to make health care decisions in certain situations, such as addiction, pregnancy, and STI care (American Academy of Pediatrics, 2007; American Academy of Pediatrics Committee on Bioethics, 1995).

On occasion, the wishes of children, families, and health care providers may differ. It is assumed that all parties will act in the best interest of the child, but best interests are in the eye of the beholder when it comes down to personally held values, such as "What makes a life worth living?" (Kon, 2006). Although it is uncommon for parents to be overruled, there are circumstances where the courts will invoke the Child Abuse Prevention and Treatment Act, which gives the state's interest in protecting minors greater weight than the rights of parents in decision making (Holder, 1983; Kon, 2006; U.S. Code of Federal Regulations, 2006). In a 2006 case, a mother was charged with second-degree kidnapping when she smuggled her child out of a children's hospital to explore alternative treatments. In situations such as these, health care providers should respect the fact that some patients may need time to understand the situation or come to terms with concerns regarding proposed care (American Academy of Pediatrics, 2007; American Academy of Pediatrics Committee on Bioethics, 1995). Legal intervention should be the last resort, and should only occur when there is a substantial risk to the child, as state intervention can cause serious harm itself.

CARE OF CHILDREN AND FAMILIES IN THE HOSPITAL

Another issue that family nurses experience when caring for families with children is the admission of a child to the hospital. Hospital admission is a stressful event for families. Nurses and health care providers have the opportunity to take this crisis situation and make it the best it can be for the child and family by decreasing stressors whenever possible. Applying the principles of partnering, setting mutual goals with the family, enhancing family connectedness to the child, valuing the family's areas of expertise, and assisting the family to understand health care processes and procedures are all ways to help alleviate some of the stress of a hospital stay (Curley & Meyer, 2001; Franck, Wray, Gay, Dearmun, Lee, & Cooper, 2015). Family and child attendance at interdisciplinary team rounds is an ideal place to set mutual goals, and such rounds have been shown to increase patient and family satisfaction. In fact, positive feelings from the family can improve health outcomes. For example, including family as valued team members has been shown to decrease intensive care unit (ICU) length of stay of ill children (Dutton et al., 2003; Vazirani, Hays, Shapiro, & Cowan, 2005). Family-centered rounds hold a potential to create a patient-centered environment, enhance medical and nursing education, and improve patient outcomes (Cypress, 2012).

Nurses often take on the role of coordinating and maintaining communication with family members throughout a hospitalization. Identifying one or two point people to provide communication to the family helps build trust and decreases the risk for communication errors and related conflict. It opens and strengthens communication, builds trust, and lessens anxiety if a consistent, limited number of health care providers are assigned to care for the child and family and maintain regular communication with family members (Mullen & Pate, 2006).

Referring to family members as "visitors" diminishes the significance of the family relationship (Slota, Shearn, Potersnak, & Haas, 2003) and may even be perceived as insulting; it is the health care providers who are the "visitors" or temporary caregivers for the hospitalized child. Ensuring that "family" is broadly defined can make available a wide base of support

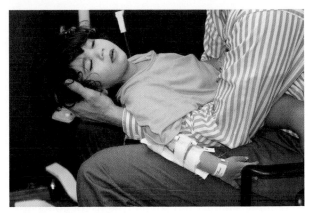

© iStock.com/jarenwicklund

from loved ones. Close friends and family members are seen as sources of security for children, and extended family members can also provide parents or guardians time for self-care and opportunities to address work and home responsibilities. The family, rather than hospital administrators, should determine individuals allowed to be part of the care of the child.

Health care providers, especially those working with critically ill children, need to be aware that parents may struggle with stress responses related to their ability to cope with the hospitalization of their child. During their study of 107 parents experiencing hospitalization within an ICU of their children, Franck et al. (2015) found that 32.7% of parents had symptoms of PTSD 3 months after their child was discharged, and 32.7% had enough symptoms to qualify for a diagnosis of PTSD. Risk factors for PTSD included being a single parent, longer stays in the hospital, previous depression and anxiety in the parent, and poorer outcomes for the child. Previous studies have found differences with other variables, such as support available for the parents, but this study failed to show significant differences between those parents receiving support versus those that did not (Franck et al., 2015). When nurses recognize the stress experienced by parents when their child is hospitalized, nurses are more able to assist parents in coping with hospitalization of their child. Offering parents resources, such as support groups or working with a social worker or in-hospital counselor, will provide options to improve parents' ability to positively cope with the stress of having a critically ill child.

The needs of siblings should also be addressed during hospitalization. Younger siblings have vivid imaginations and may believe that they caused a brother or sister to become ill or injured, or that the hospitalized child is at risk of dying. Nurses are equipped to provide parents with information, guidance, and reassurance about the appropriateness of sibling visitation for individual situations and to support these visits with appropriate preparation and support that is developmentally appropriate. Child life therapists may be available to prepare siblings for visits to the hospital and assess their readiness to visit (Mullen & Pate, 2006). In a study of critically ill children, it was found that best friends had some of the same concerns and needs as siblings (Lewandowski & Frosch, 2003). Screening siblings and young friends for contagious illnesses before visits can theoretically prevent the spread to hospitalized patients and families. There is no evidence, however, to support that sibling visits increase infection rates, even in the neonatal population (Moore, Coker, DuBuisson, Swett, & Edwards, 2003). Rather, hospital-acquired and endogenous infections pose a greater risk to the hospitalized child (Rozdilsky, 2005). Siblings do provide support to the hospitalized family member, and visits by siblings help to reduce anxiety about being separated from a family member during times of illness and stress.

Avoiding family separation from the hospitalized child is a priority. Separation increases stress for children and families and does not encourage a partnership philosophy. The Society of Pediatric Nurses and the American Nurses Association (Lewandowski & Tesler, 2003) support 24-hour parental access to hospitalized children. This access includes giving families the option to remain with their children during procedures, treatments, and resuscitation attempts, including in the emergency department (American Academy of Pediatrics Committee on Pediatric Emergency & American College of Emergency Physicians Pediatric Emergency Medicine, 2006; McAlvin & Carew-Lyons, 2014). Families benefit from this presence because it removes doubt about the child's condition, and they can rest assured that "everything" was done for the child. In the event of death, families may be comforted by the fact that the child did not die alone with strangers; the togetherness may foster a sense of closure (Bauchner, Waring, & Vinci, 1991; Halm, 2005; Mangurten et al., 2006). Nurses can assist families by supporting the decision to be present or not, assessing family reactions as needed, answering questions, helping family members to find "a place" in the room, providing instructions of what they can and cannot do, contacting spiritual support as requested, and providing comfort items such as tissues, beverages, and seating. See Box 13-3, which describes a family's experience during their child's resuscitation.

Transitions during a hospital stay can become added stressors for families. For example, those

---

BOX 13-3

Family Experiences During Resuscitation at a Children's Hospital Emergency Department

Introduction: Family presence during cardiopulmonary resuscitation has been recommended by national professional organizations, which include the American Emergency Nurses Association and the AAP.

Purpose of Study: In an effort to improve the care of families during resuscitation events, the authors of this study examined the experiences of family members whose children underwent resuscitation and their health and mental health following the episode.

Methodology: Ten family members participated in a 1-hour audiotaped interview in this descriptive, retrospective study. Data collection included both quantitative and qualitative instruments, which contained previously validated and investigator-developed items. Seven family members were present during resuscitation and three were not.

Results: Analysis of interview data revealed that families felt that: (1) they had the right to be present during resuscitation; (2) their child wanted them present during resuscitation and that they were sources of strength for the child; (3) they were reassured by seeing that all possible options to help their child were exhausted; and (4) a facilitator for information-giving would be helpful during the event, as no one was prepared to face resuscitation.

Nursing Implications: Whether present or not, all family members in this study expressed the importance of the option to be present during resuscitation. There was no indication of post-traumatic stress to family members following the event.

Source: McGahey-Oakland, P. R., Lieder, H. S., Young, A., & Jefferson, L. S. (2007). Family experiences during resuscitation at a children's hospital emergency department. *Journal of Pediatric Health Care, 21*(4), 217–225.

who have been accustomed to one-to-one nursing care for a child in an ICU may find it stressful when transferred to an acute care pediatric unit where the nurses have more patients to assist. Preparation of the families for the differences between units by use of a transfer protocol may help to prevent undue stress and increase family satisfaction (Van Waning, Kleiber, & Freyenberger, 2005).

Although families are glad to have their children discharged from the hospital, there are stressors that can accompany this transition as well. This is especially true for parents of children who have been in the ICU. Evidence shows that these individuals can experience feelings of uncertainty and unpreparedness as caregivers following discharge home (Bent, Keeling, & Routson, 1996). Adequate time for planning and preparation with families can make the transition easier. Some patient discharge situations may require collaboration with multidisciplinary team members, such as social workers, discharge planners, pharmacists, and home health providers, to ensure that the resources needed following discharge are available. Nurses often assist families in transitioning from the ICU to regular care, as well as transitioning to home care, by serving as case managers. Nurses are in a unique position to assist families in the case management role because of their education and experience working with families. According to the American Nurses Credentialing Center (2011), the specific duties of a case manager include:

- Documenting family care plans
- Working with insurance companies to assist in financial coverage of care
- Identifying risk factors that may impede access to health care
- Identifying available family resources
- Communicating care preferences between the family and other health care providers
- Advocating for families
- Developing a family-focused case management plan
- Educating the family about the role of the nurse as case manager

Case Study: Comantan Family

The following case study of the Comantan family demonstrates family nursing approaches to providing health care to a family with children. The primary patient is Carl, although other family members have health care issues as well. The focus of this case study is his health and the health of his family. See the genogram and environmental ecomap of the Comantan family in Figures 13-1 and 13-2.

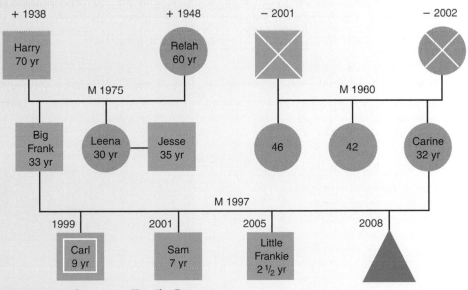

FIGURE 13-1 Comantan Family Genogram

(continued)

Case Study: Comantan Family *(cont.)*

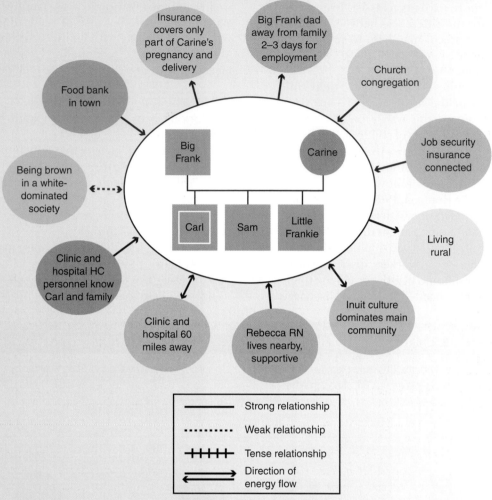

FIGURE 13-2 Comantan Family Ecomap

Setting:

Carl Comantan is a 9-year-old boy who lives with his family in a wood-frame house in a coastal, rural area of the northwest region of Alaska. He has chronic respiratory illnesses and has been diagnosed by his physician as having asthma.

Family Members:

Carl's ethnicity is Alaskan Native, or Inuit. His father and mother, as well as his maternal and paternal grandfathers and grandmothers are also Alaskan Native. His maternal grandfather and grandmother both passed away several years ago from pneumonia. The remaining family members have light brown skin and dark brown or black hair. The family speaks English and the elders also speak their native language, Inuktitut.

Carl's family consists of his mother, Carine, age 32; his father, Big Frank, age 33; and his two brothers, Sam, age 7, and little Frankie, age 2 1/2. Carine is approximately 4 months pregnant. Big Frank's sister, Leena, age 30, helps with child care. Grandfather Harry and Grandmother Relah are very involved with their children and grandchildren.

The Family Story:

Big Frank and Carine have been married for more than 11 years. The children are their biological children from this marriage. Neither has been married before. They went to high school together and met when Big Frank did business at the gas station where Carine worked. They both attend the same church.

Case Study: Comantan Family *(cont.)*

Big Frank works part-time as a professional truck driver for a trucking corporation in the region. He is often gone from home for 2 to 3 days at a time for his work. The company offers limited major medical insurance for Big Frank and his family. Office visits and care under $800 are not covered. Carine's pregnancy care and births are covered at 60% of the cost. She receives no paid maternity leave benefit from her employer.

Carine works at a local gas station that has a small grocery store attached. She manages the grocery store. The store is 5 miles from their home in the nearby village of Anokiviac. Big Frank and Carine are worried that they cannot make enough money to save, let alone pay the ongoing bills for electricity, gasoline for their vehicles, heating oil for their home, and clothing. They feel fortunate to be members of a cohesive community of family and friends, and to have jobs. Many people in their area do not have full-time employment. There are no family aid programs in the area. Monthly, they travel to the town an hour's drive away to go to the local food bank. They get a box of staples that includes flour, rice, canned vegetables, and dried milk. The food bank requires that they show bills and pay statements to prove that they qualify for the food. Sometimes the food bank has a very limited number of items.

Big Frank and Carine strongly believe in making and keeping strong relationships with the people in their family and community circles. They talk about how people have helped each other in the past and how they are always on the lookout for someone who needs help. From one conversation with a teacher, Carine learned about a summer program for first graders. She was able to enroll Sam in that 2-week-long program in the town, where he stayed with a cousin's family. In exchange for the cost of the program, she helped several evenings in their local school program during the school year.

These evening programs during the school year were also helpful for Carl, who missed several days during the school year because of his coughing and respiratory illnesses. Because of the extra time and attention, he has been able to keep up with his classmates at his school. Carine and Big Frank help the children's Aunt Leena understand how to help Carl with his studies because she cares for the children while the parents are working. Carine and Big Frank believe that if they and a few other people, such as Aunt Leena and the school teachers, know Carl well, they will notice when he starts to become ill. They believe that they have been able to avert many serious illnesses for Carl because they and the adults he is around know him well. They do not get overly worried if he wheezes a little, which they consider normal for Carl. If he gets more short of breath, however, or if his appetite wanes, then they know he is getting sick. Even his brother, Sam, knows about Carl being "fever hot" as he calls it, and worries openly about his brother when he is ill. Sam and little Frankie will bring Carl water and crackers when he is sick. The younger children also know about Carl's inhaler and will bring it to him when he is wheezing.

The physicians and nurses at the clinic in the town know that when Carine, Big Frank, Aunt Leena, or other family members call saying Carl is ill the situation is serious. They listen with high regard.

Big Frank is a partially disabled veteran of the U.S. Army. He served in an international war overseas and was injured in a tank attack. His disability involves his left leg and left arm, both of which are severely scarred from burns. He has decreased range of motion and sensation in both of these limbs. His left chest and face are also scarred; however, he did not lose vision or function of his shoulder or face. He is not overweight and is physically strong and fit.

Carine has good health but knows there is a family history of coughing spells. She is not overweight and is physically strong and fit. Both Carine and Big Frank work hard to eat well and feed their children healthy food. They eat frozen vegetables and fruits, and bread made by various family members. Their protein sources include fish that they catch and either elk or caribou from the annual fall family hunt. Occasionally they have seal, obtained courtesy of traditional hunts by Big Frank and the extended family.

Carine and Big Frank will drink an occasional beer but do not drink any other alcoholic beverages. Many of their extended family members and folks in their community drink beer, sometimes to excess, resulting in drunken behavior. Carine and Big Frank worry that their children may drink excessively as adolescents and adults. They do not allow their children to drink any beer or other alcoholic beverage. The extended family members and the folks in the community practice the same behavior. Group disapproval occurs when drunken behavior occurs and those persons are taken home.

Carl is generally healthy except for his asthma and frequent episodes of upper respiratory infections. These often progress into lengthy bouts of wheezing and coughing. He frequently wheezes in the morning on awakening and when he plays outside. He misses all or parts of days from school because of his illnesses approximately 25% of the time. He has an inhaler, but he occasionally forgets to bring it with him to school and church or out to play. He takes his antibiotics and other medications well. He says out loud, "This is for my breathing!" He also says to little Frankie, "This is not for you, this is my medicine! It is icky, you should never eat it!" Carl knows that his mother, Aunt Leena, school teacher, and Sunday school teacher know about each of his medicines. Carine and Big Frank are considering sending Carl to asthma camp for 2 weeks in the city during the summer.

(continued)

Case Study: Comantan Family *(cont.)*

The physician at the hospital has recommended Carl receive a foundation-funded scholarship at the camp because they note that he learns quickly and likes to be with other children. Also, the physician told Carine and Frank that they think Carl could benefit from the time to focus on learning more about managing his own condition.

Sam and little Frankie are both healthy. They have had occasional respiratory illnesses. Sam and Carl both had the chicken-pox, as the varicella vaccine was not available in their area at the time. Carine and the children are up-to-date on their vaccines. Big Frank has not had an influenza vaccine and does not recall when he had other immunizations since he left the military.

While Carine is at work, all three children go to their Aunt Leena's home either all day or after school, depending on their age. Aunt Leena's home is a 5-minute walk from the school. Aunt Leena has a car and has driven Carl to the emergency department several times during the last year when he has had severe bouts of wheezing and a fever. Aunt Leena lives with her husband, Uncle Jesse, who works as a truck driver and bush plane pilot in the area. Aunt Leena does not work outside her home. She is involved in the care of her brother's children and is looking forward to the next child. She occasionally takes a little gas money when her brother, Big Frank, offers. She is committed to helping her brother and his family in any way she can. She and her husband want children but have been unable to conceive.

Grandparents Harry and Relah, who are a 5-minute walk from Big Frank and his family, are also involved in watching, guid-ing, and helping their three grandchildren. Grandmother Relah has learned many treatments for illnesses over her lifetime. She studied for a while with one of the tribal shamans many years ago and maintains contact with the shaman. She makes mint and berry teas for Carl, makes steam for him in the kitchen, and feeds him dried fish for strength and healing. She talks to Carl and his brothers about the herbs she makes from various berries, bark, and leaves in their environment. She also encourages them to think about being strong and quick, wise and caring in their world. She talks to Big Frank about taking Carl to visit the shaman. They have not yet decided if they will follow through with this recommendation.

Big Frank and Carine consult extended family members, particularly the elderly parents and other elders in the area, regard-ing health and family matters of all kinds, including seeking advice regarding Carl's respiratory infections and wheezing. As the nearest clinic, hospital, or health care facility is more than 60 miles away, they are careful about taking the time and gasoline to drive there. Big Frank and Carine consider themselves equal decision makers with regard to family health matters and will consult providers and family members. Both are held in high esteem in their family and surrounding community. They are sup-ported through congregational prayer in their church, particularly when Carl is ill. Church members, especially direct relatives, often bring food to the Comantan family home when Carl is ill or when Big Frank is gone for several days on his job.

One of the Comantan family's neighbors is a registered nurse, Rebecca, who lives about 5 miles away. She works at one of the clinics associated with the hospital that is in the town 60 miles away. One time she took Carl with her to the clinic so that he could see his physician and get a renewal on an anti-inflammatory medication. She often laughs and says she is another "Auntie" for Carl and his siblings. She says she is, at least, their cousin, even though she is Salish and not Inuit.

Health Care Goals for the Comantan Family:

- Reduce the frequency and severity of Carl's respiratory illnesses.
- Reduce the number of Carl's missed school days. Maintain age-appropriate academic success.
- Increase the number of developmentally appropriate responsibilities and decision-making processes for Carl as he learns to manage his own illness.
- Prevent Carl's daily wheezing by improving management of asthma.
- Promote Carine's health during her pregnancy.
- Promote Big Frank's healthy coping with the pain and discomfort of his injuries.
- Enhance health resources for the family in its community.
- Reduce the family's barriers to health and increase its strengths for health.

Goals for Nurses Working With the Comantan Family Across Health Care Settings:

- Build a therapeutic and collaborative health-focused relationship with Carl and the Comantan family.
- Explore ways to reduce the frequency and severity of Carl's respiratory symptoms.
- Explore with Carl and his family ways to mediate and adapt to the overall impact of his illness on him and his family.
- Explore the health care resources for the Comantan family.
- Explore the main strengths and stressors for Carl and his family.

Case Study: Comantan Family *(cont.)*

- Commend the Comantan family for its current health efforts and outcomes.
- Focus on maintaining stability in the Comantan family.

Family Systems Theory in Relation to the Comantan Family:

The use of Family Systems Theory addresses the complex needs of each individual within the family, and the family as a whole. The individual concepts from the Family Systems Theory apply as follows:

Concept 1—All Parts of the System Are Connected:

Carl and his family are deeply and actively embedded in their family life and their community. Each family and community member contributes to the health of Carl and his family. When Carl is ill, connections are activated to become supportive in a focused manner, according to the needs identified.

One assumption of family systems is that the features of the system are designed to maintain stability of the system, using both adaptive and maladaptive means. The Comantan family is adaptive to Carl's illnesses in its frequent, focused interactions with family and friends. The family members realize that their situation may change quickly, for example, with finances, and that they may suddenly find themselves in financial stress. Family members also recognize that Carl's health may change quickly, and they are aware that several people should know how to monitor Carl's health and know what to do if he shows signs of respiratory distress. Their connections with Aunt Leena are part of that adaptation. They realize that with an intentional increase in the number of people who know Carl well, there is a greater likelihood that no matter where he is, he can be quickly and accurately assessed for severity and risk.

Each family member has many roles, each affecting one another. Big Frank, for instance, is a provider of financial resources, a responsible adult in his social community, a caring son to his parents, a guardian of the culture, and a caring father. These roles influence many aspects of his family. Carine is a provider of financial resources; a responsible adult in her social community, including the school; and a caring mother. These roles influence many aspects of her family.

Concept 2—The Whole Is More Than the Sum of Its Parts:

The family members consistently support each other, recognizing the strength of the whole. The Comantan family believes individuals doing their part contribute to the overall health of all and the ability of each to help at various times. The Comantan family adults focus on increasing health of all members in the long term while adapting to Carl's illness. For example, because illness sometimes forces Carl to miss school, they plan for Aunt Leena to help him. They also arrange for Sam and Carl to be in summer programs. The family adapts to the health needs of one member while taking care not to compromise the health of the other members.

The Comantan family is a cohesive unit with a lot of interdependence. This is consistent with its societal beliefs of helping each other survive and thrive. Family members believe that each person has value, yet each has responsibilities to the others in the group. They take great pride in teaching each other necessary and helpful things. This is especially true of the elders to the younger members. The elders do listen to the new ideas of the younger members, however, realizing that all ideas are worth consideration.

The entire family is happily anticipating the arrival of the new baby. They hope it is a girl, but they will be happy whether the baby is a boy or a girl. This normative, expected event may require the three boys, Carl, Sam, and little Frankie, to stay with Aunt Leena and Uncle Jesse during the birth and early postpartum stage. This will depend on the circumstances, and the aunt and uncle are prepared.

Concept 3—All Systems Have Some Form of Boundaries or Border Between the System and Its Environment:

The Comantan family stays close to family and friends, yet is mindful of the amount and types of contributions made between families. For example, if Carl needs to go to the hospital, Aunt Leena will strive to be the one who takes him, rather than asking Rebecca to do so.

The family has fairly open boundaries within its local community, and does reach out to a few resources in the town 60 miles away. The family likes the idea of Sam going to the summer program and staying with his cousins because they know the teacher and the supervisors.

The grandparents help Carl and his brothers find the boundaries of their heritage within the larger white American culture. They are teaching Carl about these boundaries and expect Carl to model these for his two younger brothers, as well as for other children in the community.

(continued)

Case Study: Comantan Family *(cont.)*

Rebecca, the nurse, who is Salish (not Inuit), is trusted and the family is open with her. The family is also open with the members of the congregation of their church.

Concept 4—Systems Can Be Further Organized Into Subsystems:

The Comantan family and the family of Aunt Leena and Uncle Jesse are an important subsystem in the Comantan family's overall functioning. Aunt Leena and Uncle Jesse contribute a lot while gaining contact with their beloved nephews. The grandparents, Harry and Relah, are also an important subsystem of the Comantan family, as are the children versus the adults.

Nursing Plan Using the Family Systems Approach:

The nursing plan for this family is more holistic if the Family Systems Approach is used.

Nurse Assessment—Noticing/Data Gathering and Interpretation:

- Explore in detail the expectations the family—including parents, grandparents, and aunt and uncle—has for Carl in relation to managing his health. Use affirmations, clarifications, respect, salutations, and honesty.
- Ask the family to share details of its health practices, including any herbal or practice treatments used by his grandparents Harry and Relah.
- Learn the history and what the family expects about the future of Carl's chronic illness.
- Explore triggers and factors that worsen his condition.
- Assess Carl's overall growth and development, his medications, what substances he has used or been given for his health, his health-related behaviors, and his interpretations of all these items. For example, determine the level of growth and development impairment the family has noticed because of his respiratory illnesses and treatment.
- Discuss the concept of illness trajectory for the Comantan family.
- Explore what the family thinks is helpful, what might be helpful, and what is not helpful.
- Explore the main adaptive features the family identifies.
- Explore additional health and health cost resources for the family, particularly for the occasions of Carl's potential hospitalizations in the future, for Carine's pregnancy and delivery, and for Big Frank's pain management.
- Explore any health care disparities the family has experienced or perceived.
- Assess the entire family's immunization status.
- Explore the impact of Big Frank's absence for 3 days at a time when he is driving his truck for work.
- Ensure that various family members have Carl's medications handy at their homes.
- Assess the boundaries of care and involvement for Aunt Leena and Carl's grandparents Harry and Relah.
- Look for trends, health patterns, illness patterns, and disease patterns for Carl's management behaviors and outcomes.

Interpretations:

- The Comantan family's strengths include their health behaviors, health actions, and beliefs. They reportedly practice health behaviors that help all members without the expense of hurting another family member.
- The Comantan family has coordinated care for Carl within its family and community. They are strong advocates for his health and well-being.
- Many members of the extended family are integral to Carl's health and the health of the entire Comantan family.
- Realize that the data so far do not support any major stressors when Big Frank is gone for 3 days at a time. This may change with Carine's advancing pregnancy and birth.
- The Comantan family career has multiple concurrent developmental needs, tasks, and transitions. For example, consider the dynamics of the transition of the new baby coming via Carine's pregnancy, Carl's chronic illness, and developmental needs of all the family's children.

Nursing Interventions:

- After assessing parents' interest and ability to read written material, bring appropriate written materials to Carl and his family about treatment and management of asthma.
- Review with Carl how to use an inhaler and talk with Carl and his family about recognizing and reducing respiratory triggers.
- Counsel and educate family members on appropriate treatment and management of asthma, reviewing treatment goals and objectives.
- Commend the family on its management of each illness episode and its overall management of family members' health.

Case Study: Comantan Family *(cont.)*

- Explore with the family members what they believe will be risky times for Carl's health, such as spring, when plants are blooming and his asthma symptoms increase.
- Support the various roles of family members and subsystems within the family, such as Carl interacting with his uncle and grandfather as adult male role models when his father is away on the road.
- Recognize the principle of honoring cultural diversity and incorporate the roles of Aunt Leena and Uncle Jesse.
- Recognize the role of the grandparents in Carl's cultural upbringing, especially learning about his Inuit culture and history.
- Recognize the strengths in the family, for example, its efforts to keep Carl successful at his grade level in school.
- Work collaboratively with the family in identifying and evaluating sources of help and support they already use.
- Discuss with the Comantan family the advantages and disadvantages of sending Carl to a 2-week residential camp for children with asthma.

Evaluation:
- Noticing how the family has coordinated many people for Carl's care: the nurse, Rebecca, Aunt Leena, and the grandparents
- Assessing how the family is doing with reducing triggers for Carl's asthma, as well as helping him when he wheezes
- Monitoring for the presence or absence of wheezing, number and duration of respiratory infections, and number of school days attended
- Considering the impact on the family if Carl is hospitalized for a severe attack, infection, or both
- Considering the question of the projected impact of Carl's illnesses on the new baby; for example, the risks of Carl's infections on a newborn infant
- Considering types and potential impact of health-illness transitions for the Comantan family
- Considering additional developmental challenges the family may face in the future, such as the increased mobility of little Frankie and the increased activity needs of Sam
- Asking if there are any additional foci for the family that have not been addressed
- Considering asking the family about their plans for financial resources during Carine's maternity leave
- Asking what additional family strengths could be engaged to assist them in the future

SUMMARY

In this chapter, family child health nursing care covered the following:

- Family child health nurses focus on the relationships between family life and children's health and illness, and they assist families and family members to achieve and maintain well-being.
- Through family-centered care, family child health nurses enhance family life and the development of family members to their fullest potential.
- The family child health concepts incorporate relevant components of family life and interaction, family careers, family development and transitions, family tasks, family communication, family routines, and family health and illness, and help nurses to take a comprehensive and collaborative approach to families.
- The family child health concepts enable nurses to screen for potentially harmful situations (e.g., risk for unintentional and intentional injury and death); instruct families about health issues and healthy lifestyles; and help families to cope with acute illness, chronic illness, and life-threatening conditions.
- The family child nurse addresses the needs of individuals within the family and the family as a whole to reach developmental and health potential. For example, siblings of children with special needs can fare well if given the guidance and support they need to develop understanding and empathy, and if included in the care of their sibling.

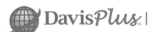 **DavisPlus** | For additional resources and information, visit **http://davisplus.fadavis.com**. References and Suggested Web sites can be found on DavisPlus.

Chapter 14

Family Nursing in Acute Care Adult Settings

Paul S. Smith, PhD, RN, CCRN, CNE

Melissa Robinson, PhD, RN

Critical Concepts

- Family nursing is the provision of care to the entire family unit and is an integral aspect of care provided by nurses in adult acute care settings.

- Families who are viewed as part of the health care team are empowered to deal with the stressors of a family member's hospitalization and are prepared to provide support, aid in recovery, or facilitate a comfortable death.

- Supportive actions by family members, as well as conflict and criticism, have an effect on patients' health behaviors, emotional well-being, immune function, and illness exacerbations.

- During the acute illness phase, nursing interventions should focus on patients and their families by providing physical care and emotional support, facilitating family communication, providing timely information, and establishing a collaborative, trusting partnership.

- Unit or hospital policies need to be updated so that patient-identified family members are not excluded. Restricted, nonflexible visitation policies add stress and trauma for both the patient and the patient's loved ones.

- Transferring loved ones from critical care units (CCUs) to the medical-surgical units is stressful for families because it creates a sense of conflict. On one hand, families are glad their loved ones are better, but they also worry that their family members may not be ready to be moved out of such intensive nurse watchfulness.

- The family member who advocates for a loved one in the hospital assumes a difficult, time-consuming, and fatiguing role: he or she often travels long distances to get to the hospital, takes time off work to be there, often stays all night in the hospital, manages the informational needs of the patient and the family, and works through a complex health care system.

- Effective communication with patients, families, and interdisciplinary health care providers improves client satisfaction, promotes positive response to care, reduces length of stay in care settings, and results in decreased overall cost and resource utilization.

- Compassionate communication provides crucial care to families as they are asked to make multiple decisions as their loved one dies in the hospital.

The concept of family can be complex and moves beyond the nuclear family to include any loving, supportive persons the patients identify as having an important role in their life without regard to social and legal boundaries (Leino-Kilpi, Gröndahl, Katajisto, Nurminen, & Suhonen, 2016; Tracy, 2014). Family nursing is the provision of care to the entire family unit and is an integral aspect of care provided by nurses in adult acute care settings. Hospitalization for an acute or critical illness, injury, or exacerbation of a chronic illness is not only stressful for patients and their families but also can be life changing and threaten the equilibrium of the family unit (McConnell & Moroney, 2015; Morton & Fontaine, 2013; Rattray, 2014). Patients and families often feel alone and unsure of their role in an acute care setting, and it is of utmost importance that the health care team engage families in this environment (Hardin, 2012; McConnell & Moroney, 2015). Family members may also have feelings of chaos and loss of control because of extreme uncertainty related to an acute admission of a family member (Beer & Brysiewicz, 2016; Page, 2015). The ill adult enters the hospital, usually in a physiological crisis, and the family most often accompanies the ill or injured person to the hospital. During this acute care admission, which is often a profound emotional experience, family caregivers will focus attention on the critically ill family member and often pay little attention to their own health (Choi, Donahoe, & Hoffman, 2016; Warren, Rainey, Weddle, Bennett, & Roden-Foreman, 2016). Simultaneously, family members continue to cope with external demands such as occupational and household responsibilities, navigate complex and often difficult financial decisions, and provide care and maintain the needs of other family members (Warren et al., 2016). Nurses and other health care providers should place emphasis on supporting family members who are particularly vulnerable and who may require special needs because of a lack of support and understanding the situation of their loved one (Frivold, Slettebø, & Dale, 2016).

Hospitalized family members worry about the effects of their illness and their potentially changed capabilities on the rest of their family (Perry, Lynam, & Anderson, 2006). When nurses provide care for and develop personal relationships with the whole family, this allows families to be included as part of the health care team, which can improve communication and care planning, prevent errors, and reduce nursing time spent on hygiene activities (Hansen, Rosenkranz, Mularski, & Leo, 2016; Wyskiel et al., 2015). Involving family members in intervention strategies not only strengthens family relationships and enhances the effects of the interventions, but it also allows family members to be more than passive bystanders by contributing to both the physiological and psychological well-being of their hospitalized relative (Cypress, 2011; Gooding, Pierce, & Flaherty, 2012; Gutierrez, 2012; Page, 2015). Close social relationships, especially family relationships, affect physical and psychological well-being, and promote adherence to disease management plans that involve changes in health behavior. When families are involved in the care of the loved one in the hospital, the patient experiences increased ability to cope with and recover from a critical illness and increased likelihood of positive health outcomes (Gooding et al., 2012; Tracy, 2014).

Since the late 1970s, progress to move to a more family-centered care model in adult critical care and medical-surgical nursing has been slow but steady (Latour & Haines, 2007). Families with members who are acutely or critically ill are seen in adult medical-surgical units, intensive care or critical care units (ICUs or CCUs, respectively), or emergency departments. The acute phase of illness or injury refers to the period immediately after the onset of the illness or the injury. During this time, family members want to be able to ask the following questions about the person who is ill or injured: Is he or she doing as well as can be expected? Is he or she getting any better? Is he or she in any pain? Has there been any change? What can I expect in the future? What can I do to help? These questions may be expressed in thousands of different ways but stem from the common concern that they fear for their loved one's well-being. Having loved ones in today's acute care hospital can be an upsetting experience at any time, but when a stay in an adult CCU unit occurs (anticipated or not), it can be especially traumatic (Kentish-Barnes & Azoulay, 2012; McConnell & Moroney, 2015). Family members and significant others of critically ill patients are integral to the recovery of their loved ones. Their involvement in providing care brings them together and assists in helping the patient feel comfortable in an unaccustomed setting, such as an acute care setting (Bhalla, Suri, Kaur, & Kaur, 2014).

The purpose of this chapter is to describe family nursing in acute care settings, including families in the CCUs and medical-surgical units. A review of literature captures the major stressors families face during hospitalization of an adult family member: the transfer from one unit to another, being discharged home, participation in cardiopulmonary resuscitation (CPR), withdrawing life support therapy, and organ donation. This chapter concludes with a family case study that (1) highlights the issues families experience and adapt to when an adult member is ill; and (2) applies the Family Systems Theory in order to demonstrate one theoretical approach for working with families.

FAMILIES IN CRITICAL CARE UNITS

In the United States, more than 5.7 million patients are admitted annually to CCUs for treatment and intensive or invasive monitoring as well as for the restoration of a stable health status or palliative care (comfort while dying) (Society of Critical Care Medicine, 2017). Approximately 20% of acute care hospital admissions are to a CCU; of the patients who are seen in the emergency department, approximately 58% are admitted to a CCU (Society of Critical Care Medicine, 2017).

The American College of Critical Care Medicine Task Force (2004–2005) developed 43 evidence-based practice guidelines for supporting and involving family in ICUs (Davidson et al., 2007). These guidelines address topics such as the "endorsement of a shared decision-making model, early and repeated care conferencing to reduce family stress and improve consistency in communication, honoring culturally appropriate requests for truth-telling and informed refusal, spiritual support, staff education and debriefing to minimize the impact of family interactions on staff health, family presence at both rounds and resuscitation, open flexible visitation, way-finding and family-friendly signage, and family support before, during, and after a death" (Davidson et al., 2007, p. 605). This section presents evidence-based practice on family nursing in CCUs, specifically addressing family needs when a member is in the ICU: visiting policies, waiting rooms, family interventions in the ICU, and ways to work with families to decrease family relocation stress and transfer anxiety.

Family Needs in the Intensive Care Unit

Family visitors in ICUs report and demonstrate symptoms of anxiety or depression after having their family members in the ICU for a few days (Pouchard et al., 2005). Family members of critical care patients may also have moderate to severe cardiac type symptoms such as shortness of breath or heart palpitations, known as cardiac anxiety, but they are physically healthy during the hospitalization of a relative (Konstanti, Gouva, Dragioti, Nakos, & Koulouras, 2016). In addition, family members are at significant risk for development of post-traumatic stress disorder (PTSD) when they have family members in the ICU (Azoulay et al., 2005). The needs of family members with loved ones in the ICU have long been studied (Al-Mutair, Plummer, O'Brien, & Clerehan, 2013). The classic work of Molter in 1979 first identified the following 10 family needs in the ICU, listed in descending order:

1. Hope
2. Health care provider caring about the patient
3. Having a waiting room near the patient
4. Being called at home for a change in patient condition
5. Knowing about the prognosis
6. Having questions answered honestly
7. Knowing specific facts about prognosis
8. Receiving information about patient once a day
9. Having explanations in understandable terms
10. Seeing patient frequently

The Critical Care Family Needs Inventory (CCFNI) is a self-report questionnaire, first developed by Molter (1979) then revised by Leske (1986), that provides a list of 45 need statements developed for family assessment and report of self-perceived needs of families in the ICU. The CCFNI is known to be a valid and reliable instrument to assess family needs and has been used in more than 50 studies (Al-Mutair et al., 2013; Paul & Rattray, 2008). The CCFNI collapsed family needs into five dimensions: (1) assurance, (2) information, (3) proximity, (4) comfort, and (5) support (Leske, 1986).

What is crucial for nurses to know about this research is that health care settings have been only partially responsive to the needs of families for information or assurance. Table 14-1 illustrates that, although nurses are providing more information to family members and that families can see their loved ones more frequently, nurses are not providing reassurance to family members or meeting the needs that families identify as important to their own health and well-being (Browning & Warren, 2006).

Table 14-1 Family Needs in the Intensive Care Unit	
Family Needs Always/Usually Met	**Family Needs Never/Sometimes Met**
• Informed about medical treatments	• Needs explanations in lay terminology
• Aware of why and what care is being provided	• Needs to have access to quality food in the hospital
• Knows somewhat about the prognosis	• Assured it is okay to leave the hospital for a while
• Allowed to visit in the ICU frequently	• To be prepared for the ICU environment before entering the unit the first time
• Understands different types of staff caring for family member	• Talks to the same nurse every day
• Knows who to call in the ICU for information	• Has feeling of hope supported
• Given directions for things to do at bedside while visiting	• Shares feelings, especially those of guilt, anger, or fear
• Called at home for condition changes	• Feels accepted by the hospital staff
• Has support of friends and family	• Discusses the possibility that family member may die
• Knows what is being done for their family member	• Visits anytime

Source: Adapted from Browning, G., & Warren, N. (2006). Unmet needs of family members in the medical intensive care waiting room. *Critical Care Nursing Quarterly, 29*(1), 86–95.

Al-Mutair et al. (2013) found that assurance followed by information were the two most reported important family member needs. Kinrade, Jackson, and Tomnay (2009) used the CCFNI in an ICU with no restriction on visiting hours to determine family needs and found that the most important family need was to have questions answered honestly and for information to be shared in a timely manner. A study by Douglas, Daly, and Lipson (2012) found that patient quality of life rarely was discussed with families when a loved one had a long stay in the ICU. (See Chapter 10 for a detailed discussion of end-of-life and palliative care.) Families with a member who had unexpected admissions to the ICU were noted to have different needs than families who had planned admissions. When a patient has an uncertain prognosis from a stay in the CCU, family needs were found to be different than when the prognosis was favorable (Prachar et al., 2010). Family members who were dealing with a poor prognosis expressed a need to talk about their feelings of what happened and wanted a religious representative to visit (Prachar et al., 2010).

Overall, families reported that they had two different sets of feelings when a family member was in the ICU (Eriksson, Bergbom, & Lindahl, 2011). First, families expressed that they fluctuated between hope and despair. They felt that information was a way to help them manage these feelings (Eriksson et al., 2011). Second, families reported that they hungered for information to help them make sense of what was happening and described themselves as being hypervigilant to even the smallest information.

The most helpful aspect of the whole experience was their interaction with the staff (Eriksson et al., 2011). Families want authentic connection with nurses who are caring for their loved ones (Nelms & Eggenberger, 2010). The family depends on the whole critical care team to provide care and keep it informed so it can make crucial decisions for loved ones (Kentish-Barnes & Azoulay, 2012).

A qualitative study conducted in Canada identified that participants described the patient/family "ICU journey" as having three phases: (1) admission to the ICU, (2) daily care in the ICU, and (3) post-ICU experience (Gill et al., 2016). Admission to the ICU was characterized by family shock and disorientation as well as presence and support of a health care provider. Five themes emerged regarding daily care in the ICU: honoring the patient's voice, the need to know, decision making, medical care, and culture in the ICU (Gill et al., 2016). Lastly, the post-ICU phase included two themes, one being the transition from ICU to a hospital ward and the other being long-term effects of critical illness (Gill et al., 2016). The participants of the study provided five suggestions for improving care in the ICU. These suggestions are:

■ Providing a dedicated family navigator
■ Increasing provider awareness of the fragility of family trust
■ Improving provider communication skills
■ Improving the transition from ICU to a hospital ward
■ Informing patients about the long-term effects of critical illness

Families are not only the primary support for loved ones in the ICU, but they can also have a positive impact on the ability of patients to cope and recover from a critical illness (Tracy, 2014). The American Association of Critical-Care Nurses' (AACN) *Essentials of Critical Care Nursing* (Tracy, 2014) identified evidence-based practice areas to assess the family's needs and resources in order to develop interventions that optimize the family's impact on the patient and the interactions with the health care team. Areas for family interventions include:

- Offer realistic hope
- Give honest answers and information
- Give reassurance
- Use open-ended communication and assess their communication style
- Assess family members' level of anxiety
- Assess perceptions of the situation (knowledge, comprehension, expectations of staff, expected outcomes)
- Assess family roles and dynamics (cultural and religious practices, values, spokesperson)
- Assess coping mechanisms and resources (what do they use, social network and support)

Patients reported knowing that their family was at their bedside supported their desire to get well (Eriksson et al., 2011). Families experience cognitive, emotional, and social stress when family members are in the ICU. These worries include:

- Information ambiguity
- Uncertain prognosis
- Fear of death
- Role changes
- Financial concerns
- Disruption of normal routines

Nursing Role Ambiguity and Conflict

ICU nurses are in the best position to support these families because they see them often, know the patient intimately, and are called to practice holistically instead of based on a biomedical model. Yet, many ICU nurses not only continue to view families as obstacles to care and consistently underestimate their professional role in meeting the needs of these families, but they also rely on personal values to guide the decision-making process as to whether or not to involve family members in patient care (McConnell & Moroney, 2015). What ICU nurses believe families need does not always match what

families identify as their needs (Kinrade et al., 2009; Maxwell, Stuenkel, & Saylor, 2007; Prachar et al., 2010). Therefore, it is important to explore why this dichotomy continues to exist given the evidence that has been known since Molter's work was published in 1979.

Stayt (2007) investigated nurses' perceptions of their ability to practice family nursing in the ICU. Two important findings in this research offer an insight into understanding these nurses' experiences: nurses express role ambiguity and role conflict. Role ambiguity is when nurses find themselves with an unrealistic role expectation. The nurses believed that it was their responsibility to "make it right" or to "take away the family members' worries" rather than to provide emotional support for families dealing with the uncertainty of outcome for a family member in the ICU. The nurses expressed that they felt guilty for not helping families. The nurses undervalued their contribution to meeting the family needs during this stressful time. Nurses identified that they felt they lacked training in how to work with families.

Moreover, ICU nurses identified two types of role conflict (Stayt, 2007). The first role conflict was difficulty in balancing the biomedical technical model of care with the holistic nursing model of care. Chesla (1997) reports a similar role conflict for ICU nurses between technical care and social-emotional care. Nurses are torn between caring for the medically unstable patient—who is their priority—yet recognizing that they are responsible for caring for the entire family. The second type of role conflict was the balance of their professional relationship and the more personal relationship the family seeks with the nurse (Stayt, 2007). In the ICU, the nurse-family relationship is established during an intense emotional time for the family. After some time, the family was described as seeking too much self-disclosure from the nurses. Nurses found keeping professional boundaries fatiguing and time-consuming. Therefore, the nurses described that they used detachment strategies to keep their relationship professional. For example, they would ask for a different patient assignment. Or nurses would physically distance themselves by focusing only on tasks when they entered the patient's room. They found ways to limit conversation with the family. They found themselves emotionally distancing themselves from the family so they would not engage on a personal level.

Nurses recognized the importance of families and wanted to work with them in the ICU, but they found it difficult to provide for the emotional needs of family members. Hospital educational programs are needed to support nurses in providing family-centered care versus patient-centered care.

Visiting Policy

Most ICUs (70%) have visitation policies to the ICU that restrict visitors (AACN Practice Alerts, 2012). Yet the evidence is clear that unrestricted visitation decreases patient anxiety, confusion, and agitation; reduces cardiovascular complications; decreases ICU lengths of stay; makes patients feel more secure; increases patient satisfaction; and enhances quality and safety (AACN Practice Alerts, 2012, p. 76). Moreover, evidence suggests that unrestricted visitation increases family satisfaction, decreases family members' anxiety, promotes better communication, contributes to better understanding of the patient, allows more opportunities for patient/family teaching as the family becomes more involved in care, and is not associated with longer family visits (AACN Practice Alerts, 2012, p. 76). The AACN suggests that there are times when family visits should be restricted, such as documented legal reasons, when a visitor has a communicable disease, or if the behavior of a visitor is a direct risk to the patient. AACN (2012) recommends that children supervised by an adult family member should be welcome in the ICU and should not be restricted by age alone.

Unit or hospital policies may need to be updated so that patient-identified family members are not excluded (Bell, 2016). Such administrative revisions need to take into consideration evidence-based data so that both nursing staff and families can be confident that patient care systems reflect these visionary professional standards even when patients cannot speak for themselves (Latour & Haines, 2007; Verhaeghe, Defloor, Van Zuuren, Duijnstee, & Grypdonck, 2005).

Debate regarding the "correct" quantity and frequency of visits in adult CCUs is ongoing (Day, 2006; Miracle, 2005). Policies that have been tried and often revisited have included 10 minutes every hour, 30 minutes several times a day, two visitors at a time, immediate family only, open visiting, closed visiting with rare exceptions, and many more versions of these options. These restrictions often are in place because health care providers feel that

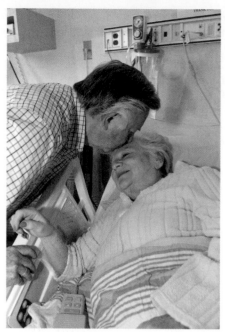

© iStock.com/JodiJacobson

having visitors interrupts patient care and also may affect the patient's well-being. However, research has shown otherwise. Following are some specifics.

Chapman et al. (2016) found that when visitation was changed from being closed during nursing report for 3 hours daily to being open at all times in a shock trauma ICU, there was not only an increase in family member satisfaction with the convenience of visitation hours and waiting room ambiance but also an improvement in nurses' perceptions of families' satisfaction. Open visitation in a neuroscience ICU and a private suite for patients' family members led to family members rating their needs as being met at a high level (Jacob et al., 2016). Family members noted that in addition to visitation, getting information about the patient and being given hope were most important (Jacob et al., 2016). When cardiac patients had unrestricted visiting hours, these patients had fewer cardiovascular complications compared with those patients who were restricted to visitors twice a day (Fumagalli et al., 2006). Liberal visiting hours not only helped patients, but benefited the staff. Family members served as historians, participated in daily rounds, and assisted with care. In addition, allowing visitors decreased unexpected calls, increased participation and engagement with staff, and increased patient and family satisfaction (Jacobowski, Girard, Mulder, & Ely, 2010). More important, unrestricted visitation reduced anxiety among patients and met the family members' needs at a high level when compared with limitations on family visitation (Gooding et al., 2012; Jacob et al., 2016).

Professional nursing organizations, such as the AACN (mentioned earlier) and the American Nurses Association (ANA), have supported the position that, despite being in critical condition, patients cannot receive adequate care when they are isolated from their families (Bice-Stephens, 2006; Latour & Haines, 2007). The Joint Commission of Hospitals recognizes the importance of visitation. In 2011, the Commission added an element to the Patient Rights Standard, which states that hospitals should permit friends and family members to be present during hospitalization in order to provide emotional support to the patient (The Joint Commission, 2010). Families are foundational to the comprehensive care of all patients, so it is the responsibility of every nurse and every health care agency to implement and regularly evaluate visitation policies and procedures that reflect this philosophy (Bell, 2016).

Cell Phones

Cell phones are an integral tool of our lives. Family members rely heavily on cell phones to remain connected to others (Eriksson et al., 2011). In many ICUs, cells phones are banned because there is concern that these devices may emit electromagnetic radiation that interferes with the functioning of medical devices (Makic, VonRueden, Rauen, & Chadwick, 2011). But newer data and voice phones do not present these issues and, in fact, are used regularly in hospitals now (Lee et al., 2013). However, there is concern that cell phones might be a source of nosocomial infections (Lee et al., 2013). Hospitals should consider assessing their policies on banning cell phones. Limiting the use of cell phones requires family members to leave and locate a designated cell phone area, which may be a challenge. Given that visiting hours and the number of guests allowed in the ICU are restricted, family members may hesitate to leave the ICU to make phone calls, considering the barriers for reentry. Reevaluating and updating cell phone policies is vital in promoting patient and family satisfaction.

Waiting Rooms

When families of critically ill patients are not in the unit with their loved ones, they are more than likely spending a significant amount of time in the unit's waiting room (Deitrick et al., 2005). Attention to the details that may help relieve family stress is critical. Little research has focused on family comfort and amenities provided in the waiting rooms adjacent to CCUs (Alvarez & Kirby, 2006). But families have consistently voiced desires to have better access to healthy food and drinks, a variety of comfortable seating options to account for all people, available computer access, and nearby rooms for private meetings with physicians, nurses, or other health care providers. Families have expressed issues with the lack of privacy because the waiting room is often shared with other families (Engstrom, Anderson, & Soderberg, 2008; Karlsson, Tissell, Engstrom, & Andershed, 2011). A room that is quiet and comfortable improves the well-being of family members (Karlsson et al., 2011). Many ICUs have been responsive to these expressed needs of families by providing a clean, organized waiting room area with several small seating sections for family conversations, adequate soft lighting, a section for computer work, private meeting rooms, and a special play area with age-appropriate toys for various children's ages. Some ICUs have dedicated sleeping rooms for family members. Providing a beeper system for the family to carry when they leave the unit or waiting room was found to be helpful to families (Deitrick et al., 2005). Receptionists in family waiting room areas are gaining in popularity (Alvarez & Kirby, 2006).

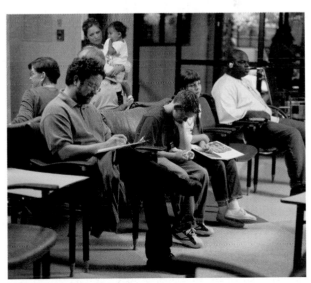

© iStock.com

Family Interventions

Aside from open visitation policies, revisited cell phone policies, and improved waiting rooms, family intervention strategies that support both nurses and families include the following:

- Helping family members feel as comfortable as possible while in the room with the patient
- Including families in the nurse-to-nurse shift change bedside report
- Including family members in the physician rounds when they discuss the progress of the patient
- Involving families in shared decision making
- Facilitating family conferences
- Offering families the opportunity to keep progress journals
- Creating a family nurse specialist in the ICU (Gooding et al., 2012)

Families are often overwhelmed and intimidated with the fast-paced, noisy, and highly technological environments that surround their loved ones in the ICU (Pikka & Beaulieu, 2004). Patients appear "lost" among all the equipment, tubes, lines, beeping, and bonging sounds, especially when interventions such as dressings or indwelling tubes around the face and head distort facial features (Maxwell et al., 2007). ICU nurses who practice from a family perspective realize how their everyday world in this fast-paced, emotionally charged setting is stressful for families. After the patient is initially stabilized on admission to the ICU, the nurses should spend time explaining the equipment and the immediate goals of nursing care, and role modeling how family members can support their loved one, including how to touch the person. Nurses should address fear of all the equipment used in this setting. This approach is helpful to decrease family stress and builds on the knowledge that family members have a strong desire to be by their loved one, particularly when there is a change in the patient's condition. They want to be an integral part of the patient's care. Allowing families to participate in the actual care of their family members likewise has been found to offer reassurance, as well as a way for family members to contribute to their loved one's recovery (Alvarez & Kirby, 2006). Family members believe that being close to the patient is their obligation and is a sign of their commitment to the patient (Eggenberger & Nelms, 2007). Fear of "not being there" if something goes wrong reinforces family members' desire to be with the patient (Eggenberger & Nelms, 2007). Therefore, nurses must see and include families as an integral part of the patient's care.

Supporting the family is another important nursing intervention. Although the nurses' priority is to the patient, families also need support. Emotional stress rises when a family member is acutely ill and families suffer with the patient during illness and treatment. They have feelings of helplessness, sadness, and fear (Eggenberger & Nelms, 2007). Some express that their emotions fluctuate similar to a "roller coaster" (Linnarsson, Bubini, & Perseius, 2010, p. 3102). They attempt to control these emotions in order to be supportive to the patient and other members of the family. In addition, many families feel the need to be watchful and protective of the patient in order to shield the patient from the emotions of the illness (Eggenberger & Nelms, 2007; Karlsson et al., 2011). Families are gatekeepers of information as they protect and shield their loved ones from emotional turmoil related to the care and the illness (Burr, 1998). It is important that the nurse support the family members by connecting with them. Nurses should spend time, provide information (good and bad), be honest, share themselves, involve families in care, and acknowledge the emotional stress they are undergoing. Families do want and depend on nurses for social support (Eggenberger & Nelms, 2007; Engstrom & Soderberg, 2007; Fry & Warren, 2007; Karlsson et al., 2011). Because nurses provide 24-hour care, they are in the best position to identify and support families.

Families often say waiting in the ICU creates tremendous physical strain. Families stay long hours in the ICU just waiting. They wait for information, to see their loved ones, and for the next thing to happen. They try to manage their personal affairs from the hospital, commute back to their homes after a long day, and take care of the patient (Eggenberger & Nelms, 2007; Higgins, Joyce, Parker, Fitzgerald, & McMillan, 2007). Family members of patients in the ICU also have been found to be at increased risk for experiencing anxiety, depression, and PTSD (Azoulay et al., 2005; Pouchard et al., 2005). Nurses can reduce some of the strain by providing and seeking information for the family members, asking how they are doing, providing a quiet place for them to rest or sleep, and determining each day how much they wish to be involved in the patient's care (Cioffi, 2006).

Timed daily family rounds with nurses and physicians decreased family anxiety and increased communication (Cypress, 2012; Gooding et al., 2012; Mangram et al., 2005). Careful and consistent information can help mitigate fears. Patients and families gain a better understanding of the plan of care when they have the opportunity to verify information, ask questions, and share concerns when they are involved in nursing end-of-shift reports (Reinbeck & Fitzsimmons, 2013; Tobiano, Chaboyer, &McMurray, 2013). Involving families and patients fosters an environment of trust, mutual respect, and understanding (Reinbeck & Fitzsimmons, 2013). When away from the bedside and the stimulation of the ICU environment, family members are able to hear more clearly and accurately the explanations and answers to their questions and concerns. Therefore, nurses should plan to spend time (e.g., a short 10-minute conference) with families away from the patient's bedside on every shift. Plans for language interpreters should be made in advance.

Shared decision making is a collaborative process in which patients and providers make health care decisions together, weighing the medical evidence of various options and considering the patient's values. Shared decision making is crucial in the ICU because patients often cannot speak for themselves and many of the treatment options are highly invasive and may have a high mortality or morbidity component to them; therefore, most treatment decisions should be made from a family perspective (Douglas et al., 2012). Refer to Chapter 5 for detailed information on family shared decision making. Ahmann and Dokken (2012) outline the following strategies nurses could use to invite families into partnership and shared decision making:

- Use "we" language that demonstrates a team approach.
- Request specific help from a family member.
- Encourage the family members to let the nurse know when they are confused by test results or what they are seeing or hearing.
- Use whiteboards in the patient rooms that include who is in the room, phone numbers, and a place for family questions.
- Give the family a journal in which to keep notes or write experiences.
- Invite the family on rounds.

Family meetings or conferences help keep all members of the health care team, including the family, focused on the needs of the loved one and the family. In addition, family meetings help health care providers communicate among team members (Ahluwalia, Schreibeis-Baum, Prendergast, Reinke, & Lorenz, 2016; Nelson, Walker, Luhrs, Cortez, & Pronovost, 2009). Unfortunately, family conferences that are not well planned in advance have hindered family learning where too many people were included, the agenda was too full, and there were time constraints (Paterson, Kieloch, & Gmiterek, 2001). The most important point made was that the health care providers should be sure not to dominate the discussion and should allow adequate time for the family to voice concerns and pose their questions. Nurses are positioned to play essential roles in family meetings and communication training. Focused attention to nurses' empowerment as well as facilitation of the nurse-health care provider relationship most likely would improve the involvement of nurses in family meetings and alleviate barriers to involvement (Ahluwalia et al., 2016).

Nelson et al. (2009) designed a toolkit for family meetings in the ICU. The toolkit helps ensure that the meetings are efficient, effective, and give all parties time to be heard in directing client care. The guide for families includes the following elements (p. 626.e13):

1. Review what you know:
   - Are you clear about why the person was brought to the ICU and what the current medical problems are?
   - What is the plan for your loved one?
   - What treatment choices are available?
   - What medical decisions need to be made?
2. Concerns or worries:
   - List what concerns you have about the current situation.
   - Identify what you are worried about the most given the current situation.
   - If the team could answer one thing for you today, what would that be?
3. If the patient can't talk to you or the team now, what would the patient say about what is happening now in his or her care? Bring any documents or papers such as a health care proxy or living will.

Encouraging families to keep a family progress journal (Kloos & Daly, 2008) or a computer family blog for extended family and friends decreased family anxiety. In their analysis of family progress journals,

Kloos and Daly (2008) found the following top three family issues addressed: the family experiencing negative emotions about the physical appearance of their loved one in the ICU, the need for more regular communication about what was going on, and the worry about the pain their loved one was experiencing. The journals illustrated that families coped with their stress through their faith and spirituality, support of family and friends, and seeing their loved one get better physically. Families wrote that the characteristics of the health care providers that were the most helpful to them were kindness, compassion, watchfulness over their loved one, and availability to answer questions.

Family resilience, or the ability of families to rebound from stressful events, is a goal of family nursing, and nurses working in the critical care environment are uniquely positioned to promote family resilience (Ellis, Gergen, Wohlgemuth, Nolan, & Aslakson, 2016). Nurses view family members as "cheerers" who are crucial in providing support by being involved in patient care (Ellis et al., 2016, p. 39). Black and Lobo (2008) identified 10 prominent protective and recovery factors of resilient families as: positive outlook, spirituality, family member accord, flexibility, family communication, financial management, family time, shared recreation, routines and rituals, and support network. Nurses identified communication as the most prominent and influential enhancer or distractor of family resilience (Ellis et al., 2016).

To meet family needs, one idea was to design a specific nursing position to work with families. This approach allowed the ICU nurses to focus on providing care to the ill person and relieved some stress of providing care to the family client. Having this clinical nurse specialist in the ICU resulted in increased family satisfaction. These nurses assessed family unmet needs and relayed information that increased family understanding, especially about tests, treatments, and condition (Nelson & Poist, 2008; Shelton, Moore, Socaris, Gao, & Dowling, 2010). Interestingly, the ICU nurses reported that they felt this position somewhat interfered with their work, and said that not working as much with the family was not as satisfying for them in the long run. Experienced ICU nurses who underwent a 2-week training period to become a family navigator facilitated family decision making (Torke et al., 2016). The feasibility of a dedicated nursing position to work with families is one that shows promise and one

that could have a direct impact on family resilience and satisfaction.

As patients improve to the point that they are stable enough to transfer out of the ICU, families experience different stressors related to relocation stress and anxiety (Chaboyer, Kendall, Kendall, & Foster, 2005).

Family Relocation Stress and Transfer Anxiety

Moving ill family members from the CCU to the medical-surgical unit is stressful for families. Even though families report relief that their loved ones are able to transfer out of the ICU, they also fear that the loss of one-to-one nurse-patient vigilance will lead to failure to detect important changes in condition (Chaboyer et al., 2005; Latour & Haines, 2007). Some families feel they were unprepared for the transfer and that they were given little information about what to expect (Hughes, Bryan, & Robbins, 2005). Families may interpret the transfer as someone throwing them out of the ICU (Engstrom & Soderberg, 2004). Patients with moderate to high care needs upon discharge from the ICU demonstrated worse depressive symptoms and high levels of anxiety (Choi, Tate, Rogers, Donahoe, & Hoffman, 2016).

Once the patient is transferred, families found that the nursing care on the medical-surgical unit is not as predictable as the ICU and families did not understand the different ratio of nurse-to-patient staffing patterns (Carr, 2002). Families also found the relocation stressful because they missed their relationship with the ICU nurses, and they struggled with changes in the environment and changes in the amount of information they received (Gelling et al., 2001).

Chaboyer et al. (2005) classified the families' emotions with relocation stress into four emotions or feelings: abandonment, vulnerability, unimportance, and ambivalence. Families felt *abandonment* when the transfer was abrupt and not planned. Families described experiencing *vulnerability* when they had to accept their new responsibility as a different kind of family caregiver within the hospital setting. For example, rather than be supportive family members from the background, they now had to provide more actual physical care for their loved one as his or her physical status improved. Their sense of vulnerability was found to be the most intense of these family emotions. The families reported having a feeling of *unimportance* because of the different staffing ratio on the medical-surgical unit. The last feeling identified was *ambivalence*. The families expressed being caught between the extremes of feeling relieved and happy their loved ones were better, and families' fears and doubts that their loved ones were well enough to leave the ICU.

Involving families in the transfer process effectively contributed to less relocation stress (Eldredge, 2004; Latour & Haines, 2007, McKinley, Nagy, Stein-Parbury, Bramwell, & Hudson, 2002). Family conferences scheduled with the health care team are a perfect opportunity for family members to express these concerns and for team members to respond to all concerns with factual, straightforward information. Ideally, both the nurse manager and supervisor of the sending and receiving hospital units should participate in this transition. A detailed and comprehensive written patient care plan helps to smooth out this important phase of the patient and family journey (Day, 2006). Family input into this care plan empowers and reassures families during this transition to the medical-surgical unit.

FAMILIES IN MEDICAL-SURGICAL UNITS

It is clear that families who have adult members in acute medical-surgical areas are stressed by hospitalization, yet this is one of the least studied areas of family nursing. In this section, family visitation, family communication needs, and family needs are explored. Family interventions relative to discharge are discussed.

Families in acute care settings reported numerous stressors and changes in their family environment, and are often desperately in need of support. Nurses are in a position to provide support in the following ways:

- Use effective communication: listen to the family's concerns, feelings, and questions; answer all questions or assist the family in finding the answers.
- Respect and support family coping mechanisms and caregiving behaviors.
- Recognize the uniqueness of each family.
- Assist the family in decision making by providing information about options.
- Permit the family to make decisions about patient care when appropriate.

- Provide adequate time to visit privately, when possible.
- Facilitate family conferences to allow open sharing of family feelings.
- Clarify information and share resources regarding support groups.
- Foster positive nurse-family relationships through all phases of care.

Family Visitation and Caregiving in the Hospital

Visitation helps to promote family cohesion and unity (Nuss et al., 2014; Van Horn & Kautz, 2007). Many of the same issues about family visitation in the ICU described previously in the chapter hold true for family visitation on a medical-surgical inpatient setting.

Many families enact a bedside vigilance that provides a close protective function (Carr & Fogarty, 1999). Families displayed both *directive* behaviors and *supportive* behaviors as family caregivers in the hospital, especially when the hospitalized family member was older (Jacelon, 2006). Family *directive* behaviors were described as follows:

- Acting in place of the ill family member by making decisions about care without consulting the ill family member, talking to health care providers, and being the organizer of care
- Acting as an advisor to the ill family member by working collaboratively with him on decisions
- Not acting in some cases; some family members were found to be available but did not become involved in any decision making.

Family *supportive* behaviors identified by Jacelon (2006) were as follows:

- Keeping the older family members going and active: families brought items from home, visited daily, and sometimes brought the family pet in for a visit.
- Keeping the older family member's life going: they did many things "behind the scenes" such as running errands, paying bills, keeping up homes, and keeping friends informed.
- Staying in the background: some family members were available but not actively involved in daily caregiving.

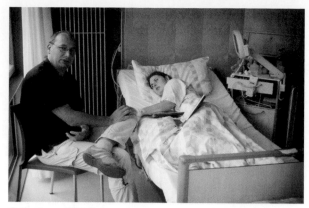

© iStock.com/Claudiad

More specifically, families helped their loved ones in the hospital in many ways that improved patient outcomes, decreased recovery time, increased reports of comfort, and decreased the length of the hospital stay (MacLeod, Chesson, Blackledge, Hutchison, & Ruta, 2005). On the other hand, health care providers on medical-surgical units did not always see families as partners in patient care in either the United States or the United Kingdom (MacLeod et al., 2005). Therefore, families reported feeling unwelcome. Families have stated that gaining access to see their loved ones was a privilege, which was extended to them by the nurses, and that they were careful not to abuse the visiting rules. While in the patient's room, they were fearful of annoying the nurses by their constant presence (Cioffi, 2006). They avoided asking any personal or emotional questions (Soderstrom, Saveman, & Benzein, 2006). For them, they were guests of the patient, not partners in the care of the patient.

The work environment can be an obstacle to allowing medical-surgical nurses to provide family-centered care. The floor nurses often carry a heavy nurse-patient caseload. Many of these patients are of high acuity, which challenges these nurses with the same role conflict mentioned earlier: balancing technical needs of their patients and practicing holistic family-centered care. Because of these work challenges, nurses may convey their stress to families and patients in unintended ways (Astedt-Kurki, Paavilainen, Tammentie, & Paunonen-Ilmonen, 2001; McQueen, 2000). Nurses may send unintended messages by saying something in casual conversation about how busy they were tonight, moving quickly and being in a hurry when they enter the room, and not addressing the family when they enter the room

but instead being very procedure focused. Nurses can work on being sure their nonverbal, inadvertent communications match their concern and caring for the client. Taking a few moments to center oneself before entering the client's room allows the nurses to slow down and focus on the client and family in the room and not on what needs to be done in the busy day.

Communication with the family is crucial for the nurses, the patients, and the families in order to improve the patients' health outcomes. The placement of whiteboards in patient rooms is routinely used in hospital settings to improve communication. These boards, typically placed on a wall near a patient's hospital bed, allow any number of providers to communicate a wide range of information such as the date; the name of the nurse, aide, and doctors on that shift; notes from loved ones to the ill person; phone numbers of the family to call in case of condition changes; patient-identified outcome goals for that specific day; questions for providers; and expected date of discharge (Sehgal, Green, Vidyarthi, Blegen, & Wachter, 2010). Including families in patient rounds with physicians and nurses helps to keep communication clear between providers and family members. Limiting the number of interruptions to the nurse while working with the patient and family would improve communication and send messages of importance to the family and patient (Darc, Lennon, & Sanders, 2013). Hospitals have moved to a limited number of overhead pagers so that patients and families are not bombarded with noise and the workings of the facility. Proactively providing information to patients' families will reduce the number of interruptions for nurses. Some hospitals send families text messages with updates on a family member that do not contain intimate details but are updated status reports (Darc et al., 2013).

Family Communication Needs

Effective communication between and with patients, families, and interdisciplinary health care providers improves client satisfaction, promotes positive response to care, reduces length of stay in care settings, and results in decreased overall cost and resource utilization (Ahrens, Yancey, & Kollef, 2003). Nurses believe that conveying information to families is essential when caring for both acute and chronically ill patients; at the same time, however, they reported refraining from doing so because they do not want to be "in the middle" or cause conflict between the family and the attending physician (Zaforteza, Gastaldo, de Pedro, Sánchez-Cuenca, & Lastra, 2005). It was found that nurses provide only basic information to family members and rarely attend to the families awaiting news in waiting rooms (Zaforteza et al., 2005). Nurses underestimate the needs of families, particularly the need for information and the need of family to be close to the patient (Higgins & Cadd, 1999; Kleinpell & Powers, 1992).

Nurses identified additional barriers to family communication that included the lack of perceived permission to share information and lack of knowledge regarding what information has already been shared with family members by the physician (Zaforteza et al., 2005). Nurses did not want to contradict physician information and expressed being worried about creating false hopes in the family. Nurses were concerned about families misinterpreting what was said because the nurses lacked training in managing the family's emotional responses, especially when the family shared negative emotions. Thus, nurses as part of the interdisciplinary team were found to avoid communication needs of the patients and the families. Rather, nurses focused their communication efforts on the needs of the institution, other health care providers, and themselves (Hardicre, 2003; Zaforteza et al., 2005).

Nurses must advocate more readily for sharing information with families. One way for nurses to advocate is to be sure to be present in the room and participate in physician family conferences. Nurses are in a position to help families understand what the physician means and they serve as a sounding board for the family. Nurses must learn to facilitate patient-family interaction and communication that will increase family support of patients at the bedside (Zaforteza et al., 2005). Clear, concise, timely information has been found to reduce family anxiety and have a calming effect (Mitchell, 2009; Zaforteza et al., 2005).

Assessment of patient care needs is integral to nursing and to providing optimal care at the bedside. It is essential to complete a thorough psychosocial and emotional evaluation to communicate effectively with patients and their families. In particular, nurses should explore each family's feelings about the uncertainty of the situation, anxiety, frustration, and fear of losing a family member (Chien, Chiu, Lam, & Ip, 2006; Zaforteza et al., 2005).

Communicating with families in an empathetic, timely, and sensitive manner is particularly effective to decrease tension, uncertainty, and distress (Zaforteza et al., 2005). Offering systematic, integrated, relevant information provides guidance to family members. Relevant information includes the nature of the illness, prognosis, treatment options, potential complications, care needs after discharge, and alternatives to continued treatment (Nelson, Kinjo, Meier, Ahmad, & Morrison, 2005). In addition, Chien et al. (2006) note the importance of communicating specific facts regarding a client's progress and expected outcomes, exploring family feelings including guilt and anger, informing family members of what was to be done for the client and why, and providing suggestions to families about actual care they could provide at the bedside to support the patient and help reduce family anxiety (Chien et al., 2006).

Family members find communication from a variety of providers to be worthwhile when health care providers are perceived as sensitive, unhurried, and honest, and use understandable language (Nelson et al., 2005). Furthermore, follow-up with written verification of information that was shared verbally at patient care conferences was found to be effective in promoting family coping (Kleiber, Davenport, & Freyenberger, 2006; Lautrette et al., 2007). Chien et al. (2006) have determined that conducting a family needs assessment and subsequent systematic education in response to identified issues is an effective means by which to facilitate both patient and family health.

Family-nurse communication is crucial during the hospital stay. Because families are key members of the health care team and will be the primary providers of care once the patient leaves the acute setting, addressing the family's educational and information needs is a critical part of the discharge process.

Family Needs During Discharge

Families and patients are excited about leaving the hospital. For some, however, it is a time when anxieties and uncertainties are high; families worry about their loved one not receiving the round-the-clock care available in the hospital. Adverse and poor outcomes are associated with poor transitions, specifically with problems in continuity of care and caregiver burden (Coleman, Parry, Chalmers, & Minn, 2006). Readmission rates to hospitals were at an all-time high, but have been noted in the last 2 years to have decreased slightly from 19% to 18.4% nationally. It is not clear what the cause of this improvement is (American Hospital Association, 2013). It is believed that approximately 75% of these readmissions may have been preventable (Medicare Payment Advisory Commission, 2009). Clearly, involving family in discharge planning is crucial for a smooth transition of care.

Families worry about adding the home caregiver role to their already overburdened load of family responsibilities. In fact, families coping with members with traumatic brain injuries reported forgetting what they were taught about what to expect, what resources were available to them, and experienced confusion in the home setting (Paterson et al., 2001). These families actually participated in extensive discharge planning and teaching, yet their severe anxiety inhibited their learning. The families told of not being able to hear the conversations during the care conferences because they were so worried about how they were going to manage at home. Other families shared that they were so overwhelmed with the complexity of the situation and the health care system that they could not pay attention in the conferences (Paterson et al., 2001).

Nurses should facilitate discharge care conferences and help families transition smoothly to providing care in the home environment. In today's health care environment, families are often caring for very ill family members at home before they are fully recovered and ready to assume their normal family roles (Bjornsdottir, 2002; DesRoches, Blendon, Young, Scoles, & Kim, 2002). Families are providing nursing care at home that is traditionally done by nurses in the hospital, such as assisting with ambulation, transfer, wound care, medication administration, and, in some cases, operating high-tech equipment. Hooyman and Gonyea (1999) call this the "informalization of health care." When families are involved in discharge planning there is increased patient adherence to treatment recommendations (Koh, Barr, & George, 2014).

The importance in providing a comprehensive discharge plan cannot be overemphasized. Discharge planning should begin when the person is admitted to the acute care setting by anticipating and identifying the patient's continuing needs. A comprehensive plan should include, at a minimum, the following: what to do when the person gets home, how to do it, and what to look for and do when a problem develops. In addition, the plan should include instructions about who will follow the care of the client in the outpatient setting and a follow-up appointment, if possible. The plan should also contain referrals to other care providers in advance of discharge. Review client management plans with families daily and update progress toward discharge with the family. Discuss possible needs the family will need to address in the home once the family members arrive there.

Given today's concern over health care costs, nurses can play a key role in helping patients maintain optimal health, and discharge planning is one key component. Interestingly, a study published in the *New England Journal of Medicine* (Jencks, Williams, & Coleman, 2012) found that about one-fifth (19.6%) of Medicare beneficiaries were readmitted to the hospital within 30 days of discharge and more than one-third (34%) were readmitted within 90 days. About one-half (50.2%) of nonsurgical hospital patients who were readmitted within 30 days did not visit a physician. The study also found that when readmitted to the hospital, these patients stayed an average of 0.6 days (13.2%) longer than those patients admitted the first time for the same problem.

As the coordinator of care, nurses can facilitate the planning of care before the patient is discharged. Establishing guidelines so that every patient has a medical appointment before discharge is essential. Nurses can make sure that patients have the correct discharge medications and receive a sufficient amount to last them for a few days. Comparing discharge medications to those medications the patients normally take at home should be part of the discharge planning. It is not unusual for a patient's medication list at discharge to be different from the medication list before admission. Unfortunately, these changes often are not conveyed to the patient's primary doctors. Sometimes patients end up taking medications from both lists or they take duplicate medications because these medications have different brand names (Alonso-Zaldivar, 2012).

Recently, hospitals have been using transition coaches to help reduce hospital readmission by targeting population groups that have a higher hospital readmission rate. These programs vary but the central tenet is to begin discharge planning while the patient is hospitalized and continue with intensive postdischarge care. Often, nurses assume the role of the transition/hospital coach. Research has demonstrated that a multicomponent intervention program—which includes early assessment of the patient's discharge needs, enhanced patient education and counseling, and early postdischarge follow-up care—is associated with reduced readmissions, particularly among older patients and those with heart failure (Coleman et al., 2006; Osborne, 2011).

Family Interventions at Discharge

Follow-up conversations with families indicate that discharge by a nurse who has been trained in transition care helps support families (Coleman et al., 2004). One in four Medicare patients returns home with an unmet need for an existing or new activity of daily living (DePalma et al., 2012), which is known to increase readmission rates. Therefore, it is crucial that nurses work with patients and families not only to address the medical discharge regimen, but also to include education or resources for how to manage the new or existing activity of daily living need, such as dressing, cooking, toileting, transportation, eating, or mobility.

In fact, patient discharge is an area that has been studied for decades. It has come more into the spotlight with the current focus in the United States on reducing health care costs and client morbidity and mortality rates by reducing hospital readmission rates. Health care systems are creating transition care programs. As a part of these programs, one intervention is to have family care transition conferences, which entail discussion on the physical care of the patient, ways to assist the family to adjust to having an ill or recuperating family member at home, and barriers to providing care at home. Concepts to include in this discharge family conference are listed in Box 14-1. Other interventions include interprofessional follow-up teams, nurse navigators, and less formalized telephone and e-mail tracking.

In a concerted effort to reduce hospital readmission rates of high-risk adults—defined as ones being discharged on 10 or more medications, having three chronic illnesses, and having been hospitalized at least twice in the last year—researchers designed an intervention, that begins even before discharge, with a follow-up interprofessional team (Hospital Case Management, 2013b). The team discusses the case and different members work to ensure that by discharge, clients and family members understand their medications, have follow-up appointments, and order any post–acute care services. The team makes follow-up phone calls to discuss care and any concerns for up to 30 days after discharge. Outcomes of this intensive program are still being determined; it is a future step in helping families care for loved ones in the home.

Specifically, nurses conducting a follow-up care phone call should address the following information, while thoroughly documenting the call:

- The client's health status since discharge and any changes that may have occurred
- Whether or not the client is taking medications correctly or following the recommendations for care correctly
- The need for, or the status of, follow-up visits
- What to do when or if a problem arises

Another intervention to help adults and families in the acute care setting is the creation of a position termed *nurse navigator*. Nurse navigators are educated in a specific area of nursing and in the hospital system, such as working with clients who have heart failure or working with clients who have cancer. They meet with patients and families, conduct client and family education, advocate on their behalf by

---

BOX 14-1

Addressing Family Needs During Discharge Conference

It is important to talk about the physical care of the family member who is being discharged home and to work with the family on its specific needs. The following points are examples of items to cover with family at discharge:

- Discuss when the family member can be left alone and for how long.
- Help the family set up an emergency call system.
- Discuss concerns about modifying the home environment.

- Facilitate setting up a family routine of care.
- Be sure the family knows when to call for help.
- Help the family learn to handle visitors, especially children.
- Talk about the balance of sleep and rest for the family caregivers.
- Provide names and numbers for personnel in the billing department for the family members to call when they start to receive insurance forms and hospital bills.

helping ensure clear communication between the client/family and their health care team, conduct medication reconciliation, and help them transition from one setting to another, such as arranging for home visits with community health nurses (Aston, 2013). Some nurse navigators work closely with families and clients in clinic or physician offices and follow clients and families into inpatient settings and back home (Case Management Advisor, 2013).

The San Francisco Medical Center experienced a 46% drop in its readmission rates for heart failure patients during the 3 years when it instituted a multipronged approach to working closely with patients and family during hospitalization and follow-up after discharge (Hospital Case Management, 2013a). Two nurse coordinators (navigators) met with clients and families for approximately 15 to 20 minutes each day during hospitalization to ensure that they understood their care needs and to work on discharge education. They followed up with families and clients via phone calls. In addition, they redesigned their patient educational materials from a health literacy perspective.

Telephone and e-mail follow-up care provided by nurses have been found to improve treatment and outcomes by developing communication and education, improving symptom management, and assisting with early recognition of complications (Mistianen & Poot, 2006). A Cochrane systematic review of follow-up phone calls or e-mails to clients recommends that these interventions should, at a minimum, include knowledge about the illness; postoperative or medical complications; self-care, including behavioral and lifestyle changes; and psychosocial evaluation and emotional support (Furuya et al., 2013).

END-OF-LIFE FAMILY CARE IN THE HOSPITAL

An important transition of care that occurs in acute care settings includes supporting the patient and family at the end of the patient's life. It is not uncommon for the goals of care in the hospital to transition from providing lifesaving or curative measures to providing comfort care at the end of life. For a detailed discussion of how to work with families in palliative and end-of-life care, including those being cared for in home and community-based settings, please refer to Chapter 10. The next section addresses considerations for working with patients and families during end-of-life experiences in acute care settings. The topics emphasize support

for families and include advance care planning, family presence during CPR, family involvement in do not resuscitate (DNR) orders, family experiences with making decisions to withhold or withdraw life-sustaining treatments, and organ donation.

Regardless of whether the death occurs in a CCU, an emergency department, or on a medical-surgical unit, families are challenged by the death of a family member. Acute care hospitalization often occurs because of a sudden major medical crisis, surgery, or because of exacerbations from a chronic illness. When the condition of their loved one becomes terminal or death occurs unexpectedly, family members experience significant stress, anxiety, and intense emotion (Gutierrez, 2012; Twohig et al., 2015). In CCUs, nurses may be challenged to support the holistic needs of patients, which includes addressing the emotional and psychological needs of their families, because of the high-technology, fast-paced orientation of the unit (Gagnon & Duggleby, 2014). While nurses are busy treating the acute physical symptoms efficiently and the rapidly changing acuity of all patients, family members may not be attended to as effectively as nurses would like. At the same time, it is necessary to provide psychological support to families that benefit from caring and supportive actions. Nurses can make a difference by advocating for patients and families, facilitating decision making, ensuring optimum pain and symptom control, and communicating consistent information with families that includes information about the patient's prognosis (Broglio & Bookbinder, 2014; Gutierrez, 2012).

Nurses work in close proximity to patients and families. Therefore, they are in the position of initiating discussions about family and patient wishes as they experience transitions in their care caused by advancing illness or disease. Advance care planning offers patients and families the opportunity to fully participate in care by identifying goals and preferences before the end of life (Simon, Porterfield, Bouchal, & Heyland, 2015). Identifying the needs of the patient and the family helps nurses facilitate decision making to support choices made by patients and families, increase the quality of care, and provide comfort during a stressful experience.

Although efforts toward advance care planning have increased in recent years, the majority of individuals do not have their wishes documented in writing. In a 2014 study of 7900 adults in the United States that addressed advance care planning, it was found that only 26.3% had a written advance directive (Rao, Anderson, Lin, & Laux, 2014). The most common reason cited for not having an advance directive was a lack of awareness (Rao et al.,

2014). Individuals who completed an advance directive were more likely to be older adults with higher levels of income and education, access to health care, and a chronic disease (Rao et al., 2014).

When asked to share their positions on advance care planning, family members described lacking knowledge of the process and experiencing differing positions among their family members, whereas others reported feeling burdened by the decisions or wanting to be involved and not excluded from decision making (van Eechoud et al., 2014). Other barriers to advance care planning involve the timing of completion of advance directives on admission to the hospital, which can be fraught with emotion and distraction, and cultural beliefs that may influence patients and families' choices and preferences for care (Johnson, Zhao, Newby, Granger, & Granger, 2012; Volandes, Ariza, Abbo, & Paasche-Orlow, 2008).

Simon, Porterfield, Bouchal, and Heyland (2015) explored the barriers and facilitators to advance care planning in a study of 12 acute-care hospitals in Canada. Based on interviews with patients identified as high-risk for dying, researchers found that advance care planning was largely dependent on the beliefs and experiences of the person who talked to them about it, that person's access to accurate information that he or she could understand, and the person's interactions and the relationship with his or her physician (Simon et al., 2015). Therefore, the following recommendations would improve the quality and quantity of advanced care planning (Simon et al., 2015).

- Assessing the readiness of the individual
- Personalizing the relevance of advance care planning
- Routinely offering scheduled family meetings for exploring individual goals and information sharing
- Ensuring systems and policies are in place within the organization
- Ensuring that providers' education includes communication for advance care planning

Advance Directives

The 1990 Patient Self-Determination Act (PSDA) encourages everyone to make their own decisions about the medical care that they would choose to accept if they should become unable to make their own decisions because of illness. The PSDA requires all health care providers and organizations to recognize the living will and durable power of attorney for health care (American Cancer Society, 2016). The legislation stimulated a host of documents related to end-of-life choices, such as advance directives, living wills, durable power of attorney for health care, DNR orders, and physician orders for life-sustaining treatment (POLST), which are described in Box 14-2.

BOX 14-2
Documents Related to End-of-Life Choices

Advance Directive

A legal document that a competent person completes. It specifies instructions and medical care preferences regarding interventions or medical treatments, such as termination of life support or organ donation, the individual would like in the event he or she is incompetent to make such decisions. The purpose is to reduce confusion and disagreement. Typically, the advance directive includes the name of the person who is the durable power of attorney for health care.

Living will

A legal document that specifically outlines medical treatments and interventions that the person does or does not want administered when the person is terminally ill or in a coma and is unable to communicate personal desires.

Durable Power of Attorney for Health Care

A legal document that designates an individual to act as a health care proxy or agent to make medical decisions in the event that a person is not able to communicate his or her own choices or make his or her own decisions.

Do Not Resuscitate (DNR) Order

A request not to have CPR in the event one's heart stops. This order may or may not be part of an advance directive or living will. A physician can put this order in a client's chart for that person.

POLST

A form (not a legal document) that states what kind of medical treatment patients want toward the end of their life. It is signed by both the patient and the doctor or nurse practitioner. This form documents the end-of-life conversation between the patient and his or her health care provider. POLST gives seriously ill patients more control over their end-of-life care. It is typically written on bright-colored (pink) paper.

Advance directives can be general or very specific, depending on the wishes of the patient. The directive can involve identifying a certain individual such as a family member or legal representative to serve as a decision maker who will carry out the wishes of the patient if the patient is no longer able to participate in his or her own health care decisions. Specific instructions about various life-sustaining therapies (LSTs) that the patient would accept or refuse may be included. Some types of advance directives define certain situations, such as the living will or the patient's choices for organ or tissue donation, or what actions the patient wants taken if his or her heart or breathing stops (American Cancer Society, 2016). The ANA Code of Ethics supports nursing care that protects patient autonomy, dignity, and rights and includes supporting patient choices for family and surrogate decision makers (ANA, 2015).

The nurse is often involved in conveying the patient's preferences to the family and other health care providers in order to facilitate the development of the advance directive. To elicit specific information about the patient's preferences and choices for the care that he or she wants, the nurse could ask the following:

1. What would you want to happen if you were to become sicker?
2. Would you want to be in the hospital?
3. Would you want to be on machines?
4. Would you want to be at home? (Perrin, Sheehan, Potter, & Kazanowski, 2012).

Preferences for where patients want to die is an important consideration when planning care for those who are near death or experiencing a decline in their condition (Perrin et al., 2012). In order to ensure that the patient's wishes can be carried out, it is important that the nurse communicate the patient's wishes with providers and families, as well as document the patient's preferences.

Family Involvement in Do Not Resuscitate Orders

The family member or appointed decision maker may be in the position of making the decision for his or her loved one to transition to a DNR order for care. Handy, Sulmasy, Merkel, and Ury (2008) investigated the experience of surrogate decision makers—durable power of attorney or next of legal kin—who are involved in authorizing DNR orders. These individuals described this experience as a process, as a cascade of decisions and negotiations, not just a single decision not to resuscitate. One of the essential elements of this process was honest, sensitive, ongoing communication with the health care team. The surrogates reported a dichotomy of emotions about feeling guilty if they authorized the order and guilty if they did not authorize the order. In the end, the surrogates reported that knowing they were alleviating their loved one's pain was crucial in their decision making.

A study of 122 women with gynecological cancers uncovered preferences for end-of-life choices. The study indicated that the women would like end-of-life discussions to occur as a routine part of their care, but they would like the discussion to be initiated by their providers (Díaz-Montes, Johnson, Giuntoli, & Brown, 2013). Patients report that they would like these discussions as they desire to have an opportunity to prepare for the end of their lives. The end-of-life preparations included assigning someone to make decisions, arranging financial matters, knowing what to expect as their health status declines, and preparing written preferences for management of their end-of-life care. The most important factors regarding end-of-life care to patients included trust in the treating physician, avoidance of unwanted life support, effective communication from the physician regarding disease status, and the ability to prepare for the end of life (Diaz-Motes et al., 2013; Heyland et al., 2006). The decision-making process of determining whether to authorize a DNR in an acute care setting is similar to the family's decision whether to withdraw or withhold LSTs.

Family Experiences of Withdrawing or Withholding Life-Sustaining Therapies

Families often become intricately involved in decisions to withdraw or withhold LSTs when no advance directive has been completed or when no previous conversations about end-of-life choices have occurred among members of the family. LSTs include, but are not limited to, advanced cardiac life support, CPR, cardiac support devices, renal support services and renal medications, blood products, artificial nutrition and hydration, cancer treatments, and surgery (HPNA, 2016). Withdrawing and withholding LSTs may also be described as forgoing treatment. Forgoing treatment includes making the decision to do without a LST that would extend the patient's life (HPNA, 2016). Withdrawing and withholding treatment are different than euthanasia or physician-assisted suicide, which are discussed in Chapter 10.

The decision to withdraw or withhold LSTs is central to advance care planning and a significant challenge for families. Nurses have a primary role in facilitating the patient and family's understanding and decision making with forgoing treatment. An important distinction for nurses to make is that the limitation of life-sustaining treatment does not mean limiting care (HPNA, 2016). It is the responsibility of the health care team to honor the decisions and advance directive in place while supporting the appropriate symptom management and personal comfort care. Family members may be affected by stress and grief during the process of making treatment decisions because of the overall poor prognosis and condition of their loved one, the weight of the responsibility, or the anticipatory grief that the family members may be experiencing.

The emotional distress of patients and family members can be reduced by effective communication and teaching to help them understand the disease process, prognosis, and various options for the high-quality management of symptoms at the end of life (Dev et al., 2013; Peden-McAlpine, Liaschenko, Traudt, & Gilmore-Szott, 2015).

Wiegand, Deatrick, and Knafl (2008) conducted research to describe the different family management styles when faced with making decisions about withdrawing or withholding LSTs. The five family management styles described are progressing, accommodating, maintaining, struggling, and floundering. Table 14-2 illustrates how families

Table 14-2	**Family Management Styles for Family Decision to Withhold Life-Sustaining Therapies**						
Family Management Style	**Severity of Condition Understood**	**Hope of Recovery**	**Verb Tense Used to Talk About Family Member**	**Willingness to Engage in Discussion of Withdrawal**	**Family Communication**	**Primary Factors Used in Decision Making**	**Family Made the Decision to Sustain Treatments**
Progressing family type	Yes	No/minimal	More past tense used	Willing	Good communication with each other and extended family	Mostly used facts and supported wishes of family member	Planned date and time of withdrawal
Accommodating family type	Yes	No/minimal	More past tense used	Somewhat willing	Fairly good communication	Mostly facts used, mixed with some emotions	Yes, with little to-moderate conflict
Maintaining family type	Yes	Very hopeful of recovery	Present and past tense used	Undecided	Varied communication, good at times and not good at times	Mixed some facts with emotions	Yes, with moderate-to-extreme difficulty
Struggling family type	Uncertain if understood	Very hopeful of recovery	Present tense used	Not willing	Most family conflict of all styles	Mostly emotions	Some unable to decide, family not in agreement
Floundering family type	No	Believe full recovery was going to happen	Present and future tense used	Not willing	Little family discussion with each other	Emotions only and not follow family member's wishes	Decided when dying was active and made with extreme family conflict

Source: Adapted from Wiegand, D. L., Deatrick, J. A., & Knafl, K. (2008). Family management styles related to withdrawal of life-sustaining therapy from adults who are acutely ill or injured. *Journal of Family Nursing, 14*(1), 16–32.

differ in their approach to making this crucial family decision. Families were found to vary in the following areas:

- Their level of understanding of the severity of their loved one's illness
- Their level of hope for recovery
- The tense (past, present, or future) with which they talked about their family member
- Their willingness to engage in a discussion about possibly withdrawing LSTs
- The overall family communication
- The prevalence of facts or emotions in making the decision
- The actual decision to withdraw LSTs

When death is approaching, it is important for families to be informed early that death is anticipated well before the final decision is made to withdraw life support. Physicians were found to prolong the withdrawal of life support systems to accommodate the needs of the families, which resulted in families' higher level of satisfaction (Gerstel, Engelberg, Koepsell, & Curtis, 2008). But in doing so, physicians felt that patients did not benefit from this prolongation because it caused nonbeneficial and sometimes painful therapies. In fact, the lack of communication between physicians and families caused slower decision making by families. If families are alerted to the possibility of the patient's death earlier in the hospital stay, when the indication for withdrawal is finally made by the physician, the families will be better prepared. Given that most deaths in critical care occur within 4 hours of withdrawal of treatment, this short time period does not allow for families to prepare for death. This short time frame puts an enormous demand on nurses as they attempt to transition care to a need for palliative care for the patient and the bereaved family (Efstathiou & Clifford, 2011; Peden-McAlpine et al., 2015). Working collaboratively with the family and the health care team during this time will help the nurse be most effective in supporting the patient's and the family's needs.

Family conferences can be an effective way to understand the primary needs and concerns of family members in a way that the nurse can prioritize the issues. In a study that examined 51 family conferences with the health care team in the decision-making process to withdraw LSTs, Hsieh, Shannon, and Curtis (2006) identified five contradictory arguments that families often talked about during these family conferences:

- If the family believed that its decision to remove LSTs was actually killing the loved one versus allowing him to die a natural death
- If the family's decision was viewed as a benefit by alleviating suffering or by eliminating a burden on the family
- If the family was honoring its loved one's end-of-life choices or following its own personal wishes
- If the ill family member expressed several differing end-of-life choices, the family had to work through which one to follow
- Determining whether one family member would be responsible for making the final decision or the family as a whole would make the decision

Regardless of which of these contradictions families discussed during the conference, information-seeking strategies used by the health care team members were found to facilitate these difficult emotional discussions. Some of these information-seeking strategies included acknowledging the contradictions, clarifying views of each person including the patient who was not present, bringing the conversation back to the point that all family members wanted to help their loved one, and reaffirming their choices even if the health care team did not agree with them (Hsieh et al., 2006).

Once a family has reached a decision to withdraw LSTs, nurses work closely with family members to guide them through this difficult procedure. A trusting nurse-family relationship is crucial to the family (Wiegand, 2006). The following nursing actions help prepare the family (Kirchhoff, Palzkill, Kowalkowski, Mork, & Gretarsdottir, 2008):

- Telling the family that the exact time of death cannot be anticipated, but that the nurse will be monitoring the situation and informing them when death appears more imminent
- Assuring the family that the nurse will continue to provide compassionate comfort care
- Giving each family member a choice to watch the actual withdrawal of the therapies
- Providing for physical and emotional intimacy needs of the family

- Informing the family of expected signs and symptoms it may see during the active dying process
- Encouraging or giving permission for the family to hold, touch, caress, lie with, talk to, and show emotion to the dying family member

Nurses need to make every effort to keep families involved and informed as death approaches. Providing the ideal level of privacy is not always possible in acute care settings; however, every effort should be made to allow for families to be with their loved ones in a private, unhurried, and quiet environment. Many families and cultures have rituals or spiritual beliefs and procedures that need to be honored. Resources such as spiritual support, social services, and palliative care can be implemented to support the patient and family, especially when death is approaching. Nurse managers need to relieve bedside nurses from responsibilities of caring for other patients, so that they can remain with families and patients who are dying.

Informing family members about what is most important to the dying patient requires communication between these two groups, and nurses can be instrumental in facilitating these discussions. For example, families sometimes prefer not to tell the patient she is dying because they fear that the patient will lose hope. Yet patients and family members have the opportunity to address personal issues and say good-bye to loved ones before they die. Therefore, it is important to assess the personal wishes of the dying patient and to facilitate open discussion between the patient and the family members. Compassionate communication provides crucial care to families as they are asked to make multiple decisions during the dying of their loved ones in the hospital. The more the nurse knows about the family, the better. The way a family deals with death is affected by cultural background, stage in the family life cycle, values and beliefs, and nature of the illness. Whether the loss is sudden or expected, the role played by the dying person in the family and the emotional functioning of the family before the illness also influence the family needs and reactions to the situation (Tong & Kaakinen, 2015).

Offering and providing emotional support to families of dying patients is one way of meeting the needs of the family. Being at the bedside, providing comfort, and offering a listening ear demonstrate that families are not dealing with the grieving process alone (Bach, Ploeg, & Black, 2009; Cronin, Arnstein, & Flanagan, 2015). Providing for privacy allows families emotional and physical intimacy. Of utmost concern to family members is to be reassured that the nurse is keeping their loved one comfortable, as pain free as possible, and is continuing to provide comfort nursing care (Tong & Kaakinen, 2015). Keeping the family informed through anticipatory guidance of the physical signs and symptoms they are likely to see is important. Giving family members the option to be present or excused during the actual death is compassionate caring. Ask the family members whether they have any special spiritual or religious rituals and ceremonies that need to be conducted at this time. For many families, spirituality provides immense comfort whereas, for the patient, it is an essential element in creating a peaceful death (Kruse, Ruder, & Martin, 2007). Most hospitals have various religious services available that can be called in to help the dying patient and his or her family. After the death, it is important to allow enough time for questions, allow the family the opportunity to view the body, and describe the events at the time of death (Tong & Kaakinen, 2015). Offering families the choice to participate in after-life preparations, such as bathing the body, is providing culturally sensitive care.

Caring for families when a member is dying is not easy. It is challenging for nurses to help families cope. Rarely do nurses in most acute care settings feel comfortable and confident discussing death with patients or families. Several issues are especially difficult for nurses and families, and are covered in more detail in the text that follows. One main component of patient and family experience and one with which many families have expressed dissatisfaction—of hospital end-of-life care is management of care before death. Factors contributing to dissatisfaction include patient suffering and pain and lack of communication with the family (Clarke et al., 2003). Part of the reason for this dissatisfaction is that health care providers, particularly nurses, are uncomfortable caring for and communicating with the dying patients. Nurses expressed discomfort when speaking with families and patients about death and felt ill-prepared in this task (Lloyd-Williams, Morton, & Peters, 2009). Therefore, nurses tend to distance themselves from the patients and engage only in practical tasks, where they are most comfortable (Shorter & Stayt, 2010), thereby missing opportunities to facilitate interactions with the family (Curtis et al., 2005). Hospitals need to provide educational opportunities for nurses so they will have the knowledge and skills to plan and deliver end-of-life care (Efstathiou & Clifford, 2011).

Mixed messages pertaining to end-of-life issues commonly arise in the acute care setting. Patients and families hear and see numerous health care providers. They receive conflicting and divergent information and opinions so that it is challenging for them to understand the care plan, thus compromising the quality of end-of-life care (Beckstrand & Kirchhoff, 2005). Because nurses spend the most time with the patient, they are instrumental in gathering the team players together to provide clarity for the patient and the family (Puntillo & McAdam, 2006).

Family Presence During Cardiopulmonary Resuscitation

Sudden life-threatening events in acute care settings can result in the possibility of administering CPR. For many years it was standard practice in CCUs and emergency departments to remove family members from the bedside during periods of cardiac arrest, as well as emergent and invasive procedures. That trend is gradually changing. An increasing number of CCUs and emergency departments allow family members to choose to remain present at the patient's bedside during CPR based on research findings that demonstrate that family presence does not disrupt patient care and actually results in positive outcomes for both family members and patients (Powers & Candela, 2016). The Emergency Nurses Association (2012) and the AACN (2016) have recommend that family presence during resuscitation (FPDR) should be offered as an option to appropriate family members and should be based on written institution policy. FPDR is supported as ethical practice in Canada with the recommendation that experienced health care professionals should accompany family members during and after the resuscitation period to address their questions and provide psychological support (Oczkowski, Mazzetti, Cupido, & the Canadian Critical Care Society, 2015).

Family members appreciate the option of FPDR as it allows them to take an active role in helping their loved one through a difficult time while providing emotional comfort and spiritual support (Powers & Candela, 2016). They can provide physical affection, talk to their loved one, and even say good-bye, all of which promote the grieving process and facilitate

healing for the family member (Powers & Candela, 2016). FPDR also reduces anxiety for the family members because they are able to see the efforts implemented to save the life of their loved one. This is particularly important to help family members with coping, considering that the survival rate for in-hospital cardiac arrest is 18% (Morrison et al., 2013).

Offering the Option of Organ Donation

The number of people who need organs far exceeds the number of donors. In the United States, there are more than 119,000 men, women, and children on the national organ transplant waiting list (Organ Donor, 2017). Each day about 80 people receive an organ transplant and 22 people die because an organ was unavailable (Organ Donor, 2017). Between January and November of 2016 there were 27,605 transplants from 13,066 donors (United Network for Organ Sharing, 2017). It has been shown that when the family knows of a loved one's intent to donate his or her organs, there are higher rates of donation than when the family is not aware of the loved one's intent (Smith, Lindsey, Kopfman, Yoo, & Morrison, 2008).

Discussing organ donation with a family whose loved one has suddenly died or with whom the decision has been made to withdraw LSTs is difficult. The discussion about organ donation should take place separately from the notification of the family member's death, and it should be done by someone who has been specifically trained in asking for organ and tissue donation (Tong & Kaakinen, 2015). Federal regulations now stipulate that hospitals are required to contact their local Organ Procurement Organization (OPO) concerning any death or impending death (Truog et al., 2001). Once contacted, the OPO sends a representative, or a local hospital representative will approach the family at the appropriate time about the option of organ donation and answer questions.

If organ donation is viewed as a consoling act, the option to elect organ donation is easier for the family (Tong & Kaakinen, 2015). Organ donation benefits the donor family, as well as the recipients and their families. Families reported that knowing that the organ of their loved one helped someone else, that a positive came out of a negative, and their family member lives on in someone else helped them cope with their loss (Tong & Kaakinen, 2015).

Many families worry that donation is disfiguring or will delay the funeral, but neither of these worries is valid and nurses should reassure families on these points. The body is not disfigured in the process of removing organs. If the body parts that are removed have the potential to disfigure the person, replacement plastic or wooden parts are inserted in the place of those removed so that the person is not disfigured. The organ donation team has a rapid response; therefore, the funeral arrangements are not delayed.

The donor family does not pay for the medical expenses once death has been declared; the costs are paid by the OPO and the recipients. The donor family receives a letter from the OPO informing it of the number of people who received organs from the deceased family member. After time, the donor family can contact the OPO to find out whether the recipient of the organs is interested in corresponding and meeting.

Case Study: Howe Family

This case study presents a family dealing with an acute exacerbation of a long-standing chronic illness and hospitalization of one of its members. The Family Systems Theory is used as the theoretical approach to the Howe family (refer to Chapter 2 for specific details of this family nursing theory and model). The Howe family genogram and ecomap are presented in Figures 14-1 and 14-2.

Glenn Howe, a 64-year-old married white male, had his first major myocardial infarction at age 41. Since that time, he dutifully embraced numerous lifestyle changes, including smoking cessation, diet modifications, and the establishment of a regular exercise regimen. In addition, he began to take numerous cardiovascular medications to control his blood pressure

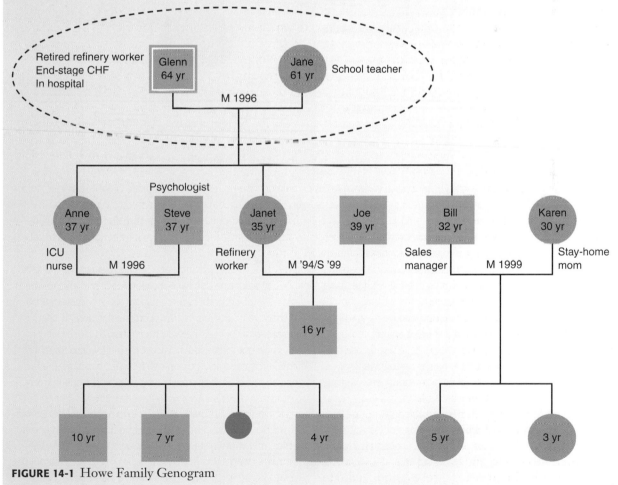

FIGURE 14-1 Howe Family Genogram

(continued)

Case Study: Howe Family *(cont.)*

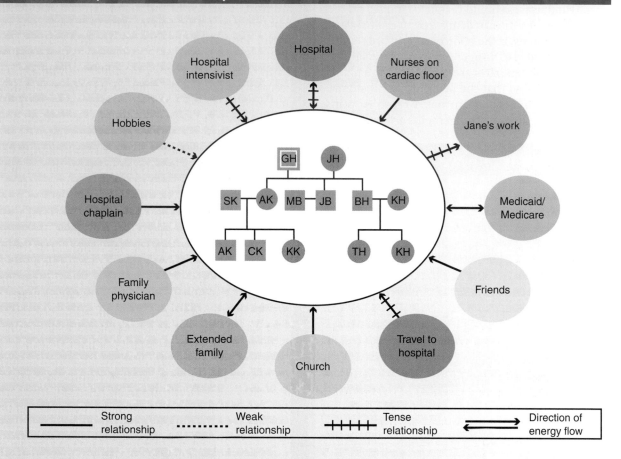

FIGURE 14-2 Howe Family Ecomap

and enhance his cardiac function. Despite his adherence to his chronic disease management program, Glenn's cardiovascular disease worsened, and he underwent coronary artery bypass surgery 10 years ago. Initial results of the surgery were positive, and Glenn continued to manage his chronic illness well. Recently, however, he experienced another small myocardial infarction, after which his cardiac function declined drastically. Therefore, physicians increased his medications, recommended more severe lifestyle modifications, and dashed his hopes for recovery.

Glenn's immediate family consists of his wife, Jane, three children—Anne, age 37; Janet, age 35; and Bill, age 32—and six young grandchildren. Glenn is currently retired, whereas Jane continues to work as a special education teacher. All family members are upper middle class and attend an Episcopal Church regularly. All family members are geographically and emotionally close to Glenn, and are quite concerned that he may not survive much longer. Since his first myocardial infarction, the family members have lived their lives in a state of anxiety, feeling as if their time with Glenn is likely to be limited, as if they are on "borrowed time." This anxiety has resulted in several benefits for the family: numerous family vacations, all holidays together, and the perspective that every chance to be together is special. After Glenn's most recent decline in cardiac function, the family experienced a heightened sense of preciousness, wanting to spend as much time as possible together and wanting every moment with Glenn to be perfect.

Before his first myocardial infarction, Glenn was a healthy, robust, active man with many interests and hobbies. After his cardiac surgery, many of his hobbies, including golf, fell by the wayside. He became increasingly short of breath with exertion and resorted to armchair hobbies, such as coin collecting, crossword puzzles, and world history. Family activities changed as well. Family vacations necessarily became sedate and wheelchair oriented, rather than activity-oriented hiking, fishing, and camping

Case Study: Howe Family *(cont.)*

trips. The family endeavored, however, to have at least one very special trip every year, the last two being a trip to Disney World with Glenn in a wheelchair and a cruise that required very little exertion.

Glenn became more and more debilitated. His cardiac function was so poor he could not eat without becoming short of breath and tachycardic. His appetite decreased dramatically, and he lost more than 60 pounds. He began to suffer from orthopnea and often tried to sleep upright in his recliner all night. As he and Jane tried to cope with his acute and chronic health care needs, their relationship changed. She became a full-time caretaker, trying anything she could to get him to eat and to make him comfortable. A normally unflappable individual, she found herself expressing her frustration at his refusal to eat more than a few bites at a time. Her outbursts were distressing to her and her children because they were so out of character. Glenn, usually a more demanding individual, became compliant and resigned as his health deteriorated. The children became hypervigilant and attentive to their parents, making frequent visits on weekends and calling every day. Family roles changed as the stressors affecting the family intensified.

Glenn had been hospitalized on numerous occasions, and he approached the impending admission to a medical-surgical unit with his usual calm and trust in his caregivers. He was being admitted for tests because his ventricular function had decreased, his weight had decreased from 200 to 140 pounds, and his urine output was declining. He called his oldest daughter, Anne, a cardiovascular intensive care nurse, the morning of his scheduled admission and asked her to meet him at the hospital. She replied that she had to travel out of town for an important meeting but would drive up later that night and be with him for the tests the next day. The other children counted on the oldest child to take care of health care needs, and because of her education and experience, it was a role she gladly assumed.

Given the chronic nature of Glenn's cardiovascular disease and the life-threatening potential for acute exacerbations requiring frequent hospitalizations, Jane and Glenn had discussed advance directives openly and honestly. Jane was well aware that Glenn did not wish for any heroic measures, especially CPR. He felt that his two cardiac surgeries were trauma enough and that his heart condition was irreparable. Jane was terrified of losing her husband, best friend, and companion, and was very concerned about having to make the decision that would honor Glenn's wishes.

During this hospital stay, Glenn and Jane renewed their close and trusting relationship with the nurses at their small community hospital. While awaiting his tests and the arrival of their daughters, Glenn experienced a lapse in consciousness with Jane at his bedside. Jane called for help, and two nurses entered the room and quickly assessed the situation. Glenn was in full cardiac arrest. One of the nurses turned to Jane and asked, "Do you want us to bring him back? We can bring him back." Jane hesitated, then shook her head no. The nurse asked again, "Are you sure? Do you want us to bring him back?" Once again, Jane answered, "No." She immediately realized the consequences of her decision to deny CPR. Glenn, her husband of 45 years, was gone; her children did not expect this hospitalization to result in his death, and she was alone at his bedside.

Jane experienced regret for her decision not to "bring him back." Her decision was so very final. She also regretted the times that she had felt frustrated at his disinterest in eating and his hobbies. Though never an angry person, she had experienced anger at her husband on more than one occasion. The children all felt a measure of guilt as well: Anne for going to a meeting instead of being with her dad at the hospital, and Janet and Bill for being at work instead of at their dad's bedside. Everyone wished they had more time together as a family.

Jane became a grieving widow, very dependent, sad, and indecisive—a person her children barely recognized. At a time when they needed a strong, supportive mother, that person was absent. The individuals best able to provide support to Jane and her children were the grandchildren and spouses. Having never experienced the death of someone so dear to them, all family members struggled with daily life for several weeks after Glenn's death.

Family Systems Theory Applied to the Howe Family:

The Family Systems Theory will be used to address the complex needs of each individual within the family, and the family as a whole. All members of the Howe family were affected by Glenn's admission to the medical-surgical unit as well as his death. Chapter 2 provides more detailed information of the Family Systems Theory.

Concept 1: All Parts of the System Are Interconnected

In the Howe case, all members of the family are affected by Glenn's declining health and eventual death in the hospital setting. Jane feels immense guilt for not "bringing him back" and all three of Glenn's children feel guilt and remorse for not being at their dad's bedside. Both Janet and Bill verbalized anger toward Anne because she was out of town for a meeting instead of being with their dad. As an ICU nurse, Anne always assumed responsibility for her dad's health care needs.

(continued)

Case Study: Howe Family *(cont.)*

Concept 2: *The Whole Is More Than the Sum of Its Parts*

In the Howe case study, it is not just the mother and children who are affected by this hospitalization and death. The spouses of Anne, Janet, and Bill and the six grandchildren are also greatly affected. A nurse working with this family would need to understand that the family is a complex system where significant changes, such as the death of a family member, would have an impact on the entire family system. Jane's overwhelming grief in addition to the family never having experienced the death of someone so dear to all them add stressors that could deteriorate the family relationships over time.

Concept 3: *All Systems Have Some Form of Boundaries or Borders Between the System and Its Environment*

In working with the Howe family, it would be important for the nurse to assess the boundaries within the family. For example, if the Howe family verbalized that they do not want to meet with a grief counselor, they may have a closed boundary. A flexible boundary would be if the family allowed their Episcopal priest to visit but no other members of their church. The nurse might want to help the family understand the value of open boundaries such as community for resources that might assist with the grief process.

Concept 4: *Systems Can Be Further Organized Into Subsystems*

The nurse would want to think of the Howe family not only as a whole but also as subsystems within the family. This might be Jane to her children, Jane to her grandchildren, Jane's children to their own children, and so forth. The nurse may work with the grief process and the adjustments of the family after the death of Glenn by focusing on the subsystems that are present within the family.

SUMMARY

When medical-surgical nurses view families as partners in the care provided to patients, they are providing unfragmented, holistic, humane, and sensitively delivered health care. When nurses practice family-centered care in acute care settings, families are empowered to manage the stressors of being in the hospital environment, which is foreign territory to most people. Families are better prepared to support their loved ones, aid in their recovery, or facilitate a comfortable death. Families are called on to support their ill family member in the hospital, make important life decisions on behalf of or in partnership with the patient, serve as caregivers, and advocate for the patient in the complex health care system.

- The stress families experience when family members are in the hospital is significant. Family members are at risk for depression, anxiety, and PTSD.
- The role of families in the hospital setting is crucial because patients have been shown to have more positive outcomes when families are involved in their loved one's care while in the hospital.
- The benefits of practicing family nursing or family-centered care in the hospital setting have been well documented. Yet health care providers in the hospital environment continue to practice patient-centered rather than family-centered care (family nursing).
- Nurses in medical-surgical environments recognize and feel responsible to practice family-centered or family nursing. Yet they struggle with role ambiguity and role conflict, as they continue to practice in settings that reward the biomedical model of health care and not a holistic nursing model of care.
- The environment for providing family-centered nursing care (family nursing) in acute care settings is dependent on hospital policies and procedures that consider the needs of families.
- Transferring loved ones from CCUs to the medical-surgical units is stressful for families because it creates a sense of conflict. On one

hand, families are glad their loved ones are better, but they also worry that their family members may not be ready to be moved out of such intensive nurse watchfulness.

- The family member who advocates for his loved one in the hospital assumes a difficult, time-consuming, and fatiguing role as he often travels long distances to get to the hospital, takes time off work to be there, often stays all night in the hospital, manages the informational needs of the patient and the family, and works through a complex health care system.

- Effective communication with patients, families, and interdisciplinary health care providers improves client satisfaction, promotes positive response to care, reduces length of stay in care settings, and results in decreased overall cost and resource utilization.

- Compassionate communication provides crucial care to families as they are asked to make multiple decisions as their loved one dies in the hospital.

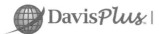 | For additional resources and information, visit **http://davisplus.fadavis.com**. References can be found on DavisPlus.

Chapter 15

Family Health in Mid- and Later Life

Diana L. White, PhD

Juliana C. Cartwright, PhD, RN

Critical Concepts

- Most older adults live and receive care in community settings. Although older adults generally are healthy and independent, the risk of chronic illnesses increases with age, causing many older adults to become more limited in activities of daily living (ADLs) with advanced age.

- Older adults have family ties that are positive, meaningful, and supportive. It is rare for older adults to be neglected or uncared for by their families.

- As is the case in all families, families of older adults are diverse. This diversity is influenced by history, race, class, and gender, as well as by individual family history and traditions. These factors influence family composition, health status, health beliefs, and capacity to support each other during times of illness or stress.

- Older adults are givers of family care, as well as receivers. Until very old age, they provide more economic, social, and emotional support to adult children than they receive; they step in to assist family members in crisis, and are key in providing child care for grandchildren. Most caregivers of older adults with chronic conditions, such as heart disease and dementia, are spouses.

- A majority of those receiving care in almost all care settings are older than 65 years. All nurses will work with increasing numbers of older adults simply because the population is aging so rapidly and because of the increased risk of chronic illness requiring nursing care with advancing age. Even nurses who focus on maternal and child or pediatric nursing are more likely now than in the past to encounter grandparents as caregivers or major support persons.

- Families are responsible for providing complex, technical nursing care, which was once only the purview of nurses. They do this in spite of often being unprepared and inadequately supported by the health care system.

- Families provide most of the care to older adults, regardless of care setting. The organization and structure of care varies. Nursing care is most effective when done in partnership with families.

- All families experience transitions over the life course, both expected and unexpected. Each transition is influenced by health status, culture, financial security, and social supports.

- Gerontological nursing takes place in all care settings, although the specific needs of older adults and their families vary.

When we think about aging clients and their families, we often think of individuals or couples who are older than 65 years. These individuals, however, are embedded within a larger family system that includes different and intersecting generations. For example, today a 75-year-old couple may be newlyweds and have living parents. They may be completely healthy with no chronic conditions, and spending some of their family time supporting themselves and others. In contrast, a 75-year-old person may be widowed and isolated from social support, have multiple chronic conditions, experience several limitations in activities of daily living (ADLs), and require significant help from others. In either case, if the 75-year-olds have children, they are likely to be grandparents and even great-grandparents, and they may be the primary caregivers to one or more of those grandchildren.

When people need help, it will come most often from family members. When older adults need care, whether at home, in the hospital, or in a range of long-term care (LTC) settings, families will be participating in that care in most circumstances. Some family members will be active leaders in that care, and others will require substantial support from nurses and other professionals. A minority of older adults will have weak social ties and may be isolated from family and friends in old age. These individuals will rely heavily on formal services.

LIFE COURSE PERSPECTIVE

The aging population is diverse, and family systems are complex. Family gerontologists (those who study aging) often use a life course perspective as a way to understand this complexity (Settersten, 2006). The life course perspective recognizes that individuals are embedded in a family system, and that individuals and the family as a whole develop and change over time. This outlook is compatible with many family and social science theories, and is often used in conjunction with other theories, including the theories that guide this book. This chapter discusses the life course perspective in relation to Family Systems Theory, Family Life Cycle Theory, and the Ecology Model of Family Development. This section describes ways the life course perspective enhances these family theories and contributes to greater understanding of the diversity of family experiences in mid- and later life.

Family Systems Theories

Family Systems Theories emphasize connections among family members. When something happens to or is experienced by one family member, others are affected in some way. The life course perspective encourages us to consider family systems broadly. Connidis (2010), for example, describes family relationships in terms of "family ties," which helps us think about families that extend beyond households and the nuclear family. Family ties include extended family members and fictive kin—those who are "like family" but are not connected through blood or marriage. As described throughout this chapter, and as is evident in Chapter 3, the character of family ties varies within and between families. Responses to life events among family members are influenced by a history of family rules and traditions that have developed over time (Hanson, 1995) and the quality and characteristics of family ties within the family system. Family breakdown may occur when rules and traditions are not adequate to cover a particular situation. For example, in some families breakdown may occur when siblings disagree strongly on how to provide support to frail, cognitively impaired parents. One may stress the importance of a parent remaining in her own home, whereas another may feel that the parent's unique health and safety needs demand nursing home care. At the same time, neither can agree on how to spend scarce resources to make either option workable. These disagreements are likely consistent with previous patterns and relationships.

Family Life Cycle Theory

The family Life Cycle Model helps to predict when normative or expected changes will occur. For example, many middle-aged and older adults experience their children leaving home and establishing their own households, a normative change. Adult children form partnerships through marriage or cohabitation. They also begin to achieve financial independence through work. Middle-aged adults who are parents can expect to become grandparents. Retirement is an expected and often desired transition for those with an adequate income and retirement savings. These types of transitions have been considered normative and for many represent "on-time" events. The life course perspective focuses on transitions, but also examines the timing of transitions, and the social circumstances, historical events, and the series of decisions that shape individual and family experiences over time. For a variety of reasons, the timing and even the occurrence of expected milestones are changing and becoming less predictable. This does not mean families or family ties are becoming less important, but these changes will affect the way that families function as well as individual and family resources and needs.

Bioecological Model

The life course perspective in conjunction with the bioecological model helps explore how societal changes are influencing the timing and context of transitions within and across families, and how societal changes both shape and are influenced by individual and family decisions. For example, it is increasingly common for young adults to leave home and then return, owing in part to difficulties finding jobs in the current economic climate. Women and men go to college in midlife to begin new careers either voluntarily (e.g., a desire for more meaningful work or a better work-family balance) or involuntarily (e.g., needing new skills after a layoff). Many couples in middle age are beginning their families, not launching them, reflecting changes in family planning norms, particularly for women pursuing professional careers. Some couples in their fifties adopt young children, sometimes their own grandchildren. Those in their seventies may seek paid employment because of a desire to work or because of financial necessity. According to Quadagno (2008), after several years of declining labor force participation by those older than 60, trends now for both women and men are to remain in the labor force longer. In the United States in 2015, 37% of men and about 28% of women 65 to 69 years continue to work full or part time. Past age 70, 16% of men and 9% of women are working (Federal Interagency Forum on Aging-Related Statistics [FIFARS], 2016). Thus, attitudes and expectations about what is normative or nonnormative, and what is on-time or off-time, are changing, resulting in much greater flexibility and diversity in family experiences. In addition, some transitions, although common, may not be expected and often cause difficulties for families. These include divorce, involuntary job loss, declining health or disability, providing care for ill or dependent family members, and death of a family member.

The life course perspective is particularly helpful in understanding the complexity and diversity of family life revealed in these examples, providing a dynamic understanding of family life across generations (Bengtson & Allen, 1993; Bianchi & Casper, 2005). As with bioecological models, the life course perspective emphasizes context, including the societal conditions in which individuals and families function as well as the actions individuals take in shaping their relationships and the trajectories of their lives (Alwin, 2012). Individuals and families are influenced by the historical times in which they live. For example, those who are currently in their late eighties and nineties and lived in the United States experienced the Great Depression as young children and many men served in World War II. Later, these children of the Great Depression were parents of the baby boom generation. The post-war baby boom represented a reversal in the trend toward smaller families, resulting in a population bulge that has dominated family life and public policy in the United States ever since. Baby boomers had a different set of challenges and opportunities than their parents and are now entering old age. Their worldview was shaped by the Vietnam War, the civil rights movement, assassinations of U.S. leaders, and the sexual revolution.

Young adults now in their twenties and early thirties have grown up in a technological and global age quite different from either their parents or grandparents. They have experienced households in which both parents were more likely to work outside the home and divorce was more common. Compared with earlier generations, young adults are more likely to form unions through cohabitation and, if they choose to marry, are marrying later than those of previous cohorts (Manning, Brown, & Payne, 2014). Young adults are increasingly postponing or even forgoing childbearing regardless of marital status (Cherlin, 2010). Today's young adults have also seen a growth in health and economic disparities among various segments of the population, came of age during the Great Recession, and, to varying degrees, experienced the Iraq and Afghanistan wars. Those pursuing higher education are incurring a huge amount of personal debt. These experiences will influence middle and late life for these individuals.

In all phases of history, societal issues related to race, class, gender, abilities, and immigration have influenced the kinds of opportunities and barriers individuals experience throughout their lives. This combination of historical events and social context must be considered in understanding how changing environments, cultural norms, economic conditions, and political circumstances affect families in mid- and later life. Such influences can be seen in work and family decisions, access to health care, and educational opportunities. Many advantages or disadvantages accumulate over a lifetime and across generations (Dannefer, 2003; Hungerford, 2007). For example, children raised in poverty are more likely to have poorer health, less likely to attend college, and more likely to experience hardships in middle and old age (Hungerford, 2007). They are also more likely to marry young, have children before age 30, and divorce (Cherlin, 2010). In contrast, those with more privileged childhoods experience better health and education, are more likely to have higher-paying jobs as adults, have adequate health care, and enter old age with adequate retirement resources. In turn, they are likely to provide their own children with a relatively privileged upbringing.

Even as we emphasize the importance of social and historical context in shaping individual and family lives, we must remember that individuals are not passive. They are active agents, even as their actions may be constrained or enhanced by broader societal circumstances (Alwin, 2012; Connidis, 2010; Settersten, 2006). There are many examples of individuals following or going against societal norms against history, and how that affected the individuals' lives. For example, in war-torn countries, the decision to leave or stay within that country influences the individual and the family for generations thereafter. The life course perspective will be used in this chapter to foster understanding of families with older adults and the family ties that influence their health. This perspective will be used to think about optimal nursing care for these families, using the nursing process. Furthermore, this approach will be used to explain current social policies influencing older adults and their families.

PROFILE OF AGING FAMILIES

Family structures and many of the functions of family are changing at a rapid pace, all of which have implications for the care needs and resources of families in mid- and later life. In this section we will explore demographic trends that influence families, including family structures and functions. We will also examine different facets of family relationships from same-generation and intergenerational relationships,

including the influence of ambivalence and conflict. Awareness of the complexity and richness of family life is critically important for nurses who help older adults and their families navigate all aspects of health, illness, and disabilities.

As we describe the most recent changes to family structure in the past several decades, it is important to recognize that the makeup of families and the individual roles within families and society has always been changing and evolving. Families are remarkably resilient even as the form of the family changes. What remains constant in families is the commitment family members, however defined, have for one another (Connidis, 2015a).

Demographic Profile

The aging of the population worldwide is unprecedented historically and has implications for all aspects of society, especially families. Globally, the number of people 60 years or older is expected to more than double by 2050 and triple by 2100, raising from 962 million in 2017 to 2.1 billion in 2050 and 3.1 billion in 2100 (United Nations, http://www.un.org/en/sections/issues-depth/ageing/index.html). More than 25 countries, including Canada, have at least 15% of their populations over the age of 65. Most of these are in Europe and Asia. Japan leads with nearly 27%, followed by Germany and Italy with well over 20% (He et al., 2016). Asia is the most rapidly aging region; South Korea, Hong Kong, and Taiwan will usurp 9% of the population (Administration on Aging, 2016). In Canada, nearly 18% of the population (35 million people) is over 65 (He et al., 2016). In the United States 10,000 baby boomers are reaching 65 every day. By 2050, numbers of older adults will have more than doubled; as a result, 25% of the U.S. population will be 65 or older (Vincent & Velkoff, 2010). Worldwide, nearly 17% of the population will be over 65. The fastest growing segment of the population in all developed nations is those in the oldest age groups (Christensen, Doblehammer, Rau, & Vaulpel, 2009). The United States will see the number of those over 85 triple between 2015 and 2040, from 6.3 to 14.6 million (Administration on Aging, 2016).

Demographers worldwide project similar increases, with the numbers of people over 80 more than tripling between 2015 and 2050 (He et al., 2016). The continent of Africa contains some of the youngest countries, with the vast majority having less than 5% of the population over 65. In African populations, this age group is not expected to exceed 7% of the population until 2050 (He et al., 2016). Although European, North American, and some Asian countries have been experiencing a growing aging population for decades, developing nations are also aging dramatically. The oldest countries had a century to transition from young to old population, but this change is occurring at a much faster pace in developing nations (He et al., 2016). Many do not have the infrastructure in place to address the emerging needs of older adults and their families.

Diversity

In the United States, 22% of older adults were members of racial or ethnic minorities, a more diverse population than in previous generations (Administration on Aging, 2016). Growing diversity is a result of demographic changes related to fertility rates and immigration. By the year 2044, fewer than half of Americans will be non-Hispanic white (Colby & Ortman, 2014). Statistically, African American and Hispanic populations have higher fertility rates than non-Hispanic whites. The older African American population will quadruple between 2000 and 2050, and the Hispanic and Asian/Pacific Islander populations will be seven and six-and-a-half times larger, respectively (Dilworth-Anderson, Williams, & Gibson, 2002).

Immigration is an additional factor contributing to growing diversity in both the United States and in Canada. In the United States, about 20% of the immigrant population is 60 years or older. Currently, over half of immigrants come from Latin America (53%), followed by Asia (28%). The majority (60%) of those who immigrate as older adults have come to join their adult children who migrated to the United States earlier (Usita & Shakya, 2012). Reasons for immigration of older adults are similar in Canada; over 93% have immigrated to join family members. The major countries of origin for all immigrants to Canada are China, India, Philippines, Pakistan, and Iran.

Minority older adults have shorter life expectancies and report poorer health throughout the life course (FIFARS, 2016). In addition, racial and ethnic minority groups tend to receive poorer quality care than non-Hispanic whites, even controlling for socioeconomic status and severity of illness or condition (Kronenfeld, 2006).

Economic Status

Globalization and various public policies have contributed to growing income inequality worldwide. In 2015, about 9% of older adults in the United States lived in poverty, although the percentage increased to nearly 14% when medical out-of-pocket expenses were included in poverty calculations (Administration on Aging, 2016). Over a third were in the highest income group. Women and people of color are disproportionately represented in the lower income groups. Women's marital status is closely linked to financial status in old age. Women, especially minority women, experience significant losses in income and net worth when their husbands die (Angel, Jimenez, & Angel, 2007). Compared with men, today's oldest women, especially women of color, have not had careers or worked in jobs with pension benefits. Those with a history of low-wage jobs, more frequent marital disruption, and fewer opportunities to accumulate assets during their working years are especially vulnerable. In the United States, 12% of older women are poor compared with 7% of older men (FIFARS, 2016). In 2013, 23% of older adults relied on Social Security for 90% or more of their income, and the majority were older widowed, divorced, or single women of color (Sullivan & Meschede, 2016). This pattern of financial vulnerability of older women is seen internationally. Financial inequality has been linked to gender in Canada (LaRochelle-Cote, Myles, & Picot, 2012) and Europe (Vlachantoni, 2012). Financial security is increasingly difficult for young adults and all adults without advanced education (Crystal, 2016).

Health Status

As a group, older adults are healthier, better educated, and more financially secure than in previous generations. People throughout the world are living longer than ever before. In Canada, life expectancy at birth is 82 years. When Canadian women reach 65, they can expect to live another 23 years; men at 65 can expect to live another 20 years. In the United States, 65-year-old women can expect to live 20.6 more years and men another 18 years (Administration on Aging, 2016). Most older adults, even those who are very old, live independently and in good health. Over three quarters of those older than 65 years report having good, very good, or excellent health (FIFARS, 2016). This is especially true for non-Hispanic whites; over 80% report being in good to excellent health compared with about 65% and 66% for African American and Hispanic/Latino older adults, respectively. These differences reflect health disparities and economic disadvantages in the United States, which are mirrored in other societies as well.

Older adults are overrepresented in all health care utilization, including hospitalization and prescription drug use. Six of the top seven causes of death in 2014 were chronic illnesses: heart disease, cancer, chronic lower respiratory diseases, stroke, Alzheimer's disease, and diabetes (FIFARS, 2016). Other chronic diseases common in old age include arthritis and hypertension.

At the same time, the prevalence of chronic disabilities in old age declined steadily in the United States between the 1980s and 2004 (Manton, 2008; Stewart, Cutler, & Rosen, 2013), and the trend continues with some conditions, such as heart disease. Unfortunately, the prevalence of other conditions common in old age (e.g., hypertension, asthma, cancer, diabetes) has increased in recent years (FIFARS, 2016). Some of this is likely a consequence of the obesity epidemic (Christensen et al., 2009). About 35% of those over 65 are obese, with highest rates for women (41%) between ages 65 and 74 (FIFARS, 2016). The lifestyle associated with obesity contributes to decreased physical activity and ultimately to poorer health, physical function, and depression (Luppino et al., 2010; Riebe et al., 2009). This trend has important implications for caregiving within families; for example, obesity increases the strain on both the caregiver and the recipient of care because of increased physical demands.

Older adults also experience sensory impairments with age, which may interfere with abilities to function or to interact socially. Nearly 75% of those over 70 years have hearing loss in at least one ear, and hearing loss is more prevalent in men than women (Goman & Lin, 2016). Hearing loss can be particularly difficult, leading to social isolation, depression, or mistaken perceptions by others that the older adult is cognitively impaired. Recent research indicates that hearing loss does contribute to cognitive decline (Deal et al., 2017). Vision loss also escalates with age, increasing risk for falls and limiting activities. For example, poor vision affects the ability to drive, thereby increasing isolation and dependency on others. Twenty-five percent of those 80 years and older have significant vision impairment (Pelletier, Rojas-Roldan, & Coffin, 2016). Major causes of blindness and severe vision loss are macular degeneration, diabetes, glaucoma, and cataracts (Pelletier et al., 2016). Senses related to smell and taste generally remain stable into old age

when one is healthy, but can be negatively affected by disease or medications. This in turn may lead to poor nutritional status, which will adversely affect health status (Maas, Buckwalter, Hardy, Tripp-Reimer, Titler, & Specht, 2001; Mattes, 2002).

More important than having a chronic disease is whether and how it affects an individual's ability to function and engage in desired and meaningful activity. Function is often tied to ADLs or instrumental ADLs (IADL). ADLs refer to basic self-care tasks such as bathing, eating, toileting, dressing, and mobility. IADLs include basic functions and activities that allow older individuals to live independently, such as using the telephone, managing money, doing laundry, maintaining one's home, shopping, and managing transportation.

At the end of the 20th century and through the first years of the 21st, rates of disabilities declined, especially those affecting IADLs (Lin, Beck, Finch, Hummer, & Master, 2012). Declines in the need for assistance with IADLs was attributed in part to use of technology, including new mobility devices. Declines in disabilities related to ADLs were tied to improved management of chronic disease, particularly cardiovascular disease (Manton, 2008). It appears, however, that the trend is reversing, with those now entering old age experiencing higher rates of disability (FIFARS, 2016; Freedman & Spillman, 2014; Lin et al., 2016). Freedman and Spillman (2014) reported that about 29% of all those older than 75 years needed some help with ADLs or IADLs. FIFARS (2016) reported even higher levels of need related to ADLs. Overall, 12% of the older adult population has limitations in IADL only and 32% have limitations in one or more ADLs (FIFARS, 2016). Limitations vary by age. More than half of those 85 to 89 and about 75% of those 90 years and older need help. Need for assistance is not always met. Estimates range between 20% and 32% of older adults who have support needs do not get the assistance they require (Freedman & Spillman, 2014; FIFARS, 2016). We will consider needs related to function, and the role of family and the health care system in meeting them, later in this chapter.

Cognitive Status

Cognitive decline is an issue of particular concern to many older adults. Neuronal and synaptic changes do occur with aging, although the range and impact of these changes vary markedly across individuals (Smith & Cotter, 2016). Although it is not unusual for older adults to have difficulty focusing on multiple tasks at once, recalling recent events, or recalling a specific word, these changes typically do not interfere with an individual's ability to lead a normal life (Smith & Cotter, 2016). However, the risk of marked cognitive decline does increase with each decade, and the prevalence of Alzheimer's disease and related dementias in the United States rises from 11% of people age 65 and older to 32% of people aged 85 and older (Alzheimer's Association, 2016). The population aged 85 and older is the fastest growing segment globally (United Nations, 2015a) and the number of people with dementia in the United States is projected to increase from 5.3 million people in 2016 to 13.8 people by 2050, with 7 million of these individuals older than age 85 (Hebert, Weuve, Scherr, & Evans, 2013).

Globally, including Canada, prevalence is projected to double every 20 years at least through 2050, also reflecting the rapidly expanding population of older adults living to 85 years and older (Manuel et al., 2016; Prince et al., 2013). Reports from several developed countries (e.g., United States, Germany, Finland) suggest a decline in dementia prevalence at the turn of the 21st century (Langa et al., 2008; Satizabal et al., 2016). Possible explanations focus on improved management of cardiovascular conditions (e.g., smoking cessation, exercise, diet, and pharmacotherapy) (Dodge, Zhu, Lee, Chang, & Ganguli, 2014; Satizabal et al., 2016). Although this trend is promising, the markedly expanding population of older adults and projected prevalence of dementia in coming decades highlight the need for nurses to understand and be responsive to the needs of people with dementia and their families. Alzheimer's disease and related dementias are now recognized as a leading cause of death, and are associated with the individual's eventual inability to perform basic functions such as swallowing, or because of complications including infections (Maxwell, 2016). We will discuss the impact of cognitive decline on individuals and families later in this chapter.

FAMILY TIES IN MID- AND LATER LIFE

We now turn to the intersection of aging and family life and its implications for nurses. With increasing life expectancy, family relationships now last for decades. It is common to see newspaper photos of couples celebrating their 60th anniversaries, and for

"children" in their sixties or seventies to have living parents. We now encounter siblings with relationships of 90 years or longer; even grandparent-grandchild relationships increasingly extend five or more decades. These long-lasting relationships with their histories of shared experiences, traditions, and exchanges of help will most often be an asset to the older adult as illnesses or functional declines occur. This portrait of ties will continue to change as society changes. We explore those in the text that follows, focusing on intimate partnerships, sibling relationships, and intergenerational relationships.

A prevailing myth in the United States is that older adults, particularly those who are part of the dominant culture, are isolated from and neglected by their younger family members, and ultimately are abandoned in nursing homes. Study after study has demonstrated that most family ties are strong and characterized by affection, caring, and many shared values (Fingerman & Birditt, 2011; Rossi & Rossi, 1990). Furthermore, families have demonstrated remarkable adaptability to social change. Although the family structure has changed in recent decades, much about family life has remained the same, including valuing families. Individuals continue to travel through life in the company of others, which Antonucci and Akiyama (1995) described as "social convoys." Some people come and go in our convoys, but many, especially family members, remain constant social companions for decades. Families value exchanges of emotional and practical support throughout the life course (Sechrist et al., 2012; Walker, Manoogian-O'Dell, McGraw, & White, 2001). We now turn to specific types of family relationships, including intimate partnerships, siblings, and intergenerational relationships.

Intimate Partnerships

Intimate partnerships refer to relationships characterized by commitment, deep feelings and expressions of caring and compassion, sharing values and goals, physical intimacy, and interdependence (Blieszner & de Vries, 2001). Marriage is probably the first type of intimate partnership that comes to mind, although cohabitation is increasingly common and other forms of intimate partnerships are emerging.

Marriage

Age at first marriage is on the rise, 26.5 years for women and 28.7 for men, an increase of 6 years since the 1960s (Manning, Brown, & Payne, 2014). These rates vary by race and socioeconomic status, with African Americans marrying later than whites and other ethnic groups. Until recently, marriage was an option only for heterosexual partners. In the United States, Canada, and many European countries, marriage is now available to same-sex couples. Before this change, cohabitation was the major option for same-sex partners. In general, older adults who are married or are in egalitarian relationships have better physical health and psychological well-being when compared with those who are single, widowed, divorced, or separated (Connidis, 2010). This is especially true for men and for couples who report high-quality relationships (Bookwala, 2012). Relationship quality in later life is influenced by retirement status, as well as by health, mental health, and caregiving roles. All these situations have the potential to influence relationships in negative ways. The way one partner responds to a stressor such as chronic illness influences how the other responds, emphasizing the importance of focusing on family and not just individuals when working with older adults.

Cohabitation

We can no longer assume that those who are single are without partners. Cohabitation was often a precursor to marriage in the past, but now more couples of all ages are choosing not to marry, especially those with less education and economic stability (Manning et al., 2014). Marriage, therefore, is increasingly connected to educational and economic status. Cohabitation as an alternative to marriage has increased in middle and later life, as many previously widowed or divorced couples choose it over marriage (Bookwala, 2012; Schimmele & Wu, 2016). Nearly 25% of cohabiting adults have one partner older than age 50 (Wright & Brown, 2016).

Cohabiting couples have historically had less stable unions than those who marry, but differences between cohabiting and married couples in the nature of the relationship appear to be diminishing. For example, in a study of cohabitation and marriage in Italy (a familistic society), Pirani and Vignoli (2016) found more similarities than differences in family function and relationship satisfaction when the percentage of couples cohabiting in a community reached 15%. Wright and Brown (2016) compared psychological well-being of older adults who were unpartnered, dating, cohabitating, or married.

Psychological well-being as measured by depressive symptoms, perceived stress, and loneliness was not related to partnership status for women. Men had a different pattern; both cohabiting and married men had more positive well-being than unpartnered or dating men. Examining comparisons of marriage and cohabitation only, cohabiting men were less likely to report depressive symptoms or stress than married men. Unpartnered men reported higher levels of perceived stress.

Living Apart Together

"Living apart together" (LAT) is an emerging form of intimate relationship, especially in old age (Bookwala, 2012). LAT couples live in different households but consider themselves to be intimate partners in all other ways. This type of relationship is appealing to older adults who desire companionship and emotional support, but value autonomy and want to avoid obligations associated with marriage. This may be particularly important for women who typically have more caregiving responsibilities than their partners. Benson and Coleman (2016) found that LAT couples varied in their definitions of their relationship, but consistently expressed commitment to one another. Whether this commitment includes caregiving responsibilities as one or both partners age is an ongoing area of study.

Never Married

With the rise in cohabitation and LAT relationships, the group of "never married" is becoming more diverse. Women who have never married tend to have high levels of well-being, second to those in satisfying partnerships and ahead of those in dissatisfying relationships. Because those who have never formed partnerships often have a history of living alone, they typically have higher levels of life satisfaction than those who are widowed, divorced, and separated. This is because most have created satisfying and robust social networks, typically including close friends, siblings, and other family members. Indeed, unpartnered aunts and uncles provide significant parent support and are actively engaged in the lives of their siblings, nieces, and nephews (Allen & Pickett, 1987).

Sexuality

Sexuality is central to intimate partnerships regardless of gender or partnership status. Women and men continue to desire sexual relationships well into late life, with many reporting increased freedom to explore sexuality because of decreased concern over procreation and decreased family responsibilities. Older adults with partners tend to rate sex as important; most couples who have been sexually active in middle age tend to remain so in old age. Greater emotional and physical well-being is associated with being sexually active (Bookwala, 2012; DeLamater, 2012). Sexual activity is dependent on physical health, quality and availability of relationships, change in role from procreation to pleasure and validation, attitudes toward sexuality, societal influences, and previous sexual experiences (DeLamater, 2012; DeLamater & Moorman, 2007). DeLamater and Moorman (2007) emphasized the error of viewing sexuality from only a biological or medical perspective, noting that attitude is more salient in predicting continued sexual desire and behavior than presence or absence of chronic illness or age. Nevertheless, advancing age is associated with decline in sexual activity for many people. Schmall (1994), however, emphasized that sexuality involves much more than sexual intercourse, highlighting the importance of intimacy, touch, affection, body image, and one's identity as a sexual being. Sexuality in intimate, same-generation partnerships, therefore, continues to be an important part of life in spite of increasing frailty and dependence. Loss of a partner through widowhood often means the loss of all these different facets of sexuality, facets that often are unrecognized or unacknowledged. DeLamater's (2002) integrated model of accessing sexuality in later life can aid nurses in understanding the role of sexuality in the lives of older adults. The model includes the following:

- *Biological influences*: physical health (i.e., presence of chronic conditions that impact sexual function or desire, or both), age, hormonal levels, medical treatments that may impact sexual function
- *Psychological*: attitudes toward sexuality, role of sexual relationships, knowledge, past experiences, mental health
- *Social*: availability of partner, including duration and quality of relationship, societal views and influences on sexuality in later life, socioeconomic status

Intimate Partner Dissolution

Intimate partnerships end through divorce, breakups (in the case of cohabitation or LAT relationships),

or widowhood. These are among the most stressful transitions in family life. In the text that follows we describe the demographic characteristics associated with dissolution. It is beyond the scope of this chapter, however, to fully explore the psychological, social, economic, and health impact of these transitions on women and men. This is due in large part to the heterogeneity of experiences. As indicated by life course perspective, the impact will be shaped by gender, the nature and duration of the intimate partnership, the roles played by each partner, the specific causes of the dissolution, the availability of social supports, economic resources, and personal agency. Furthermore, the historical, cultural, and societal context in which the dissolution occurs will also shape response.

Divorce rates increased dramatically during the 20th century, more than doubling between the 1960s and 1980s before stabilizing in the 1990s (Cherlin, 2010). Although risk of divorce is beginning to decline, the lifetime probability of divorce remains between 40% and 50%. Therefore, those entering old age now experienced higher rates of divorce than previous age cohorts. Most divorces still occur in young adulthood, although it has become more common in middle and late adulthood (Carr & Pudrovska, 2012; Lin, Brown, Wright, & Hammersmith, 2016). In 1990, these "gray divorces" accounted for 10% of divorces in the United States, rising to more than 25% by 2010 (Lin et al., 2016). Reasons for divorce in later life are similar to divorce in younger couples, including marital quality and economic resources. According to Lin and colleagues (2016), the divorce rate for older adults is 2.5 times higher for those in remarriages compared with those in first marriages. Schimmele and Wu (2106) examined the prevalence of union dissolution and repartnering of Canadians older than 45. They found the major reason for dissolution for women was widowhood (67%) compared with men (38%). In contrast, the main reason for unions ending for men was divorce (46%) compared with women (25%). Repartnering patterns also differ. After 10 years, 5.8% of women had cohabited compared with 20% of men, and 7.8% of women had married compared with 30% of men (Schimmele & Wu, 2016). Divorced people were more likely to repartner and to do so sooner than those who were widowed or whose cohabitation union dissolved.

Differences in longevity and the tendency of women to marry or partner with men who are older puts women at greater risk of widowhood, especially in the oldest age groups: 73% of very old women (those 85 years and older) and 34% of very old men are widowed (FIFARS, 2016). Living arrangements show a similar pattern, with men more likely to live with their spouses and women more likely to live alone or with other relatives in advanced old age. Men are much more likely than women to be married in old age because of greater longevity for women and somewhat higher rates of remarriage after widowhood or divorce for men. For example, more than 74% of men 65 to 74 years old are married compared with 58% of women. By the time they reach old age, the disparity is even greater; 59% of men 85 years and older are married, whereas only 17% of women in that age group are married (FIFARS, 2016). Marital status varies by ethnicity, with a greater proportion of African American and Hispanic adults widowed or divorced when compared with non-Hispanic whites (Connidis, 2010).

Siblings

Siblings represent important but often overlooked same-generation family relationships (Bedford & Avioli, 2012; Walker, Allen, & Connidis, 2005). They typically are the family tie of the longest duration and, for the most part, siblings share the same historical and social context. As with all family relationships, identifying siblings can be complex. They may include full biological relationships, siblings through adoptions, half or step siblings, and fictive relationships. With divorce, there can also be relationships of "former siblings." In adulthood, family ties expand through sisters- and brothers-in-law, and nieces and nephews, relationships made possible through sibling ties. Although often intense during childhood, many sibling relationships become inactive in young adulthood as people focus on their partners, children, and career development. During middle and late life, sibling ties are often reactivated as they have more time to devote to the relationship and as their aging parents require increasing assistance. This illustrates both the voluntary and the obligatory aspects of the sibling tie (Walker et al., 2005). Siblings tend to feel obligations to work together in support of aging parents and also respond to each other in times of need. Conflicts, when they do arise, appear to have roots in family history, and may be related to differential treatment as children. Of course, many siblings remain emotionally close and interact

frequently throughout their lives. Siblings are most likely to report being close to a sister. Throughout the life course, those who are unmarried, without children, and live in close proximity retain active ties to siblings. Having sibling relationships is associated with less loneliness in old age (Bedford & Avioli, 2012). As the birth rate declines and more people have no or only one sibling, an important family tie in old age is likely to become increasingly rare.

Intergenerational Relationships

Intergenerational relationships include a wide range of family ties, including parent-child, stepparent and stepchildren, grandparents and grandchildren, aunt/uncle and niece/nephew, and a host of intergenerational relationships that are "like family" but not related by blood, marriage, or adoption (that is, "fictive kin" as mentioned earlier). Nurses need to be aware of the multiple ways that adult children and parents or stepparents have a shared history and how that might influence mutual affection, exchange, and caregiving. Intergenerational relationships are increasingly taking on a voluntary quality influenced by affection, commitment, and a wide range of contextual factors. Assumptions about the quality of relationships cannot be made based on gender or type of relationship. Following are some things to consider.

Similar to same-generation relationships, the characteristics of intergenerational family relationships are changing because of demographic trends related to fertility and longevity as well as changes in the social structure. Fertility rates have declined worldwide in the past decades, with rates falling at or below replacement levels in Europe, North America, and Eastern Asia (United Nations, 2015a). In 2005, 19% of U.S. and 22% of Canadian women 45 years or older had no children (Connidis, 2015a). Fertility varies among ethnic groups in the United States, with the highest levels among Hispanic populations with Mexican origins. Fertility is linked to economic conditions, with lower rates during times of economic hardship. For example, during the 20th century, the rates of childlessness were highest in the United States during the Great Depression (Connidis, 2010). Similarly, marriage and the birth of a first child is occurring at older ages. This means that parents and grandparents experience these roles at later ages. The number of children born into a family has declined in the United States, resulting in more families with one or two children. Although parents can provide more individual attention to fewer children, this has implications as parents age and have fewer family members available for support and adult children have fewer siblings to share parent care responsibilities.

During the last several decades, the number of children born outside of marriage has increased, accounting for nearly half of all births in the late 2000s (Lichter, Sassler, & Turner, 2014). Households with single parents are much more prevalent in the United States (40%) than in Canada (16%; Connidis, 2015a). Although many aspects of marriage and cohabitation are becoming more similar, cohabitation remains less stable than marriage, particularly for couples with fewer economic resources. This has implications for intergenerational family ties in old age, particularly for parents who have a history of serial cohabitation.

Accompanying the reduction in fertility rates and the choice not to marry is the increase in childlessness (sometimes called "child free") across all Western countries (Ivanova & Dykstra, 2015). In 2006, 20% of U.S. women aged 40 to 44 did not have children, up from 10% in 1970 (Blackstone, 2014). The trend is continuing in younger age groups. Reasons for childlessness vary and are generally categorized as involuntary (e.g., a result of infertility) or voluntary (e.g., active choice not to have children). Increasingly, childlessness is a voluntary state. The reason for being childless and how women feel about childlessness are related to satisfaction and well-being, especially if childlessness is a result of choice and the person has low levels of childlessness concerns (McQuillan, Greil, Shreffler, Wonch-Hill, Gentzler, & Hathcoat, 2012). Overall, compared with parents, marital satisfaction is higher for childless couples, income levels are higher, and childless women have richer and more diverse social networks. Those who are childless contribute more to charitable and voluntary work, and have important relationships with nieces and nephews and other family members. With widowhood, poor health, and frailty, however, a childless person has fewer social resources and must depend more on the formal service systems. Those who have had children who have died or who have become estranged are sometimes considered childless. These situations pose a whole new set of issues for the older adult.

Parent-Child Relationships

The strongest intergenerational tie is the parent-child relationship, and these relationships are particularly strong for mothers and daughters. Most older adults have one grown child who lives within an hour's drive. This has remained relatively constant despite the often-cited geographical mobility of younger generations. At the same time, adult children with college degrees are more likely to live farther away (Uhlenberg, 2004). Contact between generations is common, with the majority of adult children reporting contact with their parents at least once a week. Contact with mothers is more frequent than contact with fathers, and contact between mothers and daughters is the most common intergenerational interaction, reflecting that the strongest intergenerational tie is between mothers and daughters. The amount of contact by adult children is influenced by parental marital status, with the lowest contact being with fathers who are widowed, divorced, or remarried, and with remarried mothers.

Relationship quality is more important than contact. Feelings of closeness between generations are the norm, with most adult children reporting feeling very close to parents, especially between mothers and adult daughters (Sechrist et al., 2012). Adult children are more likely to experience strains in relationships with fathers compared with relationships with mothers (Lendon, Silverstein, & Giarrusso, 2014). The older generation reports even more positive feelings toward their adult children than their children express toward them. Exchanges of help and support between generations occur throughout the life course and are motivated by affection as well as by a sense of obligation. Until late old age, older adults provide more help to adult children than they receive in all areas of support, including caring for family members, financial support, and instrumental support (Sechrist et al., 2012). We explore exchanges of support among generations in our discussion of caregiving later in the chapter.

Parent-child relationships exist in many different family forms, including those headed by same-sex couples. Children in these families may have accompanied his/her parent from a prior heterosexual relationship, resulting in stepfamily relationships. Overall, same-sex families have received growing acceptance in Western cultures. In addition to step relationships, children of same-sex couples are now arriving more frequently through adoption, surrogacy, or artificial insemination. Current research suggests that well-being of children raised by same-sex couples is similar to those raised by heterosexual couples: children do best in a loving, stable, and supportive environment regardless of the sexual orientation of the parents (Connidis, 2015a).

The impact of divorce on parent-child relationships varies. Cause and timing of a parent's divorce; their ability to provide stable, loving, and supportive environments to young children; and financial and educational resources all influence the long-term consequences for adult children and their parents. Bucx, van Wel, Knijin, and Hagendoorn (2008) reported less contact by adult children with divorced mothers and fathers. Divorce, particularly for men, often results in strained relationships with adult children, placing them at greater risk of isolation in old age (Connidis, 2010). They may have fewer ties that connect them to informal care and may rely more on formal services, such as nursing homes, than their married counterparts. Adult children are less likely to have strong ties or provide support to divorced, aging fathers. Although relationships with divorced mothers may be strained, adult children typically maintain relationships and provide support as needed (Sechrist et al., 2012). Delay in marriage by young adults has been attributed in part to the desire to succeed in marriage where parents have failed. An adult child's divorce also affects parent-child relationships. Parents often provide financial and child-care assistance in the immediate aftermath, particularly for adult daughters. Thus, these parent-child relationships are often strengthened.

Stepparent-Stepchild Relationships

Those now entering old age are likely to have complex family systems that include stepchildren because of divorce and remarriage, or cohabitation. As in much of family life, the nature of these relationships varies widely. Schmeekle and her colleagues found that perceptions of stepchildren that their stepparents or former stepparents were family varied from "not at all" to "fully." Being considered "fully family" is associated with the stepparent being married to the stepchild's biological parent (as opposed to cohabiting), a history of coresidence, and the stepchild's general attitude in support of family obligation (Schmeekle, Giarrusso, Feng, & Bengtson, 2006). A similar pattern was noted more recently in Germany. Although biological parents and their children appeared to have closer relationships than stepparents and their stepchildren overall, differences in the quality of relationships diminished when stepparents were married to biological parents, the relationship between stepparents and stepchildren was of long duration, and familistic values were shared (Becker, Salzburger, Lois, & Nauck, 2013).

Grandparent-Grandchild Relationships

Significant intergenerational family relationships include grandparents and grandchildren. Contact between grandparents and grandchildren is similar to that between parents and adult children, with 66% of grandparents living within an hour's drive from at least one set of grandchildren. The strongest predictor of grandparent-grandchild relationships is the quality of relationships between parents and grandparents, especially between mothers and grandparents (Monserud, 2008; Sims & Rofail, 2013). Grandparenting is a role that is contingent on the actions of adult children for timing, number, location, and amount of contact (Hayslip & Page, 2012; Thiele & Whelan, 2006). In the past, almost all older adults with children were likely to become grandparents. This will be less likely if projected rates of childlessness continue. As with parenthood, becoming a grandparent is occurring later in the life course. In Canada, for example, more than 60% of women were grandmothers in their 50s in 1985, but only 29% were in 2011 (Morgolis, 2016). With the aging of both grandparents and grandchildren, the nature of relationships will change. Older grandparents, for example, are more likely to provide money and gifts as grandchildren get older rather than direct care (Thiele & Whelan, 2006).

Although grandchildren are expected to have many years of relationship with grandparents because of increased longevity, there will be a much greater age gap than in the past with implications for the nature of those relationships. Sometimes called a "roleless role," grandparents often create their role within the family based on the family's stage in the life course and the family history of grandparenting roles. Grandparents are influenced by experiences with their own grandparents and with their parents as grandparents. Also, relationships with grandchildren are strongly shaped by the quality of relationships grandparents have with their adult children and children-in-law. When the grandparent-parent relationship is strong, grandparents and grandchildren are most likely to enjoy strong connections. The strength of these connections remains strong even as grandchildren enter adulthood (Monserud, 2010). If the role is perceived to come too early, as in the case of teenage pregnancy, the transition to grandparenthood may be altered by disappointment, anxiety, and emotional and financial distress. Parent-grandparent roles also may be strained, often related to divorce in either of the generations. This may result in limited or no contact between grandparents and grandchildren. This occurs most frequently with paternal grandparents when their sons do not have custody or for grandfathers who themselves are divorced (Sims & Rofail, 2013).

As in other family relationships, the ways that grandparents relate to grandchildren vary widely among families (Silverstein & Marenco, 2001; Stelle, Fruhauf, Orel, & Landry-Meyer, 2010; Thiele & Whelan, 2006). Most older adults find grandparenting meaningful and experience the role with both satisfaction and pleasure (Hayslip & Page, 2012). Grandparents are often an important resource for their adult children. For example, grandparents are a major provider of child care when grandchildren are young (Luo, LaPierre, Hughes, & Waite, 2012; Vandell, McCartney, Owen, Booth, & Clarke-Stewart, 2003). This is particularly true of older adults who have immigrated to the United States to be with family (Usita & Shakya, 2012). In Europe, 49% of grandfathers and 58% of grandmothers who have grandchildren 15 years or younger regularly provide some kind of care for grandchildren. Rates are highest in more conservative regions of Europe, especially when formal child-care options are limited (Jappens & Van Bavel, 2012).

Ambivalence and Conflict in Families

Family gerontology researchers have increasingly focused on the complexity of family life. The concept of ambivalence has received increasing attention, recognizing that family members simultaneously hold positive and negative feelings about one another, often because of contradictory roles (Connidis, 2015b; Connidis & McMullin, 2002; Katz, Lowenstein, Phillips, & Daatland, 2005; Pillemer & Suiter, 2004; Sechrist et al., 2012). With respect to mixed feelings, Fingerman (2001) found adult daughters tended to express more ambivalence about their mothers than mothers expressed about their daughters. Pillemer and Suitor (2004) report that the majority of parents felt "torn in two directions" about their adult children. They found that ambivalence was frequently related to their adult children's achievements, particularly achievements of their oldest child. More ambivalence was expressed toward those who did not attain normative adult statuses, such as completing college,

getting married, or becoming financially independent. Peters, Hooker, and Zvonkovic (2006) conclude that ambivalence is a normal part of family life. In their study, older adults experienced ambivalence surrounding their adult children's busy lives and boundaries related to communication (e.g., holding back on opinions and feelings about being left out). Older adults had uncertainties about the availability of help from children should they need it, though Peters and her colleagues found that those who needed help received it. Connidis (2015b) stresses the importance of thinking about ambivalence beyond individual feelings and emphasizes how societal level conditions and expectations affect individual and family life in contradictory ways. Igarashi and her colleagues (2013) used this framework to explore ambivalence as those in midlife sought to support both younger and older family members within a culture that values independence and autonomy and a society that provides limited supports (Igarashi, Hooker, Coehlo, & Manoogian, 2013).

Though less common than ambivalence, family conflict or negative social interactions can have serious consequences for family relationships. Newsom and his colleagues have reported on a growing body of research that describes the disproportionate effect of negative social exchanges on physical and psychological health when compared with positive social exchanges (Newsom, Mahan, Rook, & Krause, 2008; Newsom, Rook, Nishishiba, Sorkin, & Mahan, 2005). They found that failure of those in one's social network to provide help when it was needed was evaluated most negatively. Umberson, Williams, Powers, Liu, and Needham (2006) examined marriage quality and health during the life course, finding that poor marriage quality was associated with accelerated health declines in old age. This is especially true for women. They suggested that stress related to marital conflicts undermines immune functioning and has a cumulative effect on health over time. Conflicted families are less likely to provide assistance to each other throughout the life course and may have little contact, share few values, and generally are more detached. As such, they are less likely to be resources to older family members in need (Scharlach, Li, & Dalvi, 2006).

An extreme form of family conflict is elder mistreatment. Elder mistreatment (often referred to as elder abuse) includes physical pain or injury, psychological anguish, neglect or abandonment, and financial exploitation. Estimates of prevalence of all types of mistreatment range from 1.3% to

10% of older adults (Fulmer, Guadagno, Bitondo, & Connolly, 2004; Teaster, Wangmo, & Vorsky, 2012). Types of abuse that are reported most frequently are neglect, emotional abuse, and financial exploitation (Roberto, Teaster, & McPherson, 2015). Most perpetrators are adult children, although other family members, paid caregivers, and predatory acquaintances may be abusers. Causes of mistreatment remain poorly understood, but risk factors include unhealthy dependency of the perpetrator on the victim; disturbed psychological state of the perpetrator; frailty, disability, or impairment of the victim; and low income, lack of social support, and isolation of the family (Lachs & Pillemer, 2015; Wolf, 1996). Women are more likely to be victims. People with dementia are especially vulnerable to psychological abuse and neglect (Downes, Fealy, Phelan, Donnelly, & Lafferty, 2013). Mistreatment is often associated with dementia-related behaviors coupled with limited emotional and psychological abilities of caregivers to provider support. Beach, Schulz, Castle, and Rosen (2010) also found that African American older adults were at greater risk for both financial exploitation and psychological mistreatment. Most abuse occurs in domestic settings; those living alone are at greatest risk for financial exploitation (Teaster et al., 2012). Abuse is an issue in the Brown family case study later in this chapter. Older adults may have been perpetrators of abuse earlier in their lives, which can make it difficult for adult children, who were their victims, to provide support. Nevertheless, there is evidence that adult children do provide instrumental if not emotional support to their abusive mothers in old age (Kong &Moorman, 2016).

Frail older adults are also at risk for mistreatment by care providers. Nurses and other health care providers have a responsibility to screen and assess older adults for abuse. Fulmer (2012) reviewed and evaluated several assessment tools. One of the recommended tools is the Elder Mistreatment Assessment Instrument, which can be found on the *Try This* section of the Hartford Institute for Geriatric Nursing (HIGN) Web site: https://consultgeri.org/try-this/general-assessment/issue-15 (Fulmer, 2012).

As illustrated by the discussions on ambivalence and conflict, it is evident that many family relationships are complex and the strengths of association may vary considerably over time. To add to the complexity, levels of ambivalence and conflict vary within families (Sechrist et al., 2012). An individual may have conflicted feelings about one family member and close, affectionate feelings about another. Both ambivalence and conflict may be apparent for nurses and other health care providers when an older adult needs care. Nurses should be aware that the families vary considerably with respect to the quality of relationships and the availability of family resources in times of crisis and health decline. Nurses must be sensitive to underlying tensions and be able to provide support in nonjudgmental ways, remembering that the current family dynamics are embedded in a lifetime of relationships and actions.

FAMILY CAREGIVING

Family life is characterized by exchanges of help and support throughout the life course. Until very old age, parents are more often givers than receivers in this exchange, regardless of income. They provide financial assistance to younger adults in college or starting their careers. They often assist those who are making major purchases such as cars or homes (Bengtson & Harootyan, 1994; Connidis, 2015a). Older adults also provide child care for their adult children, often leaving the workforce early to assume this role. They provide child care for their grandchildren while their adult children work or are unable to care for their children because of illness or planned absences (e.g., vacations).

Regardless of the type of care provided, family caregiving grows out of ongoing family relationships and refers to support given to those who are dependent on that support for everyday functioning (Pruchno & Gitlin, 2012; Waldrop, 2003). The transition from the normal and mutual aid to support that is defined as caregiving is often a gradual process. Many wives, for example, do not describe what they do as caregiving, because the work they do in support of their increasingly dependent husbands is part of their ongoing family roles related to meal preparation, housework, and laundry. Walker, Pratt, and Eddy (1995) noted that adult daughters do similar things for dependent mothers as they do for mothers who are more self-sufficient, including running errands, preparing meals, and assisting with housework. Caregiving may simply mean "keeping an eye on" an older adult to monitor well-being (Messecar, 2016). As dependency increases and more time is spent on providing support, the family member and now caregiver recognizes that the care recipient is no longer able to perform these tasks without help.

Care partner is a term that is gaining favor to better reflect family views about caregiving.

In contrast, transitions to caregiving and care receiving can happen suddenly if an otherwise healthy older adult has a traumatic injury, or experiences a stroke or cardiac arrest. For many older adults, a health crisis may signal a sudden end to independence or ability to live alone. In this case, a variety of decisions are made regarding family care and formal care services. Messecar (2016) reports that between 22.4 and 52 million people provide some care to family members every year. More than 17 million are providing care to someone older than 65 years (Schulz & Eden, 2016). Estimates of the prevalence of caregiving range widely depending on how caregiving is defined. The definition of providing "unpaid care to a relative or friend 18 years or in order to help them take care of themselves" was used in the recent *Caregiving in the U.S.* report (National Alliance for Caregiving & AARP Public Policy Institute, 2015), which further specified that caregiving included helping with personal needs or household chores, managing finances, arranging outside services, or visiting regularly. Using this definition, more than 43 million caregivers were identified in 2014. About 34 million provided care to an adult older than age 50. Nearly 60% of care recipients had a long-term physical condition and 26% had a memory problem (National Alliance for Caregiving [NAC] & AARP Public Policy Institute, 2015). The U.S. federal government defined caregiving as "people of all ages who, in the last month, helped with one or more self-care household, or medical activities for a Medicare enrollee age 65 or older who had a chronic disability." They reported nearly 18 million caregivers, with daughters accounting for 29% of caregiving, spouses 21%, and sons 18% (FIFARS 2016). Most provided transportation (86%), followed by mobility (72%), medical or health care (57%), and assistance with self-care (49%; FIFARS, 2016). Most caregivers are middle-aged or older and are most likely to be wives and daughters. Research has shown consistently that women provide more personal care, more hours of caregiving, more housekeeping, and spend more years in caregiving, whereas men provide financial assistance (such as money management), make arrangements for formal care, and do home and yard maintenance work. Although these historically gender-specific roles are becoming less distinct, particularly for the oldest caregivers, these differences remain (Schulz & Eden, 2016).

Duration of caregiving may last for days or decades, with the average length of time 4 years. Yet, 25% of caregivers have been providing care for 5 years or longer. Caregivers spend an average of 24 hours a week with caregiving tasks (e.g., 59% doing ADL care, 43% helping the recipient get in and out of beds and chairs) (NAC & AARP, 2015). Caregivers often are providing assistance to more than one older adult at a time, balancing caregiving tasks with other family responsibilities such as supporting children through school or filling their own grandparenting roles (Igarashi et al., 2013; Neal & Hammer, 2007). The Hooper family case study illustrates such multiple caregiving demands as Maria provides care to both her parents and her mother-in-law.

Estimates of the value of unpaid family care are difficult to determine but are estimated to approach $400 billion (Pruchno & Gitlin, 2012; Schulz & Eden, 2016). Costs include out-of-pocket medical expenses and lost income and retirement benefits including Social Security income if spouses and adult children leave the workforce early to care for older family members. Those who maintain their jobs often lose time, which negatively affects wages, promotions, or other job opportunities. The loss of income may be particularly difficult for those with low incomes at the start.

Family Caregiving Roles

Family roles, such as family structure, have shifted across time. Major changes in mid- and late life frequently include an increase in caregiving. Experiences vary by family role. We begin by a focus on caregiving for older adults by spouses and adult children, followed by caring for grandchildren and care for disabled adult children. This section also covers ways in which nurses can support caregivers. This section ends with a discussion about the specific challenges of providing care to a person with dementia.

Caring for Older Adults

Spouses are generally the first line of caregivers for older adults. Because women live longer than men, wives are more likely than husbands to become caregivers. Spouse caregivers, in particular, may have their own health concerns that are exacerbated by strains related to caregiving. It is not unusual for partners to support each other; they are both caregivers and care recipients. These situations are often tenuous but can work for a while. Spouses typically experience greater burden and depression than adult children who provide care (Messecar, 2016). Spouses are more likely to experience chronic illnesses and frailty themselves. Because spouse caregivers typically live with the care recipient, they are at risk for not getting rest, not having time to recuperate from illnesses, and experiencing health declines. This is particularly true if the person they are caring for has Alzheimer's disease or some other kind of dementia (Schulz & Eden, 2016).

Adult children, especially daughters, experience the stresses of care in other ways. More than half of adult daughters are working outside the home while providing care for a parent and have to make a range of adjustments to be successful in both roles. This may include going to work late or leaving early, or cutting down on hours worked (Schulz & Eden, 2016). Grandchildren may participate in providing care to their grandparents as they age, especially if their mothers are primary caregivers. The ways that grandchildren cope with this caregiving role are influenced by their previous relationships with their grandparents (Stelle et al., 2010).

Caregiving is influenced by culture. Nurses need to be aware of and sensitive to possible ethnic differences in caregiving experiences and resources. At the same time, it is important not to stereotype or make assumptions based on race or ethnicity. More differences are found within ethnic groups than between them. With that caution, Dilworth-Anderson et al. (2002) argued that "culture affects caregiving experiences. Findings on values and norms provide evidence that individuals and groups use explicit rules and guidelines that influence who provides care to elders as well as interactions between caregivers, family members, and social institutions" (p. 264). From their review of the literature, it appears that minority caregivers often have a more diverse group of extended helpers than do non-Hispanic white caregivers. But although more people might be involved in providing care to a dependent family member, minority caregivers are no more likely to feel supported by their social network than are caregivers from the dominant culture. Non-Hispanic whites are more likely to care for a spouse, which is related to whites having more married couples in later life and a longer life expectancy for men. African Americans may be more likely to receive assistance through church connections. They are also more likely to have a network of kinship relationships that assist with caregiving. African Americans and Hispanics are least likely to use formal services and yet are most likely to express the need for assistance with caregiving responsibilities. Cultural values do influence who takes on the leadership role of caregiving within a family (Dilworth-Anderson et al., 2002). These values are affected by a sense of filial obligation and a sense of responsibility, cultural norms regarding who provides care (i.e., daughter or daughter-in-law), values of giving back, culturally based illness meanings (e.g., a view that disease is normal or that there is a stigma), and larger belief systems such as religion. Because of poorer health status found in most minority populations, caregiving often begins at a younger age, but the duration is shorter.

Grandparents Caring for Grandchildren

Many older adults are primary caregivers of younger members of their families. Unlike caregiving for older adults, which often evolves over time, grandparents may suddenly find themselves in the role of raising their grandchildren. This may occur when teenagers have children or because of traumatic circumstances surrounding the parent generation, including divorce, substance abuse, incarceration, child abuse or neglect, or death (Hayslip & Page, 2012). The number of grandparents who were raising their grandchildren increased dramatically by the end of the 20th century. By 2006 U.S. census data revealed about 2.4 million grandparents (11% of grandparents) had assumed parenting roles (Goodman, 2012; Lumpkin 2008). Grandparent-grandchild families are more likely to live below the poverty line. Some grandparents leave the workforce to care for grandchildren and others postpone retirement for financial reasons. Grandparent caregivers are most often women who are in poorer physical health; have poorer mental health, including higher levels of depression; and have more financial strains than other grandparents (Doley, Bell, Watt & Simpson, 2015; Whitley, 2016). Hayslip, Blumenthal, and Garner (2015) found that poor health and depression can be mitigated to some extent through social support from friends and other family members. Ongoing conflict with adult children (parents of their grandchildren) is common, with accompanying feelings of disappointment, resentment, feeling taken advantage of, and grief. If parents have been substance abusers, grandchildren may have physical and behavioral problems that cause further anxiety for grandparents (Hayslip & Kaminski, 2005).

As with caregiving in general, grandparents and their grandchildren experience many benefits when a grandparent is raising a grandchild. Grandparents are often a stabilizing influence, and their grandchildren generally do well in school, are less likely to be on welfare, and have fewer negative behaviors. In spite of their grief and the burdens associated with care, grandparents report benefits such as realizing their inner strength, close relationships with their grandchildren, and a sense of accomplishment and purpose (Hayslip & Page, 2012; Waldrop, 2003). After following grandmothers who raised grandchildren longer than 9 years, Goodman (2012), found that grandmothers had a close relationship with their grandchildren and were not found to have many of the reported negative consequences described earlier, suggesting that interventions to support these relationships are particularly important.

Older Adults Caring for Adult Children

Gilligan and her colleagues found that mothers well into their eighties provided both instrumental (e.g., help with regular chores) and emotional support to their adult children with a serious health condition (Gilligan, Suitor, Rurka, Con, & Pillemer, 2017). Over 50,000 soldiers, mostly young, have been injured in combat in recent years (Cozza, Holmes, & Van Ost, 2013). Although very little attention has focused on the role of parents caring for injured soldiers (Ramchand et al. 2014), it is likely that many parents have assumed a primary caregiver role or are assisting caregiving spouses.

Sometimes caring for dependent children into old age reflects a lifelong role. The consequences of a lifetime of caring for an adult child with intellectual or developmental disabilities are significant. Seltzer, Floyd, Song, Greenberg, and Hong (2011) found similarities to parents of children with no disabilities with respect to health, attainment and life satisfaction in midlife. They did find, however, that parents of those with disabilities had lower employment levels for women and lower social participation rates. These patterns continued as parents entered their sixties. This was especially true for those who continued to co-reside with their children. Challenges included higher rates of depression, divorce, widowhood, and poorer physical health and functional status when compared with other parents whose children did not have disabilities. Adults with intellectual and developmental disabilities are living longer and often experience chronic physical illnesses. Most older adults with an intellectual disability live at home and about 25% have a parent caregiver who is older than 60 years (Heller, Gibbons, & Fisher, 2015). Supports for both caregivers and the adult children who are also aging are needed. The Administration for Community Living has developed important initiatives to improve supports to these families (Hahn, Fox & Janicki, 2015).

Nursing Role in Assessing and Supporting Family Caregivers

Because many family caregivers are unprepared for their roles, they are at risk for negative outcomes. The degree of risk is influenced by the context of caregiving that includes family history and dynamics, nature and extent of the care recipient's limitations (e.g., physical care needs, behavioral expressions), and personal and financial resources. Messecar (2016) identified eight evidence-based strategies for working with family caregivers. To be effective, these strategies must be based on a thorough assessment and tailored to the individual caregiving situation. Yet, needs of caregivers are not assessed routinely; caregivers remain at risk for burnout and care recipients are at risk for not receiving appropriate care, either at home or in another setting.

When nurses assess family caregiving situations, they tend to focus on ADLs (bathing, dressing, eating, toileting, hygiene, and mobility) and IADLs (shopping, managing finances, meal preparation, driving, and managing medications). ADLs are useful for determining how much physical assistance a care recipient may need from the caregiver. IADLs may determine whether an individual can live independently in the community. For example, a person may have significant mobility problems, but if she has the ability to plan and direct care through execution of IADLs, it may be possible to remain at home. In any event, Kelly, Reinhard, and Brooks-Danso (2008) recommend that assessments be done both for families as clients and for families as providers of care. As Pusey-Murray and Miller report, assessments must go beyond a listing of care recipient needs related to ADLs and IADLs because:

Those concepts do not adequately capture the complexity and stressfulness of caregiving. Assistance with bathing does not capture bathing a person who is resisting a bath. Helping with medications does not adequately capture the hassles of medication administration, especially when the care recipient is receiving multiple medications several times a day, including injections, inhalers, eye drops, and crushed tablets. (Pusey-Murray & Miller, 2013, p. 115)

Families are often very involved in helping older adults manage multiple and chronic illnesses. Surveying 1677 family caregivers, Reinhard, Levine, and Samis (2012) found that 46% reported being responsible for "medical/nursing" tasks such as care coordination among multiple providers, managing or administering multiple medications including intravenous fluids, providing wound care and other treatments, or using medical devices or monitors. These activities were in addition to providing support with ADLs and IADLs. Most caregivers reported that these tasks were learned primarily through experience (Reinhard et al., 2012). Clearly, there is great need for nurses and other care providers to rethink how families are supporting older adults with frailty and/or chronic conditions, and to initiate systematic and periodic assessments and interventions that address specific caregiver roles and tasks.

Domains to be included in assessments are context; caregiver perception of health and functional status of the care recipient; caregiver values and principles; well-being of the caregiver; consequences of caregiving, skills, abilities, and knowledge to provide care; and potential resources that the caregiver could choose to use (Family Caregiver Alliance [FCA], 2006). Various caregiver assessment screening tools exist. The Preparedness for Caregiving tool (Zwicker, 2010) is brief, addresses the domains recommended by the FCA, and provides a starting point for understanding caregiver needs related to both their care activities and their own health. The HIGN's "Informal Caregivers of Older Adults at Home: Let's PREPARE!" (Atkins, Kowalski, Keefer, Silver, & Lewis-Holman, 2010) uses a checklist to identify tasks commonly required when caring for an older adult with a range of medical conditions, and could be used to evaluate caregiver competence to monitor changes in condition or perform specific tasks such as wound care or medication administration. However, this tool does not address consequences of caring for the caregiver. The Modified Caregiver Strain Index (Onega, 2008) facilitates screening for adverse effects of caregiving in multiple domains including financial, physical, and psychological strain. Screening assessments should happen periodically along the care trajectory.

Multiple interventions have been developed and tested to address the needs of caregivers, both as clients and as providers. Pinquart and Sorensen (2006) identified six types of interventions: (1) psychoeducational, (2) cognitive-behavioral therapy (CBT), (3) counseling/case management, (4) support—training the care recipient, (5) respite care, and (6) multicomponent interventions (combinations of more than one type of intervention). Outcomes of interest included reducing burden, depression, care recipient symptoms, and institutionalization of the care recipient, as well as increasing subjective well-being and caregiver knowledge and ability. The largest effects were with CBT, which helped to reduce depression and, to a lesser extent, helped reduce feelings of burden. CBT concentrates on helping caregivers identify and modify beliefs related to the situation, and develop new behaviors to cope with caregiving demands. Psychoeducational programs contributed small-to-moderate effects related to decreasing burden, depression, subjective well-being, and care receiver symptoms. Only care receiver education and multicomponent interventions were successful in reducing institutionalization. Other interventions that show some promise in reducing stress include moderate intensity exercise programs, yoga, and meditation activities (Messecar, 2016).

Pinquart and Sorensen (2006) suggest that more effort needs to be given to designing multicomponent interventions that target individual caregiver needs. For example, teaching caregivers to provide care and helping caregivers attend support groups can be powerful interventions that contribute to feelings of mastery. Those with high mastery have more positive experiences with caregiving and more positive health behaviors (Reinhard, Given, Petlick, & Bemis, 2008). They are also more likely to provide safe care and develop critical thinking skills. Unfortunately, many interventions are not covered by health insurance and providers are often unaware of local resources, although the National Academy of Science is calling for policy remedies to address this coverage gap (Schulz & Eden, 2016). Community-based nurses are in an excellent position to connect caregivers to support resources and to advocate for policy changes that cover the needs of caregivers.

Gaugler, Potter, and Pruinelli (2014) recommend a partnership-based approach to care management that fully acknowledges the family caregiver as well as the care recipient. This approach is based on respectful two-way communication among providers, patients, and families in an environment where families and patients are comfortable asking questions and expressing different perspectives or opinions on treatments or goals of care. Nurses can engage in partnership-based care by actively listening to families to understand their values, concerns, and goals; advocating for family and patient participation in care discussions; and being transparent in talking with families and patients. As the Internet is increasingly a source of information for families, nurses can also develop and share a list of trustworthy, evidence-based, consumer-friendly digital caregiving resources on various caregiving topics.

In the United States there has been a recent movement to legislate increased communication and collaboration between caregivers and providers. The *Caregiver Advice Record and Enable Act* (Escobedo, 2016, July 7) has been enacted by more than 30 states. Nurses have a critical role in implementing this law that mandates hospitals must notify the patient-identified family caregiver in advance of a discharge date and involve the caregiver in hospital discharge planning (Coleman, 2016). Hospitals must also offer discharge instructions to caregivers on "medical/nursing" tasks that will be needed by the older adult after discharge. This activity is clearly within nursing's domain, and nurses need to develop evidence-based teaching skills and strategies that go beyond providing a discharge handout to families on specific care tasks. Basic principles include learner assessment, providing information in formats beyond text descriptions, and using the "teach-back" and "show me" methods for instruction (AHRQ, 2015).

Caregiving and Dementia

As an illustration of the demands of caregiving and ways that nurses can provide information and support, we turn now to one of the most challenging caregiving situations: caring for someone with dementia. Families provide 83% of care (Friedman, Shih, Langa, & Hurd, 2015) to people with dementia, making these diseases truly a "family affair." Families often notice early cognitive, memory, or behavioral changes in the person with dementia, and may approach providers with their concerns. Encouragement for the older adult and his or her family to seek care that screens for early detection is critical, particularly to rule out treatable conditions that affect cognition. Early diagnosis can help the person with dementia and his or her family prepare for long-term management and

receive therapies that may delay onset of memory loss or other symptoms. The Alzheimer's Association, with chapters in many countries, is an outstanding resource that provides a vast and current array of information about the disease and its management, self-care, and specific places to go for more help. In the United States, the Web site is http://www.alzfdn.org/ and in Canada http://www.alzheimer.ca/en.

Budson and Solomon (2016) identified three points in the disease experience when caregivers are in particular need of education and support: (1) time of initial diagnosis; (2) when the intensity of care, including behavior management, increases; and (3) when residential care placement is being considered. At initial diagnosis, families need information about the disease and its progression, introduction to community resources, and referral for information about advanced care and legal-financial planning for the future. Families, along with the person with dementia, need emotional and practical support as they respond to a dementia diagnosis.

Disease progression varies by type of dementia as well as other, poorly understood factors. Nurses, particularly in dementia specialty and primary care settings, can develop a trust relationship with family members, coordinate services delivery, and provide anticipatory guidance, education, and resources to support families along the disease trajectory. As the disease progresses, families need to know what to anticipate and how to maximize the person with dementia's physical and cognitive function and dignity; strategies for preventing or managing difficult behaviors, with an emphasis on behaviors as responses to unmet needs; environmental modifications to enhance safety and independence; and how to manage concurrent frailty and multimorbidities in the person with dementia. The care requirements across the dementia trajectory are great, and many caregivers are in this role for 6 or more years (Maxwell, 2016.)

Although primary responsibility for care generally resides with one person, typically the spouse or an adult daughter, a network of both informal and formal care supports for the primary caregiver is associated with lower levels of perceived burden despite heavy care requirements (Sutcliffe, Giebel, Jolley, & Challis, 2016). Ongoing assessment of the caregiver is critical. Multi-component interventions that appear to positively influence caregiver morale while reducing strain are caregiver education, emotional support and counseling, practical training, and respite (Gitlin, Marx, Stanley, & Hodgson, 2015). Despite a body of research on interventions to support the caregiver, few systematic efforts have been made to translate findings to wide-scale practice, as funding has been insufficient. Therefore, governments and care delivery systems continue to rely on families to provide the bulk of care (Gitlin, Marx, Stanley, & Hodgson, 2015).

Most people with dementia do eventually transition to some type of LTC setting. The placement decision can be a time of great stress for caregivers as this decision may generate feelings of guilt or failure as a caregiver (Gaugler, Mittelman, Hepburn, & Newcomer, 2010). Further, there may be major financial implications associated with placement (Mausbach et al., 2014). We now turn to public policies that shape health care of older adults and the caregiving experience of family members. This is followed by a description of various long-term services and support options and the roles of nurses in these settings to support older adults and their families.

PUBLIC POLICIES RELATED TO AGING FAMILIES IN THE UNITED STATES

In both the United States and Canada, few public policy supports exist for family caregivers despite the extensive and increasingly complex roles that families assume and that delay costly institutionalization at the government's expense. The U.S. Family Medical Leave Act (1993) enables some caregivers to take time off from work for their care responsibilities; the details of how this act is implemented vary by state. In Canada, employment insurance compassionate care benefits (Canadian government, n.d.) guarantee unpaid, job-protected leave for up to 26 weeks to provide physical, emotional, or coordinating care to an older adult relative. Provinces vary in their implementation of this benefit (Canadian government, n.d.). Under certain conditions in both the United States and Canada, family caregivers may be able to deduct care expenses on their taxes.

In the United States, Medicare, Medicaid, and the Older Americans Act programs are public programs that shape the majority of health and medical care and long-term services and supports. These programs were originally passed by Congress in 1965 and each program has been modified with additional services added over time. We highlight specific policies that influence support for older adults and their families.

Medicare

Medicare is the U.S. government's health insurance program for older adults and some younger people meeting specific disability criteria. Medicare coverage focuses on primary, acute, intensive, rehabilitative, and hospice services. Not covered by Medicare are assistance with personal care and other ADLs such as toileting, bathing, or medication management. As described earlier, these uncovered services, sometimes called nonskilled care services, are critical for many aging adults, particularly aged 80 and older, as they experience comorbidities, cognitive decline, and physical frailty.

Individuals are eligible for Medicare at age 65. Those who delay enrollment are penalized through higher annual premiums. Medicare has four parts. Parts A and B refer to traditional Medicare. Part A covers portions of hospital and rehabilitation services, and Part B covers outpatient services. Part D covers prescription drugs. Medicare does not cover all costs, requiring most older adults to purchase additional, supplemental insurance to address gaps in coverage. An alternative Medicare option, Medicare Advantage (Part C), allows individuals to enroll with a private insurer that provides all services provided in traditional Medicare for one monthly premium. However, the enrollee cannot go to providers outside of the insuring organization for covered care. Although Medicare provides critical coverage to older adults who no longer receive insurance through their employer, selecting a plan that is a good fit with the individual's care needs can be challenging and confusing. To help older adults or their families select coverage, all states provide free Medicare counseling services through a federally funded State Health Insurance Program (SHIP).

The Affordable Care Act (ACA) provides several benefits to Medicare enrollees including no-copay screenings (e.g., mammography), annual wellness checks, and reduced prescription costs for individuals who exceeded the cap established for prescription payments when Part D was first implemented. Whether these benefits or the current Medicare plan will continue with new presidential leadership in 2017 is not clear. Current, detailed information on Medicare is found at https://www.medicare.gov/.

Acute Care

We discuss acute care here, because it is largely paid for through Medicare in the United States. Although most nurses who work in acute care do not consider themselves gerontological nurses, a high proportion of acute and critical care patients are over age 65 (Balas, Casey, Crozier, & Happ, 2016; Steele, 2010). Older adults are also commonly seen in emergency departments, where they account for up to 25% of trauma admissions (Cutugno, 2011). Although older adults vary greatly in terms of their general health, cognitive abilities, and functional status, in the hospital they are at particular risk for age-specific conditions or geriatric syndromes (Inouye, Studenski, Tinetti, & Kuchel, 2007). Examples of geriatric syndromes include falls, pressure injuries, delirium, incontinence, and deconditioning. These conditions are not normal with aging, and nurses must resist stereotyping these conditions as 'just part of growing old' (Parke & Hunter, 2014). Hospital-based nurses should be current in best practices to prevent, recognize, and manage geriatric syndromes. These conditions are costly in terms of human suffering, care resources, complicating sequelae that lead to increased mortality and morbidity rates, and re-hospitalizations after discharge. Additionally, older adults may present atypically, making difficult the ability to recognize early signs of infection or heart failure. Families can help the nurse to identify the older adult patient's baseline condition, including any assistive devices (e.g., glasses, hearing aid, walker) or routines (e.g., sleeping) that are normally used by the patient.

Models of Care

Models of elder-supportive acute care exist in some hospitals to prevent or minimize geriatric syndromes and facilitate a successful post-hospital transition. Common features of these models include interdisciplinary communication and care based on evidence-based geriatric and gerontological practices, environmental modifications that are "elder friendly" (e.g., lighting, sounds, layout of rooms), early and ongoing assessments that screen for risk factors, involvement of patients and their families in making treatment decisions that consider quality of life, and proactive discharge planning that represents collaboration among staffs at the hospital and transition locations with each other and with the patient and their family (Capezuti, Parks, Boltz, Malone, & Palmer, 2016). One model is the Acute Care for Elders unit (ACE unit). An interdisciplinary team, educated in evidence-based care for older adults, works with patients and their families. The team includes geriatricians and geriatric advanced

practice nurses. Units are designed to accommodate age-related changes and support cognitive orientation as well as functional independence and mobility by the patient along with family involvement. A body of research on ACE units demonstrates positive patient outcomes and reduced costs compared with non-ACE units (Barnes et al., 2012; Flood et al., 2013; Fox et al., 2013).

Another approach uses a geriatric care consultation program to maximize health outcomes and minimize risks of geriatric syndromes and their sequela. With this model, an interdisciplinary team with geriatric expertise is available to consult on older adult patients and make recommendations regarding hospital-based care as well as discharge plans. The consultation model used by the U.S. Department of Veterans Affairs (Phibbs et al., 2006) is associated with positive outcomes including less functional decline and less nursing home placement by veterans.

Nurses Improving Care for Healthsystem Elders (NICHE) is a nurse-led approach that emphasizes system-wide best practices in the care of older adults. NICHE promotes an environment and equipment that are particularly elder-friendly, evidence-based practice protocols in caring for older adults across all disciplines, use of geriatric resource nurses, and unit champions to develop gerontological competency for all staff. As with the other two programs, NICHE has demonstrated positive patient and staff outcomes (Capezuti et al., 2016). Nurses have a critical role in advocating for elder-friendly and elder-competent care organizations and for educating families on the advantages of seeking out elder-friendly hospitals in their community.

In all aspects of care of older adults, including hospitalization, it is important to emphasize that older adults vary significantly in their levels of independence, and family members vary in the nature of their relationship with an older adult. Hospitalization and the associated discharge transition may represent temporary family involvement in the older adult's life, or these events may be part of ongoing caregiving by families. Regardless, families are often asked to give input on treatment decisions and discharge planning. Families spend energy seeking information from myriad providers and struggle to get information on the transitional care plan, whether the plan is for discharge to home or to a care facility, and posthospitalization care needs of the older adult (Digby & Bloomer, 2014; Coleman, Roman, Hall, &

Min, 2015). The Caregiver Advise, Record, and Enable (CARE) Act (Coleman, 2016) acknowledges the significant role of families during hospitalization and transition, and will hopefully lead to families feeling empowered and competent to support their older adult after discharge. Nurses are the provider most likely to be responsible for assessing families and providing needed resources, education, and referrals to maximize successful transition on discharge.

Medicaid

Medicaid is the shared federal-state government health insurance plan for people of all ages with limited incomes. A very small number of older adults also qualify for Medicaid (Congressional Budget Office, 2013), although a significant number of those in need of long-term services and supports will "spend down" their resources and then qualify. Nurses need to know that Medicaid is the primary payer for nursing home care for older adults after they have spent down their personal assets. Some states have Medicaid waivers that allow older adults to use this benefit to pay for care in assisted living, adult care homes, and other home and community-based care programs. Some states participate in the Cash and Counseling or similar programs that allow public funds to pay family members for their care services under specified conditions. Information on Cash and Counseling is available at http://www.rwjf.org/en/library/research/2013/06/cash---counseling.html.

Older adults who qualify for both Medicare and Medicaid are considered "dual eligible." An innovative program for dual-eligible older adults is the Program of All Inclusive Care for the Elderly (PACE). PACE programs provide and coordinate all care services for enrollees through interdisciplinary care teams and close monitoring of each enrollee's health. PACE strives to keep enrollees living independently in their community despite often advanced comorbidities. Nurses have leadership roles in PACE as care and/or case managers, run clinics, visit enrollees at home, and supervise other staff in providing direct care to enrollees (Madden, Waldo, & Cleeter, 2014). Information about PACE is available at https://www.medicare.gov/your-medicare-costs/help-paying-costs/pace/pace.html.

National Aging Network Services

In the United States, the service system developed through the Older Americans Act to support a range of programs for older adults is the National Aging Network. The National Aging Network helps seniors remain at home as long as possible. With some exceptions, services are available to people who are age 60 years or older. Older Americans Act services are grouped into five large categories: (1) access to services, (2) nutrition, (3) home- and community-based LTC, (4) disease prevention and health promotions, and (5) vulnerable elder rights protection. Each state and community delivers these services according to community needs and resources. Two agencies within the National Aging Network that are important for nurses to know are the Aging and Disability Resource Centers (ADRCs) and Area Agencies on Aging (AAA) (Niles-Yokum & Wagner, 2011). To locate a local ADRC or AAA, use the national State Unit on Aging/Area Agency on Aging Finder and select your state and county.

ADRCs are available in most states and are designed to be a single access point for connecting people to a wide range of services and supports. Nurses in all settings can make referrals to ADRCs and use these organizations to enhance their own knowledge of home and community-based services and supports. The goal for ADRCs is to provide people with information and assistance regardless of age, income, or disability. Person-centered options counseling is a core function of most ADRCs. Options counselors are knowledgeable about public and private resources and assist older adults, people with disabilities, and their families to access needed services. Services are designed to meet individual values and preferences, and options counselors emphasize self-determination. Person-centered options counselors are important partners for nurses as they can work with older adults and families to ensure that needed supports are in place for a successful transition from hospital to home, a nursing facility, assisted living, or another residential care setting.

The AAAs and the organizations that subcontract with them (e.g., senior centers, adult day service, meal programs) administer the many Older Americans Act services. We highlight the Family Caregiver Support program. Established in 2000, it is the only federal program that specifically services family caregivers, including grandparents raising grandchildren. Core services provided are: information to caregivers about available services, assistance to caregivers in accessing supportive services, individual counseling and support groups to support informed decision making and solving problems, respite care for caregivers, and some supplemental services to complement caregiver support (Lewin Group, 2016). AAAs can be found through the Eldercare Locater Web site, which provides local contact information. Additional information about National Aging Network services can be found at http://www.healthinaging .org/resources/resource:aging-network-services/. In Canada, two resources that link to provinces and territories are the Canadian government (http://www .seniors.gc.ca/eng/index.shtml) and the Alzheimer's Association of Canada (http://www.alzheimer.ca/en).

Besides nationally sponsored services, resources for older adults and their caregivers include organizations associated with a variety of health problems, such as the American Heart Association and the Arthritis Foundation. Such organizations contain a wealth of consumer information on their Web sites, including tools for monitoring chronic health problems, guides for caregivers, and links to local resources.

LONG-TERM SERVICES AND SUPPORTS

Long-term services and supports encompass a wide range of services, both paid and unpaid. These services are most often provided by family with support through the National Aging Network, Medicaid, the Veterans Administration, and the private sector. Although the term *long-term care* is sometimes used interchangeably with *nursing home care*, nursing homes represent only one type of LTC service. A variety of community-based care services are available, including in-home care, supportive housing, adult day care, and a range of residential care settings. Our exploration of care settings begins with community-based care, where older adults receive care. Particular attention is given to the unpaid LTC system, which occurs mostly in the older adult's or a family member's home. Next is a discussion of LTC in residential settings, such as assisted living, adult foster care, and nursing homes.

Home- and Community-Based Care

Most older adults live in community settings with no or minimal support to manage their personal and health needs. Nurses may encounter these older adults where they receive their primary health care or to help them learn to manage chronic health problems. A variety of home- and community-based programs

have been developed to support the preference of older adults to remain in their homes. Many older adults and their families, however, have limited knowledge about what might be needed to continue living at home, the range of service options available in their communities, and how to access them. Health care providers also have limited knowledge about services outside of their own agencies.

One of the major reasons older adults prefer to remain in their own homes is to maintain autonomy and control over their lives. Yet family members are often more concerned about safety. Nurses can play an important role in working with families to identify ways to balance safety and risk related to mobility and cognitive problems such as dementia. Nurses can also help caregivers understand the normal aging process, including recognition of changes that should prompt an evaluation for potential problems. For example, Keyser, Buchanan, and Edge (2012) designed a program to teach caregivers about recognizing risk factors and signs of delirium in community-dwelling older adults with a goal of early intervention. This intervention, in turn, helps caregivers feel more capable and competent, and keeps care recipients safer by addressing treatable conditions more quickly and successfully.

Technology

Technology in the home is a strategy to support autonomy and safety in older adults, and to facilitate family caregiving. A range of technology innovations hold promise for older adults to age-in-place in their home and as strategies to facilitate family caregiving. The Centre for Policy on Ageing (2014) in the United Kingdom (UK) describes technology applications that nurses are or soon will be using or encountering in home-based caregiving. Assistive technologies include devices to help older adults with personal ADLs and IADLs. Examples include programmable pill boxes, utensils that prevent spills by accommodating hand tremors (e.g., Google spoon), "smart" hearing aids that adjust to external conditions, a wearable, invisible exoskeleton that stabilizes gait even on stairs, online assistants that support bill paying, and sensors that turn off unused stove burners (Jordan, Cory, Sainato, & Lehmann, 2016).

Telehealth applications monitor and generate physiologic trend data and enable providers to adjust treatments accordingly without requiring an office visit. Telecare via phone, Internet, or video interactions uses physiologic data to trigger emergency responders or phone contact by providers through sensors that automatically generate prescription refills or grocery lists or monitor movement within the home environment. Phone, video-conferencing, and e-mail communications between providers and older adults already supplement some face-to-face visits. Although research is limited on the use of these alternative ways of interacting, there is evidence that these types of "visits" are actually supplemental to rather than substitutes for face-to-face visits, and patient-provider relationships can be enhanced using these technologies (Pols, 2010). These applications have particular relevance for aging adults in rural and frontier regions.

Technology applications have significant implications for family caregivers, particularly if they do not live with the older adult. Already, families use Skype, Facetime, and other technologies for social interactions that provide visual as well as auditory information about the care recipient, and some older adults enjoy ongoing contact with friends to play games or chat via the Internet. Interactive technologies may be valuable in reducing social isolation (Jordan et al., 2016).

Although research to date is limited and based primarily on small samples, technology offers promise as an additional tool to support aging-in-place and family caregiving. Abrahms (2012) reported that older adults are willing to give up some privacy for the opportunity to remain in their homes with technology supports, including ongoing video connectivity with their adult children. A YouTube video illustrates one way that families across generations can support older adults aging-in-place apart from their children (LeadingAge, 2006). This video is over 10 years old with some technologies that are now commonplace, yet their application within the context of health care and family caregiving is still a work in progress. The overall message represents a reality that may be possible in the not too distant future.

Physical, social, and economic challenges exist to integrating technology as a support mechanism for community-living older adults. Early older adult adopters tend to be well educated and financially well off with resources to purchase and use smart devices and bandwidth (Smith, 2014). Most present-day devices are not user-friendly for people with physical or disease conditions that impair vision or fine motor dexterity. Older adults with limited Internet or smartphone experience need help envisioning how technologies might have a positive impact on their

health or lives. Also, older adults identify a need for assistance in learning to use new technologies, yet few technology-savvy care providers are available to support learning by older adults. However, globally, research is strong in technology as a way to improve quality of life and support care for the expanding population of older adults (Centre for Policy on Ageing, 2014). Nurses will need to understand how to use burgeoning technologies, the features that make equipment user-friendly for older adults, how to support older adults and their families in using technologies and interpreting transmitted data, and how to sustain inter-disciplinary teams while coordinating technology-based and face-to-face care for the ongoing goal of maximizing provider-patient/family caregiving relationships for the older adult's quality of life.

Grass Roots Models of Age-Friendly Community Initiatives

Increasingly, older adults are creating new geographical models to facilitate aging-in place. Families may partner with the older adult in learning about and participating in these approaches to community-based care. The Village model exists primarily in the United States although communities exist in Australia and there is global interest in the concept (Scharlach, Graham, & Lehning, 2012; Village to Village Network, n.d.). Two other models are Naturally Occurring Retirement Community Supportive Service (NORC) Programs and the Robert Wood Johnson Foundation's Community Partnerships for Older Adults (CPFOA) program (Greenfield, Oberlink, Scharlach, Neal, & Stafford, 2015). In these models, geographic neighborhoods create a formalized structure with participation by older adult members, volunteers, and paid staff that organize and provide a range of services to meet the specific needs of older adults desiring to safely and successfully age-in-place in their homes and community (Greenfield et al., 2015). Social, instrumental, health, and personal services may be provided, and meaningful member engagement in the community is encouraged as one way to prevent social isolation. Although these models are fairly new and research is just being published about the nature of the communities, targeted older adults, service impacts, and sustainability, nurses are participating in these models as care and case providers. Variations on these programs exist globally, and some have formal partnerships with governmental agencies (Greenfield et al., 2015). The concept will evolve in coming years (Lehning, Scharlach, & Davitt, 2015), and nurses have a responsibility to advocate for models that embrace health promotion through palliative care services by engaging with older adults and their families.

Residential Care Settings

Residential care options include assisted living, board and care homes, continuing care retirement communities, and home care services. In both the United States and Canada, states or provinces regulate these settings, although nursing homes are also federally regulated in the United States.

Financing for these services is primarily the individual's responsibility in the United States and Canada, although some European countries provide these services as part of universal health or social insurance coverage (AARP, 2006). In the United States, Medicare provides limited coverage for short-term rehabilitation in a nursing home, and private health insurance may provide no coverage. Although LTC insurance has been available for several decades in the United States, these policies are expensive, often provide limited coverage, and are owned by fewer than 10% of older adults (Andrews, 2010). Continuing care retirement communities include elements of both independent living and supportive care provided through home care, assisted living, and/or skilled nursing services.

Typically specified in regulations governing residential care are eligibility criteria for admission or discharge, minimal educational requirements for the staff, staff-client ratios, and care service requirements. General descriptions of residential LTC options are presented as follows. Families continue to be integrally involved in all these care settings, and nurses play a vital role in assessing residents, managing and coordinating care with an interprofessional team, ensuring that the facility complies with regulations, ensuring ongoing quality improvement, and advocating for older adults and their families. This section focuses on two aspects of LTC: assisted living and nursing homes. Throughout this discussion, we examine the changing role of LTC nurses and their partnerships with LTC residents, their family members, and other LTC providers.

Assisted Living

Assisted living was developed in part as a response to the institutional environment of nursing homes, which was considered unresponsive to the quality-of-life needs of residents. In contrast, assisted living is often described as providing a social model of care that serves as an extension of "home." Assisted living is generally viewed positively by consumers as a more home-like option to nursing homes, and viewed positively by funders because costs are significantly lower compared with that of nursing home care (Grabowski, Stevenson, & Cornell, 2012). Currently, the number of assisted living and similar communities exceeds the number of nursing homes, although the nursing home population remains higher (Harris-Kojetin et al., 2016). However, there is wide variation by region of the country.

With this growth has come increasing divergence in the definitions of assisted living and the services associated with it. Some states emphasize private units and others do not. Types of services vary widely from simple medication reminders to a full range of ADLs and dementia care services. Commonly included services are the presence of staff 24 hours/day, availability of modified special diets, assistance with personal care, housekeeping and laundry, transportation, and medication management and health monitoring (Mitty et al., 2010; Oregon Department of Human Services, 2011). Depending on the organization, additional services may be available for additional fees. Each state has its own definitions and regulations that influence how assisted living is implemented. Financing varies greatly, although most AL residents pay privately for their care. In recent years, numerous states have obtained a Home and Community Based Care Services Medicaid Waiver to support low-income clients in using assisted living, adult care homes, and other community-based care services (Centers for Medicare and Medicaid Services, 2014). The waiver stipulates that assisted living must demonstrate person-centeredness in care, provide access to the greater community, and additionally provide for privacy, independence, respect, autonomy, and freedom from coercion for residents.

Although staff is available 24 hours per day, a licensed nurse typically is not on duty at all times. Unlicensed staff can perform most care activities, including those that might be considered nursing care, such as medication administration. Similarly, training requirements for resident assistants are less standardized or rigorous as compared with nursing assistants in nursing homes.

Many people who move into assisted living apartments expect to remain there for the rest of their lives. Because of the gap between needs and services that exist in many facilities, however, individuals may be asked to move to a nursing home or perhaps a foster care placement. Some facilities have strict admission criteria that residents must meet to remain in the assisted living community and discharge criteria that will require relocation. For example, in a review of research on assisted living, Stone and Reinhard (2007) found that a sizable number (75% in one study) of facilities would not keep residents who required nursing home level care for more than 2 weeks. In contrast, they described another study that suggested that as residents become increasingly frail and dependent, assisted living can and does become a substitute for nursing home care, providing additional services as the need arises. These different findings demonstrate the difficulties of providing care in the least restrictive environment whenever possible, while at the same time ensuring that residents receive the care they need to avoid jeopardizing their health and experiencing unnecessary transitions. When working with older adults and their families, it is critical that they understand the characteristics of assisted living related to admission and discharge criteria, staffing mix including RN presence, and available services so they can make informed decisions. See Davis*Plus* for a list of Web sites that provide resources for evaluating assisted living facilities.

Roles and Responsibilities of Assisted Living Nursing:

The role of the nurse in LTC residential settings is evolving and expanding. It is as variable as are the models of assisted living, in part because residents are generally less disabled and the availability of nursing services is lower than in nursing homes. Some assisted living communities include full-time or part-time registered nurses as part of their staff, some do not employ nurses, and still others contract with nurses to provide assessment of residents' health and self-care needs and other services (Madden, Waldo, & Cleeter, 2014).

As a general matter, important roles and responsibilities of nurses in assisted living include assessment of resident needs including whether prospective residents meet admission and/or discharge criteria, communication with residents and families to help them understand what services and care are available, and participation in developing plans of care including needed medical services. Nurses may also provide staff education. Some states permit nurses to delegate nursing tasks such as insulin administration to staff. In these situations the nurse must understand and follow the state (or province) delegation rules. These generally include initial and ongoing assessment of the resident, the task, and the staff. If nurses function in a consultation role, they are not direct supervisors of staff and need to consider different strategies to encourage staff to adopt their recommendations for care. Additional nursing activities include monitoring residents for changes in condition, communicating with other providers regarding resident status, maintaining ongoing communication with nurses from home health or hospice agencies who visit specific residents, teaching unlicensed staff what to expect in caring for residents, implementing evidence-based care practices, practicing ongoing quality improvement, and ensuring advocacy, monitoring, and support for residents and families by establishing long-term, trusting relationships. The complexity of residents in assisted living has markedly increased since the concept was introduced in Oregon in the 1980s. State and national surveys between 2010 and 2014 reported that 52% of residents were over age 85 (Carder, Kohon, Limburg, Zimam, Rushkin, & Neal, 2016), almost 40% had a dementia diagnosis, 23% had been diagnosed with depression, and almost 17% had diabetes. Individual requirements for assistance with multiple ADLs, polypharmacy, and comorbidities were common (Carder et al., 2016; Harris-Kojetin et al., 2016). These resident characteristics contribute to increased demand for nurses with excellent assessment, prioritizing, communication, and leadership skills who are comfortable and competent to practice independently.

Nursing Homes

Although a very small proportion of older adults live in nursing homes, the likelihood of spending some time in a skilled nursing facility has increased. This is because shortened hospital stays have resulted in nursing homes increasingly being the location for rehabilitation and recovery from surgery and acute illness. The number of older adults who permanently reside in nursing homes has declined as more residential care alternatives have become available (Stone, 2006). Yet, with the rapidly expanding population of people age 80 and older, 13% over age 85 lived in a nursing home in 2010. Costs of care are high, $6235 per month for a semi-private room on average in 2010 (Administration on Aging, 2017), and are the responsibility of residents unless they qualify for Medicaid. Moving to a nursing home represents considerable losses for an older adult, including loss of health, privacy, independence, choice, quality of life, and autonomy. Because of space limitations, they may not be able to bring many personal possessions with them.

Most older adults and their families consider nursing homes to be undesirable and the option of last resort, largely because nursing homes have a poor image and a reputation for providing poor quality of care. The Nursing Home Reform Act of 1987 (Department of Health and Human Services, n.d.) attempted to address shortcomings by changing practice and systems of care. Practice changes included reducing restraint use (both physical and chemical or medications used to manage behavior symptoms), addressing psychosocial and physical care, and developing a national data system known as the Minimum Data Set (MDS) (Sloane & Zimmermann, 2005). Although there have always been nursing homes where excellent, nurturing care is provided, and although extensive federal and state regulations have attempted to address shortcomings, the prevailing public view and experience of nursing homes for many older adults, their families, and nurses has remained negative.

The Pioneer Network (1997) was established by a group of LTC innovators who initiated the culture change movement. It is focused on person-directed care, a way of thinking about care that honors and values the person receiving care, with an emphasis on both quality of care and quality of life so that the individual is not lost in the process of providing care. Research suggests that nursing home culture is changing, even though improvements are still needed (Doll, Higgins, McBride, & Poey, 2017; Miller et al., 2010; Rahman & Schnelle, 2008). More research is needed regarding how best to assess resident preferences and outcomes over time, particularly for people with dementia, and how caregivers perceive, value, and enact person-centered care (Kolanowski, Van Haitsma, Penrod, Hill, & Yevchak, A., 2015; Reamy, Kim, Zarit, & Whitlatch, 2013).

Roles and Responsibilities of Nursing Home Nurses: Nurses historically have played major roles in nursing home care, but similar to their counterparts in assisted living, their role is evolving and expanding in these settings. Care is increasingly complex and residents in skilled and rehabilitation units resemble hospitalized patients of the not too distant past. As in assisted living, nursing home nurses must be able to work independently, assume leadership roles, and possess strong assessment and prioritizing skills. They must be able to work effectively and collaboratively on interdisciplinary teams consisting of direct care workers, administrators, other staff who support residents (e.g., social services, rehabilitation, dietary), and other providers who may not be on staff but are critical to the well-being of residents, such as hospice teams, physicians, pharmacists, options counselors, and other home- and community-based care providers.

Best practices in caring for older adults are constantly evolving. Nurses need to stay current in areas such as falls prevention, pressure ulcer prevention and treatment, pain assessment and management, dementia care, use of restraints (physical, pharmaceutical, or electronic), and mental health care. Further, nurses must know how to implement best care practices with staff that have limited formal education in caring for older adults. The most skilled nurses are needed for these settings.

Many nurses are participating in efforts to promote culture change care in residential care settings. Person-directed care is consistent with nursing values, in that nursing strives to individualize care and put the individual and his or her family ahead of the task (Koren, 2010, Robinson & Rosher, 2006; Talerico, O'Brien, & Swafford, 2003). Common elements include personhood, knowing the person and his or her family, autonomy/choice, including family members in decision making, comfort, and valuing relationships (White, Newton-Curtis, & Lyons, 2008). Regulations from the Centers for Medicare and Medicaid Services support culturally and family-directed care practices. The Pioneer Network and leaders in gerontological and LTC nursing developed "Nurse Competencies for Nursing Home Culture Change" (Pioneer Network & Hartford Institute for Geriatric Nursing, 2010). These and other resources are available on the Pioneer Network Web site: https://www.pioneernetwork.net.

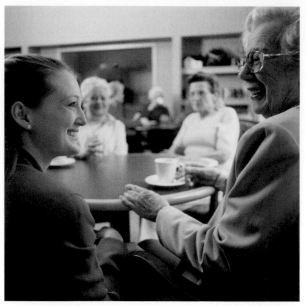

© Ryan McVay/Digital Vision/Thinkstock

Family Involvement in Residential Care Settings: Contrary to prevailing myths, families typically do not abandon their older members once they move into facility-based care, nor do they cease providing care, although the nature of that care is different (Keefe & Fancey, 2000). Decades of research in nursing homes reveals that family members continue to visit and provide emotional support, as well as some types of informal care, after transition into a nursing facility. Families typically desire to work in partnership with facility staff to provide support (Bauer & Nay, 2011; Pillemer et al., 2003). Nurses and other staff members can inadvertently set up barriers that decrease the ability of family members to participate in the life of the resident, such as by limiting visiting hours, limiting family knowledge or involvement in care, or discounting or discouraging family input into care decisions. Developing a successful relationship actually begins before a resident is admitted, when a family member makes an initial visit to the facility. In addition to evaluating the physical environment, families begin to consider the quality of care provided, and whether they can trust the staff to become partners in caring for their family member (Legault & Ducharme, 2009). During the pretransition phase, nurses are in a unique position to provide guidance and resources on types of residential care options and how to evaluate prospective facilities. Two resources for families are the Medicare Web site, Nursing Home Compare, which uses a five-star

system to rate facilities on specific quality indicators, and the Centers for Medicare and Medicaid guide, *Your Guide to Choosing a Nursing Home or Other Long Term Care Services.* Additionally, state and province offices that regulate regional nursing homes can provide recent survey information on quality of care. In the United States, each state also has an ombudsman service that can provide information on complaints that have been received about specific facilities. Nurses and other staff, therefore, can assist to strengthen the staff-family partnership through communication, making family members feel comfortable and welcomed, and providing assurance that the staff is competent and providing good care.

Family members want staff to gain knowledge about the resident, often striving to be role models in demonstrating how to give care to the individual (Duncan & Morgan, 1994). Partnerships between families and staff help staff members to know residents in meaningful ways. Families are key resources with respect to individuals' history, likes and dislikes, personality, routines, and what is and has been important to them (Austin et al., 2009; Boise & White, 2004; Iwasiw, Goldenberg, Bol, & MacMaster, 2003; Legault & Ducharme, 2009; Logue, 2003; Reuss, Dupuis, & Whitfield, 2005). This knowledge is critical, particularly when residents have dementia and cannot clearly communicate this information themselves. Family members can provide insight into resident actions, which in turn can help the staff respond more quickly to resident needs as conveyed through their behavior.

Families provide considerable psychological support to residents through their visits. Families are key members of the resident's social network, contributing to identity, dignity, and quality of life (Boise & White, 2004; Iwasiw et al., 2003). Another important role of family members is in monitoring the quality of care and advocating for the resident if needed (Friedemann, Montgomery, Maiberger, & Smith, 1997). In addition, family members continue to provide hands-on care, including helping a family member eat, attending activities, and handling personal care. Families help residents to maintain connections with the larger community by taking them to public events such as concerts, parks, shopping, and to family gatherings.

Palliative Care and End-of-Life Care in Residential Care Settings

Across developed nations, anticipated deaths are increasingly happening outside of the hospital. In the United States in 2009, 28% of Medicare recipient deaths occurred in nursing homes although in Minnesota and Rhode Island the rates approached 40% (Teno et al., 2013). Among residents in assisted living, approximately 30% die in the assisted living setting (Overview, 2009), although in Oregon the death rate ranged from 45% to 51% depending on the type of assisted living facility (Carder et al., 2016). These rates in these settings are expected to increase because of the aging population (Davidson, 2011; Kelly, Thrane, Virani, Malloy, & Ferrell, 2011). End-of-life care in these settings has its own challenges, in part because of limited staffing and staff knowledge. Additionally, nursing homes emphasize resident rehabilitation and assisted living emphasizes independence and autonomy, goals that aren't congruent with care at the end of life (Cartwright, Miller, & Volpin, 2009).

As noted in Chapter 10, palliative care and end-of-life or hospice care are often considered synonymous. To clarify for the discussion here, the focus of palliative care is to improve the quality of life for persons with chronic, life-limiting illnesses through careful identification and management of symptoms. These symptoms may include pain, shortness of breath, fatigue, constipation, nausea, loss of appetite, problems with sleep, and side effects of medical treatments (National Institute of Nursing Research, 2011). Palliative care may continue for years; ideally, it begins when the chronic condition is first identified. The focus of end-of-life care, on the other hand, is the immediate time around death.

Most long-stay nursing home residents have multiple chronic illnesses and are ideal candidates for palliative care. Yet palliative care is underutilized in LTC settings for several reasons. Even among providers there is confusion about the meaning of palliative care, and health care team members may not initiate discussion about services until the person is close to the end of life. Lack of education of staff, high turnover, and low reimbursement rates act as barriers to palliative and hospice care services in these settings, as does the dual and seemingly conflicted mission of nursing homes as organizations that provide rehabilitation and short-term care for persons recovering from acute illness with the goal of returning home as well as care for people at the end of their lives (Davidson, 2011; Kelly et al., 2011). Another challenge is the high proportion of nursing home residents who have dementia, which is often not recognized as a terminal condition by families or staff, including physicians. Dementia also has a less predictable trajectory or pattern of transition to end of life compared with other chronic conditions, making it more difficult to identify when changes are likely to happen and when additional resources such as hospice may be appropriate.

An important part of palliative care is working with older adults and their families to prepare advance directives, such as a durable power of attorney for health care or a living will. The process of preparing these documents provides an opportunity to discuss and understand values and preferences to guide decisions when the older adult is not able to directly communicate. Advance directives provide guidance regarding what treatments the individual wants as well as does not want. Besides advance care planning, in the United States there is a trend to endorse use of Physicians Orders for Life-Sustaining Treatments (POLST) or Medical Orders for Life-Sustaining Treatments (MOLST) with adults who are seriously ill or for whom death would not be unexpected. The POLST converts patient wishes to actual medical orders that facilitate these wishes. Physicians and/or nurse practitioners complete the POLST after reviewing and discussing the advance care plan with the patient and/or his or her surrogate decision maker. The POLST is a legally binding medical order that applies across medical settings to guide care by emergency responders, in emergency departments, and other settings including assisted living and nursing homes. Although over 43 states have some form of the POLST, regulations vary by state (Kim, Ersek, Bradway, & Hickman, 2015).

In Canada the term *palliative hospice care* refers to services that "aim to relieve suffering and improve the quality of living and dying" (Canadian Hospice Palliative Care Association, 2013). The services are targeted to individuals and families, and use a broadly holistic perspective in assessing and managing the spiritual, psychological, social, physical, disease-related, and practical dimensions of illness that may be life-threatening. Services are provided by an interdisciplinary team across a range of settings, with home-based and acute care settings being most common. Palliative hospice care may be provided concurrently with disease-modifying treatments (Canadian Hospice Palliative Care Association, 2013, p. 7). The nature and structure of palliative hospice care services vary across the provinces although there is a movement to create a national model of care for these services (Williams et al., 2010).

Nurses participate in palliative hospice care through direct patient and family care in home-based, acute, or LTC settings and by educating families on advance care planning, including the importance of family communication regarding individual wishes for a "good death." Nurses also participate in demonstration models of palliative hospice care, particularly in rural areas that lack adequate services; lead quality improvement initiatives to foster best palliative hospice care practices; and advocate for public policies that support practice standards and funding requirements to support palliative hospice care.

Although often associated with a location or service, hospice is, most importantly, a philosophy of care provided at the end of life. In the United States, most hospice care is provided at home, although assisted living and nursing home residents qualify as "home" for hospice as a Medicare benefit. Cartwright et al. (2009) found that quality end-of-life care was greatly influenced by the assisted living staff's commitment to the resident dying in the assisted living home and by the collaboration of multiple care providers, including assisted living nurses, direct care workers, family members, and the hospice team. Hospice also provides continued support to family members after the death. The culture change initiative in nursing homes has the potential to facilitate provision of palliative and end-of-life care through person-centered care by understanding behavior as a way of communicating needs, individually tailoring comfort care, and honoring values and preferences of older adults and their families (Long, 2009).

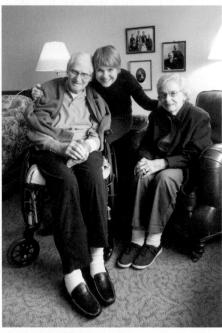

© iStock.com/iofoto

Case Study: Hooper Family

Using the life course perspective illustrated by Maria Hooper and her family (Figure 15-1 depicts the Hooper family genogram), we explore transitions that families experience because of declining health and increasing dependency common in old age. From a wider perspective, we take in the intersection of older families with the health care system.

Maria, age 60, is the oldest of four siblings. She has two brothers, James and Paul, and a sister, Ruth. Maria always counts Jane as her sister, too. Jane is a year younger than Maria and is the daughter of one of her mother's closest friends. When Jane needed a home as a young teenager, Maria's parents, Sarah and Louis, took her in, and Jane lived with them for 5 years. She and Maria became especially close, and now Jane and her family participate in all Maria's and her extended family's gatherings.

Sarah, age 82, and Louis, age 84, have lived in their community since their marriage 60 years earlier. They enjoy good health, except for Sarah's arthritis and mild hearing loss, and Louis's diabetes and hypertension, which are well controlled. They experience no limitations in ADLs, although both complain that it takes them longer to get things done. Still, they both volunteer for several different organizations and spend time with their friends. Maria lives 40 miles away from her parents, closer than the rest of her siblings. Maria and her parents talk on the phone about twice a week and they get together for dinner every couple of weeks.

Maria was divorced when her children, Jason and Kyra, were in elementary school. She still maintains connections with her ex-mother-in-law, Carol, who is now 87 years old. Carol has been widowed for 40 years. When Maria and her husband were divorced, Carol was determined that she would not lose contact with her grandchildren, as she had seen that happen with some of her friends. Maria had always been on good terms with Carol and felt it important that her children know their paternal

Case Study: Hooper Family *(cont.)*

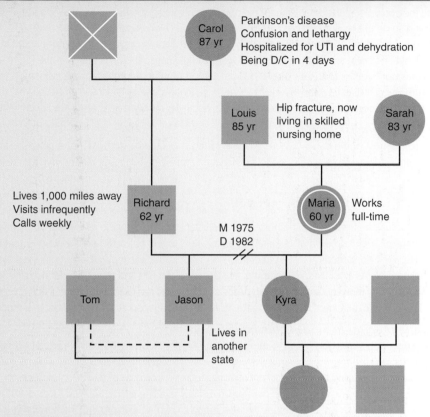

Carol
87 yr

Parkinson's disease
Confusion and lethargy
Hospitalized for UTI and dehydration
Being D/C in 4 days

Louis
85 yr

Hip fracture, now
living in skilled
nursing home

Sarah
83 yr

Lives 1,000 miles away
Visits infrequently
Calls weekly

Richard
62 yr

M 1975
D 1982

Maria
60 yr

Works
full-time

Tom

Jason

Lives in
another
state

Kyra

FIGURE 15-1 Hooper Family Genogram

grandmother, so both Maria and Carol made the effort to maintain contact. Carol lived about an hour away, but Maria and her children would spend at least one Saturday a month with her until the children entered into high school and were involved with multiple activities. Their visits became more sporadic, but Carol would come and watch her grandchildren's games and music concerts whenever she could.

When Carol was diagnosed with Parkinson's disease about 10 years ago, Maria became part of a community support system. Her role was to visit monthly, purchase groceries, and do some housekeeping. In addition to Parkinson's disease, Carol began to have problems with her memory and could no longer live alone. With some reluctance, she moved into an assisted living residence in her community. Maria has continued to visit her nearly every month. Carol usually knows Maria, but sometimes forgets she is divorced from her son. They mostly reminisce about the grandchildren.

Maria's life is quite busy. She is the office manager of a small business; in addition to her parents and mother-in-law, Maria is also involved in her children's lives. Jason and his partner live several hundred miles away, but Maria talks with him every couple of weeks. Maria often spends her vacations with them. Kyra is married and has two children of her own. Because Kyra lives close, Maria frequently babysits and delights in having each child spend the night about once a month. Maria enjoys being a grandparent, yet feels badly for her sister, Ruth, who has had sole responsibility for raising her own grandchildren for the past 2 years.

Discussion:

Maria's family is reflective of many older families. At 60 years, Maria is part of the postwar baby boom, and similar to many in her generation, she has several siblings who represent potential support systems for both Maria and her parents. This includes Jane, who is fictive kin and has a close and family-like relationship with Maria and her parents. Typical for most families, Maria lives relatively close to her parents and is in regular contact with them. Generally, they have a good relationship, characterized by affection, a history of mutual exchanges of help, and many shared values. Maria and her children are especially close to

(continued)

Case Study: Hooper Family *(cont.)*

her parents because they provided considerable support as Maria was going through her divorce. Support included temporary housing, child care, and some financial assistance. Now, Sarah and Louis (Maria's parents) are close to becoming the "old-old" generation, that is, those older than 85 years. Although they are independent, engaged in their community, and consider themselves in good health, both have several chronic illnesses that could cause them problems in the future. Maria's former mother-in-law, Carol, has not been as fortunate. She was widowed "off-time" in her forties and has lived alone since her son grew up and left home. Her activities have been limited for many years because of Parkinson's disease and, more recently, cognitive impairment. She has resided for several years in an assisted living facility that accepts Medicaid clients.

Transition 1—Louis Home to Hospital:

Sarah (now age 83) spent most of the day at a friend's house. When she returned home about 4 p.m., she found her husband, Louis (age 85), on the floor in the garage. He told her that he tripped on the stairs while carrying a chair that needed repair; this occurred about 9:30 a.m. He tried to get up or crawl up the three steps from the attached garage to the kitchen, but he could not move because the pain was too great. Sarah called 911, and Louis was taken to the emergency department. Fortunately, it was a relatively uncomplicated fracture of his hip. He was able to have a surgical repair the next morning. Because he experienced some confusion after surgery, the nurses were reluctant to give him pain medication, believing the medication would cause more confusion. He started physical therapy the day after surgery but could participate only to a limited extent because of the pain. He was also started on insulin to control his diabetes (he previously took an oral medication).

Louis's needs are common. As an older adult, Louis was at a greater risk for falls and related injuries even though he did not have other risk factors. Hospital care by those unfamiliar with the needs of older adults can exacerbate rather than prevent negative outcomes. For example, knowing that untreated pain can increase confusion and delay successful rehabilitation is important for nurses.

Transition 2—Louis Hospital to Skilled Nursing Facility:

After 4 days in the hospital, Louis was discharged to the skilled care unit of a nursing home for additional rehabilitation, with the goal of returning to his own home. The timing of the discharge came as a surprise to Sarah and Maria, giving them little time to visit and select a skilled nursing facility or for other siblings to arrive from out of town to provide support. Fortunately, Sarah and Louis had friends who had had a good experience in a skilled nursing facility that was located about 30 minutes away. It had space available; Maria stopped by to look at it and thought it would work. At the skilled nursing facility, Louis's pain was finally controlled and he was eager to begin physical and occupational therapy so that he could go home. Although attention was focused on Louis, it was important to pay attention to his caregivers and conduct an assessment to determine their strengths and needs. Sarah needed support to bring Louis home as quickly and successfully as possible. See Figure 15-2, the Hooper family ecomap. One spouse's response to stress affects the way the other spouse experiences stress. During this transitional period, it was important to be cognizant of the stress levels and needs of both Sarah and Louis. For example, nurses and others helped them consider changing their home environment to prevent future falls and provided instruction in managing Louis's pain while his hip healed. Louis's diabetes needed to be monitored and assessed to determine whether he would continue to need insulin injections or be able to return to managing the disease through oral medications.

Without including Sarah in the transition planning, Louis was likely to spend a longer time in the skilled nursing facility or return home without sufficient support. Without support, Sarah was likely to experience greater levels of stress and caregiver burden in her expanded role as caregiver. Because of her hearing loss, Sarah did not always understand what the physician, nurses, and other staff told her. Maria noticed that providers tended to treat her mother as if she had dementia and often did not include her in conversations. Therefore, Maria felt the need to be present as much as possible. Caregiver assessment also needed to include Maria because her caregiving responsibilities had also increased. She missed a lot of work, was worried about losing her job, and could not afford to take more time off. Fortunately, nurses at the skilled nursing facility were aware of these constraints and were able to arrange a care conference with Louis, Sarah, and Maria after regular business hours to begin planning for Louis's discharge to home. Maria and her parents were aware that Medicare was funding rehabilitation services, but were surprised to learn that these benefits would run out sooner if Louis did not keep progressing toward independence.

Transition 3—Louis Skilled Nursing Facility to Home:

Once again, discharge came quickly with little time to locate a home health care agency. The skilled nursing facility discharge coordinator provided a list of agencies and Maria selected one. The therapists at the skilled nursing facility gave Sarah and Maria a list of adaptive devices (e.g., raised toilet seat, grabber, elastic shoestrings, a device to help Louis put on his socks,

Case Study: Hooper Family *(cont.)*

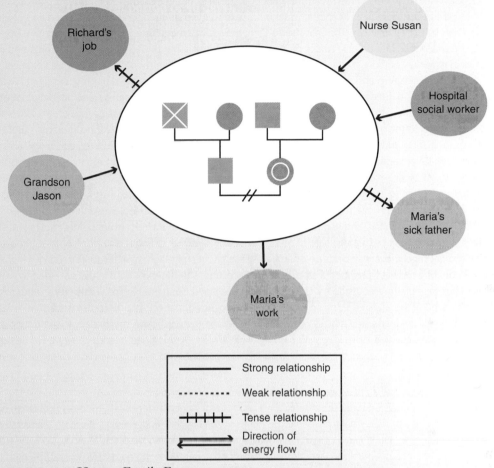

Strong relationship
Weak relationship
Tense relationship
Direction of energy flow

FIGURE 15-2 Hooper Family Ecomap

walker) to purchase before Louis's discharge. Because Louis still qualified for Medicare services, he was able to see a physical therapist, an occupational therapist, and a nurse once a week at home. These three providers collaborated to complete a home safety assessment to identify potential risks and strategies to eliminate or reduce the risks. A home health care worker also came to the house to assist with Louis's shower twice a week.

The social worker at the nursing facility had suggested that the family contact the ADRC in the community. An options counselor from the ADRC met with the family in the nursing facility and again once Louis was home. She was able to provide information about services beyond those provided by the home health agency. Once Medicare benefits ran out, she provided them information about home care workers. Sarah and Louis hired a worker to continue to help him with showers and to do a little light housekeeping, which they paid for out-of-pocket. The options counselor also identified an organization that put a grab bar in the shower and, if needed in the future, could build a ramp into the house. Because Sarah was exhausted, the options counselor helped arrange for home-delivered meals. With time, Louis recovered; although he used a cane, he resumed most of his community activities. His diabetes was once again managed through diet and oral medications and Sarah soon decided that they no longer needed the home care worker and meals. They kept the phone number of the options counselor on their refrigerator in case they needed assistance in the future.

Transition 4—Carol Apartment to Assisted Living:

Recall that Carol, Maria's former mother-in-law, had been living in an assisted living community for several years. She moved there because her worsening Parkinson's disease made it impossible to remain at home in her apartment. In the community,

(continued)

Case Study: Hooper Family *(cont.)*

Carol's main support system came from friends and neighbors, with Maria and her children helping when they could. Richard, Carol's son and Maria's ex-husband, lived in another state but would visit two or three times a year to fix things around the apartment and to handle Carol's finances. The year before Carol moved into the assisted living community, she began losing weight because she was not able to prepare meals. In response, Maria and some of Carol's friends often prepared meals and froze these meals in individual portions. Maria also did grocery shopping during her monthly visits. A local volunteer organization provided some house cleaning, and friends from Carol's church would take her to lunch or bring her dinner at least once a week. At Maria's urging, Richard arranged for meals-on-wheels from a local community center. Carol often did not eat the food from this service, however (her reasons included "It's not like my own cooking," and "It all tastes the same"). Several times, when the volunteer delivered the meal, she found Carol on the floor because she had fallen. Concern about Carol's safety prompted Richard, her friends, and Maria to convince her to move to the assisted living community, which was also closer to Maria's home. Although Carol had limited income from Social Security, the assisted living community accepted residents receiving housing subsidies as a Medicaid benefit.

Carol was initially reluctant to move to the assisted living community. She was not familiar with assisted living and thought her family wanted her to move to a nursing home, which she strongly opposed. She changed her mind after visiting a few assisted living communities and learned that she could still have her own apartment. After moving in, she discovered she enjoyed the opportunities to participate in many of the activities. Her strength also improved; at her apartment, it had been difficult to get regular exercise because of limited space and a short flight of stairs to get outside. At the assisted living community, the long hallways provided a safe walking space, and with the elevator she did not need to worry about stairs. Therefore, she was able to go outside more often. Carol developed close friendships with several other residents during the time she lived at the assisted living community. She recognized that she had become somewhat isolated in her apartment because of her increasing difficulty with mobility. As she received three meals daily in the dining room, her weight improved. She also received assistance with bathing twice a week. Bathing had been a challenge in her apartment because she had only a tub and shower combination, and the owner would not allow her to have safety bars installed in the bathroom.

Transition 5—Carol Assisted Living to Hospital:

After living successfully in the assisted living community for 3 years, Carol gradually developed memory problems; her physician was not sure whether it was Alzheimer's disease or dementia secondary to the Parkinson's disease. The assisted living staff frequently had to go find her at mealtimes. Similar to many older adults, Carol took several medications, both prescription and over-the-counter drugs. She had been able to take them safely and accurately once the med-aide had set them up for her in a pill box, but now when Maria visited, she found Carol had not taken about half of the doses. When cleaning her apartment, the staff also noted clothes soiled with urine in her bathroom. One morning, when she did not come to breakfast, the resident assistant found her still in bed. She was very difficult to wake up, she had been incontinent, and she could not stand even with the help of the resident assistant. When the assisted living nurse came on duty, she assessed Carol and suspected she had an infection. She contacted Richard, who lived several hundred miles away. He called Maria, who arranged to take time off work and took Carol to see her physician. The physician determined that Carol was dehydrated and had a urinary tract infection (UTI). He had her admitted to the hospital for treatment.

Incontinence is not "normal" for older adults; development of incontinence may indicate a change in health status. For example, it may be a sign of a UTI. Other changes in urinary elimination, such as burning or frequency, may also be signals that further evaluation is warranted. Because of her memory problems, Carol may not have remembered to mention these symptoms to Maria or the assisted living staff. If identified early, the UTI could probably have been successfully treated with oral antibiotics, thereby avoiding hospitalization.

Unlike nursing homes, assisted living communities do not have nurses available 24 hours per day; other staff members may have limited training and experience working with older adults (unlike nursing homes, training requirements for direct care workers are limited). Nurses can provide staff training focusing on normal aging- and health-related changes. Staff should also understand the importance of reporting changes in the resident's usual condition, such as a change in continence, to the nurse, who will then follow up with additional assessments and evaluations. For example, although Carol had memory problems, she was usually awake and alert, so the resident assistant finding her difficult to awaken represented a significant change.

Case Study: Hooper Family *(cont.)*

Transition 6—Carol Hospitalization:

Carol was admitted to a general medical-surgical unit of a community hospital later that afternoon. The hospital recently implemented a NICHE model. The nurses implemented use of SPICES and FAMILY as frameworks for assessing both the older adult and her family. Susan Jones, the admitting nurse, obtained the information from Maria and also from the assisted living nurse because Carol was still quite lethargic when she first arrived at the hospital:

- *Sleep disorders*: No problems.
- *Poor nutrition*: Carol had a history of problems, but over the past year her weight had been stable and within the ideal range for her height.
- *Incontinence*: As noted earlier, this was a recent development. The bathroom in Carol's apartment had safety bars and was arranged in a manner that made it easily accessible for persons with mobility problems.
- *Confusion*: The admitting nurse recognized that Carol was experiencing the "hypoactive" form of delirium as demonstrated by lethargy (it was difficult for the resident assistant to get her to wake up) and was at risk for it worsening.
- *Evidence of falling*: Carol had a history of falls but none in the past year. She had not sustained any serious injuries from falling.
- *Skin breakdown*: No problems.

The nurse continued to collect information using the FAMILY acronym:

- *Family involvement*: Carol had regular contact with Maria, who provided assistance with a variety of needs. Carol also considered her close friends at the assisted living community to be part of her family. Her son Richard called about once a week but visited infrequently. Susan learned that Maria was also involved with her own parent care activities and that her father Louis was recovering from his hip fracture. Maria had used most of her vacation days providing parent care and cannot afford to take many days without pay.
- *Assistance needed*: Because of her current mental status changes, Carol needed extensive assistance with eating and drinking, changing position, hygiene, and other activities. Because Carol had missed some doses of her anti-Parkinson's medication, her mobility was not as good as usual, and she had lost some function even from this relatively short illness. She may require more assistance than her family or the assisted living staff can provide.
- *Members' needs* (what family members need from staff to be able to continue to provide care): Maria needed to be updated regularly about Carol's condition so she could keep other family members informed (particularly Carol's son, Richard). She also needed to know whether Carol would be able to return to the assisted living community, and if not what options were available. At the same time, Maria expressed some resentment to Susan about Richard's apparent lack of willingness to step up and take more responsibility for the care of his mother. She reported feeling pulled by the needs of her parents, Carol, her grandchildren, and her sister, who was raising her grandchildren.
- *Integration into care plan* (inclusion of family in planning and teaching activities): Susan gave Maria a business card for the unit social worker; she also shared Maria's contact information with the social worker. The team made plans to meet the following day to evaluate Carol's situation. She will probably be in the hospital for 2 to 4 days; therefore, it was important to start planning for discharge as soon as possible.
- *Links to community support*: Before the team meeting, Susan followed up with the assisted living nurse to learn what care could be provided after discharge. One option could be for Carol to return to the assisted living community and receive home health care from an outside agency for additional support and follow-up.
- *Your intervention*: On admission, Susan completed the Confusion Assessment Method (Waszynski, 2007). She knew that Carol had a diagnosis of dementia. Carol was too lethargic to participate in any structured assessments of ADL or IADL function. Susan will reassess her in the morning. By then, Carol should have improved hydration and will have received a few doses of the antibiotic to treat the UTI and may be alert enough for further assessment. This will be important information to gather before the team meeting.

Transition 7—Carol Hospital to Nursing Home:

Carol's condition did improve by the next day, but she was not able to return to the assisted living community because she needed more assistance than could be provided in that setting. She was transferred to the rehabilitation unit of a nearby

(continued)

Case Study: Hooper Family *(cont.)*

nursing home with the long-term goal to return to the assisted living community. She received physical therapy twice daily. Another important aspect of her care was to get her reestablished on her medication regimen to manage the symptoms of her Parkinson's disease to improve her mobility. The nursing staff also used scheduled voiding to help Carol regain continence.

Although Carol experienced some improvements, it was clear that she would not return to the assisted living community. Richard reviewed Medicare's Nursing Home Compare Web site. Maria recommended he call an options counselor and was directed to a Web site about choosing a nursing home (e.g., https://www.nia.nih.gov/health/publication/nursing-homes, https://www.medicare .gov/Pubs/pdf/02174-Nursing-Home-Other-Long-Term-Services.pdf, http://www.aarp.org/home-family/caregiving/info-05-2012/ caregiving-resource-center-asking-right-questions.html). Finally, they found a guide to help them select a nursing home that was committed to culture change and person-centered care. At his children's insistence, Richard made several visits; after discussion with the administrator and staff, he selected a facility he thought would best meet his mother's needs. Because of her frailty and dementia, he opted not to move her closer to him. Maria and her daughter planned to continue visits, but this became unmanageable when Maria's father broke his hip.

Case Study: Brown Family

Helen Brown and her family illustrate the family lives of people who have never married and/or have no children in their social networks. Family lives of these individuals are often rich, but many experience challenges in old age, particularly with declining health and abilities, that those with children and spouses may not encounter. The life course perspective also informs our understanding of Helen and her family's resources, although we will focus mostly on the intersection with social services, LTC financing, and community-based care.

Discussion:

Helen just celebrated her 90th birthday. She enjoyed the gathering of friends and family and felt quite special. Helen never married; instead, she cared for her disabled mother when she was young and middle-aged. Her father died when she was 6 and her brother was 3. Her mother supported the family as a seamstress. Later, Helen supported her mother and herself as a school teacher, with her brother occasionally helping out. Helen retired shortly before her 65th birthday but continued teaching piano lessons well into her eighties. Her mother died shortly after Helen's retirement, after a brief illness. Helen then became involved in many volunteer activities, which she found fulfilling. Although she has "retired" from most of her volunteer activities, Helen still enjoys being out of doors and always has had a garden full of vegetables and flowers. She has many close friends and feels very much a part of the community through her long involvement as a teacher and community member. She never regretted not getting married; although she wondered how it would have been to have children of her own, she found satisfaction with her students and nieces and nephews. All in all, Helen feels she has had a full and rich life.

It is only in the past year that Helen has begun to feel somewhat vulnerable. She lives in the two-story home that she shared with her mother. Most of the neighbors she was close to have moved away, although she has made efforts to meet some of the new ones as they move in. She describes herself as in good health, but has had increasing difficulties with balance. This began after a bout with the flu 3 months ago. With great reluctance, she started using a walker when she leaves her home, which she tries to do every day when the weather is good. She also has much less energy than she used to have and finds housework and meal preparation daunting. She is no longer able to go up or down stairs without a lot of effort. Still, she is adamant about remaining in her own home and is determined to get her strength back. She has a modest income, mostly Social Security and a very small pension, totaling about $2200 per month. She had trouble paying her heating bills last winter. She frets over her garden. When she got sick, she began paying one of her youngest great-nieces to help keep it weeded, but her niece will be moving away to attend college soon.

Helen has two relatives of her generation who live nearby and have been central to her social network (Figure 15-3, the Brown family genogram). Both have her very worried. Her younger brother Roy, 87, is widowed and is dealing with prostate cancer, now at stage three. His children are attentive, but are debating among themselves about his living situation. Two of his children feel he needs 24-hour care in a nursing home, and the other two feel that he needs to be in familiar surroundings

Case Study: Brown Family *(cont.)*

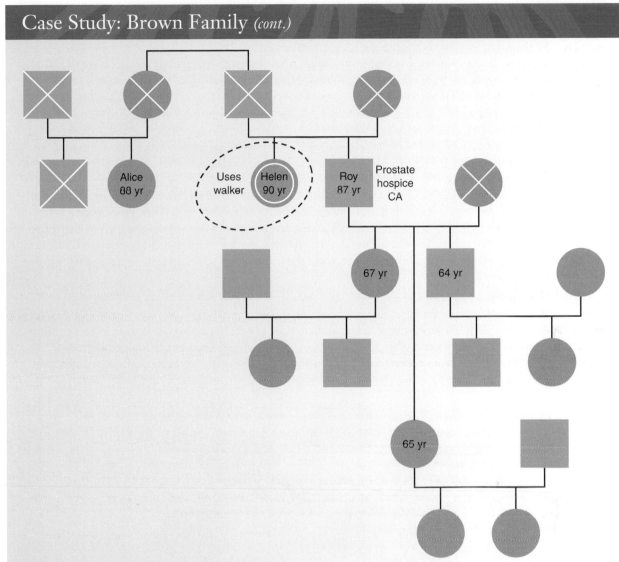

FIGURE 15-3 Brown Family Genogram

without a lot of strangers around. His physician has suggested that they consider hospice care. His children are all over 60 and only two live close by.

　　Mostly, Helen is fearful for her cousin and best friend, Alice, who is 88. Similar to Helen, Alice did not have children of her own. She did marry, however, and her husband, Charles, had several siblings. Charles and Alice doted on their many nieces and nephews and their home was often a fun-filled destination for these children, and later for their children. Alice's husband was a successful businessman and Alice had a lot of money after he died. She was glad to help out her nieces and nephews as they went through school, got married, and had children of their own. As Alice's health began to decline, Beth, one of her nieces, offered to move in to help her out. It seemed to be a good idea, but now Helen hardly talks to or sees Alice. When she does, Alice's manner has changed: She is no longer upbeat, she is not keeping herself carefully groomed, and she seems quite distracted. She has also lost weight. One of Alice's nephews told Helen that many of the family photos have been removed from Alice's walls. Helen noticed that Beth is driving a new car, has very fashionable clothes, and recently went to Europe with her boyfriend and her daughter. Helen hates to think that Beth is stealing from Alice, but she can't come up with an alternative explanation. Because Roy is so sick, she is not sure who she should talk to.

(continued)

Case Study: Brown Family *(cont.)*

Transition 1—Independence to Supportive Services:

As she has begun to "slow down," as she puts it, Helen is increasingly worried about her ability to maintain her independence (Figure 15-4, the Brown family ecomap). She tried to save money for "a rainy day" because she has no children to provide support, but knows her funds are limited. Through friends and the local senior center, she made a connection with an options counselor to help Helen make a plan for herself. The options counselor learned that staying at home and in her neighborhood is very important to Helen. Helen has important strengths that make this possible. She is capable of making decisions for herself and she is successfully managing her health. Importantly, she is determined to get better and stay well and is doing the things that will make that possible. She is engaged in her community and has good relationships with others, and at least one great-niece is likely to provide short-term assistance should she need it.

The options counselor helps Helen to come up with strategies that will keep her active. This includes taking advantage of a low-cost transportation service to visit the senior center where she can continue volunteer activities and participate in an exercise group. The van also stops at the grocery store twice a week. She also learned that she can afford to use the services of a small nonprofit gardening organization that teaches children to garden. The staff of this agency will work with children in Helen's garden in exchange for sharing in Helen's harvest. Finally, she learned about an energy assistance program that will reduce her monthly payments.

Transition 2—Transition to Hospice:

Health care providers have an important role in communicating with and supporting families as the end of life approaches (see Chapter 10). In this case study, health care providers will have to be sensitive in working with Roy's children. Although hospice care is provided in residential care settings, nursing homes, and at home, Roy needs to be involved as much as possible regarding the location of services. Health care providers can help families explore pros and cons, alleviate fears and

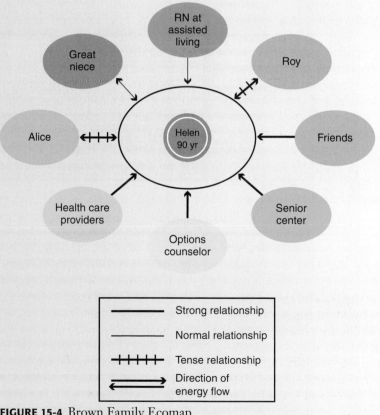

FIGURE 15-4 Brown Family Ecomap

Case Study: Brown Family *(cont.)*

uncertainties, and help to identify services that will support the family, as well as Roy. By including Roy in discussions with his children, hospice workers helped Roy's children come to agreement that hospice care at home was a feasible and desirable option for Roy. They helped establish a schedule and a list of tasks so that each child and grandchild could be present in a way that was comfortable for them and for Roy. They were able to supplement with paid caregivers to assist family members who were not comfortable being alone with Roy in case he needed help they did not feel comfortable providing. One of his children made sure that Helen was able to visit with Roy during the last days of his life. Roy's symptoms were well managed and he died peacefully at home.

Transition 3—Transition to Assisted Living:

At her most recent visit to her nurse practitioner, Helen began to describe her worries about her cousin. The nurse practitioner listened carefully and took down Alice's name, address, and contact information. After Helen left, the nurse practitioner contacted Adult Protective Services and reported this potential abuse. The agency followed up with Alice and did find evidence of neglect and financial exploitation, and worked with the family to recover some of Alice's funds and to get appropriate help into her home. (Helen could also have alerted her options counselor to the possibility of abuse and the options counselor would have made the referral to protective services.) Because of their investigation into Alice's situation, the protective service worker suggested that Alice be evaluated for dementia; older single women with dementia and living alone are at high risk for financial exploitation.

The situation with Beth caused considerable tension and conflict within the family. Beth denied that she had taken funds inappropriately and insisted that Alice, as she had in years past, insisted on giving Beth money. Beth felt she earned those funds because of the increasing difficulty in taking care of Alice as her health and cognitive status declined. Some were supportive of Beth, but other family members blamed Beth for isolating Alice from other family members, keeping her deteriorating cognitive status from other family members, and taking advantage of her previous generosity. Not all family members agreed with the dementia diagnosis.

As the extent of Alice's condition became clear to the extended family, the only area of agreement was that Alice could not remain at home without assistance. As a consequence, Alice was moved into an assisted living residence with a memory care unit. Although Alice did not yet need to live on the memory care unit, no one in her family felt comfortable with any other alternative. Living with another family member was not an option because no one wanted to worry that decisions they made would be second guessed or criticized by other family members. Because Alice still had financial resources, her family felt confident that she had the resources needed to stay in the assisted living community for the rest of her life, and that she could pay out of pocket for additional charges should they arise. Once her nieces and nephews agreed that an assisted living placement was appropriate, they consulted an elder law attorney who helped to manage Alice's assets for her care.

Alice was not happy with the decision and had a difficult adjustment period. Helen visited regularly at first, but she found that Alice was becoming more confused and kept asking to leave and return to her home. Over time, Helen's visits became less frequent because transportation was difficult to arrange and Helen felt distressed by these visits. Helen continued to call Alice at least weekly and often sent notes and cards.

SUMMARY

As stated throughout this chapter, older adults and their family members can be quite complex. They vary in structure, size, and a lifetime of experiences and relationships. All will influence how individuals and their families navigate late life, especially caregiving. This chapter has described the aging population in the United States and Canada, and provided an overview of family ties of older adults.

- Using the life course perspective, we discussed the diversity of family structure in later life and how it has been influenced by societal trends, such as increasing life expectancy, increasing divorce rates, changing fertility patterns, greater ethnic diversity, and changes in economic status and work patterns.
- Most older adults are embedded in social networks in which kin are important sources of emotional and instrumental support.

Given the diversity of family life, many configurations of "family" exist. In most families, individuals enjoy strong and affectionate relationships and can count on family members to provide care and support when needed. Nonetheless, it is also common for families to have both positive and negative feelings toward one another because they are providing support. In some families, negative feelings may predominate, which will have consequences for health, well-being, and availability of support.

■ Older adults, especially those of advanced years, have unique health care needs that must be addressed whether in clinics, at home, in hospitals, or through a variety of LTC services.

■ Nursing and other professionals in gerontology have developed evidence-based assessment tools and interventions that are the basis for optimal care. Nurses must be familiar with these tools and apply them routinely and appropriately.

■ Health care providers must also recognize that older adults, including many care recipients, are also providers of care to their spouses, children, grandchildren, or friends. In fact, family members deliver the majority of care.

■ As the population ages, it is increasingly important that nurses develop expertise in geriatric care, regardless of setting. Nurses with strong leadership skills are needed, especially in community-based care and NH settings.

■ In all settings, nurses must partner with older adults and their family members in designing and providing care that addresses unique needs and supports relationships.

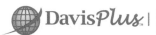 **DavisPlus** | For additional resources and information, visit **http://davisplus.fadavis.com**. References and Suggested Web sites can be found on Davis*Plus*.

Chapter 16

Family Mental Health Nursing

Laura S. Rodgers, PhD, PMHNP-BC

Critical Concepts

- All parts of the family system are interconnected; therefore, all members are affected when a member has a mental health condition.

- The family of a person with a mental health condition needs to be involved in treatment because it enhances the effectiveness of the health care treatment.

- Comorbidities are frequently present when someone has a mental health condition (e.g., depression often coexists with eating disorders or anxiety disorders; substance abuse and alcohol and substance use disorders commonly occur with mood disorders). Therefore, mental health conditions typically require integrated and complex treatment.

- Psychoeducation and participating in formal and/or informal support groups are effective interventions for family members who have a member with a mental health condition.

- People with mental disorders, as well as their families, are stigmatized in many world cultures, including North American societies.

- Nurses must examine their personal attitudes and prejudices toward persons and families who have a member with a mental health condition and seek additional education and training to challenge the negative stigmas so they can then serve as effective advocates for these families in both community and acute care settings.

- Nurses must use nonjudgmental and nonblaming communication interactions with families who have a member with a mental health condition in order to establish a therapeutic professional relationship with the family.

Previously, *mental health* was defined as a state of well-being such that an individual is able to perform mental functions that allow her or him to adapt to change and cope with adversity in order to function well in society while being mostly satisfied with life in general (American Nurses Association [ANA], American Psychiatric Nurses Association [APNA], and International Society of Psychiatric-Mental Health Nurses [ISPN], 2007). More recently, *mental health* has been redefined as "emotional and psychological wellness; the capacity to interact with others, deal with ordinary stress, and perceive one's surroundings

realistically" (ANA, APNA, & ISPN, 2014, p. 89). A person who can cope with the normal stress of family, work, and friends; can work productively; realizes her or his own potential; and is able to make a contribution to the community (World Health Organization [WHO], 2016a) would represent someone in a state of psychological, emotional, and social well-being.

By contrast, a disturbance in thoughts or mood caused by a mental disorder or mental illness can lead to maladaptive behavior, inability to cope with normal stresses of life, and interference with daily functioning (ANA, APNA, & ISPN, 2007). More specifically, *mental* disorders are defined as "any condition of the brain that adversely affects a person's cognition, emotions, or behavior" (APA, APNA, & ISPN, 2014, p. 89). The diagnoses of mental disorders are based on diagnostic criteria from either the American Psychiatric Association's (APA's) (2013) *Diagnostic and Statistical Manual of Mental Disorders, Fifth Edition (DSM-5)* or the *International Classification of Diseases–10 (ICD-10)*, which is endorsed by the WHO (2010). New editions are released only after much discussion and typically with many years between editions. For example, there were 13 years between the fourth and fifth edition of the *DSM*, and the *ICD-11* is scheduled to be released in 2018. Each set of criteria describes mental disorders as conditions characterized by alterations in a person's thinking, mood, or behavior that (1) cause an individual distress, (2) impair his or her occupational or social functioning, and/or (3) place the individual at significant risk for experiencing death, pain, disability, or a loss of freedom.

Rather than describe an individual who has been diagnosed with a mental disorder as "mentally ill," the term used throughout this chapter will be "an individual with a mental or behavioral health condition," or a person with a mental health condition (MHC). Although mental disorders have discrete diagnostic criteria, there are some mental disorders that consume a larger burden of care in the community and often have the most negative and intrusive effects on an individual's life and on family members' lives. Individuals with these disorders will be noted as persons with a serious mental illness (SMI). The Substance Abuse and Mental Health Services Administration (SAMHSA, 2016) has defined persons with SMIs as individuals 18 or older who currently or at any time in the past year have had a diagnosable mental, behavioral, or emotional disorder (excluding developmental and substance use disorders) that causes serious functional impairment and has substantially interfered with one or more major life activities. Examples of SMI include schizophrenia, major depression, bipolar disorder (BD), and other mental disorders that cause serious impairment. On the other hand, examples of disorders that typically do not cause significant social, emotional, or behavioral disability include generalized anxiety disorder, adjustment disorder, and dysthymia.

This chapter covers mental health family nursing. The chapter begins with a brief demographic overview of the pervasiveness of MHCs in both Canada and the United States. The remainder of the chapter focuses on the impact a specific mental health condition can have on the individual with the MHC, individual family members, and the family as a unit. Although the chapter does not go into specific diagnostic criteria for various conditions, it does offer nursing interventions to assist families. Note that the impact and treatment of substance use disorder is discussed within the Johnson family case study.

MENTAL HEALTH CONDITIONS IN THE UNITED STATES AND CANADA

The global burden of mental health conditions is so serious that the WHO Executive Board (2012) called for a comprehensive and coordinated response to the challenge. In Canada, 20% of adults (those 18 and older) will personally experience an MHC (Canadian Mental Health Association [CMHA], 2016). Mental illness affects all Canadians either directly or indirectly, as those who do not personally have an MHC will be affected through a family member, friend, or colleague (CMHA, 2016).

Similarly, 18% to 19% of adults in the United States have an MHC, with almost 50% of adults developing at least one MHC during their lifetime (National Institute of Mental Health [NIMH], 2014a). This section addresses the prevalence of MHCs in the United States and Canada, comorbidities associated with MHCs, general approaches being taken toward those with MHCs, and the stigma associated with having an MHC.

Prevalence of Mental Health Conditions

Mental disorders are the leading cause of disability in both Canada and the United States (Institute for Health Metrics and Evaluation, 2015; WHO, 2014) and of all diseases, with the exception of heart disease, account for the most years lived with a disability (NIMH, 2014a). In the United States, adult outpatient mental health services are paid for by private health insurance (37.9%), self-payment, or payment by a family member living in the household (33.7%), Medicare (15.2%), Medicaid (11.9%), or an employer (11.9%) (SAMHSA, 2012a).

Only about half of the 43.6 million adults in the United States with MHCs received mental health services in 2014 (NIMH, 2014b). Financial costs are one of the barriers to many people who need care, as well as lack of transportation to services and availability of services in the area consumers live.

In 2014 in the United States, the percentage of persons 18 or older who had any diagnosable mental, behavioral, or emotional disorder (excluding developmental and substance use disorders) of sufficient duration to meet *DSM-V* diagnostic criteria within the past year was 18.8% of the total population, and 15.6% among Hispanics, 13.1% among Asians, 6.3% among African Americans, 19.2% among whites, 7.1% among persons reporting two or more races, 27.1% among Native Hawaiians or other Pacific Islanders, and 1.2% among American Indians or Alaska Natives (NIMH, 2014b). Although MHCs are pervasive across the general population in Canada and the United States, some groups experience a greater impact of poor mental health. In Canada, families in the lowest income group are three to four times more likely to report poor mental health than those in the highest income group (Statistics Canada, 2013). Likewise in the United States, the number of persons with an MHC is highest among low-income families (SAMHSA, 2012a).

Mental Health and Comorbidities

It is common for someone with an MHC to have another condition, either mental or physical; the coexistence of multiple conditions is termed *comorbidity*. For example, depression often coexists with eating disorders such as anorexia nervosa and bulimia nervosa, or anxiety disorders, such as post-traumatic stress disorder (PTSD), obsessive-compulsive disorder, panic disorder, social phobia, and generalized anxiety disorder (Schwartz, 2011).

Likewise, the coexistence of substance use disorders and mood disorders has been documented among the U.S. population (Conway, Compton, Stinson, & Grant, 2006). The word *addiction* is no longer used because it also carries a stigma: It promotes marking people who use substances to relieve the symptoms of their mental disorders as bad or of weak character. The APA advocates using the term *substance use disorder* to emphasize that excessive use of alcohol or other substances is a disorder in itself and is often the result of using substances to cope with the symptoms of mental disorders

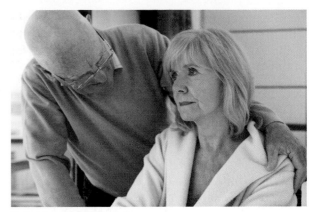
© iStock.com/Dean Mitchell

(APA, 2013). Women are more prone than men to have a coexisting anxiety disorder at the same time as depression, and men are more likely than women to exhibit alcohol and substance abuse or dependence when depression is diagnosed. In general, people with mood or anxiety disorders are twice as likely as the general population to suffer from a drug use disorder. The use of alcohol or other substances of abuse by people with mental disorders is in many cases an attempt to self-medicate the distressing symptoms of mental illness (National Institute on Drug Abuse, 2010). The term *dual diagnosis* rather than *comorbidity* is used to describe a person with both a substance use disorder and another mental disorder, so it is common in substance use disorder treatment. Given the prevalence of comorbidities, it is important that nurses take a holistic view of the person with an MHC and approach interventions from multiple perspectives, rather than simply focusing on a single MHC.

Serious general medical illnesses may accompany, and even be exacerbated by, a mental health condition. For example, heart disease, stroke, cancer, human immunodeficiency virus/acquired immune deficiency syndrome (HIV/AIDS), diabetes, Parkinson's disease, thyroid problems, and multiple sclerosis are some of the conditions that often coexist with depression. There is evidence that when depression accompanies a serious physical illness, both conditions tend to show more severe symptoms, medical costs increase, quality of life is decreased, mortality rate is increased, and people have more difficulty adapting to the physical condition compared with those with the MHC (Kang et al., 2015). Treating the depression along with the coexisting physical illness is imperative. In addition to treatment for the general medical condition, clients require individualized integrative and collaborative care that includes depression treatment. This comprehensive approach will improve the outcomes for both conditions (Kang et al., 2015).

Mental Health and General Approaches Toward Those With a Mental Health Condition

Recovery from a mental health disorder is the major goal for mental health care. SAMHSA (2012b) has established a set of principles for recovery and has defined recovery as "a process of change through which individuals improve their health and wellness, live a self-directed life, and strive to reach to their full potential" (p. 3). Health, home, purpose, and community have been identified as the four major areas that contribute to maintaining a life in recovery. The 10 guiding principles of the Recovery Model are as follows:

1. Hope
2. Person-driven
3. Many pathways (nonlinear)
4. Holistic
5. Peer support
6. Relational (interactions with others, both formally and informally)
7. Culture
8. Addresses trauma
9. Strengths/responsibilities
10. Respect

Unlike previous views of MHCs, especially in relation to the more severe conditions, that some MHCs are chronic and very difficult if not impossible to manage, part of the recovery model is the assertion that there are no limits to the potential for an individual to recover from any MHC (Till, 2007).

Another recovery model with a similar philosophy has been implemented in Canada. Called the Tidal Model, it also emphasizes a shift in how nurses think about the care provided to people with an MHC. Rather than focusing on disease and illness, this model stresses the importance of the individual with an MHC actively participating in decision making related to care and including family in the overall care (Caldwell, Sclafani, Swarbrick, & Piren, 2010). The Tidal Model was developed by nurses in collaboration with other mental health care providers and has transformed nursing practice in mental health care settings (Brookes, Murata, & Tansey, 2006, 2008).

At the center of both the Recovery Model and the Tidal Model is the philosophy that nurses recognize the uniqueness of each individual with an MHC and that nurses must collaborate not only with these affected individuals to provide person-centered care, but also with their families and the rest of the collaborative care team, including physicians, social workers, community services, and mental health care providers. There are improved outcomes when this collaboration takes place, such as reduced morbidity and mortality rates in persons with MHCs and improved preservation of the psychological and physical health of their family members (Goodrich, Kilbourne, Nord, & Bauer, 2013). In line with this philosophy, the President's New Freedom Commission on Mental Health (2003) final report (Box 16-1) recommended six national goals to move mental health care in the United States toward a recovery-oriented system, with the overall goal of improving mental health care for Americans.

BOX 16-1

Goals Identified by the President's New Freedom Commission on Mental Health

Goals identified by the President's New Freedom Commission on Mental Health in 2003 were as follows:

■ Americans understand that mental health is essential to overall health.
■ Mental health care is consumer and family driven.
■ Disparities in mental health services are eliminated.

■ Early mental health screening, assessment, and referral to services are common practice.
■ Excellent mental health care is delivered and research is accelerated.
■ Technology is used to access mental health care and information.

Source: President's New Freedom Commission on Mental Health. (2003). *Achieving the promise: Transforming mental health care in America.* Rockville, MD: U.S. Department of Health and Human Services. Retrieved from govinfo.library.unt.edu/mentalhealthcommission/reports/FinalReport/toc.html

Also in line with this philosophy, there has been an international trend to provide care to persons with an MHC in the community rather than in an institutional setting. Past practice had been to institutionalize persons with an MHC, often for a lengthy period of time; however, the recovery approaches shift both the focus and the locus of care provision. Large inpatient, mental health care institutions have been downsized or eliminated in most areas, but many governments have not provided funding for other resources to deliver the care that persons with an MHC might need. This change has resulted in the transfer of care from the institutional to the family level. The stress and burden of care experienced by these families has been well documented. Families often suffer financial and social deprivations when providing care to family members with an MHC. Family caregivers may become exhausted by a lack of respite from their affected family member who requires so much energy for care and supervision, and they often live in fear that the family member with an MHC will cause disruption to family life because of a recurrence or exacerbation of the MHC. Common needs for families living with a family member with an MHC are support including affordable respite care, information, skills training, advocacy, and referral courses (Vermeulen et al., 2015).

More than ever, families are an integral and instrumental resource for recovery for individuals with an MHC and especially those individuals with an SMI. One qualitative Canadian study examined the role of family in supporting recovery for people with an MHC who lived in structured, community housing (Piat, Sabetti, Fleury, Boyer, & Lesage, 2011). The researchers found that, even though the mental health consumers lived apart from their families and relied heavily on formal services, the residents identified their families—more than mental health professionals, friends, or residential caregivers—as those who most believe in them and in their recovery. These same mental health consumers stated that their recovery was supported by their families' affection, emotional support, and active involvement. Families offered more hope in recovery than health care providers. It is evident that nurses and other health care providers must engage the families of individuals with an MHC in their recovery.

Mental Health and Stigma

Stigma has been defined as labeling, stereotyping, separation, status loss, and discrimination. Western society singles out mental illness as undesirable and devalues the person who possesses an MHC (Burke, Mohn-Brown, & Eby, 2016). Society's stigma influences how individuals feel about themselves, which can lead to self-stigma and can both exacerbate mental health conditions and cause affected individuals to avoid treatment. Providers may even hesitate to include the diagnosis of MHCs in medical records, especially those of children, because of the stigma. The media are responsible for perpetuating misconceptions about persons with an MHC (Mental Health America, 2016b), often by sensationalizing crimes in which persons with an MHC are involved and using pejorative terms to describe the individual with the MHC.

Stigma affects both the individual with the MHC and the family members. As family members become responsible for providing more and more care to individuals with an MHC, they are reporting their perceptions of caregiving as stressful and stigmatizing (Dalky, 2012). For example, families may perceive that their family reputation has been disgraced because a member has a mental illness; they may be embarrassed at the behavioral outbursts sometimes associated with MHCs (Dalky, 2012). Stigma can cause individuals with an MHC and their families to become isolated and feel ashamed, or stigma can make individuals and family members engage in denial or a wish for things to appear normal, which may then discourage them from talking about their needs and seeking help (Abrams, 2009). Although family members living with a family member with MHC frequently experience rejection, shame, and avoidance by others, they also can develop effective coping strategies that evolve over time to counter society's stigma (Karnelli-Miller et al., 2013).

Stigma and discrimination toward persons with an MHC can prevent care and treatment from reaching people with mental illnesses. For example, stigma toward a parent who has an MHC, or who is providing care to a child with an MHC, may prevent the parent from obtaining community support because of her fear that others may assume she is not a fit parent; she may not access care because she fears losing custody of her child (Obadina, 2010). People with MHCs also may fear workplace reprisals if they seek mental health care through work-provided insurance.

In fact, the stigma can be quantified. Just more than 50% of Canadians say they would tell a friend or coworker that a family member has an MHC, compared with 72% who would discuss a cancer diagnosis or 68% who would discuss diabetes in the family (Canadian Medical Association, 2008). Only 12% of Canadians would hire a lawyer who has an MHC; just 49% would socialize with a friend who has an SMI; and many Canadians (46%) think that people use mental illness as an excuse for bad behavior (Canadian Medical Association, 2008). The proportion of Americans who believe SMI is associated with violent and dangerous behaviors doubled between 1950 and 1996 (Phelan, Link, Stueve, & Pescosolido, 2000), and in 2013 a national public opinion survey conducted after a nationally televised story about a multiple killing by a person with an SMI found that 46% of Americans believed that people with SMIs were far more dangerous than members of the general population (Mental Health America, 2016b). Unfortunately, nurses and health care providers are not immune to demonstrating stigma toward individuals with MHCs and their families. For example, nurses providing care to a mother parenting a child with attention deficit-hyperactivity disorder (ADHD) may blame poor parenting for the child's behavioral challenges.

But there is some cause to hope for decreasing stigma toward those with an MHC. For instance, in 2006, 67% of the public agreed that depression had a neurobiological cause compared with only 54% in 1996 (Pescosolido et al., 2010). Personal contact with someone with an MHC has been shown to decrease one's stigma toward persons with an MHC (Schafer, Wood, & Williams, 2010). In addition, peer-led interventions have been shown to be effective in reducing family self-stigma (Perlick et al., 2010). Education of health care providers about specific disorders and their treatments can also help reduce or prevent behaviors or discrimination caused by stigma. Increased understanding about the symptoms and behaviors arising from an MHC allows health care providers to provide optimal care. For instance, instead of blaming poor parenting, nurses working with a mother whose child has ADHD can focus on identifying those behaviors that are ADHD-related and work with the mother to develop targeted interventions that compensate for the executive function deficits and emotional dysregulation issues associated with this condition.

Nurses can help decrease stigma in several ways. Words matter. The words used by the general public to refer to people with mental disorders include: *crazy, nuts, mad, loony, one-fry-short-of-a-happy-meal, weirdo,*

psycho, and *his elevator doesn't go all the way up*, to name a few. These expressions may resemble an attempt at humor to some people, yet they have disrespectful intent. When a person asks, "Am I crazy?" and the nurse answers, "No, you have a mental disorder called schizophrenia," a small step is taken toward treating mental disorders equal to general medical disorders. When nurses discourage others from demeaning people with mental disorders, just as one would discourage racist, sexist, or homophobic speech, another step is taken in the direction toward what the culture and society will not tolerate (Burke et al., 2016).

FAMILY MEMBERS OF INDIVIDUALS WITH A MENTAL HEALTH CONDITION

The whole family may be affected by and involved in care of the member who has an MHC, or individual relationships and responsibilities may be more pronounced. For example, a spouse may be providing care to his or her partner. Parents may be providing care to young or adult children. In some cases, the parent has the MHC and so a child takes care of the parent. Siblings may provide care for siblings, and so on. The "normal" relationships and dynamics within the family may be disrupted. Nurses need to pay attention to family dynamics and to the potential burdens faced by individual members and the family as a whole when a member has an MHC. This section focuses on the general burden of family caregiving, spousal caregiving, role changes within the family, children living with a parent or sibling who has an MHC, and parenting a child who has an MHC.

Burden of Family Caregiving

Family caregivers often take on their role because of a sense of responsibility, as well as a perceived lack of available resources or services. When a family member has an MHC, remaining members may feel marginalized and distanced from the care planning process. Common themes across international studies include family feelings of isolation, lack of information, lack of recognized role, and not feeling listened to or taken seriously by health care providers (Eassom, Giacco, Dirik, & Priebe, 2014). Families also commonly report a belief that health care providers use the need for confidentiality as a way to avoid sharing important information about the identified client's condition and treatment (Eassom et al., 2014). Financial stress related to insufficient resources, educational level, and the age of the caregiver also affects the caregiver's burden (Tan et al., 2012). Single, divorced, separated, or widowed caregivers have more depressive symptoms than married caregivers (Kamel, Bond, & Froelicher, 2012). Women are typically the providers of care, with estimates ranging from 56.6% to 69% of caregivers (Zauszniewski, Bekhet, & Suresky, 2008). Each year, 54 million Americans are affected by an SMI, and though the women who provide care to their family members with an SMI are resourceful, the overall burden causes many of these women to experience depression, poorer quality of life (Zausniewski et al., 2008), and lower levels of subjective well-being and physical health than men who are caregivers (Moller, Gudde, Folden, & Linaker, 2009; Pinquart & Sorensen, 2006). Regardless of the relationship of the caregiver to the person with the MHC, formal (professional therapy) and informal (social, including support groups) support has been shown to buffer the caregiver's symptoms of depression (Chen & Lukens, 2011).

A small qualitative Canadian study (Veltman, Cameron, & Stewart, 2002) confirmed the paradox that family caregivers report not only negative impacts of providing care to a relative with an MHC but also beneficial effects, such as feelings of gratification, love, and pride. Most respondents in the study believed that caregiving made them stronger, more patient, and more appreciative of time with their families, as well as less judgmental of others (Veltman et al., 2002). Family caregivers also report being more secure (Foster, 2010) and sensitive (Chen & Lukens, 2011), and having more hope (Tranvag & Kristoffersen, 2008). Many family caregivers gain a deep respect for their family member's struggle, as portrayed in this mother's comment about providing care to her son who has schizophrenia: "He's always on my mind, I'm always worried about him, it breaks my heart, I wish he had friends, I wish he had a job, but he tries the best he can, the best he knows how, struggling every day, I don't know how he does it, but I'm proud of each of his accomplishments, no matter how small" (Veltman et al., 2002, p. 112).

Caregivers express worries about the deterioration of their family member's general health over time as the care recipient ages (Corsentino, Molinari,

Gum, Roscoe, & Mills, 2008). Moreover, caregivers frequently mention that their own physical health as they age is a major issue for them. But what caregivers fear the most is what happens to the individual with an MHC if the caregiver is no longer able to provide care (Corsentino et al., 2008).

In their international quantitative study commonly known as C4C, Vermeulen and colleagues (2015) found that caregivers experience burdens in the following life domains: emotional (through the constant anxiety of caring), social (feeling isolated and lonely), physical (fear that the identified patient will relapse such that the caregiver's safety may be at risk and that the caregiving itself makes their own health worse), financial (worries about the financial situation of the person they care for), and finally the domain of relationship (fear that the person with the mental disorder will continue to be dependent on them in the future). Some of the caregivers studied felt that they are treated differently because of the mental illness of the person they care for, suggesting that stigma extends beyond the identified patient to family members. On the other hand, the researchers also found that caregivers stated they had become more understanding of others with problems and had discovered inner strength of their own. Finally, almost all the caregivers felt the need for additional support in their caregiving role. Some were able to use other family members for respite care, but only 6% to 8% had access to paid respite care.

Spousal Caregiving

Many family caregivers for those with MHCs are caring for a spouse or partner. Care is typically provided in the family home and the most common tasks performed on a daily basis are providing companionship, providing emotional support during a crisis, and monitoring symptoms. Other aspects of care include providing or monitoring medications, paying bills, advocating for the person to receive help, arranging and coordinating services and appointments, assisting with personal grooming, taking more responsibility for child care and household chores, and going to appointments with the person who has an MHC (American Psychological Association, 2017). These tasks and aspects of care are common to anyone who has an MHC, regardless of whether the person is the spouse, child, sibling, and so on.

Spousal care providers may feel angry about the changes that they see in their spouse because of the onset, exacerbations, and remissions of the

MHC (O'Connell, 2006). Spouses may find themselves blaming their spouse for having a character flaw rather than understanding the cause of and treatments for the MHC. Additional financial and parental responsibilities can also increase the stress and negatively affect the relationships between family members. Couples and family therapy and spousal support groups can help these families adapt to the demands of the MHC (O'Connell, 2006).

Family Role Changes

It is not unusual for family caregivers of persons with an MHC to change their relationships or roles within the family (Ali, Ahlstrom, Krevers, & Skarsater, 2012). For example, an adult younger brother may find it challenging to maintain his role as younger brother while also being caregiver and guardian to his older sister who has an SMI. On the other hand, Aldridge (2006) contended that children as caregivers to parents do not necessarily change their status. Rather, the child may take on some parenting roles—such as providing personal and emotional care to a parent, engaging in household chores, providing care to brothers and sisters, administering medication to parents, or providing crisis support to a parent during an acute psychotic episode or self-harming—but not others (Aldridge, 2006). Thus, parents may maintain their role as parents, though there might be some interdependence between the child and parents. Being a child (under the age of 18 years) in the caregiver role to a parent can have a positive effect on the child's development, including improved family relationships, but it can also negatively affect the child's development and overall childhood experience (Aldridge, 2006).

Role changes may not be welcomed by the family. For instance, some family caregivers describe feeling obliged to provide care to their relative with an MHC, whether the obligation is willingly accepted or suddenly pushed on them (Rowe, 2012). They may find themselves needing to learn about their legal and moral roles in the new caregiving situation. Family care providers often struggle with unexpected and unfamiliar expectations placed on them in their new roles. Legal and moral rights related to providing care to the family member with an MHC often cause conflict between the family caregiver and the health care providers. Frequently, health care providers neither appreciate nor understand the legal needs and moral rights of the family caregiver but, rather, focus on the legal and moral rights of the person with the MHC. For example, health care providers may pressure a parent to take his adult child home with him because they believe that the person with the MHC will benefit by being cared for at home. But the parent may not feel that he has the capacity to care for his daughter, or he may have made a decision not to attempt to provide care because of previous negative consequences to the family when the daughter has been at home. This difference in perspectives can cause barriers between health care providers and family caregivers (Rowe, 2012). It is important to note, however, that family caregivers and families in general want to be included and supported in the treatment and care decision making for their family member.

Children With a Family Member With a Mental Health Condition

When an adult with an MHC accesses care, it is imperative that nurses ascertain whether there are children in the family, because research has shown that children living with a family member with an MHC are at increased risk for developing psychopathology; developing emotional and behavioral problems (Korhonen, Pietila, & Vehvilainen-Julkunen, 2010; Mental Health America, 2016a), including anxiety or personality disorders (Mental Health America, 2016a); suffering abuse and neglect (Mahoney, 2010); and being involved in accidents (Obadina, 2010). Mental health care providers often overlook children who live with a family member with an MHC; they focus their attention solely on the individual who has the MHC. Unless a child shows signs of abuse or neglect, or is in the custody of child protective services, children tend to be invisible to the health care providers who are treating the child's parent (Gladstone, Boydell, & McKeever, 2006). Even though one in six Canadian children younger than 12 years of age live with a family member who has an MHC (Bassani, Padoin, Phillip, & Veldhuizen, 2009), nurses who provide care to adults with an MHC inconsistently ask if there are children in the family (Foster, O'Brien, & Korhonen, 2012). One recommendation to avert omission of this important information is to change the hospital assessment forms to include a section that asks about children living in the home. Regardless, nurses should make it standard practice to ask the question.

Not only should nurses determine if there is a child in the family of a person with an MHC, but nurses need to understand that children may perceive their own role in a negative way. Strained relationships between family members are not uncommon and can lead to a chaotic family life (Foster, 2010). Appropriate assessment and intervention are important to ameliorate any negative consequences for a child who is living with a person who has an MHC, regardless of whether that person is the child's parent or sibling or has another relationship with the child. At the same time, nurses should remember that, in spite of the associated risks, many of these children remain emotionally and mentally healthy.

Nurses need to be aware that children living with a family member with an MHC often believe they caused the MHC and may have feelings of guilt, anger, or anxiety (Mental Health America, 2016a; Obadina, 2010). In addition, the children may feel alone (Foster, 2010). Nurses must initiate a conversation with the child and not wait until a child asks for help. It is important for nurses to tell the child that she did not cause the parent's illness or strange behavior nor is she responsible for taking care of the family member; nurses should reinforce that there are health care professionals who will provide care to the family member (Obadina, 2010). Providing age-appropriate information about the parent's MHC and treatment decreases the child's feelings of guilt and also decreases the child's negative feelings toward the MHC (Obadina, 2010). Developing a relationship with the child ameliorates the feelings of being isolated and alone. If there are several children of different ages in the living situation, the nurse must remember to provide teaching and answers to each child, appropriate to the child's developmental and cognitive ability. Children who are knowledgeable about a parent's illness are able to understand the parent's behaviors better in relation to the specific illness (Mental Health America, 2016a). Children need to be provided thoughtful, developmentally appropriate information about their parent's illness and treatment. Children who are not given the whole story are left to make up their own explanations, which only adds to their emotional confusion and possible self-blame for parental symptoms. Support for family relationships and other networks must be part of the care that nurses provide to parents in any setting (Korhonen, Vehvilainen-Julkunen, & Pietila, 2008).

Although a primary role for a nurse who is providing care to an adult with an MHC is to identify the presence of children living in the family and to offer support and education to those children, the nurse also needs to perform a family-centered assessment of the children's needs (Korhonen et al., 2010), followed by referral to relevant services (Mahoney, 2010). Once needs are identified, nurses can develop a plan for assisting the child. For example, with parental consent and within the limits of confidentiality, nurses can contact a child's school to apprise teachers or administrators of the family situation affecting the child (Mahoney, 2010). Nurses can facilitate access to other professional services and family support, such as family and/or individual therapy. Therapy that teaches children and youth how to communicate easily and have fewer arguments with their parents may be beneficial as those factors have been shown to contribute to improved mental health among adolescents ages 11 to 15 years in a very large cross-national study involving 43 countries, including 26,078 young Canadians (Freeman, King, & Pickett, 2011). In addition, it is important to provide services that can enhance a child's coping skills, because children with effective coping skills are less likely to have behavioral or emotional problems (Gladstone et al., 2006).

Although the majority of professional services for family members with an MHC are in the community, there are times when a family member may be hospitalized. Nurses need to remember to ask the hospitalized family member if there are children. Children whose family members are hospitalized want and need information about the hospitalized family member (Foster et al., 2012) and appreciate having a nurse talk with them about visiting the psychiatric facility and having someone take a genuine interest in explaining what is happening to their family member (O'Brien, Anand, Brady, & Gillies, 2011). Nurses are encouraged to "view children as complex young persons who are competent to express their views and recount their experiences" (Gladstone et al., 2006, p. 2547), rather than as children who are too young to understand what is happening. Simple words and explanations can be used even with very young children and toddlers and may alleviate a lot of the child's anxiety.

Children Living With a Parent With a Mental Health Condition

In addition to the more general areas noted previously, nurses also must recognize that specific issues may arise when a child is living with a parent with an MHC. Children growing up with a parent with an MHC may express anger toward the parent with the MHC because their parent is not similar to other parents and they may experience extreme sadness when they remember a time that the parent was healthy (Mental Health America, 2016a; O'Connell, 2006). These children also frequently worry, often needlessly, that they will inherit and develop the MHC, but they will only share this concern with another person after the person has gained their trust (Foster, 2010). Circumstances such as maternal depression can have a negative impact on the child's normal development and on his likelihood of developing a mental health problem. Therefore, nurses need to pay particular attention to specific risks when the parent is the person with an MHC.

Risks to Normal Development

Several disorders, including depression, schizophrenia, and BD, not only affect an adult's ability to parent, but also can have an impact on a child's growth and development. It is estimated that about 14% of women of childbearing age have depression (Farr, Bitsko, Hayes, & Dietz, 2010). The impact of maternal depression on children from infancy to adolescence has been observed in clinic and community settings; maternal depression can have negative effects on a child (Bagner, Pettit, Lewinsohn, & Seeley, 2010). Problems with language development and intelligence, behavior, development of depressive symptoms, sleep patterns, physical health, parent/child relationship, and attachment have all been identified by researchers.

Parents with depression may communicate pessimism and sadness to their infants, as well as laugh less and demonstrate less affection, tenderness, and responsiveness. Decreased close and continuous contact with infants can have the most harmful effects on infants (Brockington et al., 2011). A child's mental health and social competence is predicted less by illness variables and categorical diagnosis than by multiple contextual risks (Brockington et al., 2011). The Australian Maternal Health Study found that psychoeducation for parents, when the mother had been diagnosed with depression, reduced depression relapse incidence in the mothers and reduced incidence of sleep disturbances in infants. The psychoeducation program included individual meetings with nurses about parental concerns, group meetings with other new parents, brief parenting education, information about normal infant sleeping and crying patterns, and

follow-up calls to the primary caregivers when the baby was 4 and 12 weeks old (Brown, Woolhouse, & Gartland, 2014).

Children benefit by consistency in parenting behavior. Similar to children of parents with depression, children of parents with BD are at increased risk for parenting disturbances related to the cyclical nature of the disorder. Inconsistent parenting behavior can be related to the parent's depression, manic/hypomanic or mixed state, chronicity of episodes, suicidality/suicide attempts, risky behavior associated with mania, problems with adherence to treatment, withdrawn/irritable behavior during a depressed mood, relapse in spite of treatment, and/or recovery time between episodes (Nadkarni & Fristad, 2012). Parenting difficulties in themselves can be challenging stressors for any parent, but parents who have BD may experience exacerbation of the bipolar symptoms with increases in stress (Calam, Jones, Sanders, Dempsey, & Sadhnani, 2012). Nurses can provide assistance to these parents by collaborating with the parent, child, family, and other health care providers to address the health needs determined by the family needs assessment.

Nurses, teachers, and family members may not recognize the concerns and issues that children who are living with a parent who has an MHC can face unless the child demonstrates a learning or behavior problem in school or a parent requests specific support for the child. Therefore, children of parents with an MHC should be routinely assessed for parent/child relational problems and possible developmental delays so that appropriate interventions can be implemented in a timely manner.

Risks of Developing a Mental Health Condition

It has been estimated that one in five children have a parent with an MHC and that they are more likely than their peers to develop a mental health problem (Mayberry, Goodyear, & Reupert, 2012). Children's development of depression may be influenced by genetic factors, environmental influences, marital or partner stress or violence, or even disruptions in parenting. Not only are children who live with a parent with an MHC at elevated risk for developing a mental health problem, including being developmentally delayed, but they are also at increased risk of being abused and neglected (Mahoney, 2010). Children of parents with an MHC should be routinely assessed for potential mental health concerns and, where warranted, appropriate interventions should be implemented. Accumulating evidence demonstrates the effect of early life stress and trauma on mental and general medical health throughout the life span. The evidence indicates that increased investment in the health of young children, especially those with known risks, is the most effective strategy for reducing inequalities in health outcomes and breaking intergenerational cycles of social adversity (Brown et al., 2014).

Other Risks

Disruption of relationships within the family and increases in risky behaviors can be an issue, particularly for youth. Adolescents often give up hope of being able to live in a family that does not have a parent with an MHC. They may struggle with the stigma associated with the MHC and may opt out of a relationship with the parent and instead use maladaptive coping mechanisms that can lead to risky behaviors or problems with the justice system. Nurses need to be cognizant of this possibility, make sure to assess teenagers for adaptive and maladaptive coping mechanisms, and then intervene as necessary.

Some children have parents with an MHC, such as schizophrenia, major depressive disorder (MDD), or BD, that is more likely than other MHCs to lead to hospitalization. These children often worry about what will happen to them if a parent is hospitalized. A foundational, small-scale Canadian study (Garley, Gallop, Johnston, & Pipitone, 1997) found that the children's biggest fear was parental separation because of a parent's illness. The children worry that they may be removed from their home and placed in foster care or another unknown living situation; they worry about what is happening to their parent who is hospitalized; and they become anxious when their daily rhythms are disrupted by their parent's hospitalization. The children become worried and stressed when no one tells them how their parent is doing—often leaving them to their own thoughts and feelings, wondering what is happening to their parent (Ostman, 2008). Nurses can alleviate some of the concern and uncertainty by assisting these families to develop a crisis intervention plan and inviting the entire family to participate (Reupert & Mayberry, 2007). This plan should include a contact person if the parent is ill or in the hospital, someone with whom each child might stay, and who should be told if the child is staying with another friend or family member (Reupert & Mayberry, 2007).

Nurses also must remember to dispel the myth that parents with an MHC are unfit parents. Rather, nurses must emphasize that a parent with an MHC can be a very competent, effective, nurturing, and loving parent. Children and parents will benefit from continuous assessment of the child's needs and ongoing professional support and treatment for the parents. There are many effective psychotherapeutic and psychological interventions available, including family therapies, mother and infant psychotherapies, and brief cognitive therapy appropriate to the age and stage of child development (Brockington et al., 2011). Nurses can provide support to parents who have an MHC by actively listening to the parents' concerns about parenting, providing realistic information about parenting skills, and assessing for the need for interventions to support the children (Mahoney, 2010).

Adult children who grew up living with a parent with an MHC may remember negative experiences caused by their parent's illness and the lack of information and support from mental health services. They may remember worrying about their parent's well-being, wondering if their parent was going to commit suicide, being fearful that the parent was not getting the care needed (Knutson-Medin, Edlund, & Ramklint, 2007), and being anxious about coming home from school because they did not know how their parent was going to respond to them (Foster, 2010). These adult children may remember having to approach either the parent without the health condition or a health care provider to get information about their parent's condition, rather than the health care provider offering them this information. Sadly, some may recall growing up not being able to distinguish between the parent and the MHC (Foster, 2010). Children are not in a place to seek information; rather, nurses must offer and provide this information to children so that they do not grow into adults with negative memories about their experience.

Children Living With a Sibling With a Mental Health Condition

Sibling relationships have a profound impact on the development of a child. The sibling relationship provides the connection for a child to learn how to interact with others, manage quarrels, handle rivalries, share secrets, and try on different roles (Abrams, 2009). Siblings share a common genetic and social background, early life experiences, and a family cultural background that can last a lifetime. Brothers and sisters also share unique private information about their parents and families

(Abrams, 2009). The common bond siblings experience can be a source of support and companionship for the sisters and brothers. But an MHC in one sibling can interfere negatively with sibling relationships. Some siblings experience guilt for not being the brother or sister with the MHC. Abrams described situations where brothers or sisters would tell friends they were an only child or would refuse to answer questions about the sibling with the MHC because of the shame or guilt they felt toward the sibling with the MHC. Unfortunately, these kinds of actions often lead to more silence and isolation for the unaffected sibling.

Sisters and brothers who have a sibling with an SMI, such as schizophrenia or BD, often struggle to understand what has happened to the affected sibling and the impact the condition has on their relationship with their affected sibling, as well as the entire family. For example, siblings who observe an affected sibling experience his first psychotic episode may feel haunted the rest of their life. Unfortunately, too often siblings of individuals with an SMI have their needs met by mental health care providers at only the lowest level (Ostman, Wallsten, & Kjellin, 2005). Yet, these siblings want more help; for example, they want health care providers to be available to answer their questions and to clarify their role in the future care of their sibling (Friedrich, Lively, & Rubenstein, 2008). When they get older, siblings may also have problems developing and keeping intimate relationships because they are fearful of passing on any genetic deficiencies to their own children (Abrams, 2009).

Sibling participation in a support group specifically for siblings who have a brother or sister with an MHC has been shown to decrease the siblings' feelings of being alone, and helps them gain information about their sibling's MHC and learn ways to support their affected sibling (Ewertzon, Cronqvist, Lutzen, & Andershed, 2012). One study suggested that the top-ranked coping strategies for supporting siblings of persons with schizophrenia are education about the illness, a supportive family, and having their sibling suffer less because the symptoms are controlled (Friedrich et al., 2008). Providing education to siblings can clarify misperceptions about the MHC and its treatment (O'Connell, 2006). Although it is important to address the needs of the brothers' and sisters' current experiences with their affected brother or sister, nurses must also be future-oriented and provide education and support

to these siblings in preparation for becoming future primary care providers to their sibling.

Nurses also need to be aware of other ways in which the dynamic in the family might be problematic when one sibling has an MHC and the other does not. For example, parents may focus their time and energy on the sibling with the MHC, leaving the unaffected sibling feeling neglected and resentful of the attention given to his sibling. It is important that the needs of healthy siblings are not ignored, no matter how unintentional the neglect by parents may be. Nurses can work with parents to help them shape how the unaffected sibling perceives the affected sibling and the MHC, as well as identify ways in which the parents can provide the needed attention to healthy siblings. Family assessment is critical, followed by appropriate psychoeducation, discussions about how parents might relate to the unaffected sibling, and referral to supports as needed.

Parenting Children With a Mental Health Condition

Parents provide care to children with an MHC on a regular basis in what can often be a long-term, ongoing activity; they frequently are the caregivers for their adult child with an MHC. Parents often experience grief, isolation, and stigma when their child has an MHC or blame themselves for their child's MHC. They may face health care providers who are suspicious of parental involvement and do not allow parent participation in the care of the child, especially when the child is hospitalized. In addition, grandparents are assuming a caregiving role for their adult children who have an MHC and also have children.

Grief and chronic sorrow are common experiences that parents encounter after being told their child has an MHC. Parent caregivers tend to experience more grief than sibling caregivers (Chen & Lukens, 2011) and this grief can affect the parent's psychological well-being, health status, and the parent-child relationship (Godress, Ozgul, Owen, & Foley-Evans, 2005). The grief can be prolonged as the parents may experience grief differently across the life course of their child's illness. Chronic sorrow, pervasive sadness that is permanent, periodic, and potentially progressive in nature (Olshansky, 1962), also enhances parental grief. Parents may experience grief for the loss of the child that they can no longer have or may even feel they have a different child from the one they started with (O'Connell, 2006); parents grieve for their future losses, for what their child may not be able to accomplish. Some parents may feel the need to provide regular care for their child well into adulthood and, thus, they grieve not seeing their children grow up into independent individuals. They also may grieve losses in their own lives, such as not becoming empty nesters.

Parents who have a more secure affection bond and a more positive relationship with their child may experience less grief than other parents (Godress et al., 2005). On the other hand, parents who have a more ambivalent and anxious relationship with their child may experience more grief and greater negative relationships with their affected child. In one small landmark study, parents of children diagnosed with either BD or schizophrenia reported experiencing chronic sorrow that was often triggered by their unending responsibilities to provide care to their child (Eakes, 1995). Nurses need to recognize and validate the grief and sorrow parents experience and provide interventions that decrease their emotional distress and life disruption (Godress et al., 2005).

Some parents of children with an MHC experience isolation and stigma from family, friends, teachers, and school administrators. Many parents are forced to leave work to meet with teachers or administrators, which may cause them to lose their jobs or change to a less demanding job, thus adding further to the financial strain they may already be experiencing (O'Connell, 2006). Many parents of adult children with an SMI experience significant frustration as they try to navigate a health care system that they perceive as full of obstacles (O'Connell, 2006).

Parents who have a child with BD, for instance, often blame themselves for their child's MHC (e.g., because of childhood adversity, bad parenting, or substance misuse; Crowe et al., 2011). Such parents may request family interventions including psychoeducation, communication enhancement, and problem-solving skills training to help the family understand and manage the disorder (Crowe et al., 2011; Nadkarni & Fristad, 2012). Nurses should offer such interventions even if a family does not request them.

Parents want to be involved at an early stage in the treatment of their child with an MHC and it is important to them that their opinions and experiences are heard (Nordby, Kjonsberg, & Hummelvoll, 2010). Yet, many health care providers are suspicious of parental involvement and do not allow parent participation in the care of the child (Jakobsen &

Severinsson, 2006). Although trust and honesty are critical elements in relations between health care providers and family, trust does not develop naturally (Piippo & Aaltonen, 2004). Collaboration between health care providers, parents, family members, and other disciplines enhances trust among everyone involved.

Many parents experience the hospitalization of their child with an MHC. Parents report that the admission process can be very difficult for them and that they often feel in crisis; they want nurses and other health care providers to understand these challenges. They typically need written and verbal information related to their child's care, such as an up-to-date handbook that tells them who to call for information about their child, what to expect during the hospitalization, hospital costs, what the child can or cannot do, what they should be doing about school, and a list of nearby inexpensive lodging during the hospitalization, as well as easy access to the child and better access to care before, during, and after hospitalization. Parents welcome practical tips and timely, accurate, situation-specific information that is communicated to them in a clear and honest manner. In addition, parents strongly suggest that they be recommended to a parent support group and also be given a list of parents who have undergone a similar experience and are willing to talk with them. Many parents experience guilt and shame related to their child's hospitalization and find it helpful when nurses talk to them about their guilt and shame in a nonjudgmental manner.

Some parents whose child has an SMI and never achieves independence may need to assume the responsibility of caring for their grandchildren (O'Connell, 2006). A small Canadian study (Seeman, 2009) described the role of the grandmother as one with divided loyalties: the toll of providing care to their grandchildren but also the rewards that come with raising their grandchildren. In the United States in 2008, 5.7 million children, 8% of all children, lived with a grandparent. Mental disorders in the parent of the child was one of the 11 reasons why the grandmother was raising the child (Davey, Kissil, & Lynch, 2016). Caring for grandchildren involves physical exertion and dedication over time. If the grandparent is also caring for her adult child with MHC, the physical and mental toll can be overwhelming. A particularly vulnerable time for the grandparent is when the grandchild approaches the age at which the child's mother or father began developing symptoms (Seeman, 2009). Nurses should be aware of such dates and offer support to grandparents rather than waiting for the grandparents to request help. Although grandparents often provide the daily care for their grandchildren, nurses must recognize that typically it is the child's parent who is recognized as the legal guardian. This situation can present problems for the grandparent and cause negative caregiving experiences (Seeman, 2009). The grandparents may view the parent's influence as not beneficial to the child's well-being and so they may feel tempted to minimize visitations, though many do try to sustain a relationship between the parent and child. Grandparent caretakers sometimes are put into adversarial conditions with the parent and may even have to sue for custody of the child (Seeman, 2009).

And finally, as children with a chronic MHC begin to transition from child/adolescent mental health care providers to adult mental health care providers, it is important to assist the parents to not disrupt continuity of care for their child (Lindgren, Soderberg, & Skar, 2013). It is not unusual to have a child's eligibility for mental health care services change to different systems. Even though the young adult is assumed and expected to be responsible for managing his or her own health care needs, it is not uncommon for these young adults to continue to depend on their parents' assistance for accessing their mental health care (Lindgren et al., 2013). Giving the parents ample time to prepare for this transition can facilitate smooth transition without interrupting continuity of care.

FAMILIES OF INDIVIDUALS WITH A SPECIFIC MENTAL HEALTH CONDITION

Several mental health conditions warrant specific discussion in this chapter, either because of the stigma associated with these disorders or the serious impact these disorders can have on family function and well-being. The following five disorders will be discussed:

- Schizophrenia
- MDD
- BD
- Dementia
- ADHD

The diagnostic criteria for these disorders can be found in the *DSM-5* (APA, 2013). This section will discuss the impact these specific disorders can have on families and will include implications for nursing practice. Note that substance use disorder is a common comorbidity with these conditions, so it too needs assessment and intervention. The Johnson family case study, later in the chapter, discusses assessment and treatment for substance use disorder.

Schizophrenia, BD, and MDD should be considered potentially terminal illnesses for persons with these disorders. It is estimated that 40% of females and 60% of males with schizophrenia attempt suicide and 10% to 15% of those are successful (Schizophrenia.com, 2010). Approximately two-thirds of people with MDD consider suicide and about 10% to 15% of them complete suicide (Sadock, Sadock, & Ruiz, 2017). These high rates of attempted and completed suicides are cause for nurses consistently and diligently to assess for suicidality/suicidal ideations in these populations. Several suicide screening tools are available on the Internet (e.g., integration.samhsa.gov/clinical-practice/screening-tools), and the agencies where nurses work should have an identified suicide assessment screening tool available.

Schizophrenia

Schizophrenia is a chronic condition of disturbed thought processes, perceptions, and affect that can lead to severe social and occupational dysfunction and sometimes hospitalization. It has a life prevalence of 1% in Canada (Statistics Canada, 2012b) and the United States (NIMH, 2014b). It is most often diagnosed when an individual experiences psychosis for the first time in the late teens or early twenties, but there is an attempt to diagnose schizophrenia earlier by the recognition of subtler, earlier signs and symptoms, which would enable improved outcomes for affected individuals (NIMH, n.d.). Schizophrenia is a severe disorder characterized by distorted thinking and perception and inappropriate emotions. False, fixed beliefs not based on reality (delusions), as well as hallucinations, social withdrawal, and amotivation, are additional features of this disorder that can cause significant individual and family dysfunction. A person with schizophrenia may demonstrate disturbed behavior during some phases of the disorder, which can lead to unfavorable social consequences for the individual and family.

There is complete symptomatic and social recovery in about 30% of persons with schizophrenia. Up to 80% of individuals with schizophrenia may have a MDD at some time in their life, which is conjectured to be linked with the 20-fold increase in suicide over the general public (Sadock et al., 2017). Globally, schizophrenia decreases the person's life span by an average of 10 years (WHO, 2016b), with the most frequent causes of premature death other than suicide being heart disease, cerebrovascular disease, and pulmonary disease (Colton & Manderscheid, 2006; Hennekens, Hennekens, Hollar, & Casey, 2005). People with schizophrenia also have a higher mortality rate from accidents and natural causes than the general population (WHO, 2016b).

Inpatient treatment for persons with an SMI such as schizophrenia is more likely to be limited to days rather than weeks or months (Gerson & Rose, 2012). This approach means that treatment and symptom management tend to occur in the community. Some individuals with schizophrenia live with their families, but many do not. Some live on their own, others live with roommates or in a group setting; still others are homeless. Because they are adults who are considered competent when their condition is at least fairly well managed, it can be very challenging for families to help the person obtain the care he or she needs, especially if the person with schizophrenia is not managing well and is refusing care.

Regardless of whether the person with schizophrenia lives with the family or not, families need help with understanding how to manage the situation. Individuals with schizophrenia and their family members state that their greatest need from mental health care providers is to receive more general information about schizophrenia and guidance on how to cope with the symptoms of schizophrenia, including communication and social relationships (Gumus, 2008). Psychological distress is a significant predictor of family functioning, and having a family member with schizophrenia is a major stressor for the family. Being informed and knowing what to look for can help family members recognize early signs of changes in the individual's symptoms and behaviors that may need professional involvement (Chen & Lukens, 2011); if changes are addressed early, it is possible to avoid hospitalization and reduce family stress. For example, families need information about how to interact safely with a family member who may be having command hallucinations, especially

if the hallucination is commanding the individual to harm herself or others. Nurses need to inform family members that it is not appropriate to argue or disagree with the person who is actively hallucinating or having a delusion. Rather, family members should have a plan already in place to implement. If there are children in the household, the behavior the person is exhibiting may be frightening to them. Children should have a safe, prearranged place to go, such as a nearby neighbor, or have contact information to call a trusted person to come be with the child. Nurses should engage in open discussions with family members about how to interact with their family member who may be hallucinating or having a delusional thought, preferably before the experience.

Families who have a family member with schizophrenia need nurses to understand the frustration and exhaustion they frequently experience; they also want to feel respected by health care providers. On the other hand, nurses need to remind family members to be patient with the affected family member. Family members may be aware of the positive symptoms (i.e., hallucinations and delusions) and negative symptoms (i.e., anergy, amotivation, apathy, avolition) of schizophrenia. Still, many family members complain that the person with schizophrenia is lazy, manipulative, socially inept, or even incompetent, rather than realizing that these are manifestations of the illness (Muhlbauer, 2008). Even though most individuals with schizophrenia do not live with a family member, when the person who has schizophrenia does live at home, the tasks that family caregivers typically provide on a daily basis are similar to those needed when anyone has an MHC: providing companionship, providing emotional support during a crisis, monitoring symptoms, assisting with personal grooming, and so on. The nature of this condition can make it difficult for families to provide the care they perceive the person needs, especially when the medications are not effective (or the person with schizophrenia has stopped taking them). Nurses need to provide assistance to these families in managing the individual's illness, including living arrangements, job placement, day-to-day activities (Fortinash & Worret, 2007), and medications. The family's coping ability and family functioning are enhanced when appropriate social support systems are in place, and such supports can even buffer the family from the emotional distress that can occur when providing care to a family member with schizophrenia (Caqueo-Urizar, Gutierrez-Maldonada, & Mirnada-Casatillo, 2009). Nurses need to remind families that there are limits to what they can do for their family member and refer families to appropriate resources and support groups, including the National Alliance on Mental Illness (NAMI).

Medication adherence is a major part of treatment for managing the symptoms and behaviors of schizophrenia, but adherence is variable and frequently less than optimal. The side effects of medications can lead the person with schizophrenia to stop his medication, resulting in exacerbation of the condition. It is important to engage the individual and appropriate family members in administering medications and in monitoring the effects and effectiveness of the medications (Fortinash & Worret, 2007). Many of the medications have serious adverse effects. Neuroleptic malignant syndrome and extrapyramidal symptoms, including akathisia and tardive dyskinesia, which affect the muscles are serious and life-threatening complications that can be caused by typical and atypical antipsychotic medications. The individual and appropriate family members need to know what to do and who to call should they observe a dangerous or life-threatening side effect, such as difficulty in swallowing or breathing, and they should have the emergency information readily available. Selective serotonin reuptake inhibitors (SSRIs; e.g., sertraline and citalopram) can interact with some antipsychotics and cause another significant medical problem, *metabolic syndrome*, a term to describe a group of risk factors (central obesity, insulin resistance, elevated blood pressure [BP], and abnormal lipid profile) (Grundy et al., 2005) that are thought to be highly predictive of risk for heart disease. The atypical antipsychotics, such as olanzapine and risperidone, that are used to treat schizophrenia and other mood disorders, can lead to metabolic syndrome. There is no treatment for metabolic syndrome (Ganguli & Strassnig, 2011). Rather, there are interventions to decrease the risk of coronary heart disease, such as reduction of weight, treatment of high BP, and treatment of elevated lipid levels (Ganguli & Strassnig, 2011). In addition, interventions to prevent metabolic syndrome, such as eating healthy foods and participating in regular exercise, can help to maintain a healthy body and decrease the risk for developing this syndrome.

Hospitalization is not uncommon, partly because of the challenges of nonadherence to medication regimens, and it is a stressful time for the individual and family. Family members often do not understand the use and purpose of physical restraints or seclusion and may need to be taught this information by nurses in a nonjudgmental and positive manner, making sure the family understands the temporary use of these safety measures. Related to issues of hospitalization is the topic of involuntary commitment. Nurses need to be familiar with their state/provincial involuntary commitment statutes and inform families about what is involved in these laws so that families and individuals do not become overwhelmed or frustrated should involuntary commitment occur. Involuntary civil commitment means that an individual is admitted to a mental health unit against his or her will. The three main reasons for involuntary commitment are mental illness, substance use disorder, and developmental disability. Being dangerous to oneself, including being unable to provide for one's basic needs, or to others usually defines the typical commitment standard for mental illness. Most jurisdictions provide for a hearing, the right to counsel, and a periodic judicial review.

Family members of people with schizophrenia or BD may be in the position of seeking involuntary commitment for their mentally ill family member, which can be a very stressful process. People with major mental illnesses often do not understand their disorders and disagree about receiving treatment even when they feel like acting out violently. Before police or emergency mental health intervention can be called in, the mentally ill person under most state laws must be already violent. Family members may see the situation escalating, but may not receive help until treatment is no longer focused on the person's mental disorder, but on the violence. Many people have been arrested and charged with crimes of violence during exacerbations of mental disorders (Robertson & Walter, 2014). Family members and caregivers are often significant members of the decision-making process to commit a person with schizophrenia and often find themselves in a position of role conflict, confusion, and misunderstanding (Arya, 2014).

Two final comments about schizophrenia are worthy of consideration for nurses. First, persons with schizophrenia should not be labeled or called "schizophrenics" but rather identified by their names. It is more professional and respectful and less pejorative to identify the person by name and not by illness. Second, the number of children born to parents with schizophrenia has increased because of improved medications and deinstitutionalization; the fertility rate is close to that for the general population (Sadock et al., 2017). First-degree biological relatives of persons with schizophrenia have a greater than 10-fold risk for developing schizophrenia compared with the general population (Sadock et al., 2017). The aforementioned statements have teaching and education implications for nurses working with families who have a family member with schizophrenia.

Major Depressive Disorder

MDD, also called major depression or clinical depression, is a medical condition that causes a persistent feeling of sadness and loss of interest; it affects how someone thinks, feels, and behaves and it can lead to emotional and physical problems. People with MDD often have trouble doing normal day-to-day activities and they may feel as if life is not worth living. MDD, a chronic illness that usually requires long-term treatment, affects 11% of Canadians (Statistics Canada, 2012a) and about 5% to 8% of Americans (Kessler, Chiu, Demler, & Walters, 2005; NIMH, 2014b). Based on detailed interviews with more than 89,000 people from 18 countries, including the United States, Bromet et al. (2011) illustrated that people from high-income countries were more likely than those from low-/middle-income countries to experience depression during their lifetime (15% vs. 11%), with 5.5% having had depression in the last year. Women were twice as likely as men to suffer depression. The number of major depressive episodes was higher in high-income countries (28% vs. 20%) and especially high (more than 30%) in France, the Netherlands, and the United States (Bromet et al., 2011). MDD is the leading cause of disability in the United States (WHO, 2014), the fourth leading cause of burden among all diseases (WHO, 2014), and the 10th leading cause of death in the United States (NIMH, 2014b). In Canada, about one-fifth of boys and one-third of girls (ages 11 to 15) feel depressed or low on a weekly basis or more (Freeman et al., 2011).

Sadock et al. (2017) asserted that the life event most often associated with development of depression is the loss of a parent before a child is 11 years old, and the environmental stressor most associated with onset of a depressive episode is the loss of a spouse. Nurses should assess for depression using a variety of evidence-based assessment tools, such as the Patient Health Questionnaire–9 (Spitzer, Kroenke, & Williams, 1999), which is in the public domain and available online. Adults with depression experience the following: anhedonia (the inability to experience pleasure from activities normally found to be enjoyable), anxiety (Sadock et al., 2017), decreased energy, feelings of guilt, and changes in appetite or sleep. Depression often coexists with eating disorders or anxiety disorders (Schwartz, 2011), as well as substance use disorders such as alcohol/drug addictions (Conway et al., 2006) and physical medical conditions (NIMH, 2017). MDD interferes with social, occupational, and interpersonal functioning. Older adults may manifest depression with somatic symptoms. Unfortunately, many health care providers underdiagnose and undertreat older persons with depression because they assume that MDD is a natural part of aging—which it is not.

MDD can jeopardize marriages and lead to marital discord. More than 50% of spouses report that they would not have married their spouse or had children had they known that their partner was going to develop a mood disorder (Sadock et al., 2017). Family and couples therapy are important strategies to help families and they can be effective in improving the psychological well-being of the whole family.

Psychotherapy and psychopharmacology are common treatments for persons with depression. SSRIs and serotonin-norepinephrine reuptake inhibitors (SNRIs) are two common types of drugs used to treat depression. Individuals who are prescribed these medications and their families need to be aware of a potentially life-threatening drug interaction that can occur if inadvertently taken with other drugs, or in the case of overdose: serotonin syndrome. Serotonin is a chemical produced by the body that allows nerve cells and the brain to function. Too much serotonin may cause mild symptoms such as shivering and diarrhea, but severe serotonin syndrome may lead to muscle rigidity, fever, and seizures, which can be fatal if not treated. Herbs, such as St. John's wort; stimulants, such as methylphenidate; and opioids, such as hydrocodone, can interact to produce serotonin syndrome. Families need to be educated about the signs and symptoms of serotonin syndrome and receive information on how to contact the health care provider or emergency support services. Nurses should be familiar with the classification of drugs that are prescribed to their clients, such as SSRIs, SNRIs, or norepinephrine-dopamine reuptake inhibitors (NDRIs), as well as the neurotransmitters and parts of the brain these drugs affect. Drugs are used to treat symptoms and behaviors and not to treat diagnoses. There are numerous psychopharmacology textbooks, as well as many excellent online resources, available for nurses to learn more about these drugs.

Children and Depression

Depression is not always easily recognized in children because many everyday stresses, such as the birth of a sibling, can cause changes in a child's behavior. It is important to be able to tell the difference between typical behavior changes and those associated with more serious problems. Symptoms of depression in children may be demonstrated by excessive clinging to parents or by phobias, and adolescents often exhibit poor academic performance, substance abuse, antisocial behavior, sexual promiscuity, or truancy, or they run away (Sadock et al., 2017). Other behaviors to pay special attention to include problems across a variety of settings, such as at school, at home, or with peers; changes in appetite or sleep; social withdrawal; fear of things the child normally is not afraid of; returning to behaviors more common in younger children, such as bed-wetting, for a long time; signs of being upset, such as sadness or tearfulness; signs of self-destructive behavior, such as head-banging, or a tendency to get hurt often; and repeated thoughts of death (NIMH, 2009).

Children who live with a parent who has MDD are often aware of the parent's depression and are both emotionally affected and inappropriately involved in managing everyday life, such as taking over daily living or financial tasks that are normally completed by an adult (Ahlstrom, Skarsater, & Danielson, 2007). Even though children want to help their parent, they do not feel capable, which often can lead to feelings of guilt. Guilt is a feeling that children living with a depressed parent experience more often than other children. Some children worry that their depressed parent may attempt or complete suicide while they are away from home. It promotes children's health when the family as a whole learns about depression and learns how to talk more openly about it. It is important for nurses to help children understand that they did not cause the parent's depression and also to help the parents convey this message to their children (Ahlstrom et al., 2007). Nurses also need to include the family in discussions. For example, a mother with MDD who had two children (ages 19 and 11) stated that she herself had received invaluable support and help from her mental health care providers but that this made no difference when the family members were excluded (Ahlstrom et al., 2007). The 19-year-old son thought that finances and untidiness were the cause of his mother's depression, whereas the 11-year-old daughter linked the depression to family arguments that frightened her. The family members reacted differently to depression. It is important for nurses to develop strategies that assist all members of the family to participate actively in the care of the parent with depression—the child's experience of living with a depressed parent must be included in the overall treatment and management of the depressed parent. In addition, family group cognitive-behavioral interventions that focus on improving positive parenting (e.g., use of praise, scheduling pleasant family activities) contribute to the benefits for the children and the family (Compas et al., 2010).

Bipolar Disorder

BD affects about 2.6% of adult Americans in any given year (Kessler, Chiu, et al., 2005) and worldwide the prevalence is around 0.4% (WHO, 2016b). Bipolar I disorder, a subdiagnosis of BD that is characterized by one or more manic episodes, is more common in divorced and single persons than among married people (Sadock et al., 2017). BD is a recurring, treatable but incurable MHC that causes cycles of mania and depression. Episodes of mania or depression can last from 1 day to months, with euthymic (normal mood) periods between these mood shifts. It is these dramatic shifts in moods that can disrupt family function and cause damage to relationships, academic problems, financial problems caused by loss of jobs, and even legal problems, including confrontations with the police. Family members can find it very difficult to interact with a family member who is demonstrating manic symptoms—euphoria, reduced need for sleep, excessive talking, irritability, overactivity, overconfidence, impaired concentration, increased pleasure-seeking or risk-taking behaviors, and elevated surges of energy. Children especially can become disturbed when living with a family member who is manic. The child's safety can be in jeopardy and the child may feel afraid being near someone who is behaving irrationally. On the other hand, it can be equally disconcerting for families to live with or provide care to someone who is depressed and demonstrating hopelessness, extreme sadness, and loss of energy (Kessler, Berglund, et al., 2005).

Families with a member who has BD are continually challenged by the fickleness and unpredictability that this MHC can have on the family and the individual. They live with uncertainty, not knowing which mood to expect at any given time or when a change will occur. Parents of adult children with BD have more compromised mental and physical health and more difficulties in marriage and work life than comparison families (Aschbrenner, Greenberg, & Seltzer, 2009). Additionally, parents who already have an MHC before the onset of their child's BD are even more vulnerable to problems with mental health issues, psychological well-being, and work life than parents who do not have an existing MHC (Aschbrenner et al., 2009). Consequently, obtaining the history of MHC in parents and the immediate family is important to inform the nurse's interventions in promoting the well-being of each member of the family.

Family history of BD conveys a greater risk for BD disorders in general (Sadock et al., 2017). Nurses need to teach families about the genetic implications of this MHC and educate families on the signs and symptoms so that families can recognize the early signs and symptoms and initiate early professional treatment. BD is a difficult MHC to diagnose accurately, yet it is important that this MHC be differentiated from MDD, personality disorders, substance use, anxiety disorders, and schizophrenia (Sadock et al., 2017), because the treatments can be significantly different. Although BD typically emerges in young adulthood, the range of onset of BD can occur as early as 5 to 6 years of age to 50 years of age or older.

Because children and adolescents can manifest symptoms of mania and depression differently from adults, they are often misdiagnosed as having antisocial personality disorder or schizophrenia rather than BD (Sadock et al., 2017). Child and adolescent symptoms of mania can include substance abuse, irritability that can lead to fights, academic problems, suicide attempts, obsessive-compulsive symptoms, somatic complaints, and antisocial behaviors. Misdiagnosis has tremendous implications in young people. Making differential diagnoses in children and adolescents is difficult, and it is important for

nurses to advocate for additional assessments as new signs and symptoms emerge in children and adolescents so that they are treated appropriately and so that they can avoid unnecessary treatments and complications.

Just as misdiagnosis of BD in the younger population is problematic, it is also problematic for the older population. Older adults with BD are more often misdiagnosed as having schizophrenia, with older minority persons being misdiagnosed twice as frequently as white older persons or younger minorities (Luggen, 2005). Older adults are also more likely to be diagnosed with depression rather than BD, which can result in them being prescribed antidepressant medications that inadvertently place these older persons at higher risk for having a manic episode (Luggen, 2005). Equally important, many of the medications that are used to treat symptoms of depression and mania can have significant adverse effects on the older person, thus making it even more important for accurate assessment and treatment among this vulnerable population. Some of the medications used to treat these symptoms, such as the second-generation antipsychotic drugs, may place an older person at higher risk for death or cerebrovascular event (Stahl, 2011).

Mental health care providers have typically done a less than adequate job in assessing the needs of spouses who have a family member with BD and in providing information to these spouses (van der Voort, Goossens, & van der Bijl, 2009). Yet, it has been shown that caregivers who receive both psychoeducation and health promotion interventions have significantly less depression, improved health, and less subjective burden of care and role dysfunction (Perlick et al., 2010). Not only might the caregivers receive benefit from these two interventions, but the family member with BD may demonstrate a decrease in mania and depression, due in part to the improved health of the caregiver (Perlick et al., 2010).

Caregivers of persons with BD often have felt overlooked by health care providers and report that if health care providers would offer support, then it would decrease their burden of care (Rusner, Carlsson, Brunt, & Nystrom, 2012; Tranvag & Kristoffersen, 2008). Caregivers who provide care to a family member with BD identified two main themes that would make their caregiving experiences more positive (Maskill, Crowe, Luty, & Joyce, 2010). First, they would feel more supported if the mental health nurses showed understanding of the complexities associated with BD and were nonjudgmental and noncritical of the family. Second, they identified the importance of caregivers collaborating with mental health staff. Health care providers should recognize the uniqueness of the caregiver and the recipient of the care. Caregivers also encourage mental health care providers to be honest with them about the fact that BD is not curable, but to maintain hope nonetheless (Maskill et al., 2010).

Although BD is treatable, the condition can cause significant social and economic stress for families. Educational interventions for family members living with a person with BD reduce stress for the family members, increase family members' understanding of the condition, and enhance family members' ability to remain socially functional (Jonnson, Wijk, Danielson, & Skarsater, 2011). It is essential that nurses teach family members to observe for early signs of relapse into mania, such as provocative dressing, unrestrained buying sprees, hypersexuality, being more talkative than usual, or grandiosity (APA, 2013); or signs of relapse into depression, such as increased sleeping, problems sleeping, problems with concentration, anhedonia, or recurrent thoughts of suicide. It is important that family members monitor these changes in their family member who has BD (Sorell, 2011) and notify the appropriate health care provider when there are changes.

Dementia

Dementia is a syndrome that affects memory, thinking, behavior, learning capacity, judgment, and the ability to perform daily activities; it is one of the major causes of disability and dependency among older people worldwide (WHO & Alzheimer's Disease International, 2012). Globally, approximately 35.6 million people have dementia; these numbers are expected to double by 2030 and more than triple by 2050 as the population ages (WHO & Alzheimer's Disease International, 2012). In the United States, about 5% of the general population older than age 65, and 20% to 40% of those older than age 85, has dementia. Alzheimer's disease is the most common type of dementia (approximately 60% to 70% of dementia cases). People can live for many years with dementia; thus, with appropriate support, many can remain engaged in and contribute to society. There is currently no cure or treatment to alter the progressive nature of the condition.

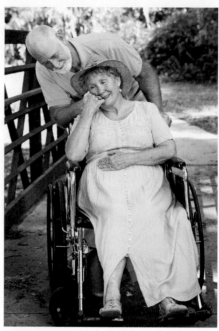

© iStock.com/lisafx

Dementia can dramatically affect the lives of individuals with dementia and their families, not only health-wise but also economically, socially, and legally. Providing care to a family member with dementia can interrupt the normal family activities. Depending on the severity of the dementia, families may need to take on responsibility for tasks ranging from paying bills to ensuring the individual attends medical appointments to full personal grooming. Discussions about power of attorney and substitute decision making (living wills, advance directives) need to take place, preferably soon after diagnosis.

The majority of care to persons with dementia is provided by family and informal community support services, though some individuals receive long-term, institutional care. Women typically provide family home-based care to persons with dementia. Emotional and physical stressors are not uncommon among caregivers. The loss of the ability to interact meaningfully with a loved one who no longer, or perhaps intermittently, remembers you is a source of grief and stress for many families. Caregivers have a very high prevalence of depression (Cuijpers, 2005) and may have a compromised immune system. Psychoeducation programs have been shown to decrease depression and stress among caregivers (Gallagher-Thompson et al., 2012) and are one source of support that nurses can help families obtain. These caregivers need strong support from health professionals; assessment and intervention are critical. More detailed information about dementia assessment and intervention is available in Chapter 15.

Despite the commonly held societal belief, dementia is not a normal part of the aging process; dementia is much more than slight memory loss. A family's cultural-based beliefs about dementia can be a barrier to accessing care (Gallagher-Thompson et al., 2012). For instance, families can view dementia as a medical illness, a mental illness, or as part of normal aging. When conducting a family assessment, the nurse should explore each of these views. In addition, it is important that the nurse listen to each member of the family's story. These stories can be used to map the journey of the person with dementia and the family's journey as it lives this experience (Doherty, Benbow, Craig, & Smith, 2009). Other sources, such as extended family members, other informal caregivers, health care records, and formal health care providers should also be used to obtain information. Information collected from a variety of sources can be used to develop effective family-focused interventions.

Although the family member with dementia may have increased confusion and decreased ability to communicate, it is important that nurses not treat this person as a child. The person with dementia is an adult and should still be treated with respect as an adult. Speaking to an adult as if she or he were a young child is demeaning to the individual and to the family members. There may be some similarities between a young child and an older person with dementia, such as incontinence or inability to dress oneself. Nevertheless, the adult should be treated as an adult who has a cognitive deficit and not as a child. For example, it is important to use normal conversational pitch and words when talking to an older adult, rather than affecting a high-pitched voice or using words that are appropriate to a child's developmental level rather than that of an adult.

New technologies are being used to assist family caregivers who are caring for persons with dementia. Telehealth, for instance, allows family members to communicate with their health care providers via the Internet, and smartphones and new applications provide information to family members about dementia, caring for a person with dementia, and support sources for the family. These technologies can be used to inform families on how to handle daily problems, such as wandering, falling, decreased memory, and eating problems (Gallagher-Thompson et al., 2012).

A new multidisciplinary field, gerontechnology, has developed to interface between technology and older people. The mission of the International Society for Gerontechnology (IGS) is to "encourage and promote technological innovations in products and services that address older peoples' ambitions and needs on the basis of scientific knowledge about ageing processes including cultural and individual differences" (gerontechnology.info/about.html). The IGS values not only meeting the needs of older people, but also supporting the caregivers. Developments such as gerontechnology offer exciting possibilities about how to provide needed support to caregivers of persons with dementia.

Attention Deficit-Hyperactivity Disorder

ADHD is one of the most common MHCs among children and adolescents (Foley, 2010), with more prevalence in boys, ranging from 2:1 to as much as 9:1 (Sadock et al., 2017). The underrepresentation of girls may be attributed to underdiagnosis, however, because girls often present with the inattentive rather than hyperactive type of ADHD and are overlooked. In the United States, the presence of ADHD varies from 2% to 20% among grade-school children, and the incidence of the symptoms of ADHD persisting into adulthood is about 40% to 50%, or 4% of the adult population (Sadock et al., 2017). Children, adolescents, and adults with ADHD typically demonstrate diminished sustained concentration, increased levels of impulsivity, hyperactivity, and problems with social interactions. Other people may view them as lazy, stupid, reckless, or uncaring because of how the symptoms affect the person with ADHD. Some children, especially girls, may be inattentive rather than hyperactive, and the hyperactivity in adults is often internal rather than external. ADHD has a genetic component (Foley, 2010) and so it is not uncommon to have more than one family member with ADHD, including one or both parents (Singh et al., 2010). Diagnosis is complex and requires collaborating with many key adults in the child's life, including teachers, parents, friends, and other community adults with whom the child may interact. Diagnosis in adults often follows a diagnosis for one of their children.

Young people who are diagnosed with ADHD often endure stigma from their peers, teachers, family, and society. Examples of stigma include teachers and peers thinking that a person with ADHD chooses to be inattentive in class or that the person with ADHD has a character trait flaw rather than an MHC. Many young people struggle with the negative assumptions that others have toward them and that they have toward themselves (Kildea, John, & Davies, 2011). They often experience a lack of empathy and understanding from key adults in their lives (Singh et al., 2010). Young people with ADHD frequently feel that the diagnosis itself gives them a bad reputation, including thinking that others consider them stupid (Singh et al., 2010).

Parents of children with ADHD often report feeling blamed by professionals, their families, and society for their child's behavior (Kildea et al., 2011). Families of children with ADHD have a higher level of dysfunction than other families; thus, earlier identification and intervention with these families can result in healthier family function and child outcomes (Foley, 2010). For instance, families who received eight to twelve 50-minute sessions that included psychoeducation about ADHD, behavioral principles, and specific parenting skills and strategies demonstrated improved parenting behaviors and less parenting stress for mothers (Gerdes, Haack, & Schneider, 2012). Examples of parenting skills and strategies include having regular and consistent daily routines, such as mealtimes (Tamm, Holden, Nakonezny, Swart, & Hughes, 2012), praising positive behavior, ignoring mildly negative behavior, consistently using time out, and giving effective instructions (Gerdes et al., 2012). It is also recommended that families eliminate computer/screen time before bed to decrease sleep problems (Becker, Goobic, & Thomas, 2009). Parenting skills should include supervision and provision of assistance to the child so he can remain organized and focused when doing homework; short movement breaks at regular intervals also are helpful (Becker et al., 2009).

Although it is very beneficial for parents to learn about and use home management skills, it is also important that the parents request appropriate neuropsychological and psychoeducational evaluations for their child to determine if the child might benefit from school-based supports, particularly if their child has academic difficulties, a learning disorder, or executive functioning difficulties (Becker et al., 2009). For example, in the United States some children with ADHD qualify through a federal law, the Individuals with Disabilities Act, to receive an Individual Education Plan (IEP) that is unique to the child and supports the child's educational needs. Another plan, the 504 Plan, is provided by a civil rights law that protects children with ADHD from being discriminated against because of their MHC; therefore, some children who may not qualify for an IEP may receive additional educational support under the 504 Plan. IEPs are also common in Canada after appropriate assessment and evaluation.

Treatment for ADHD may include medications, psychotherapy such as behavioral therapy, psychoeducation including lifestyle changes, coaching, and other interventions to decrease the number and severity of stressors in the individual's and family's life. Family therapy will help to maintain and promote healthy family functioning. Family therapy is also indicated if the condition jeopardizes the marriage, for example, if a spouse whose partner has ADHD is considering leaving the marriage (Sadock et al., 2017). Family therapy is especially recommended if a child and a parent have ADHD, because it may be difficult for a parent to recognize her own disorganization, inconsistent responses to the child's behaviors, and/or impulsivities and the impact they can have on the family (Singh et al., 2010).

Medications are often used to treat ADHD, in conjunction with other interventions, but the decision to use these medications needs to be based on the benefits of taking the medication versus the consequences of not taking the medications. The parent or adult needs to make these decisions without outside pressure from family or media who may be misinformed. Parents of children with ADHD often experience misgivings about administering a stimulant to their child, based on feedback they get from their family, friends, or the media (Jackson & Peters, 2008) even though stimulants are the recommended treatment. Much of the information parents obtain about treating ADHD with medications is secondary and not evidence based. Nurses have a responsibility to provide accurate information to parents so the parents can make a thoughtful and informed decision about whether or not to treat their child with medication. Amphetamine-containing formulations of stimulants are the most commonly prescribed ADHD medications in Canada and the United States (Berman, Kuczenski, McCracken, & London, 2009). Though stimulants have been used successfully for decades, there has been a link to slower bone growth in children taking amphetamines and to psychosis in adults taking amphetamines (Berman et al., 2009). The child and adult who are prescribed a stimulant require regular checkups. Just as many clinical settings contact patients for follow-up visits, such as for diabetes management, these settings should likewise designate a nurse to be the point person to provide this service to persons with ADHD and their families (Van Cleave & Leslie, 2008).

Medication adherence and behavior modification can be problematic for individuals with ADHD and their families. It has been suggested that health care providers approach ADHD as a chronic health condition, which includes long-term therapy (Van Cleave & Leslie, 2008). Nurses should educate families that medication neither cures ADHD nor necessarily eliminates the impulsive behaviors a child or adult may be exhibiting. Families should be aware of the advantages and disadvantages of taking medication several times during the day versus taking a long-acting stimulant.

ROLE OF THE FAMILY MENTAL HEALTH NURSE

In order to establish a collaborative relationship with the family, nurses must have a nonblaming and accepting attitude toward family members. Families value interactions with health care providers that demonstrate openness, cooperation, confirmation, and continuity (Ewertzon et al., 2012). As family members increasingly have assumed the role of primary caregivers for mentally ill individuals, it is more important than ever to include them as partners in the delivery of mental health care. Care delivery systems that involve family members acknowledge the effect mental disorders have on entire family systems. They seek to prevent the return or exacerbation of a disorder, and they alleviate pain and suffering experienced by family members. To fulfil these goals, researchers (Dixon et al., 2001) have identified 15 evidence-based principles that continue to be relevant and can be incorporated into family nursing interventions for families of individuals with a mental illness (Box 16-2). This section briefly examines a few areas of focus for mental health nurses within care delivery systems: prevention of MHCs, psychoeducation, family recovery, crisis plans, and providing culturally sensitive care.

Prevention of Mental Health Conditions

Arguably, the most important role for the nurse in mental health care is to engage in professional activities that *prevent* mental health conditions. Stress during childhood, especially before 3 years of age when synapses are still being formed, can trigger the expression of genes that may otherwise have remained unexpressed (Grayson, 2006). Neglect and abuse are negative experiences that can cause serious hormonal

---

BOX 16-2

Evidence-Based Principles for Working With Families of Individuals With a Mental Illness

Following are evidence-based principles for health care providers who work with families that include an individual or individuals with mental illness:

- Organize care so that everyone involved is working toward the same treatment goals within a collaborative, supportive relationship.
- Attend to both the social and clinical needs of the primary patient.
- Provide optimal medication management.
- Listen to family's concerns and involve them in all elements of treatment.
- Examine family's expectations of treatment and expectations of the primary patient.

- Evaluate strengths and limitations of the family's ability to provide support.
- Aid in the resolution of family conflict.
- Explore feelings of loss for all parties.
- Provide pertinent information to patients and families at appropriate times.
- Develop a clear crisis plan.
- Help enhance family communication.
- Train families in problem-solving techniques.
- Promote expansion of the family's social support network.
- Be adaptable in meeting the family's needs.
- Provide easy access to another professional if current work with the family ceases.

Source: Adapted from Dixon, L., McFarlane, W., Lefley, H., Lucksted, A., Cohen, M., Falloon, I., . . . Sondheimer, D. (2001). Evidence-based practices for services to families of people with psychiatric disabilities. *Psychiatric Services, 52*(7), 903–910.

and chemical changes in the brain and interrupt normal brain development (Grayson, 2006). The "physical connections between neurons formed in childhood are not 'hard-wired' or 'unchangeable'" (Grayson, 2006, p. 1). Genetics influence brain development and exposure to significant stress can affect the way specific genes are expressed. There is a polymorphism (genetic variation within a population) in the 5-HTT gene that results in the occurrence of MDD only if the gene carrier experiences a major life stressor (Burke et al., 2016). Stress itself, such as physical, emotional, and sexual abuse; famine; and natural disasters can also profoundly affect the emotional, behavioral, cognitive, social, and physical functioning in children. Secure attachments and ample nurturing not only allow for a positive environment for the brain to build neural connections to integrate the brain systems but also strengthen an infant's ability to cope with stress (Grayson, 2006). When babies cry and their needs are taken care of, such as through food or attention and comfort, their neuronal pathways are strengthened and they learn how to get their needs met both physically and emotionally (Grayson, 2006). On the other hand, babies who are abused or neglected learn other lessons that can be damaging and may interfere with a child's ability to self-regulate. For instance, the child whose needs are not met and who endures repeated painful disappointments may abandon crying for help, resulting in problems with hyperarousal or dissociation.

Maltreatment at an early age may have enduring effects on the development and function of a child's brain. Child maltreatment can manifest internally—depression, anxiety, or suicidality—or outwardly, with aggression, impulsiveness, hyperactivity, delinquency, or substance abuse. There is an association between maltreatment in childhood and a person being diagnosed with borderline personality disorder. Borderline personality disorder is characterized by seeing others and situations in black-and-white terms, having unstable relationships, having feelings of abandonment, exhibiting self-harm, having problems with anger, and escaping through substance abuse. The limbic system plays a key role in regulating emotion and memory of one's experiences. Research has shown that abuse in children can cause permanent damage to the neural structure and function of the brain. People with borderline personality disorder often have reduced integration between the left and right brain hemispheres, a smaller corpus callosum, and limbic electrical irritability (Hockenberry, Wilson, & Rodgers, 2017).

There is also some evidence that a mother smoking and drinking alcohol during pregnancy affects the growth of neural pathways and can contribute to the development of conditions such as ADHD (Nigg, 2006). Healthy lifestyle behaviors, including diet, exercise, stress-reduction strategies, and nonconsumption of alcohol, cigarettes, or illegal substances, seem to play a role in reducing the risk of developing an MHC. Nurses should put effort into encouraging and supporting healthy lifestyles, whether prenatally or for children, youth, or adults.

Nurses must, of course, advocate for good parenting and must offer parenting support in a nonjudgmental way. Nurses should be at the forefront of ensuring that childhood maltreatment does not take place. Early assessment and intervention is important to help prevent serious repercussions for children. Nurses can provide resources for caretakers of children so they learn the necessary skills to provide responsible care, support, and nurturing to their child. Moreover, nurses should be active in local, state, and national policies that affect child welfare.

Persons with SMI tend to die earlier, up to 20 to 30 years, compared with the general population because of preventable diseases (Walker, McGee, & Druss, 2015) and suicide (WHO, n.d.). These premature deaths can dramatically affect families because of burden of physical care, financial costs, and role changes. Mental health nurses play a significant role in addressing the physical health care needs of persons with SMI and must be able to assess and address the physical impact that the person's lifestyle (such as nutrition, exercise, and sleep), psychotropic medication adverse effects, and living environment can have on preventing cardiovascular, metabolic, and respiratory diseases among this population (De Hert et al., 2011).

Psychoeducation

A major role for a professional nurse in working with families who have a member with an MHC is to provide psychoeducation. Psychoeducation includes teaching clients about the cause and treatments of the MHC, while being attuned to each of the family members' unique needs. Family psychoeducation is a term used to describe various family programs that incorporate the following three elements:

- Family education
- Training in coping skills
- Social support (Schock & Gavazzi, 2005)

The time commitment and emphasis on each of these elements is what differs among the diverse psychoeducational models. Currently, these interventions may continue for months or years. Because psychoeducational programs are multifaceted and involve such long-term relationships, they are typically delivered by teams of health care providers working together. Nurses' training and education make them well suited to participate in such interdisciplinary teams that emphasize client and family education, enhance coping skills, and develop supportive networks.

The educational element of these programs involves providing information to relatives regarding diagnoses, cause of mental illness, prognosis, and treatment. Skills training may include coping skills for family members and social skills training for the family member with the MHC. In addition, the entire family may work on developing communication skills so members can communicate more effectively with one another. Nurses can enhance social support for the family by actively including relatives as members of the treatment team and by helping to establish connections to other families with similar experiences. Through networking with one another, families can find support and share problem-solving strategies. A local chapter of the NAMI is one support and advocacy organization that families may find helpful.

Nurses can teach individuals and family members about no-cost relaxation techniques to reduce stress (e.g., breathing techniques and exercises, guided imagery, yoga, and progressive muscle relaxation) and provide pet and/or music therapy. Nurses have the skills to help families cope with feelings of anger and disappointment as they go through the grief process after learning about the MHC of one of their family members. It is important to realize that it may take time for families to accept the diagnosis and the level of acceptance will vary between members of the family (O'Connell, 2006). A variety of family intervention strategies are outlined in Box 16-3.

Family Recovery

The phases of the recovery process of families who have a family member with an MHC (Spaniol & Nelson, 2015) involve four fluid phases that may not be the specific process for each individual: (1) shock, discovery, and denial; (2) recognition and acceptance; (3) coping; and (4) personal and political advocacy. Mental health nurses who are aware of these phases can provide specific interventions to these families in each of the phases.

Family members and relatives of persons with an MHC often experience challenging ethical dilemmas that affect the lives of everyone (Weimand, Hall-Lord, Sallstrom, & Hedelin, 2013). For example, when should a family member make a decision on behalf of (1) him/herself, (2) the person with the MHC, or (3) the entire family? It is often appropriate for a family member to encourage individual freedom and autonomy for the person with an MHC, but allowing this freedom can also have negative impacts

---

BOX 16-3
Family Intervention Strategies

Family intervention strategies include:

- Coordinate information and treatment plans across settings and with multiple health care providers.
- Ensure that communication is bidirectional from health care providers to families and from families to health care providers.
- Provide validation for commitment and work being done by all family members.
- Create ways for families to manage treatment plans that affect everyday routines.
- Identify realistic ways that the mentally ill family member can participate in and contribute to the family.
- Articulate an action plan to implement during times of crisis.
- Negotiate ways to manage specific problem behaviors.
- Connect with appropriate social resources (individual/group therapy, support groups, extended family, friends, religious organizations).
- Provide diagnostic and treatment-related family psychoeducation.
- Encourage self-care behaviors for all family members.
- Identify effective coping skills for individual family members.
- Advocate for policy changes that benefit individuals with mental health conditions and their family members.
- Challenge detrimental stereotypes and stigma of persons with a mental health condition and their families.

on the family, such as not "making" a person take her psychiatric medication but then knowing that the possible emergence of psychosis will cause increased stress for all family members. Prioritizing among oneself, others in the family, and the person with the MHC can cause guilt for family members, such as deciding when to exclude a person with an MHC from a special family event. Mental health nurses can provide support to these families by listening nonjudgmentally and providing hope as families struggle to balance their lives with providing care to the person with an MHC.

A large Canadian study (Aldersey & Whitley, 2015) found that the family itself can be a positive influence on the recovery of the family. Family members "being there" for each other, such as listening, making telephone calls, and providing verbal encouragement, fostered family recovery. Practical support, such as providing financial assistance for housing and treatment, also facilitated family recovery. Lastly, families who provided motivation to recover assisted the recovery process.

Crisis Plans

Violence against family members who provide care to relatives with a severe MHC experience a rate estimated to be between 10% and 40% higher than the general public (Solomon, Cavanaugh, & Gelles, 2005). Yet, these family caregivers frequently feel guilt, embarrassment, and hopelessness about experiencing violence from a family member. Moreover, it is a topic that is difficult for family members to raise with health care providers and others. One major way to support families so they can manage violence is to include relatives as valuable sources of information (Kontio, Lantta, Anttila, Kauppi, & Valimaki, 2017). For example, ask family members about how they have managed violence in the past and what signs/symptoms they have observed that indicate a family member's escalation of violence. Family members may feel guilty about having a family member involuntarily admitted to a hospital, especially if the police are involved.

Nurses are integral in assisting families to develop a crisis plan that is put in place before the need for such a plan; it is more challenging to manage a crisis when you do not have a predetermined plan to follow. Part of this plan may include a visit to the local police precinct to ascertain the best way to deescalate a violent situation (Nadkarni & Fristad, 2012).

Nurses should suggest that families have a binder/notebook available with the following information:

- A list of health care providers, emergency professional contact names, and telephone numbers
- Suicide hotline telephone numbers
- Insurance information
- Details about the best route to the appropriate emergency department or health care facility, including specific directions to get to the sites
- Safe locations where children or other members of the family can go during escalation times

This binder should be readily available to family members and needs to be updated regularly (Nadkarni & Fristad, 2012). Also included in this binder should be advance agreements set up with the person who has an MHC when she was well; these agreements should specify the individual's preferred treatment and note with whom information can be shared during periods of exacerbation of the MHC (Gray, Robinson, Seddon, & Roberts, 2008). Finally, nurses should provide information for families to obtain support by participating in local support groups such as through the NAMI in the United States and the CMHA in Canada.

Providing Culturally Competent Care

Nurses must remember that cultural norms and beliefs shape family members' perceptions of coping and managing care for relatives with an MHC (Dalky, 2012). NAMI's informative Web site (NAMI, n.d.) includes mental health fact sheets for different ethnic groups in the United States (African American, American Indian and Alaska Native, Asian American and Pacific Islander, Latino/Hispanic). Nurses are encouraged to review these fact sheets to become more informed about facts that will help them in practice, and so they can decrease myths and stereotypes about different ethnic groups. For example, American Indian and Alaska Native languages do not include the words *depression* and *anxious*, nor does the word *depression* exist in some Chinese languages. Somatization of mental health conditions may be more common in African American and Asian cultures than in white counterparts.

NAMI also has fact sheets about depression among the following groups: veterans, lesbian/gay/bisexual/transgender, seniors, women, men, and children/

adolescents. Misdiagnosis and undertreatment are not uncommon among some cultural groups; improved understanding about various cultural groups will enhance nursing practice. In addition, because psychiatric medications are a significant part of treating MHC, it is important for nurses to know which populations may be fast metabolizers and which might be slow metabolizers in order to avoid overmedicating or undermedicating a specific individual. At the same time, it is important not to stereotype individuals or families based on their cultural identity but rather to use cultural identity as one aspect of the nursing assessment to take into consideration when developing a nursing plan for the entire family.

Case Study: Johnson Family

The following case study of the Johnson family demonstrates the assessment, diagnosis, outcome identification, planning, implementation, and evaluation for care of a family with a member who has been diagnosed with BD and substance use disorder.

Setting: Inpatient acute care hospital, cardiac intensive care unit (ICU).

Nursing Goal: Family will identify a family-oriented community resource for people with family members with mental disorders or substance use disorders that they are willing to attend by the time the client is discharged. Tony will engage in a change conversation (Miller & Rollnick, 2013) in which he lists his own reasons to adhere to his mood stabilizing medications, and at least one strategy from his own life for making adherence possible/easier.

Family Members:
- Steve: father (now married to Debbie), 49 years old, small business owner
- Mary: mother (now married to Harold), 49 years old, server at a restaurant
- Debbie: stepmother, 54 years old, schoolteacher
- Harold: stepfather, 60 years old, successful building contractor
- Tony: identified patient, 23 years old, oldest child, son, unemployed, sleeping on couches of friends
- Susie: younger daughter, Tony's sister, 17 years old, overachiever and "perfect" child
- Thomas: Mary's father, 86 years old, wealthy businessman
- Emma: Mary's mother, 85 years old, substance use disorder

Johnson Family Story:
Tony Johnson is a 23-year-old man who was admitted to the hospital through the emergency department in acute cardiac distress from an accidental methamphetamine overdose. He arrived at the emergency department by ambulance from his drug-free friend Doug's single-room occupancy hotel room. Tony is currently homeless. For the past 2 weeks, he has been sleeping on Doug's floor.

   When he was 12 years old, Tony was diagnosed with ADHD by his pediatrician who was consulted about his disruptive behavior in school. He took methylphenidate (Ritalin) prescribed by the pediatrician, which made him feel "more quiet," in his words. When he was 13 years old and his sister was 7, his parents divorced. His father, Steve, left the home and started living with Debbie, whom he later married. Steve kept his children on his company health insurance. Tony felt responsible for the divorce because of all the arguments his parents had concerning how to manage his behavior and poor school performance. During the turmoil in their relationship, his parents did not take him back to the pediatrician, nor to the recommended psychologist, but continued to refill his prescription for methylphenidate. He continued to take it in high school. By this time, Tony stated that the medicine made him "feel energetic, like I didn't need as much sleep." When he was emotionally stable, Tony did well in school.

   Tony had several episodes in high school during which he was unable to go to school. He felt angry and irritable yet tired; he was unable to concentrate mentally, had nightmares, and had difficulty with goal-oriented behavior (mealtime, personal hygiene, doing homework, and meeting friends, which he used to be able to do).

   Tony started drinking alcohol at age 16. He stole his father's liquor, as well as money from his parents to buy beer illegally or alcohol from friends. During these irritable episodes, he increased his drinking in an attempt to feel better. When he was

(continued)

Case Study: Johnson Family *(cont.)*

arrested for driving under the influence of intoxicants at age 18, the court mandated an alcohol use disorder program that had a family counseling component. His father Steve was angry about the arrest and about how this might affect Steve's relationship with his new wife, Debbie. Steve told Tony that if his behavior had a bad effect on Debbie, he would never speak to him again. Although his entire family was encouraged to participate in the program, only Tony's mother Mary, his sister Susie, and his grandfather Thomas (Mary's father) attended. His father, Steve, and stepmother, Debbie, accepted the family teaching literature but did not attend the group counseling sessions. The prescription for methylphenidate was stopped.

Tony stayed in the treatment program because of the legal requirement, but did not believe that he had a problem with alcohol. He stated, "I can quit any time I want to." His sister wanted to protect him, so she minimized the impact of his illness when she described it in the group. His mother did not mention the stealing of money or liquor from the home. His grandfather said, "Boys will be boys. He's healthy and high-spirited. If he says he can control his drinking, he can."

Tony spent the next 2 years having episodes of either agitation or lack of energy and depression. He spent the night sleeping at the houses of various friends and occasionally at his mother's or later his step-father's house. He used alcohol in an attempt to solve his problems and eventually started stealing prescription painkillers from his grandmother Emma. He also bought drugs from a dealer and continued to steal from his family, friends, and their families, and burglarized one family's home while they were away. He stole credit cards and shoplifted at stores to pay for drugs and alcohol.

When his stepmother caught him stealing her jewelry, Tony promised to try rehabilitation again at a facility financed by his father's insurance; this program was a dual diagnosis program. There he was diagnosed with BD and substance use disorder. He was prescribed new medications for mood stabilization. His parents and both stepparents, as well as his sister, participated in the family portion of the program. The family continued in the group portion of the program, even after Tony quit the program early.

Tony stopped taking his mood-stabilizing medications approximately 2 weeks ago when his most recent binge use of methamphetamine started. Currently, his mental health care provider is withholding the mood-stabilizing medications until the methamphetamine is no longer affecting Tony's major systems.

Family Members:

The admitting nurse and the social worker have gleaned the following familial information from Steve, Mary, Debbie, and Harold. The Johnson family genogram is illustrated in Figure 16-1 and the family ecomap is illustrated in Figure 16-2.

Steve is very concerned about his son's health and reminds him that the health care providers have said his son will not survive another year if he continues to use methamphetamines. Steve recognizes his son's depression and anger and feels guilty that he did not notice sooner that Tony was depressed and "self-medicating" with alcohol and drugs. He blames himself for the divorce, which he believes precipitated Tony's alcohol and drug abuse. He also regrets working so much during Tony's

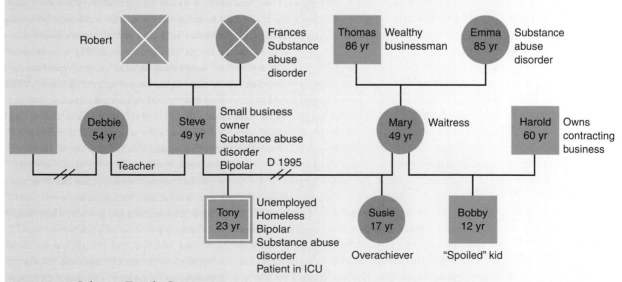

FIGURE 16-1 Johnson Family Genogram

Case Study: Johnson Family *(cont.)*

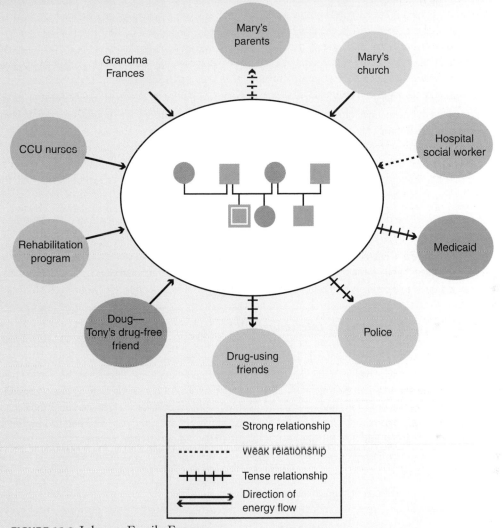

FIGURE 16-2 Johnson Family Ecomap

early years and for ignoring Tony's alcohol use and stealing. Mary initiated the divorce when she discovered Steve was having affairs and using cocaine. Steve was diagnosed at the time of the divorce as having BD, with a manic episode that resulted in his hospitalization. He had also been drinking excessively for years and has alcohol use disorder. He has been clean and sober for 8 months, during which he has been regularly attending Alcoholics Anonymous. His BD is being managed by medications and is stable.

Mary, Tony's mother, became a stay-at-home mom when she gave birth to Tony. She resented that he was not a good student. She went back to work as a server in a restaurant shortly after Susie was born.

Susie has been under pressure all her life to "be good, not like Tony." Unlike Tony, she excels at school and is obedient to her parents and all authority figures. Despite all the comparisons to Tony, she loves her brother and wants to protect him. She does not tell her parents when she knows he breaks the family rules.

Debbie is a better limit-setter than Steve and is often more practical about recognizing and addressing Tony's needs. She is influential with both Steve and Mary in making decisions about Tony. There are no members in her extended family with substance use disorder.

(continued)

Case Study: Johnson Family *(cont.)*

Harold, Tony's stepfather, is 11 years older than Mary and, in many ways, is a father figure for his wife. He dotes on his 12-year-old son and largely ignores his stepson, Tony, and stepdaughter, Susie; he does brag about Susie's successes. He is a successful building contractor and is able to provide a luxurious life for his wife and son.

Susie, 17 years old, is bright and well behaved. Tony calls her the "perfect" child he never was. She is an honor student, talented in music and art, and well-liked by her fellow students and by adults. She worries about Tony and has always tried to please him.

Steve's mother, Frances, died 10 years ago of complications from a liver transplant. She had substance use disorder, which the family never admitted to anyone, even to themselves. Steve's father died when Tony was young. His parents owned a grocery store that they ran as a family.

Mary's parents, Thomas and Emma, live nearby. Thomas is a wealthy but distant businessman who believes that each person is a "master of his own destiny" and should just change behavior if it is a problem. Emma was a stay-at-home wife and mother; she has substance use disorder, mostly alcohol, but takes excessive prescription pain medications as well. Thomas is aware she drinks too much, but protects her every way he can.

Discharge Plans: Tony will be discharged in 3 days, with the discharge diagnosis of acute methamphetamine poisoning resolved.

Family Systems Theory in Relation to the Johnson Family:
The health event the Johnson family is managing will be viewed through the lens of a nurse who used Family Systems Theory as the foundational approach to working with this family. A more detailed discussion of this family nursing system can be found in Chapter 5.

Concept 1—All Parts of the System Are Interconnected:
In the Johnson case, all members of the family are affected by Tony's dual *DSM-5* diagnoses of substance abuse disorder and BD, and his dramatic overdoses and near-death experiences. His father feels enormous guilt and is afraid to confront and set limits with his son for fear of sending him to his death. Steve is humiliated that his son knows that he himself misused drugs. He is much more concerned about the stigma of drug use than that of alcohol use. He is trying to understand what role BD plays in the problems that both Tony and he have. Tony's mother, Mary, believes that she can help Tony change his self-destructive behavior. Tony's stepmother is more realistic because she is not as emotionally attached to Tony, but she worries about the effects of Steve's drug use, and she fears a relapse of Steve's own bipolar symptoms.

Concept 2—The Whole Is More Than the Sum of Its Parts:
In the Johnson family case study, the complexity of the blended family increases the interconnectedness and interdependence of the family members. It is not just parents and children or grandparents and parents, but a complex system involving different permutations of the family relationships that can deteriorate over time as the stress of Tony's illness takes its toll on the entire system.

*Concept 3—All Systems Have Some Form of Boundaries or Border
Between the System and Its Environment:*
In the Johnson family, the normal boundaries of self and others, and of family and outsiders, are dysfunctional. Spousal boundaries are violated by infidelity; parent-child boundaries are violated by theft. When Steve drank alcohol with his son Tony then parent-child boundaries were violated. Some of the boundaries are closed by distant, aloof parents and spouses.

Concept 4—Systems Can Be Further Organized Into Subsystems:
The Johnson family has many subsystems: parent, parent-stepparent, parent-child, grandparent-parent, sibling, grandparent, and in-law. Each of these subsystems can be mobilized to help with the goals defined for the family. Specifically, the mother-father-stepmother-son subsystem will probably prove most influential in discharge planning.

Family Impact:
In the Johnson family, objective impact includes the financial costs of treatment, physical strain and damage, effects on the health of other family members, and disruption in the daily lives of many of the family members. The subjective impact is the enormous guilt and fear felt by the family members, the damage to Tony's mental and social health, the disruption felt by other children in the family, the strain placed on the marriages, and the disrupted family routines, such as regular mealtimes and leisure time.

Case Study: Johnson Family *(cont.)*

Social Support and Stigma:

The Johnson family has been moderately successful in previous generations at hiding the substance abuse and dysfunction. Although more acceptable now than in previous generations, some social stigma is attached to divorce, remarriage, substance use disorder, and mental illness—all of which affect the Johnson family. Methamphetamine use carries a large social stigma today. Family and health care providers need information that is evidence-based to increase the understanding of the immense physical, mental, and social impact this combination of problems has on the family. Providing family members with accurate information about the disorder and the treatments and medications can improve family functioning.

Coping and Resiliency:

The Johnson family is in need of intervention to teach it more successful ways of dealing with Tony's and others' behaviors, and with feelings of worry and concern. Most mental health care providers would suggest that they attend 12-step meetings for families affected by substance use, such as Alcoholics Anonymous and Al-Anon, and that they have family counseling with Tony. All subsystems need help learning more effective coping strategies, from those who remain aloof from the problems to those who become overly enmeshed in the lives of other family members.

Assistance From Mental Health Care Providers:

The Johnson family needs referral to a treatment facility that focuses on the dual diagnosis approach to treatment for the identified client and family members. In addition, the extended family needs counseling concerning the impact of these disorders and the maladaptive coping styles being used. Tony needs treatment for both his substance use disorder and his BD at the same time. These disorders are intertwined and respond poorly when treated in isolation.

Family psychoeducation for the Johnson family would include education about substance use and BDs; coping skills for Tony and the family members, especially in dealing with grief and anger; and effective communication skills to express feelings constructively. Tony would also receive medication teaching about his mood stabilizer.

Mental Health Care Nursing From a Family Systems Perspective:

This section will identify the needs of each member of the Johnson family and address the family as a whole by looking at the family from a Family Systems perspective.

Assessment:

The nurse and a social worker conduct the assessment of the Johnson family with Tony, Steve, Mary, and Debbie. It includes the following:

- *Perception of and understanding of the illness*: The Johnson family has some experience with substance abuse and BD. The diagnosis of BD is newer, and they have a poorer understanding of it alone and combined with substance use. The nurse assesses whether the knowledge is accurate and current.
- *The primary complaint, symptoms, or concerns*: The Johnson family believes that Tony's illness is the family's "problem." In reality, the dysfunctional family dynamics are more central needs. Since this crisis has arisen, the family's biggest concern is Tony's safety. They now fear that Tony will either end up dead or in prison.
- *Physical, developmental, cognitive, mental, and emotional health status*: The Johnson family is in a great deal of emotional pain and is in a crisis state at this time. The family's stress level is at an all-time high.
- *Health history:* The Johnson family has a history of mental health problems but appears to be physically healthy otherwise.
- *Treatment history:* Tony has a history of unsuccessful treatment attempts, with brief periods of abstinence from alcohol and drugs, and minimal treatment for his BD. Tony takes mood-stabilizing medication intermittently but has not had a long-term relationship with a psychiatrist since he was 17.
- *Family, social, cultural, racial, ethnic, and community systems*: The Johnson family systems have been described and are reflected in the ecomap of the family (see Fig. 16-2). Mary is involved with church activities. Tony is in contact with friends from high school in addition to his friends who use drugs.
- *Activities of daily living and health habits*: These activities are seriously disrupted for Steve, Debbie, Mary, and Susie. The stress, worry, and concern they have for Tony, and the time and energy they are using to help Tony find a place to live and get into treatment, are affecting their own abilities to spend time focusing on their own health and well-being.
- *Substance use:* The Johnson family has alcohol, cocaine, and methamphetamine abuse in its history.

(continued)

Case Study: Johnson Family *(cont.)*

- *Coping mechanisms used*: Although some healthy mechanisms are used by the Johnson family, they also use rationalization, projection, denial, and substance use as ways of coping. Susie is coping by making everyone else happy. She is compliant with the demands of everyone else, and may not be making the personal growth during adolescence that she needs to move into a healthy adulthood.
- *Spiritual and religious beliefs or values*: The Johnson family members state they are Christians, but the only family members to attend services or admit to spiritual practices are Steve, Susie, and Mary. Steve uses meditation to maintain focus in his life but has been unable to do so for many months because of his increased time spent on attempting to keep track of Tony.
- *Economic, legal, or other environmental factors that affect health*: Steve's finances have been strained by Tony's illness. Harold and Mary refuse to accept any of the monetary burden of his care, saying that "he needs to take care of himself," but they remain emotionally involved.
- *Health-promoting strengths*: There is obvious love between Tony and his father, and between Tony and his grandfather; this can be mobilized to promote healthy family behaviors and communication.
- *Complementary therapies used*: Tony's friends have recommended acupuncture for his substance use disorder, but he has not been clean long enough to try it. Debbie is trying meditation to ease the stress and is trying to get Steve to join a yoga group with her.
- *Family conflicts*: Numerous unresolved family conflicts continue in the Johnson family.
- *Familial roles and responsibilities*: In the Johnson family, Mary alternates between being overprotective and harsh and critical with her children. Steve is an enabler and unable to set appropriate limits. Susie is pseudomature in her relationship with Tony.
- *Treatment goals*:
  - In the short term, the goals are for the family to identify a family-oriented community resource for people with family members with mental disorders or substance use disorder that they are willing to attend by the time Tony is discharged. The nurse wants Tony to engage in a change conversation (Miller & Rollnick, 2013) in which he lists his own reasons to adhere to his mood stabilizing medications, and at least one strategy from his own life for making adherence possible/easier.
  - The longer-term treatment goals for the Johnson family are to admit Tony into a short-term residential treatment facility and to find a long-term treatment program for families with a member with dual diagnoses. The family desires social support from others with similar experiences, education regarding Tony's ongoing treatment options, and skills training that will help them communicate better with one another and teach them to manage the impact of these disorders on the family in between these intermittent crises.
- **The person's ability to remain safe**: Without long-term treatment and medication management, Tony is at great risk for harm.

Diagnosis:

Tony's dual diagnosis of BD with substance use disorder helps determine the best treatment approach for Tony as an individual. His dual disorder probably began when he was an adolescent. For Tony, he describes the feelings of depression and hopelessness preceding his misuse of drugs.

Family Diagnoses:

It is often said that the "mentally ill" patient is just the "delegate to the convention" for the family; most experts advocate for the inclusion of the family in treatment. In addition to the plan of care that staff nurses have established to address Tony's individual nursing diagnoses, family diagnoses for the Johnson family include the following:

- Compromised family coping related to situational crisis as evidenced by Tony's overdose and hospitalization, the family's disruption in their daily activities, and the increased need for support.
- Dysfunctional family process related to drug abuse, as evidenced by familial conflict and ineffective problem solving.

Case Study: Johnson Family (cont.)

- Ineffective family therapeutic regimen management related to decisional conflict (discharge decision), economic difficulty, and excessive demands on family as evidenced by verbalization of desire to manage Tony's treatment and prevent the negative sequelae of his methamphetamine abuse and untreated BD.

Outcome Identification:

For the Johnson family and Tony, treatment attempts have failed to date, and it appears that Tony will need to aim for abstinence and control of his mental illness to survive. The desired outcomes for the Johnson family include but are not limited to Tony's recovery from his methamphetamine substance use disorder and control of his BD. Outcomes for the family include identifying familial support systems in the community, exploring financial options for paying for Tony's treatment, making a family decision regarding the best treatment option available for Tony, facilitating Tony's acceptance into a residential treatment facility, expressing anger appropriately, discussing openly substance abuse and other "family secrets," setting limits on inappropriate and enabling behavior, and honoring individual and family boundaries and needs.

Planning:

For the Johnson family, an integrated program in the community is most appropriate but not easy to find and often quite expensive. Discharge planning for the Johnson family includes the following: The family will be given information about appropriate referrals for residential care, the family (and Tony) will seek out and accept an appropriate referral, and Tony will be discharged to the referral facility. The family will also be given referrals to the Meth Family and Friends Support Group, as well as the NAMI. The family will also be referred for counseling to a therapist/counselor who is available through Steve's insurance plan so family members may work on their communication and coping skills, develop more appropriate boundaries with one another, and address some of their own needs.

Implementation:

Tony and his family accepted a referral to a Volunteers of America drug-free facility/treatment program in which family members participate on a regular basis. This program is free to Tony as long as he continues to work at the facility. He was willing to accept this placement, and it did not burden Steve economically. Other discharge plans were also effectively implemented.

Evaluation:

Follow-up is necessary to determine the effectiveness of the referral in assisting the family to function more appropriately, helping Tony to be drug free, and providing treatment for Tony's BD.

Benefits of Involving Family:

In the Johnson family, Tony is reaching out for help from his family. He has been unsuccessful in receiving and accepting treatment on his own, and he needs the resources of his family (insurance and finances) to get the treatment he needs. The family needs him healthy to improve its self-image and its own successful functioning.

Barriers to Involving Family:

Many of the barriers to involving the Johnson family are a result of the family dynamics that the family exhibits. The family has a pattern of blaming Tony for family problems and then rescuing him during periods of crisis and has difficulty setting appropriate limits and insisting that Tony take responsibility for his actions. The family members tend to become overly involved during some periods and remain aloof at others, resulting in inconsistent participation. They are in need of long-term partnership with a treatment team. Tony's lack of commitment to treatment hinders any type of healthy long-term relationship being established with his family. In addition, Steve may experience a sense of guilt that Tony may have inherited the BD from him, and he may need counseling to express some of these feelings. The stress of Tony's illness and recent crisis may exacerbate Steve's own disorder.

Case Study: Anderson Family

The following brief case study illustrates how a school nurse's interaction with a student led to psychoeducation and support for members of the entire family. The Anderson family consists of a grandmother and the two older children she is raising. See Figure 16-3 for the family genogram.

Karen, age 14, has an older brother, Tom, who is 21 and still lives at home. Tom was diagnosed with paranoid schizophrenia when he was 17. Their grandmother, Ellen, is raising Karen and Tom because both of their parents were killed in a motor vehicle accident 5 years ago. Ellen is 67 and is a retired schoolteacher with a limited income. Karen seldom brings friends to the house because she does not want to be embarrassed by her brother. Tom has been acting paranoid and frequently mumbles sentences under his breath that don't make any sense to Karen. Karen is aware that the psychiatric mental health nurse practitioner (PMHNP) is in the process of regulating his psychiatric medications but she thinks that things will just never get better. Karen is afraid that she's going to develop the same traits as her brother when she gets older and worries that her grandmother won't be able to take care of both of them. Karen's grandmother takes Tom to his psychiatric medication appointments and also to individual therapy and is preoccupied with the thought that she is going to have to take care of Tom for the rest of her life—she loves Tom but had been looking forward to living independently and doing things with her friends.

The school nurse was aware of Karen's living situation and asked Karen to come and see her after school. The nurse did a brief assessment (see Figure 16-4 for the family ecomap) and was able to help Karen voice her fears and concerns about her brother's disorder. She spent some time teaching Karen about schizophrenia and treatments. Karen felt relieved to be able to talk to someone and learn more information that helped her understand why her brother did and said things that did not make sense to her. The nurse was aware of a local NAMI chapter that had a separate parent and sibling support group for families who had a family member with schizophrenia. Reluctantly, Karen went to a meeting where she was relieved to hear the stories from other kids her age and was surprised to learn that they had similar experiences. Karen's grandmother hesitatingly went to a support group—she had driven Karen to the NAMI meeting and sat in the car and eventually decided to attend a meeting herself. Karen and her grandmother eventually began to talk more openly about their worries and concerns.

Tom's PMHNP learned from Tom that his sister and grandmother were attending NAMI support groups. The PMHNP asked Tom if it would be okay if Karen and his grandmother could come to one of his appointments and he agreed. The PMHNP spent time explaining the purpose and adverse effects of the medications Tom was taking and encouraged Karen and Ellen to

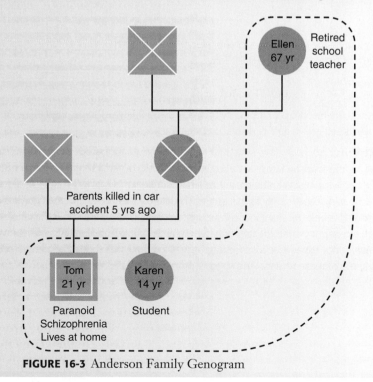

FIGURE 16-3 Anderson Family Genogram

Case Study: Anderson Family *(cont.)*

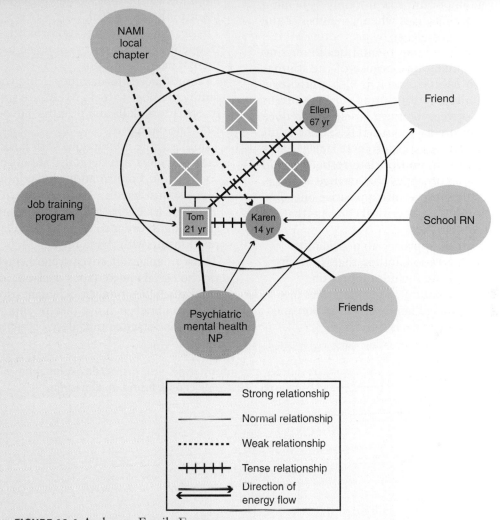

FIGURE 16-4 Anderson Family Ecomap

contact her if they noticed changes in his behavior that might suggest his symptoms were increasing or he was having a side effect from the medications.

As Tom became stabilized on his medication he began to be more involved in communicating with his sister and grandmother. Eventually, Karen became more comfortable bringing her friends to the house. Ellen was able to learn more about community training programs that Tom could attend during the day to learn a skill that could eventually lead to a job. The job-training program was part of a community grant and so did not add a financial burden to Ellen. Ellen was now able to do more things during the day with her friends. Psychoeducation decreased not only the family stress as a unit, but also Karen and Ellen's stress. The school nurse was instrumental in providing psychoeducation, which led Karen and Emma to peer-led support groups.

SUMMARY

Nurses play an important role not only by helping families manage their lives when a member of the family has an MHC, but also by preventing MHCs from occurring. Providing mental health nursing care may be challenging because of the stigmas associated with MHCs, but it is also a privilege. The nurse-family relationship is very important in effecting positive outcomes: Nurses can reduce stigmas; correct myths about MHCs; offer family-centered interventions that promote family health, including referrals to appropriate resources; and provide nursing approaches that change a potentially negative experience into a positive one. The following points highlight critical concepts that are addressed in this chapter:

- A family-focused approach to providing mental health care to families, that is, viewing the family as a unit, includes supporting families in their natural caregiving roles in ways that encourage family collaboration and choice in treatment decisions.

- There are improved outcomes for the person with an MHC if the health care provider collaborates with families when providing treatment to the individual.
- Physical and/or mental comorbidities are frequently present when someone has a mental health condition.
- Common needs for families living with a family member with an MHC are support, information, skills and training, advocacy, and referral sources.
- Families value interactions with health care providers that demonstrate openness, cooperation, confirmation, and continuity.
- Nurses must have an attitude toward family members that is perceived as nonblaming and accepting in order to establish a collaborative relationship with the family.
- There are many effective psychotherapeutic and psychological interventions available, including family therapies, mother and infant psychotherapies, and brief cognitive therapy appropriate to the age and stage of child development.

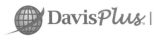 | For additional resources and information, visit **http://davisplus.fadavis.com**. References and Suggested Web sites can be found on Davis*Plus*.

Chapter 17

Families and Community and Public Health Nursing

Linda L. Eddy, PhD, RN, ARNP

Annette Bailey, PhD, RN

Dawn Doutrich, PhD, RN

Critical Concepts

- Community is a mind-set, not a place.
- Transitioning from individually focused nursing care to care of families and communities is a process.
- Community and public health nurses care for families in a variety of settings.
- Community and public health nurses view families as subunits of the community or as clients in the context of the community.
- Community and public health nurses aim to meet the holistic needs of families and communities while targeting prioritized health needs.
- Healthy families contribute to healthy communities.
- Community and public health family nursing is grounded in social justice and culturally safe, ethical practice.
- Rather than blaming families for their situations, community and public health nurses think upstream to consider how social, political, economic, and environmental conditions affect families' health choices and outcomes.
- Using a combination of relational collaboration and health promotion strategies and principles, community and public health nurses strive to partner with families to assist with all levels of healthy change.
- Nurses foster interconnectedness among families in the community.
- Family interventions in the community are targeted toward primary, secondary, and tertiary prevention.
- The nurse-family relationship is central in interventions at all three levels of prevention.
- Community and public health nursing are evidence based and policy driven.
- Interventions for families are planned, implemented, and evaluated from a health promotion perspective.
- Population health goes beyond the traditional definition of public health by focusing on the distribution of health within a defined group and considering ways in which a variety of health determinants affect those populations.
- Community and public health nurses are advocates for improving population health, partnering with families and communities to develop data-based programs designed to improve population health outcomes.

What does health mean to you? What are the indicators you use to conclude that you are either healthy or unhealthy? Different people will apply different indicators of health. A definition of health set by the World Health Organization (WHO) in 1948 is that health is "a state of complete physical, mental, and social well-being and not merely the absence of disease or infirmity" (WHO, 1948, p. 1). This definition implies that achieving health is much more than treating diseases. Health is not just physical, it is also emotional and social. Community and public health nurses understand that creating a balance in the various dimensions of people's lives—culture, society, economic, politics, and their physical environment—is crucial in helping them to cultivate health (WHO, 1986). Community and public health nurses recognize that disease patterns are a result of interactions between human beings and their environments and this understanding guides their actions. Community and public health nursing practice is based on an understanding of population health. Population health adds to the traditional public health perspective of responsibility for overall health by examining the distribution of health outcomes within particular groups (Kindig, 2007). This more holistic understanding of our practice demands that we engage communities and populations in envisioning what health means to them. But how do community and public health nurses transform this understanding of health into health promotion for families?

A broad definition of *family* guides community and public health nurses toward inclusiveness in working with and understanding complex family systems. Family, for purposes of this chapter, comprises two or more individuals who depend on one another for emotional, physical, and economic support. The members of the family are self-defined.

Along with this broad definition of family, community and public health nurses utilize two prevalent schools of thought. One view sees the family as the unit of care and the community as context. The other view focuses on the community as client with the family as context. The commonality between these views is that family, and thus family health, is indistinguishably linked to community. Therefore, health promotion actions should be concurrent and encompassing for both contexts. Identifying family needs and developing a plan of care for families cannot be done in isolation from the broader context of their surroundings and experiences. When working with families, nurses need to consider environmental, psychological, and behavioral health issues, as well as those of a more physiological nature. Doing so recognizes that family health problems have contextual roots.

The social determinants of health (SDOH) have a significant impact on health outcomes (Braveman & Gottlieb, 2014; Heiman & Artiga, 2015). The WHO (2017) has defined SDOH as the conditions in which individuals are born, grow, live, work, and age. The WHO definition of SDOH goes on to state that these conditions are shaped by the distribution of money, power, and resources, globally, nationally, and locally. In short, SDOH constitute much of the individual's and family's contextual roots. It is important for nurses to understand the impact that SDOH have on the families they work with in order to include these determinants in their assessments. A more detailed discussion of SDOH comes later in this chapter.

It is important to note that for some individuals, the definition of self is wrapped up in the family (Doutrich, Dekker, Spuck, & Hoeksel, 2014). For example, *familismo* has been reported as a typical feature of Hispanic families (Smith-Morris, Morales-Campos, Alverez, & Turner, 2013). *Familismo*, according to the classic work of Sabogal, Marín, Otero-Sabogal, Marín, and Pérez-Stable (1987), includes three specific types of value orientations: (1) obligations to provide support; (2) perceived high levels of help and support from family; and (3) the perception of relatives as behavioral and attitudinal referents, meaning that one's family determines how one is perceived and perceives the world. Caring for such families will require attention to these values, and to the understanding that family is the unit of care rather than just the individual. For the community and public health family nurse, this definition of self that is inclusive of family will influence the provision of competent and culturally congruent family care.

Healthy communities are comprised of healthy families. Hence, families as units of relationship are important components of communities, and undoubtedly are heavily affected by their community's state of health. The word *community* means more than just a geographical space; it is a group of people who share similar interests, needs, and outcomes, regardless of geographical location (Young & Wharf Higgins, 2012). Community and public health nurses understand the effects that communities can have on individuals and families, and recognize that a community's health is reflected in the health experiences of its members and their families (Canadian Public Health Association [CPHA], 2010; Institute of Medicine (IOM), 2012). Issues of violence, homelessness, unemployment, unclean physical environments, unsupportive relationships, and poor access to needed resources (i.e., food, shelter) are just a few insignia of an unhealthy community. These issues are inextricably linked to the health of families. Promoting and sustaining health for families means helping them to tap into their personal strength, access social and economic resources, and cope with stressors (CPHA, 2010). Community and public health nurses use health promotion strategies, such as facilitating access to resources, to improve the health of families.

Community and public health nursing places an interest in the social, political, and economic aspects of health to help individuals, families, and communities gain a higher degree of harmony within the mind, body, and soul. A community or public health nurse who visits a new mother in her home and realizes that a bed used for the newborn baby is infested with bedbugs cannot simply focus on the physical health of the mom and baby. In the same way, it is necessary to focus on the ways that broader social contexts and political decisions create and exacerbate homelessness. Paying attention to the lack of resources caused by poverty becomes an essential aspect of the nurse's role in promoting health for families. In fact, the degree to which nurses can contribute positively to the well-being of vulnerable families in communities depends on their convictions and commitments to modify these factors, as well as society's support and recognition of the importance of their work.

This chapter offers a description of community health nursing in promoting the health of families in communities. It begins with a definition of community health nursing, and follows with a discussion of concepts and principles that guide the work of these nurses, the roles they enact in working with families and communities, and the various settings where they work. This discussion is organized around a visual representation of community health nursing. The chapter ends with a discussion of current trends in community and public health nursing.

WHAT IS COMMUNITY AND PUBLIC HEALTH NURSING?

According to the CPHA (2010), community and public health nursing involves a synthesis of nursing theory and public health science that focuses on population health promotion and primary health care with the intention of maintaining and promoting health, preventing illnesses and injuries, and developing communities. Congruently, the American Public Health Association (APHA, 2013) defines public health nursing as the practice of promoting and protecting the health of populations using knowledge from nursing, social, and public health sciences. The APHA (2013) further defines key characteristics of public health nursing practice as (1) a focus on the health needs of an entire population, including inequities and the unique needs of subpopulations; (2) assessment of population health using a comprehensive, systematic approach; (3) attention to multiple determinants of health; (4) an emphasis on primary prevention; and (5) application of interventions at all levels—individuals, families, communities, and the systems that have an impact on their health.

In 2013 the American Association of Colleges of Nursing (AACN) released an important supplement to the Baccalaureate Essentials for Nursing Education, identified as the *Recommended Baccalaureate Competencies and Curricular Guidelines for Public Health Nursing*. As the organization guiding professional nursing curricula in the United States, their recommendations are consistent with the APHA (2013) and the IOM (2012) report and focus on competencies and skills needed for community and public health nurses currently and in the future.

These definitions communicate the critical role of community and public health nurses in fostering care for families beyond a clinical perspective. In their process of work, community and public health nurses rely on various concepts/principles to promote health for individuals, families, and communities. Drawing from various health promotion frameworks and set standards of practice, these nurses enact these concepts/principles in various settings, with modifications based on families and communities' needs. This is done through a process of empowerment, with the aim of achieving improved health and empowered families. Empowerment

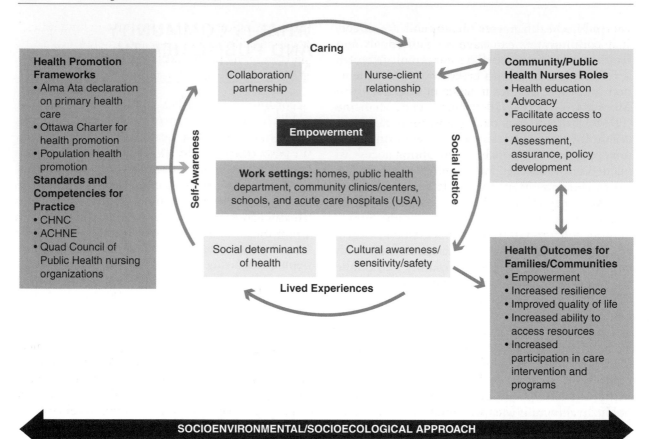

FIGURE 17-1 Contextualizing Community and Public Health Nursing

enables families to express aspirations and develop their capacity to lead a fulfilling life. This work could include developing strategies for improved engagement with clients, adopting partnership models for all work with clients, and challenging institutional and professional barriers (Piper, 2014). The model in Figure 17-1 helps to contextualize community and public health nursing.

HEALTH PROMOTION FRAMEWORKS, STANDARDS, AND PRINCIPLES

Health promotion and disease prevention are foundational to community and public health nurses' work (see Chapter 6 for more in-depth information on family health promotion). Interventions for families are planned, implemented, and evaluated from a health promotion perspective. From this perspective, nurses help to reduce health inequities by engaging

families in processes that promote their control over their own health. This includes developing families' skills, increasing participation in their care process, and improving access to resources. To prevent illness and injuries, nurses employ health education to help families modify lifestyles/behaviors (e.g., healthy eating, wearing bicycle helmets/seat belts, tobacco use prevention, and physical activity). Nurses know that for families to modify their behaviors, they must address specific barriers beyond their control, such as lack of money, lack of time, and stress. Rather than blaming families for their situations, community and public health nurses shift their thinking and focus on population health, which is concerned with changing the social, economic, political, and environmental conditions that affect families' health choices and outcomes.

The nurse can intervene in public policy at the community, organizational, and/or the individual level to help improve outcomes for individuals and families. For the most sustainable outcomes, nurses rely on the socioenvironmental/socioecological approach pictured in Figure 17-1 to guide their actions in addressing factors that impede families' choices to improve their health. The socioenvironmental/ socioecological model is based on systems theory and is grounded in an understanding of health as influenced by interrelationships between personal and environmental factors (Townsend & Foster, 2011; Young & Wharf Higgins, 2012). Focusing on these environmental factors, including the SDOH (U.S. Department of Health and Human Services, 2016), shifts the blame from the family to conditions in which they live and choices that they do, or do not, have.

The health of vulnerable families in various settings in society (e.g., homeless families, refugees, victims of intimate partner violence, and families in poverty) is affected negatively by many outside circumstances. An understanding of the factors that negatively affect family health, and strategies to modify these factors, is a priority for the role of community and public health nurses. The use of health promotion strategies is crucial to helping nurses to fulfill this priority. For example, the Breastfeeding Coalition of Oregon (2012) used the socioecological framework to outline who/what influences a mother's breastfeeding success and how public health providers can influence these influencers. Using the socioecological model, nurses are able to identify and address influences at the individual level (e.g., culture, lack of personal breastfeeding skills); interpersonal level (e.g., lack of support from family and friends, lack of encouragement from health care providers); community/ environmental level (e.g., neighborhood stress, lack of community breastfeeding accommodations, workplaces, and hospitals); and organizational level (e.g., public health organizations, pediatric groups, and the formula industry). Community and public health nurses can target these influencers using various health promotion strategies. At the individual level, nurses need to learn about cultural-specific barriers and needs and build mothers' skills in breastfeeding. At the interpersonal level, nurses can provide education and facilitate access to support services to key influencers to support mothers' breastfeeding efforts. At the community/environment level, community and public health nurses can get involved in advocacy activities such as organizing community activities during World Breastfeeding Week, disseminating breastfeeding materials at workplaces, and helping employers understand and initiate breastfeeding-friendly practices. Finally, at

the organizational level, nurses can employ advocacy, coalition building, lobbying, and program evaluation skills targeting public health organizations, pediatric groups, and the formula industry.

Health Promotion Frameworks

Whether working with individuals, families, or a community, nurses use key health promotion frameworks to guide their work: (1) the Alma Ata Declaration on Primary Health Care, (2) the Ottawa Charter for Health Promotion, and (3) the Population Health Promotion Model. Although various health promotion documents exist, the following three frameworks remain central to health promotion interventions with families and communities.

Alma Ata Declaration on Primary Health Care

The Alma Ata Declaration on Primary Health Care (WHO, 1978) laid the foundation for subsequent health promotion frameworks. It proposed five interconnected primary health care principles: health promotion, accessibility, public participation, appropriate technology, and intersectoral collaboration. The principles are based on access to health and health care, equity, and empowerment. Because families' SDOH influence how they access resources, manage chronic conditions, and engage in healthy behaviors, addressing the SDOH for families by integrating primary health care principles is an integral component of nurses' work. For example, community and public health nurses who work with families to increase access to needed resources that are cost or distance-prohibitive are practicing the primary health care principle of accessibility.

Ottawa Charter for Health Promotion

The Ottawa Charter for Health Promotion (WHO, 1986) proposed five overarching strategies: develop personal skills, create supportive environments, build healthy public policy, strengthen community action, and reorient health services. The strategies are intended to enable families and communities to increase control over and improve their health. Using these strategies, nurses work with families to address their physical, mental, and social needs, and attain prerequisites of health, such as shelter, food, sustainable resources, social justice, and equity. For example, to allow newcomers to acquire and sustain needed resources, nurses may facilitate personal skill development in resume writing, job seeking, and interviews for them to acquire employment.

Population Health Promotion Model

The Population Health Promotion Model (Hamilton & Bhatti, 1996) draws on two decades of health promotion knowledge to guide practical actions. Key assumptions of this model include the recognition of determinants of health, the use of knowledge gained from research and practice, collaboration with families about the most appropriate actions to care for them, and building relationships with families based on mutual respect and caring, rather than on professional power. In addition to incorporating these assumptions into their work, nurses applying this model are able to focus on the concerns of at-risk groups, such as youth and women in at-risk families. The population health model focuses on the specific issues that put populations at risk. Interventions to modify these issues are targeted at a broad social, political, and economic level, and tailored to meet the needs of groups at the community and family level. For example, the older adult population is victim to ageist assumptions and treatment in society that may infringe on their social engagement and integration. Knowing this, nurses can educate communities and families about ways to prevent age discrimination and promote the health of older adults.

Health Promotion Standards of Practice

To be effective in their roles, community and public health nurses integrate a broad range of competencies and interrelated standards of practice in their work. In Canada, community health nurses work within the Canadian Community Health Nursing Professional Practice Model outlined by the Community Health Nurses of Canada (CHNC) (CHNC, 2011). Seven standards are set by CHNC:

- Health Promotion, Prevention, and Health Protection
- Health Maintenance
- Restoration and Palliation
- Professional Relationships
- Capacity Building
- Access and Equity
- Professional Responsibility and Accountability (CHNC, 2011)

In addition, Core Competencies for Public Health in Canada (CPHA, 2010) provides a baseline for nurses to fulfill effective public health functions. These standards/competencies guide community and public health nurses in delivering acceptable, safe, and ethical care in an effort to protect, preserve, and promote the health of families (CHNC, 2011).

Standards/competencies are also an integral part of U.S. community and public health nursing practice. In the United States, community and public health nursing practice at the generalist and advanced or specialist level is competency based, and is divided into three tiers of practice: the public health nursing generalist, the public health nursing specialist or manager, and the public health nursing organization leader or administrator (Quad Council of Public Health Nursing Organizations, 2011). Likewise, core competencies for public health professionals are comprised of three tiers of practice (Council on Linkages between Academia and Public Health Practice, 2014). Partnering with communities, populations, and organizations is essential for public health practice at all levels and is a primary principle of public health nursing practice (American Nurses Association [ANA], 2013; Quad Council of Public Health Nursing Organizations, 2016). In addition to the previously identified core competencies, the AACN's *Recommended Baccalaureate Competencies and Curricular Guidelines for Public Health Nursing* have informed nurse educators preparing community and public health nurses for now and the future. Clearly, the role of the community and public health nurse has been an evolving one with collaboration and partnership (relational skill building including cultural sensitivity) at the core and the ability to evaluate outcomes (understanding data collection and analysis) as essential.

Public health nursing competencies include analytic and assessment skills, policy development/program planning skills, communication skills, cultural competency skills, community dimensions of practice (using an ecological perspective), public health sciences skills, financial planning and management skills, and leadership and systems thinking skills (Quad Council of Public Health Nursing Organizations, 2011).

Principles in the Process of Community and Public Health Nurses' Work

Underlying the role of the community health/public health nurse in any context is a focus on maintenance and promotion of health and prevention of illnesses and injuries. These concepts and principles include, but are not limited to, the SDOH, cultural awareness/sensitivity/safety, collaboration/partnership, nurse-client relationship, and empowerment. These principles are rooted in the values of caring, social justice, self-awareness, and honoring of families' and communities' lived experiences.

Social Determinants of Health

When working with families and communities, one of the most important concepts that influence community and public health nurses' thinking and action is SDOH.

These SDOH, or conditions necessary for living, can include factors such as education, income and unemployment, climate change, social support and status, culture, housing, childhood development, planetary sustainability, and access to health services (Divakaran, 2016; Goodman, 2016; Mikkonen & Raphael, 2010; Stamler & Gabriel, 2012). These and other determinants shape peoples' vulnerability, put them at risk for illnesses, and influence their social status and the level of respect they gain in society. For example, vulnerability to homelessness is shaped by complex and connected determinants of health such as any or all of the following issues: mental health challenges, substance abuse, precarious immigration status, and domestic and sexual abuse, intricately tied to poverty that requires global legislative changes (Mackie, 2015). Social injustice occurs when the health outcomes of individuals, groups, or communities are disproportionally affected because of differences in access and exposure to opportunities (e.g., education, employment).

The effects of the SDOH have been found to have a greater impact on health than behavioral factors, such as smoking and dietary habits (Divakaran, 2016; Goodman, 2016; Mikkonen & Raphael, 2010). Because of this significant influence on health equity, it is critical that community and public health nurses recognize and address the SDOH as the root cause of many issues faced by families and communities. For instance, community and public health nurses in Toronto, Ontario, working in the *Investing in Families Program* (Table 17-1), provide resources, mental health care, and other support to sole-parent families with children between the ages of 6 and 18 years who are receiving social assistance. For families in this program, determinants of health can be many and interrelated. So, community and public health nurses target prioritized health needs while trying to meet the holistic needs of families.

Key determinants of health needs assessed by nurses would include emotional, economic, employment, educational, housing, and mental health needs.

Cultural Awareness, Sensitivity, and Safety

Community and public health nurses will often find themselves working with a culturally diverse community. Within this diversity, often there are also inequalities between different groups. Social determinants frequently are predictors of health disparities (U.S. Department of Health and Human Services, 2016). Moreover, a report by the IOM found that ethnic and racial minority populations "tend to receive a lower quality of health care" (Smedley, Stith, & Nelson, 2003, p. 1) than the majority of populations even when access and income were controlled. And, although the IOM "Unequal Treatment" report came out in 2003, recent studies are still finding unequal treatment even when access is improved. For example, Shaw and Santry (2015) conducted a retrospective study of more than 49,000 patients dependent on ventilators at 185 academic medical centers in the United States. Early tracheostomy for these patients is associated with increased survival. Yet, patients who were women, African American, Hispanic, and/or on Medicaid were all found to be less likely to receive early tracheostomy. The reasons for this and the findings of unequal treatment related to other conditions such as diabetes (Adeola, 2012) are complex but include bias (implicit and explicit), time pressures, and lack of language and cultural understanding (Smedley et al., 2003; Wyatt, Laderman, Botwinick, Mate, & Whittington, 2016). Rectifying these inequalities is not as simple as the nurse developing cultural competencies, because each individual, family, and community will have variations in values and practices based on their unique experiences (Browne et al., 2009). That is, minority populations and diverse communities are heterogeneous. There is wide variation within groups as well as between them.

It is important for nurses working with diverse populations to reflect on similarities and differences, and to undertake nurse-client relationships from that place of understanding. Because community and public health nurses work with people of diverse cultural backgrounds in various settings, it is crucial for them to engage in continuous reflective practice that explores their values and beliefs, as well as those of the groups/families they serve. This reflection can lead to sensitive, client-centered care.

Table 17-1 Examples of Community and Public Health Nursing

Name of Program	Program Description	Role of the Community/ Public Health Nurse	Specific Example of Programming	Interprofessional Program Collaboration
Healthy Baby Healthy Children	To enable all children to attain and sustain optimal health and developmental potential in the areas of • Positive parenting • Breastfeeding • Healthy family dynamics • Healthy eating, healthy weights, and physical activity • Growth and development	Assessments Referrals and recommendations Service coordination Supportive counseling Health promotion Health teaching Advocacy	Supports families with children from 0–4 years old Assesses growth and development, mother-child attachment Links and refers to various community agencies	Family home visitors Registered dietitians Nutrition promotion consultants Community nutrition educators High-risk consultants Health promotion consultants Mental health nurse consultants Infant hearing screeners Family support worker/social workers Speech-language pathologist Program evaluators
Mental Health Promotion	To promote mental health in Toronto's diverse communities through competent clinical and consultative practice along with education, both internally to Toronto Public Health (TPH) programs and externally to relevant community agencies	The mental health nurse consultant provides consultation to a variety of internal and external programs Education and training	Using a narrative approach, the mental health promotion team focuses on suicide prevention, violence prevention, and mental health promotion	Examples of internal consultations Healthy communities Chronic disease prevention Healthy families Communicable disease control Healthy environments Examples of external consultations Children's Aid Society Parks, Forestry, and Recreation Shelter, support, and housing Toronto social services Toronto community housing cooperation
Investing in Families	To improve the economic, health, and social status of select families receiving social assistance in Toronto Overall goal of investing in family public health nursing service is to meet the health needs of select, vulnerable families receiving social assistance in Toronto To promote healthy lifestyles To increase personal resilience To improve physical and mental health To enhance social and community supports To improve the family's circumstances through greater access to employment training and supports	Assessments Referrals and recommendations Service coordination Supportive counseling Health promotion Health teaching Advocacy	Supports families with children from 6–18 years Receives referrals from Toronto Social Services Conducts detailed assessments Uses a strengths-based approach assessing the positive assets of the client	Toronto Social Services caseworker Public health nurse Health promotion consultant Mental health nurse consultant Recreationist

Table 17-1 Examples of Community and Public Health Nursing *(cont.)*

Name of Program	Program Description	Role of the Community/ Public Health Nurse	Specific Example of Programming	Interprofessional Program Collaboration
School Health	To enhance the physical, mental, social, and spiritual well-being of all the members of the school community To strengthen the capacity of school communities to achieve optimal health To enhance resilience in all school-age children and youth in the city of Toronto	Develop working relationships with all members of the school community to promote healthy schools Work with school communities to increase their capacity to identify health issues, develop and implement a plan of action, evaluate, and build on their successes Participate in existing health committees and advocate for the establishment of new school health committees Engage students and parents in healthy school initiatives Identify and consult with school communities on emerging health issues and trends Link between schools and TPH services and programs Partner with community organizations that support healthy schools	Liaison public health nurse establishes a healthy school committee that assesses the needs of the school in a comprehensive manner The work of the school health committee includes • Creating a shared vision for a healthy school • Assessing strengths and needs of the school community • Prioritizing the issues • Developing a plan • Implementing the plan • Monitoring and evaluating the plan • Celebrating success	School administration School boards Teachers Students Parent council Internal programs in TPH Community agencies

Many families that community and public health nurses care for may not speak English in their homes or have other cultural differences with providers that challenge the provision of culturally congruent care. Increasing the numbers of bilingual, bicultural, underrepresented providers is identified as one of the IOM solutions aimed at improving health disparities, and a way for institutions/organizations providing care to demonstrate cultural sensitivity. There are many benefits to promoting ethnic diversity in the health care workforce. After graduation, minority health care providers often return to work in medically underserved areas. When providers share a similar ethnic or racial background with their patients, the result is higher patient satisfaction and higher quality health outcomes (Noone, Wros, Cortez, Najjar, & Magdalino, 2016). Refugee families may comprise a subset of those with limited or no English abilities that community and public health family nurses will serve (Wojnar, 2015). It is the professional responsibility of nurses to plan ahead for visits and ensure that families understand what is going on in meetings, through the use of skilled interpreters.

Added to this context, refugee families, in particular, may have survived war, disaster, and devastating trauma such as torture, rape, and/or watching family members or others die. Often, refugee families are enduring post-traumatic stress disorder, depression, or both, which may intensify the life challenges they face. In understanding the family's context, nurses need to be aware of not only how to satisfy language deficits, but understand how both theirs and the families' cultural backgrounds and perspectives influence the caring process.

Community and public health nurses can care for culturally diverse populations through the practice of cultural safety. Originally developed in New Zealand, cultural safety goes beyond cultural sensitivity and competence to address the attitudes of health care providers, with an emphasis on discrimination, power, and the effects of colonization (Doutrich, Arcus, Dekker, Spuck, & Pollock-Robinson, 2012; National Aboriginal Health Organization [NAHO], 2009; Nursing Council of New Zealand, 2011).

Culturally safe care involves the nurse's reflection and self-awareness of his or her attitudes and beliefs with regard to "nationality, culture, age, sex, political and religious beliefs and sexual orientation" (Doutrich et al., 2012; NAHO, 2009, para 4; Nursing Council of New Zealand; 2011). This approach shifts the focus from the nurses' expertise to the expertise of the community, which defines whether the care has been safe or not (Brascoupé & Waters, 2009; Doutrich, Dekker, Spuck, & Hoeksel, 2014). Culturally safe care is provided to all within their cultural norms and values, and in a manner that garners their trust and promotes their empowerment. For example, in promoting health for Aboriginal families hurt by colonization processes, community and public health nurses would invite the families to partner with them. This process helps to build their capacity and facilitate trust (Brascoupé & Waters, 2009). Whereas culturally safe care can yield trust, open communication, and empowerment, culturally unsafe care can foster humiliation and disempowerment (Browne et al., 2009; NAHO, 2009; Nursing Council of New Zealand, 2011). Promoting culturally safe care requires that nurses are sensitive to cultural differences, aware of their own cultural values, and knowledgeable enough to engage in culturally safe practices as defined by the clients.

Collaboration and Partnership

Community and public health nurses are usually one member of a team promoting health and well-being for families and communities. They work in collaboration with other key members of a community/family team. These collaborative relationships are crucial to reaching "a common vision to deliver care" (Betker & Bewick, 2012, p. 30). Nurses' participation in such collaborations depends on the type and purpose for which they were formed. For example, nurses working on a school health team collaborate with various stakeholders—teachers, parents, school board, government officials, and others—to promote health in schools. On such teams nurses may share specialized public health knowledge, share needed resources, interface with external partners, and/or contribute to decision-making processes. The essence of these collaborations is to share knowledge and power among key stakeholders to produce solutions that no one partner could achieve independently. Collaborations are ways in which nurses honor families and community members' lived experience. They realize that health solutions are similar to large puzzles. The lived experiences, knowledge, and expertise that other members bring to the team represent an important piece of the puzzle toward better health outcomes for families/communities.

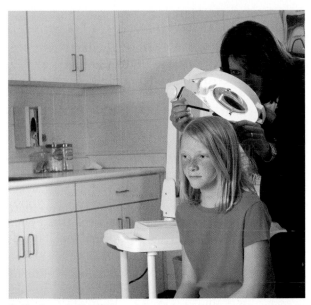

© iStock.com/beichh4046

Interprofessional collaboration refers to a collaborative partnership between two or more different health and social care professions who regularly come together to solve problems or provide services (Interprofessional Education Collaborative Expert Panel, 2011). When multiple providers and patients communicate and consider each other's perspectives they can better address several factors that affect the health of individuals, families, and communities (Sullivan, Kiovsky, Mason, Hill, & Dukes, 2015). One example of interprofessional collaboration can be found in Ontario, Canada's Family Health Teams. These primary care teams feature different professionals working in collaboration with each other and the families. These teams are in existence to address the shortage of family physicians in Ontario, increase access to and quality of care, and decrease the number of individuals visiting the emergency department for minor issues. Rather than going to see a family physician, residents of Ontario are able to receive primary care services from an entire team of health care providers in the community. A family health team might include a physician, registered nurse, nurse practitioner, pharmacist, social worker, and dietitian. Instead of being referred elsewhere, patients of the family health team are able to acquire services from this team, which collaborates on the provision of their care. As another example, the *Investing in Families Program* involves collaboration between various divisions across the city of Toronto—Parks, Forestry and Recreation, Toronto

Social Services, Children Services, and Public Health. At any point, public health nurses can collaborate with any of these partners in the provision of care for families in the program.

Supporting families in their journey toward healthy change within their lives requires the development of collaborative partnerships between nurses and individuals, families, and communities (CHNC, 2011). Because of the complex nature of the SDOH, community and public health nurses will find themselves engaging in interdisciplinary teamwork. These interdisciplinary teams feature collaboration between individuals from a broad variety of disciplines, such as sociology, economics, education, human services, government, and health sciences (Reeves, Lewin, Espin, & Zwarenstein, 2010). The collaborative relationships and partnerships with other professionals, disciplines, clients, families, and communities are critical to addressing the complexity of modern health care, because no single profession can accomplish this alone (Reeves et al., 2010).

Nurse-Client Relationship With Families and Communities

Community and public health nurses caring for families in the community rely on the nurse-client relationship as the foundation of their care (Porr, 2013). This relationship allows the nurse to maximize client involvement, recognize strengths and available resources, and ultimately facilitate empowerment at the individual, family, and community level (CHNC, 2011). Within these professional nurse-client relationships, the development of trust is critical. For example, the early phase of home visiting programs is based on the development of trust through helping clients identify problems, engage in mutual problem solving, make decisions about necessary health services, and adopt health-promoting behaviors. This trust-building phase is crucial to the success of a program such as this, because longer-term home visiting programs seem to be more effective than shorter-term ones. However, for some clients with traumatic pasts developing trust and maintaining it over time is a challenge (Dmytryshyn, Jack, Ballantyne, Wahoush, & MacMillan, 2015). In addition to developing trust, the nurse-client relationship is established for the nurse and the client/families to work as partners toward accomplishing a mutual goal in health. As partners, the expertise of both is valuable to an interactive and therapeutic process.

The nurse-client relationship is key to the success of intervention programs. In a study of relationship building between public health nurses and single mothers living on public assistance, Porr (2013) found that this interactional strategy was a key practice standard for public health nurses and was instrumental in improving SDOH in this population. Components of relationship building included engaging in a positive manner as well as offering verbal commendations.

In spite of budgetary barriers, relational practice continues to be intensely necessary for holistic, family-oriented care (Spadoni, Doane, Sevean, & Poole, 2015). Nurses working in the Healthy Baby Healthy Children (HBHC) (see Table 17-1) program, for instance, are trained in implementing principles of home visiting, which includes establishing therapeutic relationships with families. According to a mental health nurse with the city of Toronto's Public Health Department, "one of the key approaches to building relationships with families in home visiting is for nurses to stay present in the visit, and relinquish the pressing need to fill out paper work" (A. Reid, personal communication, December 29, 2012).

In an early but still relevant example of relational practice, Doutrich and Marvin (2004) paired students enrolled in a community health nursing course with local public health nurses in their clinical rotations. The students reported that they learned to value relationship building with community clients as critical to practice. They described this relationship as the key to "finding the door," getting through it, and establishing a trust relationship with clients. Other important skills these students identified included becoming aware of their own biases, getting the client's story, and not blaming or judging the clients. This ability to remain nonjudgmental usually occurred when the students were truly engaged with families and understood the family's context. For example, if issues such as poverty, discrimination, and racism are not explored as underlying factors in Indigenous people's overrepresentation in homelessness in Canadian and other societies (Patrick, 2014), we are likely to approach these families with bias and blame, hence sabotaging opportunities to establish therapeutic working relationships.

Empowerment

Empowerment can be viewed as a nurse-facilitated, strengths-based process in which nurses and families work actively to share knowledge that promotes families' capacity to find and sustain solutions for improved health outcomes (Malone, 2012). Most important, although nurses can facilitate empowerment, they cannot "give" it; it is a process as well as an outcome. Although hierarchical relationships still characterize the power dynamics within many provider-client relationships in health care, it should be the goal of all nurses to facilitate empowerment within their community and public health practice.

Facilitating healthy change can be difficult because of the complex and fluctuating nature of the family in its unique environment, and requires considerable skill in various empowerment strategies. Nurses must have the skills to build trusting, nonjudgmental relationships that allow/encourage families to tell their stories so they can jointly uncover the family's needs. Additionally, community and public health nurses must have skills that facilitate empowering families to make decisions about their health (CHNC, 2011). For example, nurses can adopt the role of mediator or coach rather than director or decision maker. The CHNC (2011) suggests a client- or family-centered approach to helping clients problem-solve by building on the strengths and resources available to them. In a study of the importance of control in chronic care self-management, Lawn et al. (2013) stressed the importance of power coming from within the client. Families who have hindrances to participating actively in empowering processes need an advocate. Community family nurses must learn to speak out and are obligated to be actively involved in issues and policies that affect their family clients. Toronto street nurse Cathy Crowe has for years used political advocacy and activism to bring attention to the social injustice surrounding access to housing. Recognizing that issues such as homelessness occur at the intersection of power, politics, and families' personal lives, Cathy Crowe has used political activism to question unjust political decisions and inactions as a moral obligation to promote equity and access (Falk-Rafael & Bradley, 2014). She has strategically galvanized the use of print, social media, documentaries, and the involvement of key stakeholders at the community and governmental levels. By doing so nurses, such as Cathy, give voice to the policy and environmental factors that affect families while also providing support for the "individual, family, group, community, and population to advocate for themselves" (CHNC, 2011, p. 19). These actions are important in transforming families and communities from a state of powerlessness to recognition of their own strengths.

SETTINGS WHERE COMMUNITY AND PUBLIC HEALTH NURSES WORK

Community and public health nurses care for families in a variety of settings, such as the following:

- In the home
- Community settings, such as schools, clinics, adult day care or retirement centers, and correctional facilities
- On the streets or in an alternative environment for homeless families
- Temporary housing, such as shelters or transitional or recovery programs
- Community-wide programs outside of a traditional "place"

Although diversity exists in settings and families specific to sociodemographics (i.e., ethnicity, age, gender, sexual orientation, socioeconomic status, and family type), geographical location, attitudes, values, and subjective well-being, nurses use health promotion concepts/principles to go between people and their interactions with their environment in order to prevent illnesses and promote health (WHO, 2012). Knowing what strategies to use with different families requires an understanding of their diverse needs. This section covers three common settings where community and public health nurses work: family homes, community nursing centers, and public health departments.

Family Homes

Community and public health nurses working with families make home visits to assess family health status, needs, and their environment in order to develop specific interventions and identify available resources. For example, community and public health nurses conduct visits with clients, usually in a client's home, after a baby is born. They visit the home to determine safety, nutrition status, emotional needs, and relationship support needs. They then provide education, counseling, and referral as needed. Nurses help new mothers set goals for making healthy lifestyle choices and fostering personal growth. In some cases, nurses meet with families and their infants to conduct genetic counseling and inform them about the different tests that are possible. In other situations, nurses work with older adults in their homes to help

them remain in their homes through case management, home care, and telehealth services. Assessment of the social, emotional, and physical development of families across the age span is a key role of the nurses in home visiting programs. Nurses assess the physical environment of the home, including safety hazards, such as availability of smoke detectors and fire extinguishers, any dangerous equipment, and the adequacy of running water and indoor plumbing.

In the HBHC program (see Table 17-1), for example, nurses promote the health of mothers and children in their homes. The HBHC program is a free public health initiative implemented in Ontario, Canada, to foster social, emotional, and physical health for vulnerable children. Families with anticipated poor birth outcomes, children with challenges to thrive, family stress, little social support, and low income are often referred to the program. In this program, public health nurses and family home visitors work together to assess families' situations (breastfeeding, nutrition, literacy, and social development, such as mother-child bonding), help them to access services and supports, and facilitate skill development of parents (Ontario Ministry of Children and Youth Services [OMCYS], 2011). Community nurses working with the Victorian Order of Nurses (VON) in Canada provide home care services to families recovering from an illness. These nurses conduct assessments, provide personal support, and facilitate links to community services (VON Canada, 2009).

Research has demonstrated the effectiveness of home visiting programs in the United States as well. The seminal work of David Olds (e.g., 2002) and his colleagues in the development and evaluation of the Nurse-Family Partnership program illustrates the effectiveness of family-centered care and community and public health nursing home visitation. Nurses visited low-income, unmarried mothers and their children. The families with home visitation had significantly improved health outcomes. The home visitation was found to contribute to reductions in the following: number of the mothers' subsequent pregnancies, use of welfare, child abuse and neglect, and criminal behaviors for up to 15 years after the first child's birth. At this early stage, there was little research about the effectiveness of this and other home visitation programs by nurses. However, a recent systematic review of home visiting in the United States from 2005 to 2015 found that nursing home and visitation intervention programs by nurses provided an effective route to empower people at risk for health disparities to avoid injury, maintain health, and prevent and manage chronic disease (Abbott & Elliott, 2016).

Community-Based Care Settings

Community and public health nurses also practice in community-based care settings. Community-based care settings, found in both rural and urban communities in the United States, offer the public access to a wide array of nursing services in a single setting. These programs typically provide services that are not available elsewhere and are likely to focus on the needs of underserved populations (King, 2008). Within these centers, nurses focus on promoting health and preventing disease; they offer health screening, education, and well-child care. In addition, such centers may offer secondary and tertiary prevention services, such as management of acute and chronic health conditions, and mental health counseling.

The model for these centers is usually multidisciplinary and strives to provide affordable, accessible, acceptable care that serves to empower individuals across the life span to meet their own health care goals. The focus on social justice in many of these centers is realized by attempts to reach out to marginalized populations and to provide comprehensive, quality, non-judgmental health care. In keeping with the community-as-mind-set concept, community-based care settings may be either physical places or they may be embedded in more traditional health care settings. Some community-based care settings provide educational experiences for nursing students and students from other disciplines, making these settings a place where

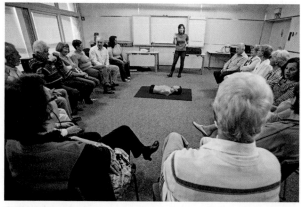

© iStock.com/vm

nursing practice, theory, and research can blend in a model that serves those who need health care the most. With the national focus on interprofessional education, nurse-led interprofessional collaborative practice teams have been integrated into many nurse-led community-based programs. These programs are often affiliated with or attached to schools of nursing, and offer practice and research opportunities for faculty as well as students (Pilon et al., 2015).

The Ontario Early Years Centers (OEYCs) is a similar model in Canada. OEYCs are government-funded, early learning drop-in programs for parents/caregivers and children that are located in communities across the province of Ontario. Community and public health nurses and other early professionals and experts from the community assist parents and caregivers to get the help they need to promote health, long-term learning, and positive behavior among children within the first 6 years of their lives. Parents, caregivers, and children participate actively in educational activities together, whereas public health nurses provide guidance and support for new parenting skills and linkages to other services in the community, such as prenatal nutrition programs (OMCYS, 2011).

Public Health Departments

Probably the most widely known and accepted model for community-based services for families is that used by county and state departments of health services. The role of governmental health departments at all levels (local, state, national) is to address public health core functions, including assessment, policy development, and assurance (Towne & Chaudry, 2017). Public health departments serve the needs of individuals and families across the life span in both health department and home-based models and, more recently, in acute care settings in the United States. These programs include services to vulnerable groups, such as pregnant and childbearing families (women, infants, and children programs [WIC]), children with special health care needs, individuals at risk for or diagnosed with infectious diseases, and those with chronic conditions. Recent health care reform and budget-reduction measures have resulted in reduced direct care clinical service provision in most local health departments (Beck & Boulton, 2016). Still, public health nurses represent the largest group of public health practitioners working in U.S. local and state health departments, in spite of administrative and educational barriers to their practice. Regardless of the type of health department, public health nurses provide essential population health services such as diagnosis and treatment, epidemiology, health promotion, disease surveillance, community health assessment, and policy development (Boulton & Beck, 2013).

Chronic pain management in older adults living in the community is a pervasive public health problem that can be amenable to public health nursing interventions aimed at individuals and families. Dewar (2006) reviewed the literature about chronic pain management by nurses in the community and found that most studies focused on pain assessment tools, with less focus on how older adults managed pain and what community resources were available to help these families with pain-management issues. An effective nurse-patient relationship is important in comprehensive assessment and management of pain in the older adult population.

Related to chronic pain management in the United States is the increasing problem of opioid addiction and overdose. In July of 2016, the Comprehensive Addiction and Recovery Act (CARA) was signed into law. It contains multiple initiatives to help address America's opioid crisis (Roberts, Gellad, & Skinner, 2016). Before the national focus, local agencies have attempted a variety of preventative interventions including the use of naloxone in the community, needle exchange programs, and "take back" medication programs. Often community and public health nurses and nursing students have been involved in these injury prevention programs. One such academic-practice collaboration was described as "service learning for injury prevention" and involved multiyear public health nursing clinical practicum with students involved with community stakeholders engaged in multiple interventions (Alexander, Canclini, & Krauser, 2014, p. 175).

Elder abuse is emerging as an area of major concern nationally and internationally, and is called out as such in *Healthy People 2020* (U.S. Department of Health and Human Services, 2010). Public health nurses are often on the frontlines in detecting such abuse in a variety of settings. In a study of elder maltreatment in assisted living facilities, public health nurses played key roles in abuse detection as well as policy and education development and delivery (Phillips & Ziminski, 2012).

Nurses also must be aware of the omission of needed support and attention as a type of abuse. Nurses need to know how to report elder abuse in their communities and be willing to take quick action to prevent further abuse. In many U.S. states, nurses are mandatory reporters of elder abuse. For example, in the states of Oregon and Washington, nurses must report abuse of older adults who sustain physical harm, financial exploitation, verbal or emotional abuse, lack of basic care, involuntary seclusion, wrongful restraint, unwanted sexual contact, or abandonment by the caregiver. Each state has an individual policy for reporting to protective services. More information about reporting elder abuse in the United States can be found at the National Clearinghouse on Abuse in Later Life (NCALL) Web site (http://www.ncall.us).

Despite the fact that homeless families are the fastest growing segment of the homeless population (Gultekin, Brush, Baiardi, Kirk, & VanMaldeghem, 2014), most research about homelessness focuses on individuals, often men. In an attempt to understand the experience of families experiencing homelessness, and to respond appropriately, these authors interviewed homeless mothers and their caseworkers to assess alignment between needs and available services. Persistent lack of social support was a key theme. Understanding how public health nurses can assist with the process of rehousing while supporting family agency and self-efficacy can lead to a rich new role for public health nurses. The authors suggest that services address practical supports, but also be trauma-informed, help build self-esteem, repair and rebuild family relationships, and develop healthy communities.

Engaging nurses and nursing students in caring for this growing segment of our population, homeless families, is challenging and creativity is warranted. Loewenson and Hunt (2011) found that participation in a service-learning clinical rotation with families experiencing homelessness suggested that the clinical experiences positively influenced students' attitudes and supported integrating service-learning opportunities with individuals experiencing homelessness into nursing curricula. Similarly, Rasmor, Kooienga, Brown, and Probst (2014) found that nurse practitioner students who completed an experience working with vulnerable families in free clinics increased their interest in working with these populations after graduation. With decreasing funding for targeted services for vulnerable populations such as families experiencing homelessness, nurses need to engage in providing care where the families can access it.

COMMUNITY AND PUBLIC HEALTH NURSING ROLES WITH FAMILIES AND COMMUNITY

In their capacities, community and public health nurses play several roles. These include, but are not limited to, health education, advocacy, facilitation of access to health resources, assessment, assurance, policy development, referrals, building capacity, and consultation. Table 17-1 illustrates some of the diverse roles assumed by these nurses. In this section we discuss community and public health nursing roles in health education, facilitation of resources, assessment, assurance, and policy development.

Health Education

Health education is essential to the promotion of health and the prevention of disease in families. Using information gained through family health appraisals/assessments, community health nurses reinforce health-promoting behaviors and provide health information and teaching in identified at-risk areas. The Centers for Disease Control and Prevention (CDC) lists five major determinants of health: (1) genes and biology, (2) health behaviors, (3) social environment or social characteristics, (4) physical environment or total ecology, and (5) health services or medical care (CDC, 2014; WHO, 2012). Community and public health nurses have a role in facilitating high-level wellness for their clients by advocating for positive changes in health determinants, including health behaviors, social environment and characteristics, physical environment and ecology, and health services.

Community health nurses use a variety of strategies to modify behaviors, characteristics, or care limitations identified in the health appraisal. Teaching and health information can be used to discuss immunizations, nutrition, rest, exercise, use of seat belts, and abuse of harmful substances, such as alcohol and drugs. Community health nurses may refer families to programs and resources that assist in their lifestyle modifications (e.g., smoking cessation classes, exercise programs). One example of this is the "Biggest Loser" intervention program that was designed to assist clients in a West Virginia county to lose weight. This intervention was developed

in response to high obesity rates and included a program based loosely on the television show of the same name. Nurses provided specific education, social supports, weigh-ins, exercise, and dietary help to the participants, although in the public health intervention no one was voted off.

Health teaching, based on appraisal of the physical environment, might also include information on child safety and prevention of falls for older adults. Other teaching might focus on psychological or social environmental problems, such as family communications or dealing with peer pressure. In some situations, community health nurses promote a healthy and safe environment by meeting with the school board to provide evidence about playground hazards or poor food-handling practices.

Facilitate Access to Resources

A major health-promotion strategy is to ensure access to health promotion and prevention services, including immunizations, family planning, prenatal care, well-child care, nutrition, exercise classes, and dental hygiene. These services may be provided directly by community health nurses, or community health nurses facilitate access to these services through referrals, case management, discharge planning, advocacy, coordination, and collaboration.

Nurses must consider access to resources within a context of what choices families realistically have. For example, eating healthy meals requires that healthy foods be available in locations that families can access easily and without expensive transportation. Also, accessing health providers and facilities requires that, in the United States, families have some type of health insurance or other means to pay. According to the 2010 U.S. census report, almost 50 million Americans (16%) did not have health insurance (DeNavas-Walt, Proctor, & Smith, 2012). The ACA's major coverage provisions went into effect in January 2014 and have led to significant coverage gains. As of the end of 2015, the number of uninsured non-elderly Americans stood at 28.5 million, a decrease of nearly 13 million since 2013, and a decrease of 21.5 million since the census report of 2010 (Kaiser Family Foundation, 2016b). There has been movement toward patient/client/family-centered care, and toward upstream thinking/prevention. Still, in 2015 according to the Kaiser Family Foundation (2016b), 28.5 million Americans remained without coverage. Although there are still some Americans without insurance, the change in coverage since the implementation of the ACA is significant. In addition to providing (and mandating) coverage, the ACA did not allow health insurance companies to deny individuals health insurance based on pre-existing conditions. The Kaiser Family Foundation found in a recent study that 52 million Americans (or 27%) have a pre-existing condition "that would likely make them uninsurable if they applied for health coverage under medical underwriting practices that existed in most states before insurance regulation change" (Kaiser Family Foundation, 2016a, para. 1).

Facilitating access to resources for families who are deprived because of race, social class, and gender requires understanding of how social injustice operates on a social level to cause such depravity. Paul Farmer, a physician and author best known for his medical work in Haiti and worldwide with tuberculosis and acquired immune deficiency syndrome (AIDS), wrote about structural violence in his book, *Pathologies of Power: Health, Human Rights and the New War on the Poor* (Farmer, 2003). Structural violence refers to historical, economic, and political roots of generational oppression. It is about unequal treatment, racism, classism, and discrimination. We see these factors dominating the experiences of gun violence victims and survivors (Bailey, Clarke, & Salami, 2015; Bailey, Hannays-King, Clarke, Lester, & Velasco, 2013). These same factors are intimately involved as predictors and facilitators in diverse homeless populations' experience (Milburn et al., 2010). Whether homelessness or structural violence, these social issues are rooted in systematized, unequal access to resources. Working toward social justice requires a partnership between families and professionals. The community and public health nurses' responses to the structural violence perpetuated by policy, the myth of meritocracy (that anyone who is hard working and deserving can succeed), and our biases make it an ethical obligation to engage in deep relational practice with the families we serve.

Assessment, Assurance, and Policy Development

Community and public health nurses are engaged in the core public health functions of assessment, assurance, and policy development. These core functions include assessing and monitoring the health of communities and populations at risk to identify health problems and priorities, ensuring that all populations have access to appropriate and cost-effective care (assurance), and formulating policies designed to solve identified local and national health problems and priorities. Assessment is facilitated by the trust that public health nurses have earned from their clients, agencies, and private providers, trust that provides ready access to populations that are otherwise difficult to access and engage in health care. In addition, these nurses have knowledge of current and emerging health issues through their daily contact with high-risk and vulnerable populations. This trust and knowledge provides the foundation for ways nurses work with communities (populations) and families and individuals in the community. Table 17-2 lists the different assessment approaches nurses can use in the community, based on the focus of the health care.

Table 17-2 Comparison of Assessment Approaches		
Community	**Family**	**Individual**
Analyze data on and needs of specific populations or geographical area. Identify and interact with key community leaders, both formally and informally. Identify target populations that may be at risk. These populations may include families living in high-density low-income areas, preschool children, primary and secondary school children, and older adults. Participate in data collection on a target population. Conduct surveys or observe targeted populations, such as preschools, jails, and detention centers, to gain a better understanding of needs.	Evaluate a specific family's strengths and areas of concern. This involves a comprehensive assessment of the physical, social, and mental health needs of the family. Evaluate the family's living environment, looking specifically at support, relationships, and other factors that might have a significant impact on family health outcomes. Assess the larger environment in which the family lives (their block or specific community) for safety, access, and other related issues.	Identify individuals within the family who are in need of services. Evaluate the functional capacity of the individual through the use of specific assessment measures, including physical, social, and mental health screening tools. Develop a nursing diagnosis for the individual that describes a problem or potential problem, causative factors, and contributing factors. Develop a nursing care plan for the individual.

Table 17-3	Assurance Activities in Community, Family, and Individual Care	
Community	**Family**	**Individual**
Provide service to target populations, such as child-care centers, preschools, worksites, minority communities, jails, juvenile detention facilities, and homeless shelters. Interventions may include health screening, education, health promotion, and injury prevention programs. Improve quality assurance activities with various health care providers in the community. Examples include education on new immunization policies, educational programs for communicable disease control, assistance in developing effective approaches, and support techniques for high-risk populations. Maintain safe levels of communicable disease surveillance and outbreak control. Participate in research or demonstration projects. Provide expert public health consultation in the community. Ensure that standards of care are met within the community (assurance).	Provide services to a cluster of families within a geographical setting. Services may be provided in a variety of settings, including homes, child-care centers, preschools, and schools. Services may include physical assessment, health education and counseling, and health and developmental screening. Provide care in a nursing clinic to a specific group of families in a geographical location.	Provide nursing services based on standards of nursing practice to individuals across the age continuum. These services may encompass a variety of programs including, specifically, First Steps and Children With Special Health Care Needs, and more generally, child abuse prevention, immunizations, well-child care, and HIV/AIDS programs. Assess and support the individual's progress toward meeting outcome goals. Consult with other health care providers and team members regarding the individual's plan of care. Prioritize individual's needs on an ongoing basis. Participate on quality-assurance teams to measure the quality of care provided.

Table 17-4	Activities That Influence Policy Development	
Community	**Family**	**Individual**
Provide leadership in convening and facilitating community groups to evaluate health concerns and develop a plan to address the concerns. Recommend specific training and programs to meet identified health needs. Raise awareness of key policymakers about health regulations, budget decisions, and other factors that may negatively affect the health of communities. Recommend programs to target populations such as child-care centers, retirement centers, jails, juvenile detention facilities, homeless shelters, worksites, and minority communities. Act as an advocate for the community and individuals who are not willing or able to speak to policymakers about issues and programs of concern. Work with business and industry to develop employee health programs.	Recommend new or increased services to families based on identified needs. Recommend programs to meet specific families' needs within a geographical area. Facilitate networking with families with similar needs or issues. Guide policymakers on specific issues that affect clusters of families. Request additional data and analyze information to identify trends in a group or cluster of families. Identify key families in a community who may either oppose or support specific policies or programs, and develop appropriate and effective intervention strategies to use with these families.	Recommend or assist in the development of standards for individual client care. Recommend or adopt risk classification systems to assist with prioritizing individual client care. Participate in establishing criteria for opening, closing, or referring individual cases. Participate in the development of job descriptions to establish roles for various team members who will provide service to individuals.

Assurance activities are the direct individual-focused services that public health nurses provide. Although the current shift in emphasis is toward assessment and policy development, critical assurance activities remain for the public health nurse. Assurance activities at the community, family, and individual levels are outlined in Table 17-3.

In 1988 the IOM compiled a report called *The Future of Public Health*. At that time the IOM articulated the Core Functions of Public Health and the Ten Essential Services of Public Health in the United States. The Core Functions identified in this report were Assessment, Policy Development, and Assurance (IOM, 1988). These remain the guiding framework for U.S. Public Health (CDC, 2012). In some areas over time this changed the focus of public health from delivering primary health care or providing safety-net services to individuals to a more population, upstream, data-driven, policy-focused organization. See Table 17-4 to review ways that

BOX 17-1
The Healthy Living Collaborative of Southwest Washington

The HLCSW is a community-driven coalition that works together on upstream initiatives that promote health equity and strengthen communities (HLCSW, 2016). Members participate from a variety of sectors including health care, public health, social services, education, a tribal nation, housing services, transportation, and more. Functions of the coalition include:

■ Supporting and advocating for health in all policies and systems

■ Facilitating decision making across sectors and policy areas for long-term change
■ Creating connections across diverse organizations and communities
■ Participating in community engagement and action to elevate community voices and strengthen the community
■ Promoting shared learning across the community (HLCSW, 2016)

BOX 17-2
Geographical Information Systems

GIS visually display, analyze, and manipulate spatial data to locate geographical areas, potential hazards, water sources, and other important information. This digital technology helps the user to understand trends and issues of concern by rendering data visually, in the forms of maps, charts, histograms, and a variety of reports. Having access to this type of detailed data in visual format allows community and public health nurses to intervene more quickly and accurately to enhance public health and safety.

policy comes about relative to public health. Though many local health departments still provide some level of health care to individuals or families, this movement toward the core functions has meant changes in what it means to be a public health nurse or provider. For example, the growing number of new cases of pertussis in the United States requires us to consider all health as public health. With most serious morbidity and mortality from pertussis occurring in infants who are too young to mount an immune response to active vaccines, community and public health nurses are actively working in acute care and long-term care facilities to vaccinate all adults to provide "herd" immunity that shields our youngest and most vulnerable family members.

Coalitions of community partners that include academic-practice partnerships, traditional public health services, council for the homeless, peer mentors, and regional acute and ambulatory care systems are joining together in some areas. Their purpose in these coalitions are to use data to influence provision of coordinated efforts to address services and craft/influence policies aimed toward "making living better—for everyone" (Healthy Living Collaborative of Southwest Washington [HLCSW], 2016, para 1).

See Box 17-1 for an example of a regional coalition/policy influencer, the HLCSW.

TRENDS IN PUBLIC HEALTH

Community and public health nursing positions in the United States, rather than growing with population needs, have declined. In the past two decades, fewer nurses are public health nurses and these nurses make up a lower proportion of the public health workforce (Baldwin, Lyons, & Issel, 2011). Similar to nurses in many contexts, those community and public health nurses with positions in public health are being asked to do more with less. Responding to workforce and economic constraints, some public health services have switched to a focus on the core functions and community/neighborhood interventions. Skills in connecting planning to SDOH, understanding the multi-perspective views of all stakeholders, and being able to translate (almost in a multilingual way) the contextual realities of clients are among the skills required (SmithBattle, 2012; SmithBattle, Lorenz, & Leander, 2013). Community and public health nurses today must become comfortable with geographical information system (GIS) (Box 17-2) mapping and epidemiology, and should know and be able to connect with the communities these representations depict. Importantly, nurses must be willing to engage in political actions to address issues not easily ameliorated at the individual level. Thus, establishing proactive policies should be an important health goal for public health/community nurses to facilitate transition in the health state of vulnerable families and groups.

Nurse Practitioner Roles in Community and Public Health Nursing

In April 2013, the National Organization of Nurse Practitioner Faculties (NONPF) released the following six nurse practitioner population-foci competencies: Family/Across the Lifespan, Neonatal, Acute Care Pediatric, Primary Care Pediatric, Psychiatric–Mental Health, and Women's Health/Gender Related. NONPF incorporated population health into nursing education programs for nurse practitioners, and into its accreditation for these programs, with the intent that all nurse practitioners be educated and competent in population health.

One example of a program employing nurse practitioners in population health takes place in Oregon. Oregon has a comprehensive network of child abuse assessment and intervention centers designed to minimize trauma to child abuse victims by coordinating the local community's response to reports of suspected child abuse. This community-based, interprofessional child maltreatment intervention model offers population-focused nurse practitioners the opportunity to prevent, recognize early, and treat families that have experienced dysfunction and/or child maltreatment in order to prevent some of the negative life impacts of these early experiences. Services include interviews of suspected victims of child abuse, medical evaluations, mental health treatment and/or referrals, provision or coordination of other victim services, and individual- and community-specific needs. This important work grew, in part, out of findings from the Adverse Childhood Events (ACES) study (Felitti et al., 1998). The study revealed the following: (1) More than half of study participants had experienced at least one of the adverse events studied (psychological, physical, or sexual abuse;

violence against mother; or living with household members who were substance abusers, mentally ill or suicidal, or ever imprisoned); (2) persons who had experienced four or more categories of childhood exposure, compared with those who had experienced none, had a 4- to 12-fold increased health risk for alcoholism, drug abuse, depression, and suicide; (3) persons who had experienced four or more categories of childhood exposure had a 2- to 4-fold increase in smoking, poor self-rated health, greater than 50 sexual intercourse partners, and sexually transmitted infection; and (4) persons who had experienced four or more categories of childhood exposure had a 1.4- to 1.6-fold increase in physical inactivity and severe obesity (Felitti et al., 1998). Findings from this foundational study have been replicated in more recent work (Gilbert et al., 2015).

Several very creative and successful community programs integrate knowledge about ACES and resilience. For example, the Walla Walla Valley's Children's Resilience Initiative in Washington State (https://acestoohigh.com/2014/10/07/childrens-resilience-initiative-in-walla-walla-wa-draws-spotlight-to-trauma-sensitive-school/) grew out of an understanding of ACES and their consequences. The Initiative is a learning community whose goal is to build a toolbox of resilience-based strategies to confront the challenges of life. This is a community-wide project that exists outside of a traditional nursing "space." Quality care for families in the community can be enhanced when rigid understandings of place and/or position of nursing care are rethought and flexed according to family and community needs.

Population-focused nurse practitioners often fill positions in inpatient and outpatient settings that focus on the care of groups of clients with particular chronic illnesses, such as diabetes or heart disease. These nurse practitioners provide primary care to these clients, as well as offer individual and group health education and other health promotion activities. Their interest and expertise in a particular health condition lends itself well to advocating for necessary resources for their population of interest, and to becoming active in health policy change on behalf of their clients.

Case Study: Davis Family

Three weeks ago, two senior nursing students participating in their community/population health clinical as members of an outreach team at a homeless outreach program were asked by one of the case managers on the team to do an assessment of the client John Davis at his apartment, as he had been refusing help from his case manager and denied offers to connect him with medical care. The students completed a physical assessment to the best of their abilities and observed the following: urine-, feces-, and blood-stained clothing; bilateral 2+ pitting edema of the lower extremities; diminished bilateral lung sounds in all quadrants; numerous open sores on his neck and upper extremities; disorientation to time; overgrown toenails that embedded themselves into the bottoms of his toes; muscle wasting; and extreme generalized weakness. It was clear to them that the client's safety was in jeopardy and they made the decision to call emergency medical services for transport to the hospital. Their decision was fully supported by the case manager and outreach team. The homeless outreach program does not provide any health services nor employ any health care providers. Nursing students do community/population health clinical rotations at this site every semester.

Following his transport to the hospital, Mr. Davis was admitted for a 3-week stay to address concerns associated with his mental illness, addiction to drugs and alcohol, severe dehydration, open skin sores, and extreme weakness. Mr. Davis is a 57-year-old male who had been estranged from his family and chronically homeless for many years until recently being placed in a Housing First scattered site apartment in a small town 10 miles from the hospital. John resembles an 80-year-old man, has a long problem list of health issues, and uses drugs and alcohol to self-medicate for an underlying chronic mental illness (see the family's genogram in Figure 17-2 and the ecomap in Figure 17-3).

A day after his discharge from the hospital and returning to his Housing First apartment, Mr. Davis was sent for treatment to the emergency room of the local hospital. His symptoms included severe shortness of breath, weakness, confusion, and chest pain. He was immediately readmitted to the hospital with a unilateral pneumothorax.

The senior nursing students who worked with Mr. Davis visited him at the hospital. They noticed a drastic decline in his neuro/mental status from the day before and were concerned that he was unable to feed himself or get to the bathroom. When they discussed these issues with the primary nurse, she mentioned that he would likely show progressive decline

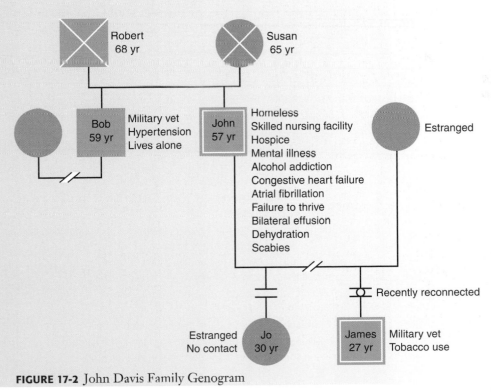

FIGURE 17-2 John Davis Family Genogram

(continued)

Case Study: Davis Family *(cont.)*

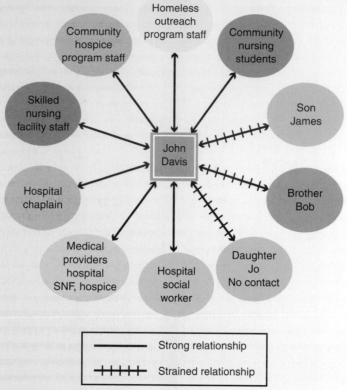

FIGURE 17-3 John Davis Family Ecomap

because of his compromised respiratory status. She also said that the social worker was in the process of contacting his family, per his request, and assisting him in the process of filling out an advance directive. During the next week, the primary nurse and social worker began making arrangements for him to be transferred to a skilled nursing facility upon discharge from the hospital. Because he continued to decline, they realized that his current needs for support and caregiving would exceed what could be provided at the homeless outreach program. The outreach team was involved with the discharge plan and agreed that Mr. Davis was no longer capable of caring for himself independently.

During the week that he was in the hospital, Mr. Davis had several visits with family members who had agreed to visit him. His son and his brother both visited and the family was supported by members of the homeless outreach program and the hospital staff including the nurses, social worker, and chaplain. With Mr. Davis's consent, his family was involved in the discussions about his declining condition and transfer to the skilled nursing facility. On the day of his discharge from the hospital, the nurse also placed a call to the local hospice program that would admit him to the hospice program once he got settled in the skilled nursing facility. In the referral to the hospice program, Mr. Davis's diagnosis list was updated to include the following: congestive heart failure, atrial fibrillation, bilateral pleural effusion, failure to thrive, dehydration, scabies, and a sacral pressure ulcer. He was now dependent on oxygen, confined to a wheelchair and hospital bed, and required 24-hour skilled care.

When Mr. Davis arrived in the skilled nursing facility, he became combative and began refusing assistance. He also refused to wear his oxygen or take his medication for comfort, which caused increased hypoxia, pain, and confusion. It is important to remember that Mr. Davis had multiple mental health issues, making his acceptance of any help very difficult. In addition, his confusion from what appeared to be oxygen deprivation increased the risk that he could become combative. Meanwhile, Mr. Davis exhibited signs of air hunger: tripod position, respiratory rate of 36, and agitation. The care team and family set up his room and called to schedule the hospice admission sooner, rather than later. His son and his brother took turns staying with

Case Study: Davis Family *(cont.)*

him and provided much of the care that he needed, including medication administration of comfort medications when he would take it. He was no longer eating or drinking and declined quickly.

Outcome:
Mr. Davis died in the skilled nursing facility 3 days after his transfer from the hospital. His son and his brother were at his bedside providing loving support and care.

Nursing Student Comment:
"The care the client received demonstrated the importance of the nurse's role in coordinating care in the hospital and community. Involving multiple services and support allowed the patient to be close to his family at the end of his life. Having an interdisciplinary team involved allowed for holistic care, including spiritual support, quality discharge planning, and coordination of care by people who knew him including the homeless outreach team. His SDOH were also addressed by considering his housing, safety, and access to care in a variety of settings. He was truly supported until his death."

Setting:
Community, Homeless Outreach Program, Home, Hospital, Skilled Nursing Facility

Health Promotion/Standard:
• Create supportive care environment.

Concepts/Principles Used by Nurse:
• Access to resources
• Holistic care
• SDOH (housing, safety, access to care)
• Nurse-client relationship
• Interprofessional care

Role Played by Nurse:
• Assessment, advocacy, support
• Facilitated access to care
• Coordination of care and support for care transitions
• Team member involvement
• Fostering support and connections with family
• End-of-life comfort care

SUMMARY

Community health nurses forge strong nurse-client partnerships as they maneuver through the maze of interventions and resources in providing family-centered nursing. They are concerned with the health of families and the ways in which family health influences the health of communities.

■ Nurses foster interconnectedness among families in the community.
■ The settings in which community and public health nurses work with families vary and include, but are not limited to, public and private health agencies, schools, and occupational sites.

■ Community and public health nursing roles vary according to whether the nurse is focusing on the family as the unit of care in the context of the community, or focusing on the health of the community with families being a subunit.
■ Community and public health nurses aim to meet the holistic needs of families and communities while targeting prioritized health needs.
■ Rather than blaming families for their situations, community and public health nurses consider how social, political, economic, and environmental conditions affect families' health choices and outcomes.

- Family interventions in the community are targeted toward primary, secondary, and tertiary prevention. The nurse-family relationship is central in interventions at all three levels of prevention.
- Interventions for families are planned, implemented, and evaluated from a health promotion perspective.

- Using a combination of relational collaboration and health promotion strategies and principles, community and public health nurses strive to partner with families to assist with all levels of healthy change.

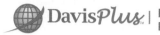 | For additional resources and information, visit **http://davisplus.fadavis.com**. References can be found on Davis*Plus*.

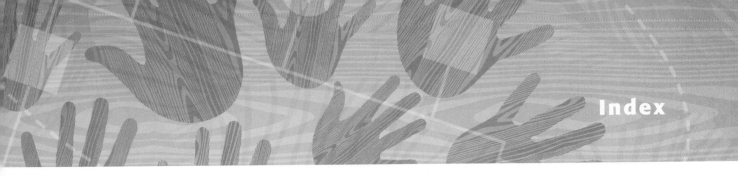

E

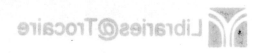